T0226523

Anomalies of Binocular Vision:

Diagnosis & Management

Anomalies of Binocular Vision:

Diagnosis & Management

Robert P. Rutstein, OD, MS
Professor of Optometry
School of Optometry
University of Alabama at Birmingham
Birmingham, Alabama

Kent M. Daum, OD, MS, PhD
Associate Professor of Optometry
School of Optometry
University of Alabama at Birmingham
Birmingham, Alabama

Illustrations by James T. Hays and Ken Norris

Photographs by Bruce Hyer and Kim Washington

Four contributors

309 illustrations and photographs

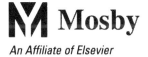 Mosby

An Affiliate of Elsevier

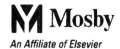

Vice President and Publisher: Don E. Ladig
Executive Editor: Martha Sasser
Developmental Editor: Amy Christopher
Project Manager: Mark Spann
Production Editor: Beth Hayes
Book Design Manager: Judi Lang
Designer: Top Graphics
Manufacturing Supervisor: Karen Boehme
Cover Art: Jen Marmarinos

Permissions may be sought directly from Elsevier's Health Sciences Rights Department in Philadelphia, PA, USA: phone: (+1) 215 239 3804, fax: (+1) 215 239 3805, e-mail: healthpermissions@elsevier.com. You may also complete your request on-line via the Elsevier homepage (http://www.elsevier.com), by selecting 'Customer Support' and then 'Obtaining Permissions'.

Printed and bound by CPI Group (UK) Ltd, Croydon, CR0 4YY
Transferred to Digital Printing, 2013

Mosby
11830 Westline Industrial Drive
St. Louis Missouri 63146

Library of Congress Cataloging-in-Publication Data
Rutstein, Robert P.
    Anomalies of binocular vision: diagnosis and management / Robert
P. Rutstein, Kent M. Daum: with illustrations by James T. Hays, with
photos by Bruce Hyer; with 4 contributors.
        p.   cm.
    Includes bibliographical references and index.
    ISBN-13: 978-0-8016-6916-3   ISBN-10: 0-8016-6916-2
    1. Binocular vision disorders. I. Daum, Kent Michael,
II. Title.
    [DNLM: 1. Vision Disorders—diagnosis.   2. Vision Disorders—
therapy.   3. Vision, Binocular—physiology.   WW 141 R9814a 1998]
RE735.R88   1998
617.7'55—dc21
DNLM/DLC   97-14847
    ISBN-13: 978-0-8016-6916-3
    ISBN-10: 0-8016-6916-2

John G. Classé, OD, JD

Professor
School of Optometry
University of Alabama at Birmingham;
Member, Alabama Bar
Birmingham, Alabama

Martin S. Cogan, MD

Assistant Professor of Clinical Ophthalmology
Ophthalmology Department
Eye Foundation Hospital
University of Alabama at Birmingham School of Medicine
Birmingham, Alabama

Kent M. Daum, OD, MS, PhD

Associate Professor of Optometry
School of Optometry
University of Alabama at Birmingham
Birmingham, Alabama

Paul B. Freeman, OD

Department of Ophthalmology
Allegheny General Hospital
Pittsburgh, Pennsylvania

Andrew Mays, MD

Clinical Instructor of Ophthalmology
Department of Ophthalmology
University of Alabama at Birmingham
Birmingham, Alabama

Robert P. Rutstein, OD, MS

Professor of Optometry
School of Optometry
University of Alabama at Birmingham
Birmingham, Alabama

To my parents, Ben and Sylvia Rutstein, who always encouraged me, and to my wife, Judy, and my son, Marc, who continue to inspire me.

—Robert P. Rutstein

I dedicate this book to Kathy, Sara, and Margaret, who have patiently loved me and taught me about life. Jeremiah 29:11.

—Kent M. Daum

Foreword

As optometry has expanded its scope of practice in recent years, it has evolved from a profession with a primary emphasis on physiologic optics to a profession that is an integral part of primary health care. Consequently, emphasis has shifted to the clinical diagnosis and management of visual problems. The optometrist must not only collect and analyze data but must be a diagnostician, problem solver, manager, and advisor.

Evaluation and treatment of binocular anomalies have long been an integral part of optometric care. The societal importance of education and the increasing number of individuals who use computers in the workplace are obvious examples of why efficient binocular vision is important to patients. Moreover, as the profession is increasingly involved in the care of patients with systemic conditions, neurologic disease, and head trauma, accompanying binocular vision anomalies will present. As a result, now more than ever, the optometrist will be called upon both by patients and other members of the health care team to be the professional responsible for the diagnosis and management of binocular vision dysfunctions. Because optometry is uniquely qualified in this challenging field of vision care, it is the optometrist's responsibility to ensure that the patient receives the best possible care.

There has been an exponential increase in scientific knowledge in the area of binocular vision with the passing of time. Drs. Rutstein and Daum have already contributed by taking an active part in a variety of clinical research projects and other activities. Now they contribute again by combining their expertise and sharing their knowledge, experience, and clinical insight in textbook form.

Thanks to extensive experience in the field, the authors have succeeded in producing a comprehensive book on a subject that deserves every optometrist's attention. There is most definitely something for everyone in this book, and it will be appreciated by students, residents, and practitioners alike. For clinicians, the book provides essential background information for the diagnosis and care of patients with binocular anomalies. This text will provide a foundation and guidance to students and individuals new to the field and is appropriate for those wishing to solidify their foundation or "brush up" on binocular anomalies. It will be equally useful as a reference book, because it is up-to-date and comprehensive in its review of the ophthalmic literature in each area.

Although the book is not a "cookbook" text, it is clinically oriented. The emphasis is on providing thorough descriptions of many distinct binocular anomalies and the testing procedures used to correctly diagnose them. Management recommendations are given, based on the authors' own clinical experience and literature consensus. The writing is clear and concise. Strengths that merit highlighting include the text's thoroughness and overall organization, the significant number of illustrations, photographs, and case studies and the comprehensive and timely references at the end of each chapter. Other appealing attributes are the clinical pearls, which emphasize major points, and the contributions of other authors in the last three chapters on medical and surgical management, practice management, and liability issues.

Drs. Rutstein and Daum have produced a textbook of considerable merit. Together, they have written a scholarly, comprehensive, and useful book that will be a valuable addition to any library. I commend Drs. Rutstein and Daum for compiling and presenting this information in a manner that will be a valuable resource for students and practitioners who regularly care for patients.

Susan A. Cotter, OD, FAAO, FCOVD

Professor
Southern California College of Optometry
Fullerton, California

It is a great pleasure and honor for me to write a Foreword for this significant book, *Anomalies of Binocular Vision: Diagnosis and Management.* One of the essential areas of optometric health care is the diagnosis and management of the anomalies of binocular vision.

The authors are well-known teachers, clinicians, and researchers. Their experience and understanding have been utilized in writing this book, and it will be of great practical clinical value and benefit to any health care practitioner or student who wants current and clinically useful information on the anomalies of binocular vision.

This book is a thoroughly readable text on this complex and broad health care area. It is written in a clear manner, based on current information, and has many excellent and informative figures and tables. The clinical value of the book is also greatly enhanced by the very thorough and complete bibliography. The text condenses a tremendous amount of clinical experience and research information into practical and usable methods and procedures with which to diagnose and manage anomalies of binocular vision. It also includes many case reports that will guide the reader toward making more appropriate patient care decisions and feeling more clinically comfortable.

The authors are interested in the training of students, residents, and all those engaged in the clinical care of patients with anomalies of binocular vision. Their efforts and enthusiasm for the topic are evident and have been exceedingly successful.

This book has reached the goals of the authors and will be an outstanding, high-quality resource for optometric students and practitioners for many years. It presents the state of the art in the care of anomalies of binocular vision. It will serve as a splendid desk reference, providing clinical information and direction to help students, teachers, and practitioners make better patient care decisions in the eye care of their patients. This clear, comprehensive, and beautifully illustrated book is an excellent contribution to the literature on the health care of patients with anomalies of binocular vision.

J. Boyd Eskridge, OD, PhD

Professor Emeritus
School of Optometry
University of Alabama at Birmingham
Birmingham, Alabama

This book grew out of our mutual feeling that a clinically oriented text on binocular vision was needed that could be used by students and experienced individuals in private practice. To date, most books in this area contain information on the various clinical techniques and their application. Their is often only the barest description of the binocular vision anomalies themselves, few references from the literature, few illustrations of patients with these disorders, and very few case studies. Other more scientifically oriented books that are available provide little practical application for clinicians.

The purpose of *Anomalies of Binocular Vision: Diagnosis and Management* is to provide thorough descriptions of the many binocular vision anomalies, describe the necessary testing procedures to correctly diagnose each disorder, and to describe the most appropriate management. We feel that the many illustrations and case studies, particularly concerning strabismus and incomitant deviations, are unique in the optometric literature. Orderly and practical approaches to diagnosis, differential diagnosis, and treatment decision making for binocular vision disorders are provided in this book. The information on the efficacy of various treatment methods is based not only on our own clinical experience but also on the consensus from the literature. This book can serve as a clinical guide and a reference volume.

The book is organized to take the reader from the base to the tip of the "pyramid" of binocular vision. Sensory anomalies are discussed first, integrative anomalies are discussed next, and motor anomalies are discussed last. The organization reflects the necessary hierarchy in dealing with binocular vision disorders and further emphasizes the logic of sequential diagnosis and management. Each chapter contains clinical pearls that emphasize the major points.

Chapter 1 describes the hierarchy of binocular vision, previews the various anomalies, and reviews the advantages of normal binocular vision and the disadvantages of abnormal binocular vision. Chapters 2 and 3 deal with the sensory anomalies of amblyopia and accommodation, respectively. Each of these chapters contains descriptions of the testing procedures necessary for the effective diagnosis and descriptions of the specific clinical features of these disorders and concludes with a discussion of the most appropriate treatment technique. Using a similar organizational structure, Chapters 4 and 5 are devoted to the integrative anomalies (aniseikonia and suppression/anomalous correspondence) and Chapters 6 to 10 are devoted to the motor anomalies (vergences, strabismus, esotropia, exotropia, and incomitant deviations). Much of the emphasis in the chapters on vergence and strabismus involves differentiating the vergence and strabismic disorders and assigning appropriate therapy. For example, infantile esotropia presents with markedly different clinical findings than does accommodative esotropia. Not only is the treatment different but so are the expectations for perfect normal binocular vision following treatment for these two types of esotropia.

Chapters 11, 12, and 13 place the optometric management of binocular vision anomalies in appropriate context. Chapter 11 was written by pediatric ophthalmologists and describes the pharmacologic and surgical treatment of binocular vision anomalies. The strabismic disorders that are amenable to extraocular muscle surgery and the appropriate type of extraocular muscle surgery are emphasized. Chapter 12 discusses the practice management aspect of binocular vision and was written by an optometrist whose practice heavily involves orthoptics/vision therapy. Chapter 13, written by an optometrist who is also an attorney, deals with the many legal aspects of diagnosing and managing binocular vision anomalies. Case studies of cases that led to litigation are included. The book concludes with an extensive glossary.

Our firm belief is that the diagnosis and management of binocular vision anomalies must be based on testing that allows a consistent diagnosis from practitioner to practitioner. Many forms of treatment may be useful for a particular anomaly, and we have tried to describe the most common and effective while also including comments about less-known but deserving alternatives. Our aim is to bring further clarification to each binocular vision anomaly and therefore allow more consistency in optometric diagnosis and treatment of binocular vision anomalies.

Robert P. Rutstein, OD, MS
Kent M. Daum, OD, MS, PhD

Acknowledgments

We acknowledge the contributions of Mr. Bruce Hyer and Ms. Kim Washington, who were responsible for much of the photography; of Mr. James T. Hays and Mr. Ken Norris for their contributions of graphic art; of Ms. Denise Chambers for her assistance in typing portions of the manuscript. We also gratefully acknowledge the support of the administrations and staff of the School of Optometry of the University of Alabama at Birmingham, including Dean Arol Augsburger and Department Chair, Dr. John Amos. We thank Drs. Ralph Garzia, Susan Cotter, and J. James Saladin for reviewing the book and providing many valuable comments. We also thank Ms. Amy Christopher for her untiring assistance in assembling the book. We thank Drs. John Classé, Martin Cogen, Andrew Mays, and Paul Freeman for their chapters. Finally, without the assistance of our colleagues here at UAB and across the country, our patients, and our many students, this book would not have been possible.

Contents

Normal and Abnormal Binocular Vision

THE BINOCULAR SYSTEM

Normal binocular vision is "the use of both eyes simultaneously in such a manner that each retinal image contributes to the final percept."[1] It requires a coordinated array of highly sophisticated optics, motor skills, and neurologic processing.[2] When this occurs, both eyes must be functional and be able to "see" similar parts of visual space. The resolution ability (visual acuity) of the eyes also must be similar and result in comparable cortical images in corresponding areas. The eyes must each be able to fixate on images, and the oculomotor system must be able to move the eyes quickly and accurately to images in different locations. Finally, the binocular system must fuse the two percepts into a single image.

HIERACHIC ARRANGEMENT OF THE BINOCULAR SYSTEM

Although the diagnosis and treatment of anomalies of the binocular visual system is a complex task, the many facets of knowledge that are required are arranged about a single, very important principle: the binocular system is hierarchically arranged. This means that some parts of the binocular system depend on others for proper function. In other words, problems in a basic area of the system may cause deficits in less fundamental areas. Merely detecting an abnormality is usually not sufficient to make a diagnosis, because the challenge diagnostically is to find not only subnormal areas of function but also the source or cause of the problem(s).

❖ CLINICAL PEARL
The binocular system is hierarchically arranged.

For example, poor binocular depth perception, or stereopsis, is a common feature of an individual with strabismus (crossed eyes). Although the poor depth perception may in fact be a problem for the patient (and probably is) the clinician must determine the source of the poor stereopsis to make a proper diagnosis. The source could be the strabismus, to be sure, but blur caused by an uncorrected refractive error also causes impaired stereopsis and could in some cases also cause strabismus. Much of the challenge of diagnosis in binocular vision anomalies is following "leads" such as poor stereopsis and determining their cause. Learning to diagnose binocular vision anomalies includes learning the sequelae of many problems that commonly affect vision, especially ones such as uncorrected (or miscorrected) refractive errors and poor focusing. Because of the hierarchic arrangement the most fundamental parts of the binocular system must be treated before the less fundamental parts.

WORTH'S LEVELS OF BINOCULAR VISION

Clinicians long have sought to simplify binocular vision and its various processes by describing this hierarchy of binocular vision. One of the first attempts was presented by Worth[3] as first-, second-, and third-degree levels of fusion. First-degree fusion is simultaneous binocular perception of dissimilar objects that are projected in the same direction, as in the projection of a star seen by one eye into a circle seen by the other eye. Second-degree fusion is single, simultaneous, binocular perception of identical, haploscopically visible targets. Third-degree fusion is stereopsis that requires fusion of disparate targets, with a resultant third-dimension percept.[1] Most patients have first-degree fusion and are able to superimpose dissimilar targets; a smaller group has second-degree fusion and is able to align targets having common borders; and a still smaller group has third-degree fusion and is able to recognize stereopsis. Although Worth's description of binocular vision does not accurately model the actual function of binocular vision, it is still used to analyze and determine the prognosis for patients with various binocular anomalies, particularly strabismus. Patients who are able to obtain all three levels of fusion have the best prognosis for clear, comfortable, normal binocular vision. Usually, if a patient has a range of several prism diopters (PD) of second-degree fusion (i.e., a vergence range), the patient will have intact binocular vision and stereopsis. This analysis is used before strabismus treatment because, with a small investment of time, the binocular

TABLE 1-1   ANOMALIES OF BINOCULAR VISION
REQUIRING MANAGEMENT

Process	Condition
Sensory process	Disease (ptosis, keratoconus, opacities in media, retinal or visual pathway disease, etc.)
	Ametropia
	Amblyopia
	Eccentric fixation
	Accommodative insufficiency
	Accommodative infacility
	Accommodative spasm
Integrative process	Disease (tumor, trauma, etc.)
	Aniseikonia
	Suppression
	Anomalous correspondence
	Horror fusionis (horror fusionalis)
Motor process	Disease (infection, vascular disease, tumor, etc.)
	Incomitancies
	Latent (phoria) or manifest (intermittent or constant) deviations of the line of sight
	Vergence quantity (amplitude)
	Vergence quality (facility)
	Nystagmus

(Modified from Eskridge JB, class notes.)

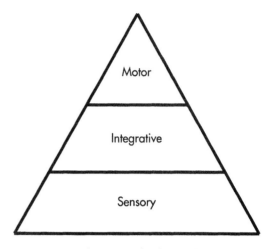

FIG. 1-1   The pyramid of binocular vision.

status of a patient can be reduced to one of three levels that are helpful in determining the probable status after treatment.

THE PYRAMID OF BINOCULAR VISION

A more comprehensive view of the hierarchic arrangement of the binocular visual system is that it is composed of three independent but nonexclusive processes: the sensory, integrative, and motor systems (Table 1-1, Fig. 1-1).[4] The most fundamental part of the system is the sensory process, followed by the integrative process, and then the motor process. The sensory process must be functioning properly for any of the remainder of the binocular system to work efficiently. Deficits in the sensory process may cause deficiencies in either or both of the remaining processes. The least fundamental part of the system is the motor process, which is at the top of the pyramid of binocular vision.

Similar to Worth's model, the concept of the pyramid of binocular vision also is artificial, although it is consistent with the anatomic and neurologic arrangement of the visual system. The sensory process includes the anatomic, physiologic, and psychologic activities involved in the collection and transmission of visual information to the cortex. The integrative process includes those activities involved in the fusion

(i.e., synthesis) of the two cortical images to form a single binocular percept of visual space. The motor process includes those activities necessary to properly align eyes at various distances and directions of gaze. Although not discussed in this book, the perceptual process at the tip of the pyramid could be considered. It includes all activities involved with the correlation of visual information with experiential information to form a final integrated perception. This process includes conditions such as dyslexia, perceptual anomalies, and problems of visual information processing. Although the pyramid of binocular vision is a very good guide to approaching the binocular visual system, some anomalies have both sensory and motor aspects (i.e., amblyopia, strabismus).

Anomalies of the Sensory Process

Because anomalies of the sensory process are at the fundamental level of binocular vision, they are extraordinarily important and can present an insurmountable barrier to good binocular vision. If in doubt about the significance of a sensory factor affecting binocular vision, always correct it before proceeding.

 CLINICAL PEARL

If in doubt about the significance of a sensory factor affecting binocular vision, always correct it before proceeding.

Ametropia

Ametropia is the refractive condition in which the far point (punctum remotum) of the optical system is not located at infinity. Emmetropia is the refractive condition in which the far point is at infinity. Myopia is ametropia with a far point located at a finite distance in front of the eye, whereas hyperopia is ametropia with a virtual far point located behind the eye.

Astigmatism is a condition in which light coming into the eye focuses at more than one point because of the toricity of the refracting surfaces. Anisometropia, usually defined as the refractive state in which the eyes differ by more than 1 D in sphere or cylinder, is the condition of unequal refractive state in the two eyes.[1] Although it is almost always important to correct any sensory deficit, myopia of 0.5 D or more, hyperopia of +0.75 D or more, astigmatism of 0.75 D or more, and anisometropia of 1 D or more are typically considered clinically significant and indicate refractive correction (different guidelines for refractive correction apply for infants and children). In certain visually demanding situations, such as the use of a video display terminal, all ametropia is frequently corrected. Although ametropia is typically corrected via spectacle lenses, there are situations in which contact lenses are superior, particularly situations involving anisometropia (because of aniseikonia) or high corrections (because of weight and the poor cosmesis and optics of high-powered spectacle lenses). Without clear imagery, however, it is pointless to be concerned with less fundamental problems, such as aniseikonia or vergence anomalies, because the patient does not have the images necessary for the problem to develop. Many binocular visual anomalies can be minimized or entirely eliminated by the prescription of the proper refractive correction.

 CLINICAL PEARL

Although it is almost always important to correct any sensory deficit, myopia of 0.5 D or more, hyperopia of +0.75 D or more, astigmatism of 0.75 D or more, and anisometropia of 1 D or more are typically considered clinically significant and indicate refractive correction.

CLINICAL PEARL

Many binocular visual anomalies can be minimized or entirely eliminated by the prescription of the proper refractive correction.

Amblyopia and Eccentric Fixation

Amblyopia is reduced visual acuity not correctable by refractive means that is not attributable to obvious structural or pathologic ocular anomalies.[1] Although reduced visual acuity is the most obvious trait, amblyopia has many other characteristics.[5] For example, eccentric fixation is the condition in which the patient with amblyopia does not use the central foveal area for fixation under monocular conditions, while at the same time the feeling is that the eye is pointed straight ahead. Although several types of amblyopia occur, eccentric fixation is overwhelmingly associated with strabismic amblyopia.

Accommodative Dysfunction

The characteristics of accommodative dysfunction include insufficient amplitude, decreased facility, fatigue, or spasm of the system. Accommodative dysfunction must be discriminated from the normal decrease with age in accommodative function; accommodative dysfunction does not occur at ages greater than the onset of presbyopia at approximately age 40. Deficiency of accommodation typically produces both symptoms and reduced performance.

Disease

Any anomaly that interferes with visual acuity affects the binocular process. Disease processes that can affect binocular vision include ptosis, keratoconus, opacities in media, and retinal or visual pathway disease, as well as many others. Disease processes potentially affect the visual ability of any patient, regardless of binocular visual difficulties. If a portion of the system is afflicted with a disease at a particular level, the problem must be eliminated before proper function can occur in the higher levels of the pyramid (and sometimes even on the same level).

Anomalies of the Integrative Process

The visual system uses extremely sophisticated neural processing in combining the images from the two eyes into a single percept. When the images from the eyes are too dissimilar, various processes are used to eliminate the resultant diplopia and visual confusion. Although these processes impede normal binocular vision, they are very beneficial in restoring a single clear image, even though this image is not the fusion of the images from the two eyes. Anomalies of the integrative process should be manipulated with caution because the consequences of their elimination are not easily reversed if the binocular fusional apparatus is not intact.

 CLINICAL PEARL

Anomalies of the integrative process should be manipulated with caution because the consequences of their elimination are not easily reversed if the binocular fusional apparatus is not intact.

Suppression

Suppression is the lack or inability of perception of normally visible objects in all or part of the field of vision of one eye, occurring only on simultaneous stimulation of both eyes and attributed to cortical inhibition.[1] Suppression typically occurs to prevent diplopia in strabismus. It varies in area and intensity and interferes with the disparity vergence system's ability to acquire information. Physiologic diplopia and stereopsis are closely related to suppression. Physiologic diplopia is the awareness that all objects in the binocular field of view, outside of a small area within which fusion occurs (Panum's area), are double. Objects except those located at the point of fixation appear double because they fall on noncorresponding points. Patients are usually unaware of physiologic diplopia because of suppression. Stereopsis is the recognition of disparities produced by the stimulation of certain noncorresponding points. Stereopsis is impaired by suppression. Although stereopsis is a major aspect of binocular vision, other factors, including a variety of monocular cues, such as visual perspective and overlay, are also very important in perceiving depth.[6] If suppression is not eliminated before treatment, the effective treatment of an associated vergence anomaly is impossible, because one of the two images necessary for the vergence system is missing. However, suppression should be treated cautiously in patients with strabismus, unless strong evidence indicates the patient will successfully fuse the resultant images.

 CLINICAL PEARL

> If suppression is not eliminated before treatment, the effective treatment of an associated vergence anomaly is impossible, because one of the two images necessary for the vergence system is missing. However, suppression should be treated cautiously in patients with strabismus, unless strong evidence indicates the patient will successfully fuse the resultant images.

Anomalous Correspondence

Anomalous correspondence (abnormal retinal correspondence) is the condition in which the foveae of the two eyes do not give rise to a common visual direction, the fovea of one eye functioning directly with an extrafoveal area of the other eye.[1] Anomalous correspondence is found in some strabismic individuals (intermittent or constant). Different types of anomalous correspondence occur. More common in patients with constant and small angles of strabismus, there are different types of anomalous correspondence. Anomalous correspondence in intermittent strabismus is usually not an important barrier; however, it does affect the prognosis for constant strabismus. Therefore, as with suppression, when anomalous correspondence is present in patients with constant strabismus, strong evidence should indicate that normal fusion can be obtained before eliminating anomalous correspondence.

Horror Fusionis

Horror fusionis (horror fusionalis) is the inability to obtain binocular fusion or superimposition of hap-

loscopically presented targets. It occurs frequently as a characteristic in strabismus, in which case haploscopically presented targets approaching superimposition may appear to slide or jump past each other without apparent superimposition, fusion, or suppression.[1] Horror fusionis carries a strong negative prognosis for normal binocular vision.

Aniseikonia

Aniseikonia is a relative difference in the size and/or shape of the ocular images. These differences generally occur in anisometropia, although they can be found in other conditions. Even small differences in image size can affect binocular function (1% or 2%), whereas larger differences (5% or more) have a profound affect on binocular vision. Generally, approximately 1% per diopter of anisometropia image size difference is assumed to occur.

Anomalies of the Motor Process

Motor anomalies are at the apex of the pyramid of binocular vision and are the last to be treated. Vergence disorders, for example, should be approached after other identifiable sensory and integrative problems have been fully treated. Motor anomalies are very common and have a significant effect on both visual comfort and performance.

Vergence Dysfunction

Anomalies of the vergence system, such as convergence insufficiency, are among the most common binocular anomalies diagnosed. Vergence dysfunction may be associated with either esophoria, exophoria, vertical phoria, or a combination of these. The anomalies may or may not lead to strabismus. Vergence dysfunction typically produces both symptoms and reduced performance, especially for tasks requiring good binocularity.

Strabismus (Comitant and Incomitant)

Comitant (concomitant) strabismus is a type of crossing of the eyes in which the amount of crossing, as determined objectively, remains stable regardless of the direction of gaze or the eye that is viewing. Comitant strabismus is common and includes many childhood and other types of strabismus.

Incomitant (noncomitant or nonconcomitant) strabismus is a type of crossing of the eyes in which the crossing varies according to the direction of gaze or the fixating eye. Much incomitant strabismus is the result of trauma, surgery, tumor, vascular disease (e.g., diabetes, hypertension, atherosclerosis, and so on), or aneurysm. Incomitant strabismus can become more comitant with time and is less frequently observed than the comitant varieties.

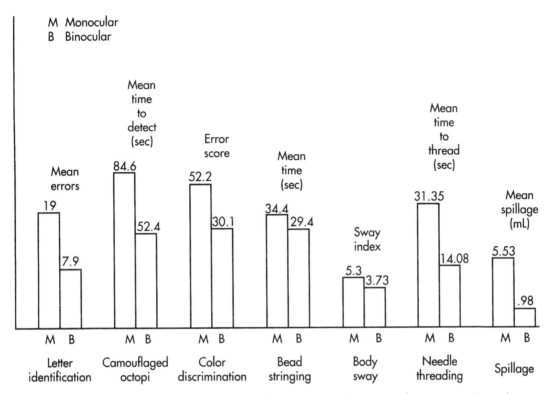

FIG. 1-2 Using two eyes improves performance on tasks not involving stereopsis, such as identifying hidden letters. (Modified from Jones RK, Lee DN: Why two eyes are better than one: the two views of binocular vision, *J Exp Psychol Hum Percept* 7:30, 1981.)

Nystagmus

Nystagmus is the rhythmic to-and-fro oscillation of the eyes. Nystagmus does not include the small oscillatory movements associated with fixation of normally seeing eyes. There are many varieties of nystagmus with various etiologies. Although nystagmus can sometimes be managed effectively, typically it carries a poor prognosis for both visual acuity and binocular vision.

ADVANTAGES OF NORMAL BINOCULAR VISION AND DISADVANTAGES OF ABNORMAL BINOCULAR VISION

Normal binocular vision provides the advantage of increased performance and efficiency in many situations.[6-8] Imagery from the two eyes provides information as a result of both concordant (matched) and disparate (mismatched) information. Disparity allows stereopsis. Crossed disparity suggests that an object is closer than the point of regard, and uncrossed disparity suggests that the object is farther away. Stereopsis can be exceptionally precise, sometimes allowing discrimination of only a few seconds of arc difference in depth.

A variety of experiments suggest that patients with normal binocular vision and the use of two eyes have superior ability in many more situations than would be the case with one eye. Identifying letters, detecting camouflaged objects, and color discrimination all favor patients with two eyes (Fig. 1-2), even though stereopsis is irrelevant to the task (p <00).[6] Other visuomotor tasks that can be specifically arranged to preclude stereopsis include bead threading or tracking a moving target using closed-circuit TV and the control of stance. In each situation, even without stereopsis, the individual with two eyes is able to perform the task much better than an individual with only one eye. Visuomotor skills that include disparity information are uniformly better with binocular vision (p <00).[6] These skills include diverse activities, such as how quickly a needle can be threaded, measuring the accuracy of pouring water into a container, assessing the accuracy of reaching toward an object with the hand visible and the same task with the hand invisible. Others have also studied performance under binocular and monocular conditions, confirming these results.[7] Additional advantages of binocular vision include increased depth perception, a spare eye in case of acci-

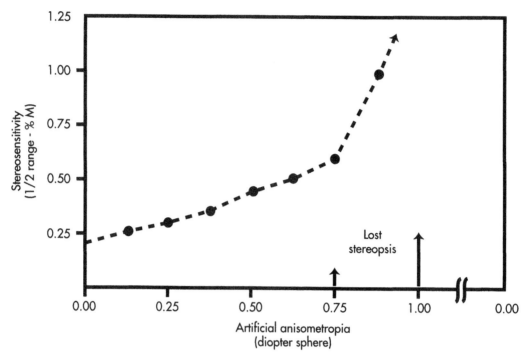

FIG. 1-3   The influence of artificially induced anisometropia (diopters sphere) on stereosensitivity (percent magnification), as measured on a space eikonometer: mean values for five subjects. (Modified from Peters HB: The influence of anisometropia on stereosensitivity, *Am J Optom Arch Am Acad Optom* 46:120, 1969.)

dents, increased visual acuity, and an increased field of view compared with one eye.

✿ CLINICAL PEARL

A variety of experiments suggest that patients with normal binocular vision and the use of two eyes have superior ability in many more situations than would be the case with one eye.

There are many significant disadvantages to abnormal binocular vision. One disadvantage is decreased performance and inefficiency, as noted above.[6,8,9] Decreased binocularity results in decreased performance.[8] Prism additions of 8 and 12 (BI or BO given to patients with normal binocular vision produce performance decrements of 3% to 6.7%.[8] This is less than the performance decrement of 20% to 30% when binocularity is denied. The decrements produced by absent or poor binocularity depend on the task; those that require depth perception are most affected. Likewise, uncorrected anisometropia commonly causes decreased stereoacuity (Fig. 1-3).[9] Abnormal binocular vision also can cause asthenopia, diplopia, objectionable cosmesis such as sometimes occurs with strabismus, and various sensomotor adaptations, such as amblyopia, eccentric fixation, suppression, and anomalous correspondence.

SUMMARY

Determining whether or not a patient has normal or abnormal binocular vision is challenging because of the many factors, both objective and subjective, related to diagnosis and treatment. This book discusses various aspects of the diagnosis and management of binocular visual anomalies in optometric practice.

REFERENCES

1. Schapero M, Cline C, Hofstetter HW, eds: *Dictionary of visual science*, ed 2, Philadelphia, 1968, Chilton.
2. von Noorden GK: *von Noorden-Maumenee's atlas of strabismus*, ed 3, St Louis, 1977, Mosby
3. Worth C: *Squint*, London, 1903, Blakiston & Sons.
4. Flom MC: The use of the accommodative convergence relationship in prescribing orthoptics, *Pennsylvania Optometrist* 14:3, 1954.
5. Ciuffreda KJ, Levi DM, Selenow A: *Amblyopia: basic and clinical aspects*, Boston, 1991, Butterworth-Heinemann.
6. Jones RK, Lee DN: Why two eyes are better than one: the two views of binocular vision, *J Exp Psychol (Human Percept)* 7:30, 1981.
7. Sheedy JE et al: Binocular vs. monocular task performance, *Am J Optom Physiol Opt* 63:839, 1986.
8. Sheedy JE et al: Task performance with base-in and base-out prism, *Am J Optom Physiol Opt* 65:65, 1988.
9. Peters HB: The influence of anisometropia on stereosensitivity, *Am J Optom Arch Am Acad Optom* 46:120, 1969.

Amblyopia, which literally translates as *blunt sight,* is an acquired unilateral or bilateral decrease of visual acuity for which no obvious structural or pathologic causes can be detected by physical examination of the eye. Amblyopia is generally considered to be a loss of visual acuity that cannot be improved by corrective lenses.[1] There is no ophthalmoscopically visible lesion of the retina, especially of the macular area or optic nerve head. Amblyopia develops in infants and very young children, beginning only during the first 6 years or so of life.[2] Once established, how-

ever, it can persist for life. If treated early, its effects are completely or nearly completely reversible. Amblyopia produces few symptoms, because the patient usually has normal acuity in the other eye. Adults have described what they see with their amblyopic eye as similar to the shimmer effect of hot air over a highway, a continuous wavy motion in the environment. The object of regard does not remain stationary; parts of it fade in and out of focus continuously.[3]

 CLINICAL PEARL

Amblyopia develops in infants and very young children, beginning only during the first 6 years or so of life.

The level of visual acuity that constitutes amblyopia ranges from slightly less than normal (20/25) to functionally blind (worse than 20/200). Light perception is always maintained.[4] Some clinicians require either more than two Snellen lines difference between the eyes or corrected visual acuity of 20/30 or worse for amblyopia to be diagnosed, whereas others only require corrected visual acuity worse than 20/20.

The visual acuity loss in amblyopia has been described as the "tip of the iceberg."[5] Amblyopia represents a syndrome of deficits, and amblyopic eyes perform much differently on many visual tasks than an ametropic eye or a diseased eye with equal visual acuity loss. Amblyopia results in an eye in which other ocular functions, including ocular motility, accommodation, contrast sensitivity, and spatial judgment, are depressed.[6-11] Amblyopia also results in decreased function in the normal eye.[12] An understanding of these abnormalities is important, because they can aid in the diagnosis of amblyopia, be monitored to follow the effectiveness of therapy, and help in understanding the pathophysiology of amblyopia.

PREVALENCE

Amblyopia is relatively common, but its prevalence in the general population has been difficult to assess. The prevalence of amblyopia varies, depending on the study population selected and diagnostic criteria used. Diagnostic criteria have included reduced visual acuity in one eye, difference in refractive error between the two eyes, presence of strabismus, and noticeable difference in behavior when one eye is occluded in infants and toddlers. The level of visual acuity selected to

TABLE 2-1   PREVALENCE OF AMBLYOPIA

Preschool and school-age children	1.0% - 4.8%
Patients seeking eye care	1.7% - 5.6%
Military personnel	1.0% - 4.0%

define amblyopia is a major factor in estimates of prevalence. If the criteria selected is corrected acuity of 20/30, 3.5% of the population has amblyopia, whereas if the criteria selected is 20/40, it drops to 1.4%.[13] Not surprisingly the highest incidence is found in ophthalmic clinical practices (Table 2-1).

The most frequent estimate for the overall prevalence of amblyopia in the United States is from 2% to 2.5% of the population, with estimates ranging from as low as 1% to as high as 6%.[4] Approximately 6 to 10 million Americans are likely to be amblyopic. The prevalence of amblyopia in other industrialized nations is similar.[14,15]

A higher incidence of amblyopia has been associated with prematurity, low birth weight, retinopathy of prematurity, cerebral palsy, and mental retardation.[16-21] Maternal smoking and the use of drugs or alcohol during pregnancy are also associated with increased risk for amblyopia.[22,23]

Data on the epidemiology of amblyopia in various subpopulations (African-Americans, Asian-Americans) is generally not available. No difference in prevalence rates between males and females has been reported. The relative importance of environment and genetic factors in the development of amblyopia is also unclear. It is uncertain whether the tendency to develop amblyopia in the presence of an amblyopiagenic factor is inherited. Heredity may be a stronger factor with strabismus than with amblyopia. A higher incidence of strabismus is found in the children of amblyopic adults. Nevertheless, amblyopia is the most common visual disability in childhood. Nearly 60,000 children per year develop amblyopia.[4] Amblyopia is also the leading cause of monocular vision loss in the 20 to 70 age group, surpassing diseases such as diabetic retinopathy, glaucoma, macular degeneration, and cataract.[24]

The toll of amblyopia is even greater because the risk for the patient with amblyopia sustaining blinding trauma to the normal eye is significantly higher (3 times that of a normal adult and 16 times that of a normal child) than for the general population.[25]

ETIOLOGY

The clinical conditions causative for amblyopia are listed in Box 2-1.

BOX 2-1   CAUSES OF AMBLYOPIA

UNILATERAL
Constant unilateral strabismus
    Esotropia
    Exotropia
    Hypertropia
Anisometropia
    Anisohypermetropia
    Anisomyopia
    Anisoastigmatism
    Aniseikonia
Visual deprivation
    Cataract
    Complete ptosis
    Opaque cornea
    Hyphema
    Vitreous clouding
    Prolonged uncontrolled patching
    Prolonged unilateral blepharospasm
    Prolonged unilateral cycloplegia

BILATERAL
Visual deprivation
    Cataracts of equal density
    High uncorrected hypermetropia
    Ametropic astigmatism
    Motor nystagmus

Modified from Dell W: The epidemiology of amblyopia. In Rutstein RP, editor: *Problems in optometry*, Philadelphia, 1991, JB Lippincott.

Although diverse, the causes of amblyopia have in common an incongruity of visual information received by the two eyes, a decrease of visual input, or a combination of both factors. The factors shared by these clinical entities is an inability to form well-defined and well-focused images in one or both eyes (form-vision deprivation) and, in the case of unilateral amblyopia, unequal vision input from the two eyes to the brain (abnormal binocular interaction).[4] The most common causes of amblyopia are strabismus and anisometropia, accounting for 90% of all cases.[1,5] Approximately 30% of all people who have amblyopia have both strabismus and anisometropia.

 CLINICAL PEARL

The most common causes of amblyopia are strabismus and anisometropia.

CLASSIFICATION

It has been customary to classify amblyopia as being either organic, psychogenic, or functional. Some contend that amblyopia should be limited to func

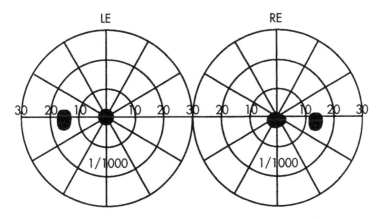

FIG. 2-1 Visual field for patient with nutritional amblyopia. (Modified from Harrington DO: *The visual fields: text and atlas of clinical perimetry,* ed 6, St Louis, 1990, Mosby.)

TABLE 2-2 COMPARISON OF ORGANIC AND FUNCTIONAL AMBLYOPIA

	Organic	Functional
Visual acuity	Often < 20/200	Usually > 20/200
Crowding phenomenon	Absent	Present in ⅔ of cases
Visual field	Absolute scotoma	Shallow, relative scotoma
Afferent pupillary defect	Can be present	Usually not present
Color vision	Defective (achromatopsia)	Usually normal
Visual acuity loss with neutral-density filter (3.0)	Significant decrease	Close to normal eye's VA
Entoptic phenomenon	Not seen	Usually seen
Laterality	Bilateral	Mostly unilateral
Onset	Any age	Before age 6
Strabismus and/or anisometropia	Rare	Common

Modified from London R, Silver JL: Diagnosis of amblyopia: emphasis on nonacuity factors. In Rutstein RP: *Problems in optometry,* Philadelphia, 1991, JB Lippincott.

tional etiologies, arguing that if organic or psychogenic factors exist, the condition cannot truly be amblyopia. Organic and psychogenic amblyopia fit into the definition of amblyopia because a reduction of best corrected visual acuity exists in an eye that is otherwise normal to clinical examination. Organic and psychogenic amblyopia occur much less frequently than functional amblyopia, have a distinctive set of signs and symptoms, and are treated differently than functional amblyopia.

ORGANIC AMBLYOPIA

Organic amblyopia occurs when the components of the visual pathway fail to develop either because of structural defects or the functioning of the normal visual pathway becomes impaired because of metabolic or toxic disturbances.[26] The absence of gross, readily detectable anomalies in the eye with reduced visual acuity does not exclude the possibility of subtle, subophthalmoscopic morphologic changes or previous pathology that may have healed. Some patients with reduced visual acuity may have malorientation of their retinal receptors, possibly as a sequel to neonatal retinal hemorrhages.[27]

The clinical features for organic amblyopia are compared with the clinical features of functional amblyopia in Table 2-2.[27]

Organic amblyopia includes nutritional amblyopia, toxic amblyopia, and congenital amblyopia.

Nutritional Amblyopia

Nutritional amblyopia is the gradually progressive and painless loss of central vision as a result of dietary insufficiencies, specifically the lack of B vitamins (B_1, B_2, B_6, and B_{12}). This nutritional deficiency is frequently associated with excessive alcohol and/or tobacco consumption.[28-39] Nutritional amblyopia occurs most frequently in middle-age and elderly men. The loss of vision can occur from 2 weeks to several years after a history of chronic alcohol abuse. Visual acuity loss usually ranges from slight (20/30 to 20/70) to severe (20/200 or less), with a usual range of 20/50 to 20/200. The resulting visual field defect is a symmetric bilateral defect of the central or cecocentral type and is more pronounced in response to color stimuli (Fig. 2-1). The peripheral field is preserved. The scotoma is irregular in shape, extending usually 2 to 5 degrees, with the area of greatest density at the point of fixation. The levels and duration of alcohol and tobacco consumption necessary to create a visual field loss have yet to be determined. Formation of a centrocecal scotoma has been associated with mean daily consumption levels between 54 and 80 g of alcohol or two packs of cigarettes.[38,39]

Temporal pallor of the optic disc is the only significant fundus finding and occurs only if the disease goes untreated for many years. Patients with nutritional amblyopia may show grossly abnormal pattern visual evoked potentials, but without evidence of demyelinization. Magnetic resonance imaging is normal for these patients.[36]

Treatment consists of (1) administration of thiamine (and/or the complete vitamin B complex), (2) the reinstitution of proper diet, and (3) the discontinuation of alcohol abuse by referral to social and/or medical services. The vitamin B complex is clearly important, because its administration often causes at least some reversal of amblyopia, despite, in some cases, the continued use of alcohol by the patient.

Krumsiek, Kruger, and Patzoid[33] report on 40 representative patients with nutritional amblyopia. All 33 men and 7 women indulged in chronic alcohol consumption of more than 80 g of alcohol per day. They were also heavy smokers. The amblyopia was the first distinct sign that led the patients to a doctor. More than half had visual acuity of 20/70 or less, with both eyes affected simultaneously. Thirty-two patients had central scotomas, and 8 had centrocecal scotomas. Color vision testing revealed deficiencies in 19 of 20 patients tested, with 16 displaying a disturbance in red-green vision. Abnormalities were also found with visual evoked potential, the amplitudes of the p-100 peaks being reduced and deformed. For the 15 patients who were followed over a period of 31 months, the visual abnormalities improved in one half of the patients, but complete recovery was never reached, despite vitamin B therapy.

Clinical studies have defined the primary pathologic defects occurring with nutritional amblyopia.[31,40] Smiddy and Green[31] report atrophy of the maculopapillary bundle (loss or reduction of the nerve fiber and ganglion cell layers) in both eyes of 25 patients at post mortem. Malnutrition, anorexia, and weight loss were common to all of the patients. Alcohol abuse had been documented in 20 cases. In those cases in which alcohol did not play a role, other factors contributed to the malnutrition. One patient had carcinoma in the gastrointestinal tract, three patients had chronic obstructive pulmonary disease, and one patient had suffered a cerebral vascular accident.

The differential diagnosis of nutritional amblyopia includes Leber's hereditary optic neuropathy, which is also characterized by bilateral visual loss and centro-

cecal scotoma.[29,30] Unlike nutritional amblyopia, which occurs mostly in middle-age and elderly men, Leber's optic neuropathy occurs most frequently in young men.

Organic amblyopia related to excessive smoking and neither alcohol abuse nor malnutrition can occur. Recovery of vision can follow cessation of smoking or after hydroxocobalamin therapy.[32,35]

Toxic Amblyopia

Toxic amblyopia is a bilateral visual loss that has been associated with methanol, quinine, ergots, mercury, and lead, as well as therapeutic use of cisplatin, deferoxamine, hexamethonium, and antihypertensives.[41-43]

Quinine is a cinchona alkaloid used in the treatment of malaria and nocturnal cramps. Visual defects can occur in 27% of cases.[43,44] In a report on 31 patients with quinine amblyopia, there were 28 adults, ages 16 to 75 and 3 children, ages 2 to 4.[43] The nature of the visual deficit and its recovery was reported in 24 patients and ranged from minor field defects to tunnel vision with reduced acuity in one eye and blindness in the other. Because quinine amblyopia has been recognized and thought to be caused by retinal arteriolar constriction, blockage of the sympathetic supply to the retinal arterioles has been recommended as treatment. However, no treatment for ocular toxicity was of benefit for these patients.

Moloney, Hillery, and Fenton[42] document the electrophysiologic and psychophysical findings over a 2-year period for a 19-year-old patient with quinine amblyopia. The patient had ingested in excess of 20 tablets of quinine sulfate (6 g). Four hours later she had light perception. The electrophysiologic tests performed were the electro-oculogram, electroretinogram, and visually evoked potential. Psychophysical tests were dark adaptometry, contrast sensitivity, and color discrimination. Visually evoked responses and the electro-oculogram were abolished early. By 2 months, the visually evoked responses and visual acuity had returned to normal. The electroretinogram, initially mildly subnormal, became virtually normal by 2 months. No recovery in cone function took place. Of the rods, 50% regained function with normal latency by 1 year, but receptor sensitivity did not return to normal until 2 years after ingestion. The electro-oculogram also became normal slowly over a 2-year period. Quinine apparently exerts a direct toxic effect on the cells of the outer retina, pigment epithelium, and ganglion cells.

Toxic amblyopia associated with crack cocaine use has been reported recently.[45,46] This complication is presumed to result from a direct vasoconstrictive effect of cocaine on the retinal vasculature.

Congenital Amblyopia

Congenital amblyopia involves reduced irreversible bilateral vision attributed to congenital or hereditary anomalies in the visual receptors or visual pathways. The visual system may fail to develop completely.[47] This form of amblyopia is usually associated with other congenital ocular defects, such as nystagmus, ocular albinism, cone deficiency syndrome, and achromatopsia. Congenital amblyopia is presumed by some clinicians to also be present when treatment is unsuccessful, even though given at the appropriate age and with good compliance.

Nystagmus associated with a central nervous system abnormality such as hydrocephalus can lead to poor vision because of the inability of the patient to maintain fixation with the fovea. A continuously moving world is clearly a cause of poor image formation on the retina. The cause of poor vision is less clear in cases of nystagmus associated with ocular anomalies such as albinism or achromatopsia. Amblyopia in children with albinism has been attributed to lack of macular development, scattering of light in the posterior pole as a result of lack of choroidal pigment, and pendular nystagmus.

The poor vision in congenital achromatopsia is most likely the result of lack of cone function in these patients. The presence of nystagmus and extreme photophobia also are likely contributing factors in the amblyopia.[48] Treatment of the amblyopia in such cases rarely succeeds because of the multiple ocular and visual system abnormalities.

Congenital amblyopia may occur with myopia greater than 10 D.[49] High degrees of myopia are frequently associated with retinal thinning and macular pigment abnormalities. Many such myopias do not achieve normal visual acuity, even when corrected with contact lenses. It has been proposed that the amblyopia is caused by an organic micropsia that results from the stretching of the retina to cover the axially elongated eye.[49] This disperses the retinal elements over a greater area, which produces a relative micropsia, reducing the potential acuity of the eye anatomically. Several investigators have also reported a relationship between peripapillary myelinated nerve fibers, myopia, and unilateral organic amblyopia.[50-54]

Some patients with amblyopia have been shown to have an abnormal Stiles-Crawford function (light that passes through the center of the pupil is perceived as brighter than a pencil of light that passes through a peripheral point of the pupil yet stimulates the same retinal point). Because of the abnormal Stiles-Crawford function, it has been suggested an anatomic anomaly or misalignment in the retinal receptors exists in these patients.[55] However, the idea of receptor amblyopia has not been totally accepted.[56]

PSYCHOGENIC AMBLYOPIA

Psychogenic or "hysteric" amblyopia is a well-recognized clinical cause of visual acuity reduction. The visual loss that occurs is of emotional or psychologic rather than physiologic origin, as is the case in functional amblyopia. Psychogenic amblyopia is characterized by the substitution of reduced visual acuity for anxiety or emotional repression. The triggering factor may be the death of a relative or pet, accident, trauma, fear of failure, sickness, sexual or peer conflict, anxiety, or poor school performance. The symptoms are not under voluntary control, such as in malingering.

The prevalence of psychogenic amblyopia varies from 0.1% to 0.4% for military institutions and approximately 1% for civilians. It may comprise as much as 5% of a typical ophthalmic practice.[57] Patients are generally children (ages 8 to 14) or young adults. Psychogenic amblyopia can occur rarely in older patients.[58,59] It is more frequent in females, the female-to-male ratio ranging from 2.6:1 to as high as 11.5:1.[60]

Psychogenic amblyopia is a diagnosis of exclusion made only after organic pathology and sensory problems have been ruled out. The clinical features include a bilateral reduction in visual acuity, usually ranging from 20/70 to 20/200 (but can be better); normal ocular health; a minor symmetric refractive error (usually emmetropia or hyperopia); normal binocular vision, with either orthophoria or small heterophoria; and abnormal visual fields. Unilateral visual acuity loss is very rare. Direct questioning of the patient, in addition to blurred vision, nearly always reveals additional symptoms, such as headache, periorbital pain, photophobia, and, sometimes, diplopia.

 CLINICAL PEARL

Psychogenic amblyopia is a diagnosis of exclusion made only after organic pathology and sensory problems have been ruled out.

If the patient is a young child, the decreased visual acuity is usually discovered by the pediatrician or school vision screening. Although the visual acuity loss may appear quite significant, these patients do not demonstrate any difficulty in walking through a room with obstacles in their path. Typically, the patient reads the visual acuity letters slowly, deliberately, and with more difficulty than is usual. In some cases, visual acuity is improved by suggestion. A first clue as to the appropriate diagnosis is the retinoscopic finding of low or insignificant refractive error.

The most important diagnostic finding is the visual field.[61-63] By convention, tangent screen visual fields are performed on each eye at 1 m, using a white

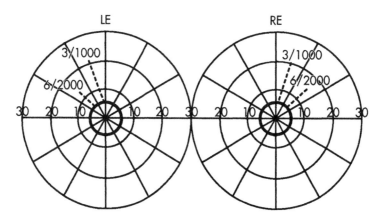

FIG. 2-2   Visual field for patient with psychogenic amblyopia. Field in each eye is constricted and remains similar in linear dimension when test distance is changed from 1 meter to 2 meters. (Modified from Harrington DO: *The visual fields: text and atlas of clinical perimetry,* ed 6, St Louis, 1990, Mosby.)

test stimulus of 3 mm. The patient is then moved to a 2 m test distance, and the measurements are repeated with a 6-mm white test target. The visual fields are constricted, usually to within 5 to 15 degrees of fixation. In addition, tubular or tunnel-shaped fields are found. The visual fields measure the same size in linear dimension, regardless of the size of the test target or the test distance used (Fig. 2-2). On the contrary, for the patient with visual loss associated with organic disease, as well as for the normal patient, if the test distance and target size are increased, the centimeter value will also increase but the angular value will remain constant.

Streff[64] describes a group of children who also had bilaterally reduced visual acuities, minimal or no refractive error, ocular alignment, and normal ocular health. We feel that this condition, referred to as the *Streff nonmalingering syndrome,* does not represent a separate clinical entity from psychogenic amblyopia.[65]

With regard to treatment, we refrain from giving glasses to patients with insignificant or nonexistent refractive errors; orthoptics/vision therapy; or nonmedical eyedrops, such as lubricants, because they may serve to reinforce the problem rather than address its true basis. Most patients can be handled by a strong dose of reassurance that no serious eye disease is found, and symptoms are likely to resolve with time. If the triggering factor is obvious and includes, for example, loss of a relative, sexual conflict, or trauma or if the patient has symptoms suggestive of a psychiatric or psychologic syndrome, referral would be appropriate.

Psychogenic amblyopia generally improves with time. However, some patients continue to manifest signs of visual loss for an extended period. Interest-

ingly, in studies that followed a total of 109 patients with psychogenic amblyopia from 6 months to 32 years, only 55 patients (50%) recovered entirely or improved, whereas 51 patients (47%) stayed the same or became worse.[58,59,66-68] Despite the continuity of the findings, few patients became socially or economically impaired by the functional visual disability. Younger patients appear to have a much better prognosis for improved visual function than older patients.[60] Apparently, adults with psychogenic amblyopia generally are more emotionally disturbed than children and adolescents who develop such symptoms. Children may also have more alternatives for conflict solution than adults. (See Cases 1 and 2.)

CASE 1

A 12-year-old girl presented for a second opinion regarding blurred vision. The patient said she could not see clearly things that were far away. She was using "reading" glasses prescribed by another clinician a year earlier. The patient was not taking any medications and had not suffered either physical or emotional trauma.

Examination revealed visual acuities of 20/200 for each eye. The patient was orthophoric at distance and near. Versions were full. Pupillary and color vision testing were normal. With the Titmus stereotest, the patient had 50 seconds of arc. Cycloplegic refraction was OD +0.75 −0.50 × 85 and OS +0.25 −0.50 × 85. Ophthalmoscopic examination through dilated pupils was normal. The visual fields as measured with the tangent screen at 1 and 2 m were constricted and tubular.

The diagnosis was psychogenic amblyopia. Both patient and parent denied any school or family problem. The parents sought evaluation by a psychologist. One year later, the visual acuity was 20/160 for each eye. The patient did not appear to be visually handicapped.

CASE 2

An 8-year-old girl complained of blurred distance vision. The parents reported that the child holds books very close. An examination 5 years before revealed orthophoria, normal visual acuity, and insignificant refractive error. The child was healthy and progressing well in school.

Examination revealed 20/200 vision in each eye. The patient was orthophoric at distance and near. Versions were normal. Pupils and color vision were normal. With the Titmus stereotest, 100 seconds of arc was elicited. Cycloplegic refraction was OD +0.50 − 0.75 × 180 and OS +0.50 − 0.50 × 180, which did not improve the vision. Visual fields done at 1 and 2 meters with the tangent screen were within 5 degrees of the fixation point and tubular. Dilated ophthalmoscopy was normal.

The diagnosis was psychogenic amblyopia. Letters were sent to the pediatrician and teacher. Over a period of 6 months the visual acuity improved to 20/20 for each eye. There has been no recurrence.

FUNCTIONAL AMBLYOPIA

In functional amblyopia the visual pathway is intact and normal at birth but fails to develop or operate normally because of an abnormality in its stimulus or use. A functional, or reversible, amblyopia may become superimposed on structural defects or diseases that cause the initial reduction in visual acuity. This visual acuity seems poorer than expected for the organic disease. Amblyopia as a result of strabismus and/or anisometropia has been described as a major cause of vision loss in juvenile glaucoma, with estimates of its incidence as high as 78%.[69,70] This has also been shown to be the case in some abnormalities of the anterior segment, retina, choroid, and optic nerve.[71-73] It is important to rule out the possible presence of a superimposed functional amblyopia in these cases. Treatment should be considered to determine whether some improvement in vision can be achieved in children with partial media opacities, macula lesions, or optic nerve abnormalities.

Functional amblyopia consists of strabismic amblyopia, anisometropic amblyopia, isoametropic amblyopia, deprivation amblyopia, and idiopathic amblyopia.

Strabismic Amblyopia

Strabismic amblyopia is a consequence of a constant and unilateral strabismus that is acquired during the period of visual immaturity. Its period of peak sensitivity probably lies between ages 9 months and 2 years. The median age of presentation in our clinic is before the fourth birthday. The cause of the amblyopia is presumably an active cortical inhibition of impulses originating from the fovea of the deviating eye. With strabismus, dissimilarly contoured images are presented to the two foveae. The perceptual conflict arising from the situation of visual confusion causes the fovea of the strabismic eye to be continuously inhibited or suppressed. The suppression over time results in loss of visual acuity. The average best corrected acuity initially for strabismic amblyopia is 20/74.[13] When coexisting with anisometropia, the average best visual acuity is poorer, at 20/94.[13] The degree of amblyopia is not correlated with the magnitude of the strabismus.[74]

Strabismic amblyopia is most commonly associated with esotropia.[75] In one study, amblyopia occurred in nearly 80% of the esotropic cases, whereas it occurred in only 16% of the exotropic cases.[76] This is because exotropia usually presents as an intermittent strabismus, whereas esotropia usually presents as a constant strabismus. Patients with intermittent strabismus bifixate sufficiently to prevent the development of amblyopia. The chance of exotropia existing with amblyopia is greater when amblyopia is either secondary to a preexisting unilateral decrease in vision, such as anisometropia or sensory exotropia, or a consecutive exotropia. Frequently it can be determined that an older patient with amblyopia who has exotropia actually developed the condition while being esotropic at an earlier age. The higher incidence of amblyopia in esotropia vs. exotropia may also be related to the nasotemporal asymmetry of the retinocortical projections. In esotropia the fovea of the deviating eye must compete with the strong temporal hemifield of the fellow eye, whereas in exotropia the fovea competes with the weaker contralateral hemifield.[77]

 CLINICAL PEARL

Strabismic amblyopia is most commonly associated with esotropia.

Strabismic amblyopia is less likely to occur in alternating, intermittent, and incomitant strabismus. It has been reported to occur in only 12% of patients with superior oblique palsy and in only 10% of patients with Duane's syndrome, who frequently manage to maintain bifoveal fusion in some position of gaze with a compensatory head tilt or a head turn.[78,79]

 CLINICAL PEARL

Strabismic amblyopia is less likely to occur in alternating, intermittent, and incomitant strabismus.

A dual amblyopiagenic mechanism has been proposed in strabismic amblyopia. Focusing of the foveal image in the deviated eye is determined by the accommodative requirement of the fixating eye. Because the object seen by the fovea of the deviating eye is at a different point in space than the object seen by the fixating eye, its image will not only be dissimilar relative to the image on the fovea of the fixating eye but also defocused, unless the object happens to lie at the same distance from the object of interest. Lack of stimulation of those cells that are tuned to only sharply focused images (sustained, or, X retinal ganglion cells) occurs, resulting in the amblyopiagenic mechanism of foveal form-vision deprivation.[80,81]

Experiments on animals have provided evidence that the deleterious effect of form-vision deprivation on geniculate cell growth can be inhibited if binocular interaction is blocked by experimentally inactivating the cells in the adjacent nondeprived lateral geniculate nucleus laminae.[82,83] With normal binocular vision, balance of interaction between the terminals from corresponding retinal points in the lateral geniculate nucleus takes place either in the lateral geniculate nucleus or in the visual cortex (see Pathophysiology). When visual experience is abnormal early in life, the deprived cells are at a disadvantage in the competition and their growth is inhibited. Clinically, this implies that the functioning of the amblyopic eye is subject to inhibitory factors elicited by stimulation of the fixating eye. Competition occurs between the two foveal images. This is the other proposed amblyopiagenic mechanism, abnormal binocular interaction, which is thought to be the primary mechanism causing vision loss in strabismic amblyopia.

It appears improbable, however, that foveal form deprivation plays a significant role in strabismic amblyopia. Given consensual accommodation, it is likely that the strabismic eye's image would be sharply focused much of the time and not cause retinal changes. Also, the fact that the depth of amblyopia is not related to the magnitude of strabismus implies that abnormal binocular interaction is likely the only amblyopiagenic mechanism.[84]

Amblyopia of Arrest and Amblyopia of Extinction

Chavasse[85] divides strabismic amblyopia into two subtypes: amblyopia of arrest and amblyopia of extinction. Chavasse believes that 20/20 vision reflects a conditioned reflex that develops with normal visual stimulation and is firmly established by age 6. If a child develops strabismus at a younger age and the visual acuity is at a certain level, there is cessation of visual acuity development in the involved eye. No amount of treatment will improve the visual acuity. Suppression occurring during the first 6 years of life arrests the full development of vision. This is the amblyopia of arrest. If the strabismus goes untreated, further deterioration of visual acuity relative to that previously attained will occur. An extinction of an unused or nonreinforced conditioned reflex could occur. This loss, according to Chavasse, is recoverable and is the amblyopia of extinction.

The clinical implication is that if a child develops

a constant, unilateral esotropia supposedly at the age of 1½ years, the level of visual acuity developed would be approximately 20/80. This is the amblyopia of arrest and supposedly represents the highest level of visual acuity possible in the strabismic eye. If the child is not examined until age 4, the visual acuity in the strabismic eye may have deteriorated further to 20/200. Therapy would be expected to improve the visual acuity to 20/80 at best.

In view of present knowledge, the views of Chavasse cannot be accepted. First, sufficient clinical evidence exists demonstrating that visual acuity can be restored to a much higher level than was present at the onset of the strabismus. Second, amblyopia depth is related more to the length of time that an eye is strabismic in childhood rather than the age of onset. Third, visual acuity develops in children earlier than previously expected. Chavasse reported the acuity level of a 4-month-old infant to be about 20/2500, whereas presently a visual acuity from 20/50 to 20/200 is considered normal, depending on the method of measurement.[86] Consequently the majority of strabismic amblyopia is of the extinction type and is potentially reversible.

Anisometropic Amblyopia

A significant difference in the refractive errors between the two eyes can cause amblyopia in the young patient.[26] This refractive difference causes a blurred image in the eye with the greater refractive error, disrupting the normal physiologic development of the visual pathway and visual cortex.[87] As in strabismic amblyopia, there is dissimilarity of the foveal images between the two eyes. The difference is in clarity, size, and contrast rather than form. Because they are usually asymptomatic and have straight eyes, children with anisometropic amblyopia tend to be examined later than children with strabismic amblyopia, sometimes not until the child is in school and vision is tested during a routine screening examination.[88] The median age of presentation in our clinic is after the sixth birthday.

Although having a wide range of visual acuities, the average best corrected acuity initially for patients with anisometropic amblyopia is 20/60.[13,82] Anisometropic amblyopia is considered the most common type of amblyopia, occurring twice as frequently as strabismic amblyopia.[26,89] It is associated with strabismus in about one third of cases. The incidence of pure anisometropic amblyopia may be overestimated, because some of these patients may not foveally fixate and actually have an ultrasmall strabismus.[90]

Amblyopia is much more likely to occur in anisohyperopia than in anisomyopia. In anisohyperopia, the amount of accommodation used will be just enough to form a clear retinal image in the less hyper

---

From *Care of the patient with amblyopia: optometric clinical practice guideline,* St Louis, 1994, American Optometric Association.

---

opic eye at all distances. Because the accommodative response is conjugate and is controlled by the accommodative requirement of the less hyperopic eye, the more hyperopic eye never receives a clear image at distance and near and becomes amblyopic. Many investigators believe that a spheric equivalent of 1.50 D or more is amblyopiagenic. However, patients with hyperopic anisometropia of 1 D (Box 2-2) have developed amblyopia.[26]

 CLINICAL PEARL

Amblyopia is much more likely to occur in anisohyperopia than in anisomyopia.

In anisomyopia the more myopic eye can be used for near and the less myopic eye can be used for distance. Sharply focused images will be available to both eyes up to their respective near points, with both eyes maintaining foveal fixation and good corrected acuity. Amblyopia in either eye is unusual in anisomyopia, unless the refractive difference between the eyes exceeds 3 to 4 D. Amblyopia existing in patients with less anisomyopia not coexisting with strabismus requires further examination by the clinician to rule out any possible organic causes for the reduced visual acuity.

Bilateral myopic shift during late childhood and adolescence may account for the rare finding of amblyopia in the emmetropic eye of an adult with unilateral myopia, which was more hyperopic than its fellow during early childhood. The high frequency of myopic anisometropic amblyopia in patients with prematurity and low birth weight should lead the clinician to suspect it in all such children, even in the absence of other signs that indicate retinopathy of prematurity.[91]

In summary, the patient with a refractive error of OD +1.00 D and OS +3.00 D who is not corrected in early childhood is likely to become amblyopic,

whereas the patient with OD − 1.00 D and OS − 3.00 D is not likely to become amblyopic. Anisometropia involving astigmatic refractive errors usually requires that the anisometropia be at least 2 to 3 D difference. Oblique astigmatic errors in one eye may lead to amblyopia if the other eye has against-the-rule or with-the-rule astigmatism.

Anisometropic amblyopia involves a dual amblyopiagenic mechanism. The fixating, or less ametropic, eye always has a clear image, whereas the more ametropic eye always has a blurred image, causing foveal form-vision deprivation. There is also active inhibition of the fovea of the more ametropic eye, its purpose being to eliminate sensory interference caused by superimposition of a focused and a defocused image originating from the fixation point (abnormal binocular interaction).

Several views exist on whether or not the degree of anisometropia correlates with the depth of amblyopia.[92-96] Helveston[92] analyzed data on 57 patients and found no relationship between the degree of anisometropia and the depth of amblyopia. Similar findings were reported by Malik, Gupta, and Choudry.[93] However, Sen[94] and more recently Townshend, Holmes, and Evans[95] found that higher degrees of anisometropia were associated with more severe degrees of amblyopia. It appears that studies that separately analyze hyperopic and myopic anisometropia tend to find a better relationship between the depth of amblyopia and the difference in refraction between the two eyes.[95] Because the severity of amblyopia cannot be consistently correlated with the degree of anisometropia, abnormal binocular interaction caused by unequal focused foveal images in the two eyes and not form-vision deprivation plays the greatest role in the production of anisometropic amblyopia.

Isoametropic Amblyopia

Isoametropic (isometropic, ametropic) amblyopia is caused by a high but approximately equal bilateral uncorrected refractive error that creates an equally blurred image on each retina. It occurs less frequently than either strabismic or anisometropic amblyopia, with an overall incidence of 0.03% of the population.[84] The amblyopia is relatively mild. Typically visual acuities are in the range of 20/30 to 20/70 in each eye when first corrected.[97] When deep bilateral amblyopia is found in a child with symmetric refractive error, especially if nystagmus exists, the possibility of an underlying organic factor should be considered. In most cases of isoametropic amblyopia, visual acuity improves once corrective lenses have been worn for a few months but usually does not improve completely. The lower the refractive error, the greater the chance for improvement after the proper correction has been worn.[98]

CLINICAL PEARL

> When deep bilateral amblyopia is found in a child with symmetric refractive error, especially if nystagmus exists, the possibility of an underlying organic factor should be considered.

The degree of refractive error necessary to produce isoametropic amblyopia differs, depending on the type of ametropia present.[99] Generally, bilateral hyperopia exceeding 5 D, bilateral myopia exceeding 8 D, and bilateral astigmatism exceeding 2.50 D are causative for amblyopia (see Box 2-2). As with anisometropic amblyopia, the uncorrected myopic refractive error must be greater than the hyperopic error because of the ability of the patient with myopia to have a clear image when viewing at near. For example, of 18 patients with isoametropic amblyopia with refractive errors between 5 D and 9 D who were treated from ages 1 to 2½, half of those with hyperopia developed amblyopia, whereas none of those with myopia developed amblyopia.[100] Isoametropic amblyopia is also unlikely to develop in the patient with high hyperopia with refractive accommodative esotropia. Of 184 children who had hyperopia exceeding 4 D in each eye, 12 (6.5%) had bilateral amblyopia of 20/50 or worse.[101] Lower degrees of hyperopia were more likely to lead to refractive accommodative esotropia (assuming absence of a low AC/A ratio), because the young child's visual system can readily compensate for the excessive accommodative demand.[102]

Unlike strabismic and anisometropic amblyopia, abnormal binocular interaction is not a factor with isoametropic amblyopia. The two retinal images are equal in clarity and size. The cause of isoametropic amblyopia is equally uncorrected refractive errors. The resultant bilaterally blurred retinal images deprive the visual system of the necessary stimulation found in focused retinal images. The only amblyopiagenic mechanism is foveal form-vision deprivation. No competitive inhibition between the two eyes occurs. This explains why the amblyopia associated with isoametropia is generally not as severe as either strabismic or anisometropic amblyopia and exhibits a lower resistance to therapy.

A form of isoametropic amblyopia, meridional amblyopia, results from uncorrected high astigmatism. In patients with simple hyperopic astigmatism, for example, one meridian, or axis, is blurred while the other meridian (at 90 degrees to the first) is in focus. Visual acuity losses only occur along the habitually blurred meridian.[103] This has been confirmed in the laboratory by contrast sensitivity functions, which have been shown to be reduced for gratings oriented to the astigmatic (amblyopic) meridian.[104] Meridional amblyopia is also observed clinically in patients who show a mild reduction in visual acuity even when the full astigmatic correction is in place.[105]

The high degree of astigmatism in infants that improves during the first year of life does not appear to be related to an equally high incidence of meridional amblyopia.[106,107] Astigmatism leads to meridional amblyopia only if it persists for 2 years or longer.[107]

Deprivation Amblyopia

Deprivation, or stimulus deprivation, amblyopia refers to amblyopia secondary to the occurrence of a constant physical obstruction along the line of sight that prevents the formation of a well-focused high-contrast image on the retina.[84] This obstruction can occur in one or both eyes. The unilateral form is often accompanied by sensory esotropia or sensory exotropia. Deprivation amblyopia has the most potential of all the types of amblyopia to cause severe visual loss. The degree to which amblyopia develops depends on the time of onset and the extent of the physical obstruction. Short periods of deprivation at any early age can have a profound effect. If present in the first 3 months of life, it frequently leads to severe and sometimes permanent reduction in visual acuity. The prognosis for improvement is less favorable in cases with complete physical obstruction, compared with cases with only partial obstruction.

Congenital cataract is the most frequent cause of deprivation amblyopia.[108] Other causes include traumatic cataract, persistent hyperplastic primary vitreous, congenital ptosis, surgical lid closure, corneal opacities, prolonged patching, uncorrected aphakia, and prolonged unilateral cycloplegia.[109-116] With ptosis the risk of amblyopia occurs only when the lid is drooping enough to occlude the visual axis (Fig. 2-3). Some children develop a chin elevation as compensation, to avoid palpebral occlusion.

The prevalence of deprivation amblyopia is low compared with the other types of functional amblyopia, accounting for no more than 3% of all amblyopias. Flom and Neumaier[117] found only 3 cases (all cataracts) in a sample of 2762 school children. However, an estimated 10% to 38% of all visual impairment in children is caused by congenital cataract.[118] The significance of congenital cataract is illustrated by a prevalence rate of 0.4% in newborns.[119] Some of these cataracts cause only partial obstruction.

Unilateral deprivation is much more detrimental to visual acuity development than bilateral deprivation because of its dual amblyopiagenic mechanism. For example, in congenital unilateral cataract, decreased optical quality of the image is received by the fovea of the cataractous eye (form-vision deprivation), and competition (abnormal binocular interaction) occurs between the blurred diffused image and the focused image received by the noncataractous eye. With bilateral congenital cataracts, both images are equally blurred and there is only form-vision deprivation. This frequently leads to the development of nystagmus, which is likely to persist and be associated with poor visual acuity despite subsequent treatment.

Detection and management is considerably more difficult when the congenital cataract is partial. The management undertaken will depend on the potential for the partial cataract to create retinal image degradation. A slit-lamp examination is necessary to evaluate the type and density of the cataract. Lamellar cataracts, if bilateral, have the best prognosis, and axial cataracts and nuclear cataracts have the worst prognosis; however, a unilateral lamellar cataract may produce significant amblyopia. The degree of visual impairment induced by cataracts differs markedly, depending on location. The more posterior and central the location, the more visually significant the cataract will be. Small anterior polar cataracts do not cause amblyopia unless associated with significant corneal astigmatism.[120] Small posterior polar cataracts frequently impair vision. A partial cataract of 3 mm diameter located along the visual axis is as equally capable of producing deprivation amblyopia as a total cataract.[121] Generally, if an adequate retinoscopic reflex cannot be obtained or the retina cannot be visualized adequately by ophthalmoscopy, the cataract is of sufficient density to be amblyopiagenic.[122,123]

Partial cataracts in young children must be followed closely, because a cataract that initially appears to be insufficient to cause amblyopia may progress. A clinical dilemma occurs when an older child presents with a cataract of unknown origin or onset. It may be impossible to distinguish between a total cataract and a total cataract that was once only partial.[124,125] Kushner[126] treated 17 children between ages 1 and 5¾ who had monocular total cataract of unknown origin and unknown time of onset. In 14 of the patients, final visual acuity in the aphakic eye was 20/50 or better. The presence of microphthalmos was associated with a poor visual prognosis and suggested that the cataract was congenital. The clinician must remember that congenital cataracts are often associated with other organic ocular disease, such as microphthalmia, and in these cases there is little hope for visual improvement.

Occlusion amblyopia is an iatrogenically induced type of deprivation amblyopia. Patching of the nonamblyopic eye or the use of prolonged unilateral cycloplegia can lead to vision loss in that eye for patients below age 5.[113,114,127] The sensitivity to develop this visual loss is especially high within the first 2 years of life.[128,129] Visual acuity of the nonamblyopic eye in the infant has been reported to decrease, with a simultaneous increase in the amblyopic eye, after as little as 2 hours of occlusion per day.[130] The likelihood of this visual loss is greatest when the visual acuity in the amblyopic eye improves in the range of 20/40 to 20/60. Fortunately, the vision loss is usually transient and readily restored by reversing the occlusion to the amblyopic eye. Infrequently, it may be permanent. Simon, Parks, and Price[114] report on two infants who developed severe amblyopia after patching of 13 and 30 days. Bilateral amblyopia persisted for one child, despite reversal of the occlusion. Our experience is that occlusion amblyopia can be avoided by the use of judicious alternating occlusion.

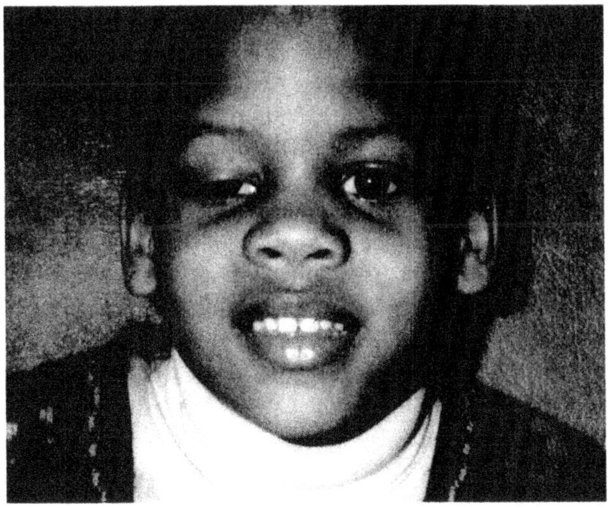

FIG. 2-3 Congenital ptosis that was amblyopiagenic.

CLINICAL PEARL

Patching of the nonamblyopic eye or the use of prolonged unilateral cycloplegia can lead to vision loss in that eye for patients below age 5.

Idiopathic Amblyopia

In 1985 von Noorden[131] described two children without strabismus, anisometropia, or a history of form deprivation who had normal stereoacuity yet were deeply amblyopic in one eye. Psychogenic visual loss and diseases affecting the afferent visual pathway were ruled out. The amblyopia responded to treatment for both patients but recurred after cessation of treatment. Because there was no known cause for the amblyopia, it was classified as being idiopathic. It is possible that binocularly provoked inhibition of the fovea of one eye was conditioned during infancy by an amblyopiagenic condition, such as anisometropia.[131,132] Clinically significant astigmatic refractive errors and anisometropia are common in infancy and usually disappear spontaneously as a child grows.[106,133] Once competition between the eyes has been established the acuities "see-saw," even if the original anisometropia is no longer present. If this is the cause, idiopathic amblyopia would be much more common. Reference to this type of amblyopia in the literature, however, is rare.[132]

We have examined a patient who could possibly be categorized as having idiopathic amblyopia. The 9-year-old girl was referred with a diagnosis of amblyopia. The previous records at that time indicated that the youngster had been treated for amblyopia of the right eye 4 years previously. Vision had improved from 20/70 to 20/30. Our examination revealed visual acuities of 20/40 and 20/20 for the right and left eyes respectively. The neutral-density filter test (see Diagnosis and Clinical Features) was inconclusive. The patient was orthophoric at distance and near. Stereopsis with the Randot stereotest was 20 seconds of arc. Visuoscopy indicated foveal fixation in the amblyopic eye. Cycloplegic retinoscopy (OD +1.00 − 0.25 × 180 and OS +0.75 D sphere) did not improve the vision in the right eye. All ocular health testing was normal, including visual fields. The fact that the visual acuity in the amblyopic eye had improved earlier with therapy and then subsequently regressed and absence of any amblyopiagenic mechanisms suggested the diagnosis to be idiopathic amblyopia.

With this case as an exception the possibility of a subclinical microtropia or another binocular vision anomaly causing inhibition of foveal function and a subclinical organic amblyopia remains a possibility for idiopathic amblyopia.

DIAGNOSIS AND CLINICAL FEATURES

The diagnosis of amblyopia includes measurement of visual acuity in each eye, determination of the refractive error, assessment of ocular alignment, and assessment of monocular fixation status.

VISUAL ACUITY

The hallmark of amblyopia is a decrease in visual acuity. Accurate measurement of visual acuity is critical to its detection and management. As indicated earlier, a commonly used diagnostic criterion is a loss of visual acuity of two or more lines on the Snellen chart while wearing the proper refractive correction. Such measurement can be difficult if not impossible at the ages when it is most necessary. It is obvious that a Snellen visual acuity measurement cannot be taken on the very young child, yet this is the most important age at which to diagnose amblyopia. Although electrodiagnostic evaluation and psychophysical testing are available in hospitals and teaching clinics, it is usually sufficient for the clinician in the office environment to make a qualitative judgment of the visual acuity in each eye. Of utmost importance is whether there is difference in visual acuity between the two eyes.

In testing visual acuity of infants and other preverbal or noncommunicative patients, we occlude one eye

---

Box 2-3	CLASSIFICATION OF BINOCULAR FIXATION PREFERENCE

Grade 0: The habitually fixating eye resumes fixation immediately on removal of the cover. There is an absolute preference for the habitually fixating eye.

Grade 1: The deviating eye can hold fixation only momentarily after removal of the cover. There is strong fixation preference for the habitually fixating eye.

Grade 2: The deviating eye can maintain fixation after removal of the cover until the next eye blink. There is a moderate fixation preference for the habitually fixating eye.

Grade 3: The deviating eye is able to hold fixation through the next blink. There is slight fixation preference for the habitually fixating eye.

Grade 4: The patient habitually alternates equally between the two eyes. There is no fixation preference for either eye.

Modified from Garzia RP: Amblyopia in children. In Scheiman MM, editor: *Problems in optometry*, Philadelphia, 1990, JB Lippincott.

---

and then the other eye and observe the patient's behavior. It is helpful to use the thumb as an occluder. Searching, unsteady, or nystagmoid fixation movements and inability to pursue a moving visual target indicate poor vision. Also, if the patient objects more strongly to the covering of one eye than the other, it is assumed that the uncovered eye has poor vision. If amblyopia is deep, it can be diagnosed by this method, but with lesser degrees of amblyopia, this finding is too qualitative. If the patient objects equally to the occluding of each eye, then the test is of no significance.

Fixation Preference

More helpful is the observation of the binocular fixation pattern, or the fixation preference. Fixation preference is the most common test for amblyopia diagnosis in preverbal children with observable strabismus. When the young child's fixation preference is tested, a target such as a small moveable toy should be used. The strength of fixation preference is estimated under binocular conditions. Monocular occlusion is best accomplished by placing the hand at the level of the child's forehead and quickly moving the thumb downward as an occluder to cover each eye alternately. If the fixating eye is covered for several seconds and then removed with the result that the child immediately returns to viewing with the formerly fixating eye, amblyopia is presumed to be present. If when the fixating eye is covered and then removed, with the result that the child now holds fixation with the formerly deviating eye, forced alternate fixation is present and there is likely to be a better prognosis for avoidance of amblyopia. Zipf[134] developed a classification of binocular fixation preference (Box 2-3). Children

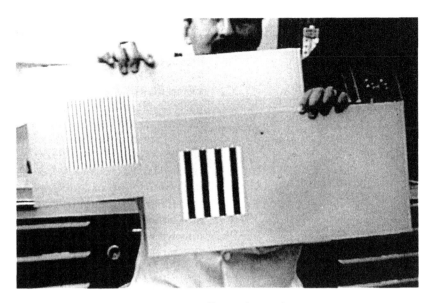

FIG. 2-4   Teller acuity cards.

with grades 0, 1, or 2 fixation preference are at highest risk for the presence of amblyopia.

 CLINICAL PEARL

Fixation preference is the most common test for amblyopia diagnosis in preverbal children with observable strabismus.

In general, the presence of a strong unilateral fixation preference is an excellent predictor of amblyopia in a young child with strabismus, whereas an alternating fixation pattern implies no amblyopia. In a study of 427 patients, standard fixation preference testing showed good sensitivity and specificity for strabismic deviations greater than 10 PD.[135] When the angle of strabismus is too small for a definitive diagnosis or there is no apparent strabismus, a vertical prism of 10 to 15 PD is held before one eye while the child fixates a toy. The test should be repeated with the prism held before the other eye. When no fixation preference exits, the child will show observed vertical alternation with each eye, which implies the absence of amblyopia.[136]

 CLINICAL PEARL

The presence of a strong unilateral fixation preference is an excellent predictor of amblyopia in a young child with strabismus, whereas an alternating fixation pattern implies no amblyopia.

Fixation preference may overestimate the incidence of amblyopia in certain cases. Some patients have normal and equal visual acuity in each eye, despite showing a fixation preference. Children with high degrees of anisometropia and strabismus may never prefer to fixate with the more ametropic eye,

even though the visual acuity may be good enough to exclude amblyopia by the standard definition. Similarly, some patients with small angles of deviation may not hold fixation with the affected eye, even though they are not in need of treatment for amblyopia. Furthermore, studies in both animals and humans have shown a variable delay between the induction of constant unilateral strabismus and its resultant amblyopia.[137-142] Thus although a preference for fixation with one eye may not necessarily indicate the presence of amblyopia, it may suggest that the patient is at risk of developing amblyopia.[141]

Preferential Looking and Optokinetic Nystagmus

Two behavioral techniques, preferential looking (PL) and optokinetic nystagmus (OKN) have been used to measure amblyopia in infants and very young children. Both measure visual acuity by means of a motor response.

PL tests measure resolution acuity and are based on the fact that young children have a greater tendency to fixate a patterned stimulus than a uniform or homogeneous field.[144] The targets used are gratings, which are alternating black and white stripes of strictly controlled size. The clinician monitors the child's looking behavior during presentation. Suprathreshold gratings are preferentially fixated compared with a uniform gray field. When the clinician can no longer tell the position of the grating by the child's looking behavior, it is assumed the child cannot see the grating. Term new-born infants will differentially respond to 20/400 gratings and to 20/20 gratings at 18 to 24 months. The Teller acuity cards are available for PL testing in a clinical setting (Fig. 2-4). The process can be cumbersome and may take as long as 10 minutes per patient. Difficulty in assessing fixa-

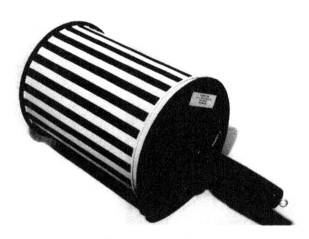

FIG. 2-5   OKN drum.

tion movements because of nystagmus or large-angle esotropia is common. In our experience, PL is rarely effective beyond 18 months, after which the child's mobility and curiosity reduce concentration.

The measurement of grating acuity in patients with amblyopia may underestimate the degree of visual loss. There is general agreement that PL is sensitive to amblyopia secondary to refractive errors and stimulus deprivation.[145-155] However, it may not be as sensitive for strabismic amblyopia.[150-152] Prospective studies of acuity development in infants with untreated esotropia, for example, show reduced acuity in the nonpreferred eye from approximately age 6 months and significant interocular differences from age 9 months.[141] Only 31% of the infants with a fixation preference were diagnosed with PL testing as amblyopic. With infants with treated esotropia, normal acuities were found until approximately age 30 months, whereupon acuity in both preferred and nonpreferred eyes dropped below average.[153] For these patients it is not clear whether more sensitive tests than PL would reveal a significant acuity deficit or whether fixation preferences are commonly seen in the absence of amblyopia in infancy.

Grating acuity testing cannot be automatically equated with recognition task acuity, such as naming pictures or Snellen letters. In patients without strabismic amblyopia, grating acuity is supposedly better than recognition acuity, and this difference is likely to be exaggerated in amblyopic cases.[154] Friendly, Jaafar, and Morillo[155] compared grating acuity and recognition visual acuity in 32 patients with anisometropic amblyopia, using 20/30 or better as the criterion for normal visual acuity. Eight eyes with visual acuities ranging from 20/42 to 20/138 were found normal with the Teller acuity cards. Mandava, Simon, and Jenkins[156] studied the value of PL in predicting eventual visual outcome. PL acuities of 64 preverbal pa-

tients considered at risk for amblyopia were measured. When these children became verbal, their visual acuities were determined using standard recognition acuity tests. Monocularly, a consistent correlation between PL and recognition acuities was not found. Apparently, PL is predictive of recognition acuity only in patients whose visual acuity is expected to remain stable. PL testing should therefore be used cautiously when measuring amblyopia. Although unequal monocular PL responses are of value in the diagnosis and monitoring of amblyopia, we support the view that treatment should be guided by clinical assessment of fixation behavior in preverbal patients with strabismus with no apparent difference in grating acuities between the preferred and nonpreferred eye.

OKN is elicited by the movement of repetitive stimuli, such as black and white stripes on a rotating drum (Fig. 2-5) across the child's visual field. The initial movement, if the stripes are seen, is a pursuit movement that follows the movement of the stimulus. This is followed by a corrective saccade. The repetitive alternation of these two eye movements results in a nystagmoid effect. Stripes of increasing spatial frequency are presented until a frequency is reached that fails to elicit nystagmoid movement. The visual angle subtended by the smallest stripe width that still elicits nystagmus is a measure of visual acuity. With OKN, infants have approximately 20/400 visual acuity at birth and 20/20 by 20 to 30 months.

Although OKN has been used to access acuity in various types of amblyopia, it is clinically useful only for tentative qualification of acuities less than 20/200.[157-159] Finer acuities require increasingly larger testing distances and/or much finer stripes that tax young children's ability to attend. Furthermore, visual acuity is only indirectly assessed by OKN. The additional pathways required to drive the motor output (occipital cortex-brain stem-extraocular muscles) create an opportunity for abnormal responses that have nothing to do with visual acuity.[160] Positive responses do not necessarily indicate form vision, because it has been elicited in patients having cortical blindness. Negative responses are also difficult to interpret. OKN must be interpreted cautiously and has little value in diagnosing amblyopia.

Visually Evoked Potential

The use of pattern visually evoked potential (VEP) has been the primary technique for electrophysiologically detecting amblyopia in patients unable to perform conventional testing.[161] The VEP is a gross response that reflects the visual input from the photoreceptors to the occipital cortex. Results obtained from a nonvariable flashing stimulus can give information about cortical responses to light but not about acuity. More sophisticated VEP testing is possible and has been used in amblyopia.[162] In very young children, chloral hydrate sedation may be necessary.[163] When a patient views either a light flash or a patterned stimulus (grating or checkerboard), small electrical potential changes occur in the occipital cortex, which can be recorded by overlying scalp electrodes and summarized to give a waveform response.[166] The light flash can be presented by using pediatric goggles (Fig. 2-6). The stimulus is presented from 50 to 200 times and repeated using gratings of higher spatial frequency. The electrical changes recorded are summated and processed by computer. The highest spatial frequency pattern that elicits an electrical potential change is the measure of visual acuity. Visual acuity of 20/20 can be demonstrated by 6 to 12 months in children with normal binocular vision. For strabismic and/or anisometropic amblyopia, the VEP response to patterned stimuli is generally reduced in amplitude and has a slightly prolonged latency. In amblyopia caused by stimulus deprivation, marked abnormalities occur in the VEP in response to luminance, and as patterned stimuli.

Because quantification is difficult, absolute amplitudes of VEP have been of little value in diagnosing amblyopia. In addition, the level of visual acuity recorded is frequently higher than that found with other methods, suggesting that amblyopia may be underestimated. More significant for the diagnosis of amblyopia is the ratio of amplitude measurements between the two eyes. If the visual acuity between the child's eyes is similar, the difference in amplitude should be close to 0, and the ratio of the two eyes should be approximately 1. By comparing the amplitudes of the two eyes, clinicians have been able to detect amblyopia and monitor its treatment.[163] Because the technique is expensive, time consuming, and difficult to administer, VEP testing for this purpose remains in the investigation stage.[165]

Graded Optotypes

For children between ages 2 and 4, we measure amblyopia using either the Broken Wheel test, tumbling E's, or pictures (Allen pictures, Lighthouse cards, Lea symbols). These tests measure recognition acuity.[166] The child is asked to discriminate and recognize one target among other similar targets.

The Broken Wheel test employs the two-alternative forced choice format.[167] Using the Landolt C as the critical distinguishing factor, the child is required to point to the card with the broken wheel (Fig. 2-7). The test distance is usually 3 meters. Four correct responses in a row are required to determine the acuity values with 94% certainty.[144] Because the Broken Wheel test requires pointing and not a verbal response from the child, it is our test of choice for measuring amblyopia in children between ages 2 and 4.

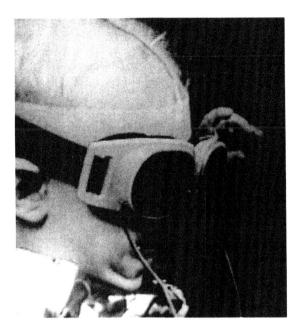

FIG. 2-6 Pediatric goggles used with VEP.

Picture testing, such as with the Allen picture cards, Lighthouse cards, and Lea symbols, is also used with this age group. However, recognition of pictures requires interpretation. With younger children, considerable patience, effort, and experience on the part of the clinician are necessary to ensure reliable measurement of visual acuity. Children's experience, familiarity with pictures, and verbal expression skills may vary and can interfere with diagnosis of amblyopia.

Snellen Chart

For most patients age 5 and older the Snellen letters can be used in the usual manner. Patients with amblyopia tend to read standard Snellen acuity charts in a unique way, showing slow and labored responses, variability in responses for apparently equivalent optotypes, and poor test/retest reliability.[26] These patients read the visual acuity chart much slower with their amblyopic eye. Patients with amblyopia are frequently able to identify the first and last letters in a given line while being unable to read the middle letters. This may occur for several consecutive acuity lines on a Snellen chart before the patient reaches threshold acuity. Furthermore, these patients rarely say that the Snellen letters are blurred but say they are too small or distorted.

The spacing between neighboring test targets on the Snellen chart or similar charts can greatly affect visual performance in patients with amblyopia. The interletter separations on the Snellen chart for visual acuities between 20/200 and 20/50, for example, are all less than one letter size. The additional stimuli provided by the surrounding optotypes causes confusion

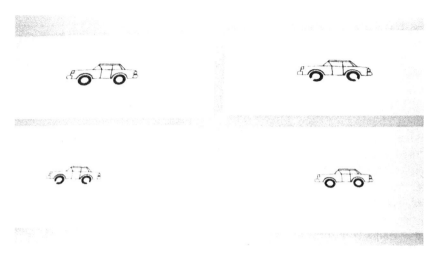

FIG. 2-7   Broken Wheel test.

in the amblyopic eye. The amblyopic eye exhibits separation difficulty and is deficient in ability to resolve closely spaced contours and recognize the patterns they form. Consequently, many patients with amblyopia will have two visual acuities, a linear and a single-letter acuity.[168] Presenting a row of symbols rather than an isolated symbol will produce a significantly lower visual acuity in many patients with amblyopia. This is more common with patients with strabismic amblyopia, occurring in 66.6% to 90% of these patients.[169] This is referred to as the *crowding phenomenon* and represents an abnormality of contour interaction between the point of fixation and adjacent objects. It is likely the result of an alteration of lateral inhibition, typical of amblyopia. The existence of the crowding phenomenon implies the presence of abnormally large receptive fields in amblyopia. Visual signals from adjacent contours interfere with one another because the summation of visual information takes place over an abnormally large area. The crowding phenomenon may also be related to the abnormal eye movements typical of amblyopia.

The crowding phenomenon is a hallmark of amblyopia, although crowding is also present to a lesser degree in people without amblyopia. It becomes more pronounced during the course of treatment (single-letter acuity improves more rapidly than does line acuity). As the end point of therapy is reached, the two types of acuity approach each other. The crowding phenomenon does not occur when the optotypes are presented in vertical rows nor is it present with organic amblyopia or deep functional amblyopia. If the reduction in vision is caused by destruction of retinal receptors or if the amblyopic process has gone so far as to make the retinal receptors at least temporarily unresponsive, improved vision cannot be expected from a different method of examination. The presence or absence of the crowding phenomenon can be used

to help differentiate organic from functional amblyopia (Table 2-2).[72]

The degree to which lack of the crowding phenomenon invalidates visual acuity tests in amblyopic eyes is substantial. For example, in one study, 44 of 847 patients with amblyopia had a visual acuity of 20/20 recorded with an isolated letter test.[3] On a subsequent visit, when tested with the linear chart, 36 of the 44 patients showed a decrease in visual acuity, with an average decrease of four lines. We occasionally examine patients in whom the visual acuity has been overestimated because the referring clinician only tested with single optotypes rather than full-line presentation, as shown in Case 3.

CASE 3

A 15-year-old boy was referred for the evaluation and treatment of amblyopia. Ocular history revealed strabismus surgery and amblyopia therapy at age 5. The referring clinician had reported the visual acuity in the amblyopic eye as 20/60. Our examination showed a 3-PD constant right esotropia at distance and near. The patient was also emmetropic. Visual acuities with the full Snellen chart were OD 20/400 and OS 20/20. Psychometric visual acuity for the right eye was 20/244. When tested with isolated letters on the Snellen chart the patient recognized all of the 20/60 optotypes.

Snellen charts have other inherent design problems, in addition to poor control of contour interaction, that limit the precision of acuity measurement in amblyopia.[170,171] The visual acuity levels on the Snellen chart at the low end are 20/400, 20/200, and 20/100. The large gaps between acuity levels can cause either gross overestimation or underestimation of acuity in patients with deep amblyopia. A patient with true 20/120 amblyopia would show a Snellen acuity of 20/200 because there are no test targets between

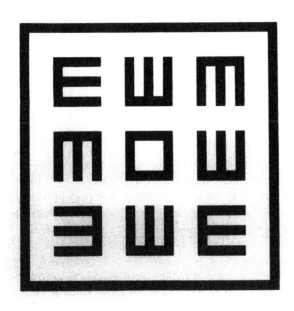

FIG. 2-8 Psychometric visual acuity card.

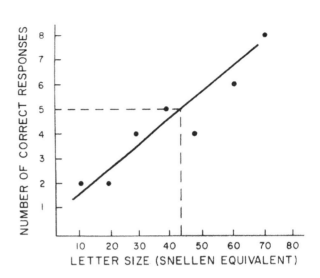

FIG. 2-9 Determination of psychometric visual acuity by graphing number of correct responses per card.

20/200 and 20/100. The visual acuity is based on only one or two letters per line at this level. Improvements, such as equalizing the ease of recognition of the specific letters chosen, supplying an equal number of letters per acuity level; using an appropriate scaling factor to size neighboring letters; and controlling the vertical and horizontal spacing between letters; would make it easier to use the Snellen chart with patients with amblyopia.

Psychometric Visual Acuity

Difficulty with measuring visual acuity in patients with amblyopia can be overcome by using psychometric visual acuity cards.[172-174] Flom, Weymouth, and Kahneman[172] designed a visual acuity test consisting of a series of 21 slides that span a range of visual acuity value from 20/277 to 20/9. Each slide contains eight Landolt Cs, and the patient is asked to identify the orientation of the gap in each C. At each of the 21 acuity levels, the interletter spacing is equal to the letter diameter, and every test letter is surrounded by an equal number of contours, thus bypassing the inadequacies of the Snellen chart.

We use the psychometric visual acuity cards designed by Davidson and Eskridge.[173] These differ in that tumbling E's are used as targets. Surrounding contours are placed one-half letter width away. Each card contains eight tumbling E's at various rotations (Fig. 2-8). The usual test distance is 10 feet. The cards prevent inaccuracies in measurement because some letters are easier to recognize than others, regardless of size. The entire card can be rotated at repeat acuity measurements to prevent memorization. The actual visual acuity is obtained by plotting the number of correct responses per card and estimating the level at which 5 of 8 responses are correct, which yields the 50% level corrected for guessing. Fig. 2-9 illustrates a psychometric visual acuity of 20/42.

Although we find visual acuities obtained with the psychometric chart to be more reliable than those obtained with the Snellen chart, we use caution with young children who may confuse left and right. Psychometric testing also takes longer than standard visual acuity testing.

Effect of Illumination

The decrease in visual acuity in amblyopia is most pronounced under photopic visual conditions and less when tested under mesopic and scotopic visual conditions.[175,176] As luminance levels decrease, the relative difference in visual acuity between the normal and amblyopic eyes becomes less.[84] The visual acuity of the amblyopic eye decreases less than that of the normal eye. Amblyopic visual perception simulates the perception of the peripheral retina of the normal eye under reduced illumination. The cone system of the amblyopic eye behaves as if a scotopic state is present, when actually photopic visual conditions exist. The improvement of visual acuity under reduced illumination demonstrates that the amblyopic eye is at its worst under the bright illumination that is necessary for optimal form vision. On the contrary, visual acuity in eyes with macular disease and other organic lesions tested at lower luminance levels decreases dramatically.

As a result of these observations, the neutral-density filter test has been used to help differentiate functional amblyopia from organic amblyopia (Table 2-2).

The neutral-density filter test involves the following procedures. The patient wears refractive correction while in a dimly lit room. The amblyopic eye is occluded, and the normal eye is preadapted with a 3 neutral-density filter for 5 minutes. The visual acuity of the normal eye is then measured. The 3 neutral-density filter is then placed on the amblyopic eye for 5 minutes, and the procedure is repeated. With functional amblyopia, the visual acuity of the amblyopic eye relative to the normal eye improves or stays the same under these conditions. For example, assume a patient has amblyopia of 20/40 in the right eye and 20/15 in the normal eye (four-line difference). With the filter before the normal eye the visual acuity should reduce to at least 20/40. With functional amblyopia the visual acuity with the neutral-density filter will likely also reduce but to a lesser extent than the normal eye, that is, to 20/60. The relative difference between visual acuities with the neutral-density filter is less (two lines vs. four lines). With organic amblyopia the relative difference in visual acuity between the eyes increases substantially.

Because of the test's extreme variability, we use it sparingly. A patient who presents with decreased visual acuity, no observable pathology, and absence of any amblyopiagenic etiologic factors is a candidate for the test. Even in this instance, we are cautious in making definite conclusions based solely on the neutral-density filter test.

REFRACTION

Reassessment of visual acuity with best refractive correction is essential to avoid misdiagnosis of amblyopia. Refracting a patient with amblyopia is an art that is critical to the successful management of amblyopia. Subjective refraction is typically unreliable.[3] Attempts to subjectively refine the refraction in one eye that has deep amblyopia can be frustrating. Many patients with amblyopia are unable to distinguish the difference between changes in increments of 1 D.[3]

Retinoscopy

We prefer to refract patients with amblyopia objectively with retinoscopy under both noncycloplegic and cycloplegic conditions. One drop of 1% cyclopentolate hydrochloride usually followed by a second drop 5 minutes later is adequate. For infants less than 6 months of age, 0.5% cyclopentolate hydrochloride is used. The retinoscopy can be performed 30 to 40 minutes later. The accompanying pupillary dilation affords an opportunity for a funduscopic examination by binocular indirect ophthalmoscopy.

A major source of error in retinoscopy on young children is that the clinician is off the visual axes. We have the child with cycloplegia look at the retinoscopic light. With strabismus, we also occlude the eye that is not being refracted. Loose lenses or lens bars are used for infants and younger children. Pediatric trial frames and loose lenses are ideal for older children. Rarely do we use the phorometer in a child under age 6. Children may tilt their head behind the phorometer, and this can also produce errors in the axis of astigmatism.

Photorefraction

Photorefraction has been used to screen for refractive errors that may be amblyopiagenic.[177-183] Photorefraction is an objective method that uses photography or video in a variety of procedures to evaluate refractive error either qualitatively or quantitatively. The clinician can either read the photographs or the film may be sent to a processing lab to be analyzed. The instrument is located from 1 to 6 meters from the child. Room illumination is low, and the child is seated in the parent's lap. Frequently, the photorefraction is done without cycloplegia. In a color photograph taken on a child who is accurately focusing on and fixating the camera fixation light with both eyes, the fundus reflex in each pupil is very dark and the corneal light reflexes are symmetric. If either eye (or both eyes) is not appropriately focused or fixating, the fundus is brighter and yellow or white. Significant amblyopiagenic conditions, such as hyperopic anisometropias of more than 1 D, high ametropias, and astigmatism, can be detected, as can strabismus and media opacities. Although photorefraction is presently being used mainly for large vision-screening programs, it should not be used as a replacement for retinoscopy.[181]

Changes Over Time

Changes over the years in the refractive error for the nonamblyopic and amblyopic eyes may not be symmetric.[184-186] Amblyopic eyes emmetropize less effectively and tend to remain hyperopic. Lepard[184] monitored the refractive error in 55 patients with esotropia and amblyopia from early childhood to about age 25. Generally, the nonamblyopic eyes became more myopic with age, relative to the amblyopic eye, whereas there was no appreciable change in the average refractive error of the amblyopic eye (Fig. 2-10). Both eyes of a control group of patients of similar age and normal distant vision and orthophoria were more myopic with age. In the control group, there was an insignificant difference in the change in refractive error of one eye compared with its fellow eye during comparable periods. In patients with esotropia who had equivalent function of both eyes (alternating strabismus), the refractive changes over the years were found to run practically parallel in the two eyes.[186] These findings support the use-abuse theory of changes in refraction, which holds that myopia increases during early school years as a result of use, as opposed to the

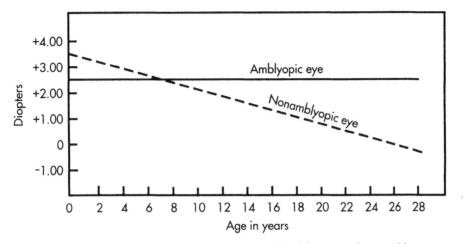

FIG. 2-10 Changes over time in the refractive error of amblyopic and nonamblyopic eye. Broken line represents least square fit to all observed refractive errors in nonamblyopic eyes; solid line represents least square fit to all observed refractive errors in amblyopic eyes. (Modified from Lepard CW: Comparative changes in the error of refraction between fixing and amblyopic eyes during growth and development, *Am J Ophthalmol*, 80:485, 1975.)

biologic theory, which emphasizes that growth and heredity are causative factors in changes in refraction.

MONOCULAR FIXATION STATUS

As many as 23% to 82% of patients with amblyopia and strabismus use an off-foveal point and do not employ foveal fixation when the fellow nonamblyopic eye is occluded.[187] Under monocular conditions, the amblyopic eye remains more or less deviated. The patient has difficulty directing the fovea at the target. This contributes to the loss of visual acuity in the amblyopic eye. Eccentric fixation is a monocular sensory adaptation to disordered binocular vision in which the normal visual axis from the normal fovea fails to intersect the target of regard.[188] It occurs even though acuity in the amblyopic eye is best at the fovea, not at the eccentric fixating point. In anisometropic amblyopia, eccentric fixation is rare. Some of these patients tend to have an ultrasmall angle of strabismus with anomalous correspondence. Eccentric fixation can be bilateral, but this is extremely rare.[189]

 CLINICAL PEARL

As many as 23% to 82% of patients with amblyopia and strabismus use an off-foveal point and do not employ foveal fixation when the fellow nonamblyopic eye is occluded.

Eccentric fixation is categorized according to its location, size, and steadiness. The location, relative to the fovea, can be nasal, temporal, inferior, or superior. It is usually nasal in amblyopia associated with esotropia and usually temporal in amblyopia associated with exotropia. Commonly, both horizontal and vertical eccentricity exist. Paradoxic eccentric fixation is the reverse of the expected situation, with temporal eccentric fixation in esotropia and nasal eccentric fixation in exotropia. Although uncommon, it can occur in consecutive strabismus either after surgical overcorrection or spontaneous reversal of the deviation.

The size is the distance in either degrees or prism diopters between the fovea and point "*e*," point "*e*" being the mean point on the retina on which the object of regard falls during monocular viewing by an eccentric fixator. This is difficult to determine precisely because in most cases the point is more an area or locus of points than a single fixed point. Eccentric fixation covers an area that becomes larger the farther it is from the fovea. A careful mental average will give a good approximation of the amount. Generally, eccentric fixation is described as being either *parafovealar* (1 to 3 degrees off fovea), *paramacular* (3 to 5 degrees off fovea), or *peripheral* (greater than 5 degrees off the fovea). In deep amblyopia, fixation can be several degrees from the fovea. We have seen patients fixate with the optic nerve head of the amblyopic eye when the nonamblyopic eye is occluded.

Eccentric fixation may be steady or unsteady. Frequently, the site used for fixation varies from time to time, even during the same examination. Averaging three locations at 1-minute intervals can be used in these instances. A descriptive sequence for a patient with amblyopia might therefore be "4 degrees, unsteady, nasal, eccentric fixation."

The magnitude of the strabismus when measured with the alternate cover test and prisms will be affected by eccentric fixation.[190] Because the cover test assumes that the patient foveally fixates with each eye, the angle of strabismus will be underestimated for a patient with esotropia with nasal eccentric fixation and, in the same case, a patient with exotropia with temporal eccentric fixation. In the rare case with equal angles of eccentric fixation and strabismus, cover testing will fail altogether to detect strabismus. Other tests that measure strabismus, such as the Hirschberg and Krimsky tests (see Chapter 7) are not offset by eccentric fixation because they do not require the patient to monocularly fixate with the amblyopic eye.

 CLINICAL PEARL

The magnitude of the strabismus when measured with the alternate cover test and prisms will be affected by eccentric fixation.

The diagnosis of eccentric fixation is made by using visuoscopy, entoptic phenomena, or afterimages or by measuring angle kappa.

Visuoscopy

The method of choice is visuoscopy using a direct ophthalmoscope with a calibrated fixation target.[191] There are several ophthalmoscopes that have been adapted for evaluation of fixation status. Most modern direct ophthalmoscopes contain a target suitable to determine the fixation pattern. The most commonly used is the Welch Allyn, in which the markings are set approximately 1 PD apart and the center circle is 2 PD in diameter. The target pattern seen by the patient in the light-transmitting aperture serves as a fixation target and casts a shadow of its form onto the fundus. The procedure is to locate the foveal reflex of the amblyopic eye, then click in the visuoscopy target. It is easier when performed with pupillary dilation. The eye not being examined is occluded to ensure that the test is monocular. The patient is asked to look directly at the center of the fixation target. The clinician notes the location of the foveal reflex in relation to the center of the fixation target. The light should be kept low, so that the eye is not dazzled. A green filter can be used in conjunction with the fixation target to facilitate observation and reduce glare. If the foveal reflex is not present, its position in the center of the darker macular area should be estimated. Fixation status in the nonamblyopic eye is generally evaluated first to allow the patient to become familiar with the requirements of the procedure and to determine if the patient understands the task.

When there is normal steady central fixation, the central portion of the fixation target surrounds or covers the fovea, which is centered in the deeper red macular region (Fig. 2-11, *A*). When eccentric fixation is

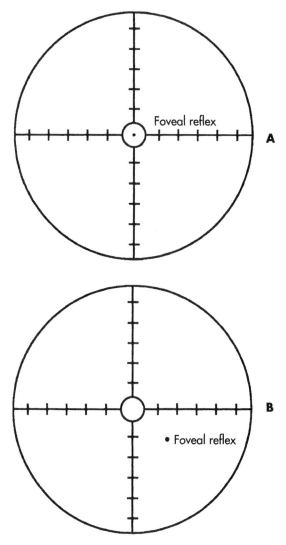

FIG. 2-11 Visuoscopic responses with Welch Allyn direct ophthalmoscope target in (**A**) central fixation and (**B**) eccentric fixation.

present, the central portion of the target is seen either to the side of the foveal reflex (Fig. 2-11, *B*) or, if no reflex can be seen, is not centered in the macular area.

When recording the position of eccentric fixation, the clinician is looking at the portion of the retina on which the fixation target falls and determining whether fixation is steady or unsteady. If the target is inferior to the foveal reflex, the patient is demonstrating inferior eccentric fixation. Combinations of horizontal and vertical eccentric fixation should be recorded separately, for example, 3-PD nasal and 4-PD inferior eccentric fixation.

Other ophthalmoscopes, such as the Neitz euthyscope and Keeler projectoscope, are specifically modified as visuoscopic instruments. The Neitz has a target with nine consecutive circles at 0.5-degree intervals,

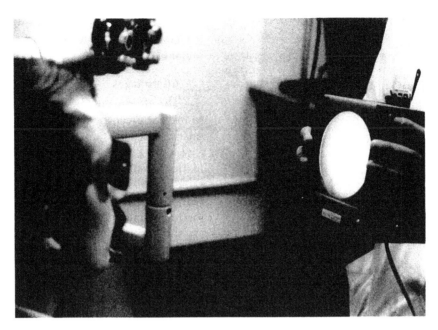

FIG. 2-12 Macula Integrity Tester.

and the Keeler uses a Linksz star grid as a target. This target consists of an open-center four-pointed star surrounded by two concentric circles subtending angles of 3 and 5 degrees. These ophthalmoscopes are rarely available. Difficulties with visuoscopy arise when the foveal reflex is not well formed and thus is not easily visible, such as with high myopia. Poor patient cooperation and photophobia can also make the test difficult.

Haidinger Brushes

The Haidinger brushes are the most frequent subjective method of measuring fixation status in amblyopia. They are an entoptically preceived pattern of closely packed radiating lines emanating from opposite sides of a common central point, forming a shape similar to an airplane propeller or bow tie.[192] The brushes are elicited by viewing a homogenous field of polarized blue light, with the meridional orientation corresponding to the axis of polarization. The brushlike pattern is derived from the macular area, with the center of the pattern corresponding to the center of the fovea. The patient monocularly looks through a deep blue filter at a rotating Polaroid filter. The instrument used most commonly for testing fixation using Haidinger brushes is the Macula Integrity Tester (Fig. 2-12).

The nonamblyopic eye should be tested first to demonstrate to the patient the expected appearance of the brushes. The patient is directed to look at a fixation point and perceive the rotating brushes. If the patient cannot perceive the brushes with the nonamblyopic eye, determination of the fixation status in the amblyopic eye with the test will not be possible. To confirm the reliability of the patient's responses, a

piece of cellophane can be placed over the target and the patient asked to report the direction of the brushes rotation to be reversed. The clinician brings a pointer in from the side and asks the patient to notice when the pointer touches the brushes. A patient who fixates centrally sees the brushes and pointer superimposed over the fixation target (Fig. 2-13, *A*). Displacement of the brushes and pointer from the fixation target is indicative of eccentric fixation (Fig. 2-13, *B*). Displacement is in the direction of the eccentric fixation. Nasal eccentric fixation is associated with nasal displacement, and temporal eccentric fixation is associated with temporal displacement. The magnitude of the eccentric fixation is determined by the following formula:

$$\text{Eccentric fixation (PD)} = \frac{100 \times \text{separation in centimeters}}{\text{test distance in meters}}$$

Assuming a test distance of 50 cm, if the patient perceives the brushes 2 cm nasally from the fixation point, 4 PD of nasal eccentric fixation is present.

The phenomenon of Haidinger brushes is dependent on the anatomic macular structure. The anatomic constituents, especially the retinal receptors and Henle's fibers, must be normal in structure and arrangement or the brushes will not be seen.[192] Patients with organic amblyopia will not see the brushes. However, even though perceiving the brushes indicates macular integrity, lack of perception does not necessarily mean macular dysfunction or organic amblyopia. The Haidinger brushes do not stand out boldly, and careful attention by the patient is necessary. Also, the subjective nature of the test frequently allows

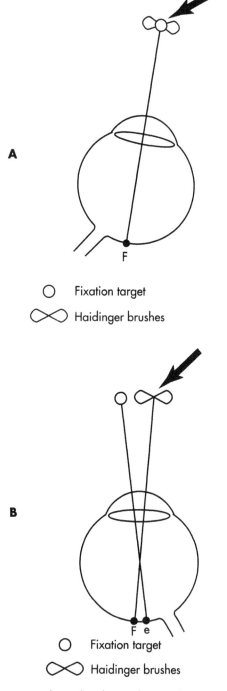

○   Fixation target

∞   Haidinger brushes

○   Fixation target

∞   Haidinger brushes

FIG. 2-13   Haidinger brushes with central and eccentric fixation. With central fixation (**A**), pointer, brushes, and fixation target coincide. With eccentric fixation (**B**), brushes and pointer are displaced from fixation target.

younger patients to make up responses to please the clinician. Rarely do we use this procedure on children under age 7.

Afterimages

The afterimage transfer technique can also be used to test for eccentric fixation.[193] The technique is based on the normally corresponding relationship of the foveae. In patients with normal correspondence, stimulation of the fovea of the two eyes gives rise to the same visual direction. An image falling on one fovea will be directionalized to the same spatial location as the image falling on the other fovea. The patient covers the amblyopic eye and looks at a fixation point blanked out in the center of a vertical light source. This creates a vertical afterimage on the fovea. The occluder is then switched to the nonamblyopic eye. The patient looks at a fixation point with the amblyopic eye while attempting to visualize the transferred afterimage. If the transferred afterimage is located on the fixation point, central fixation exists (Fig 2-14, *A*). Any offset of the afterimage from the fixation point represents eccentric fixation (Fig. 2-14, *B*). The formula that was used with the Haidinger brushes is also applicable here. For example, if the afterimage is located 1 cm away from the fixation target and the test distance is 1m away from the fixation target, 1 PD of eccentric fixation exists.

Angle Kappa

With very young children and other untestable patients, angle kappa (actually, angle lambda) can be used as a method of determining the fixation pattern. Angle kappa is the angle between the pupillary axis (the line through the center of the pupil, perpendicular to the cornea) and the visual axis subtended at the nodal point of the eye. When the patient fixates a penlight held approximately 50 cm from the patient, below the clinician's eye, the corneal light reflex in the nonamblyopic eye is positioned on the average 0.5 mm on the nasal side of the center of the entrance pupil. This is because the fovea is located slightly temporalward from the optic axis of the eye. Angle kappa is designated positive when the light reflex is positioned nasally and negative when it is positioned temporally. A large positive-angle kappa may hide a small-angle esotropia or cause pseudoexotropia, and a large negative-angle kappa may hide an exotropia or cause pseudoesotropia.

To measure fixation, one eye is occluded and monocular comparison is made between the angle kappas of each eye. When each eye has central fixation the angle kappa measured in one eye is equal in direction and size to the angle measured in the other eye. If fixation in one eye is eccentric of a large enough

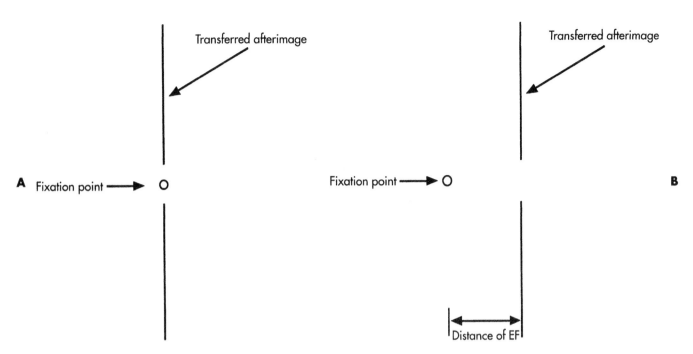

FIG. 2-14 Afterimage transfer responses with central fixation and eccentric fixation. With central fixation **(A)**, transferred afterimage coincides with fixation target. With eccentric fixation **(B)**, transferred afterimage is displaced from fixation target.

size, a difference between the two angles will be found. The eye with eccentric fixation will make no movement or perhaps only a small one when the other eye is covered, and the reflection of the light will not be centered in the pupil (Fig. 2-15).

Comparing angle kappas can only indicate large amounts of eccentric fixation. Because 1 mm deviation on the cornea is equivalent to 22 PD of eye turn, even a half-millimeter deviation (the smallest most clinicians can detect) indicates 11 PD of eccentric fixation (visual acuity of approximately 20/240 or worse).[194,195] A 2.5-degree angle of eccentric fixation results in only about a 0.125-mm difference in the location of the two corneal reflexes. This inability to detect a difference in the angle kappas between the two eyes indicates that either central fixation is present or eccentric fixation is present with an angle smaller than can be detected by this method. The real usefulness of measuring angle kappa may be more as an aid to determine unsteadiness of fixation.[27] This is accomplished by observing the stability of the corneal light reflex over several seconds.

Effect on Visual Acuity

Eccentric fixation cannot explain entirely the visual reduction that accompanies amblyopia. A loose association exists between the depth of amblyopia and the degree of eccentric fixation. Some patients with small-angle eccentric fixation show only a slight reduction in visual acuity, whereas others have much worse visual acuity than would be expected from the retinal locus of their fixation. Also, deep amblyopia can occur in the absence of eccentric fixation. We have examined patients with amblyopia manifesting either central fixation or 1, 2, or 3 degrees of eccentric fixation who all had 20/200 visual acuity. Clinicians are not able to predict eccentric fixation from the amount of visual acuity impairment but are able to predict the best visual acuity a patient can have, based on the amount of eccentric fixation present.

In nonamblyopic eyes a linear relationship exists between visual acuity and retinal eccentricity (Fig. 2-16). The visual acuity in amblyopia with eccentric fixation is not the equivalent of the visual acuity in normal vision measured at the same amount of eccentricity from the fovea.[196] The equation MAR = EF(PD) + 1 provides a good approximation of the visual acuity to be expected in amblyopia.[197] It indicates that the minimum angle of resolution (MAR, the inverse of the Snellen fraction) equals the amount of eccentric fixation measured in prism diopters plus the constant number 1. Thus a patient with 3 degrees (5.25 PD) of eccentric fixation will have an MAR of 5.25 + 1 = 6.25. This can be converted to the Snellen

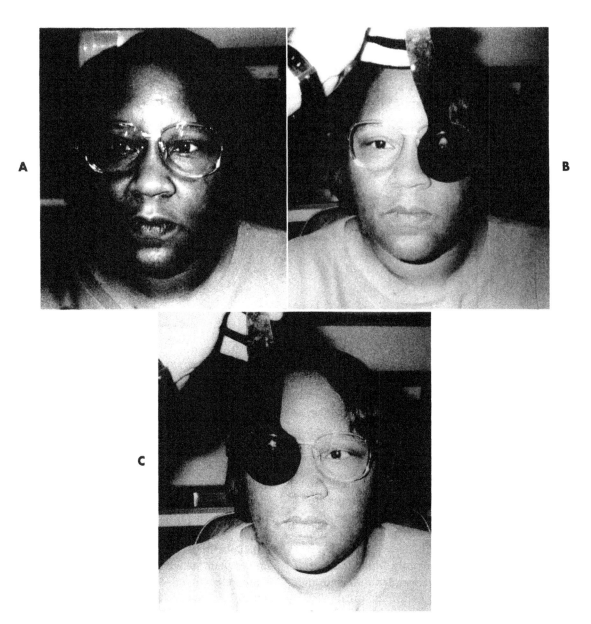

FIG. 2-15 Eccentric fixation in left eye, as diagnosed by measuring angle kappa in each eye. **A,** Patient is esotropic and deeply amblyopic in left eye. **B,** Central fixation occurs in right eye. **C,** Eccentric fixation occurs in left eye.

TABLE 2-3 VISUAL ACUITY OF NORMAL AND AMBLYOPIC EYES BASED ON THE AMOUNT OF ECCENTRIC FIXATION

Angle of EF (Degrees)	Normal Eye	Amblyopic Eye
1	20/30	20/55
2	20/40-20/50	20/90
3	20/50-20/60	20/125
4	20/60-20/70	20/160
5	20/70-20/100	20/195

denominator by multiplying by 20. The expected visual acuity is 20/125.

As illustrated (Table 2-3), visual acuities are lower for amblyopic eyes than for nonamblyopic eyes with identical eccentric fixation because of the inhibitory influences and the unsteadiness of fixation that exist in amblyopia. When predicting visual acuity for the amblyopic eye with eccentric fixation, we use Table 2-3 in the following manner: the amblyopic eye will have no better visual acuity than the visual acuity of the normal eye with identical eccentric fixation. In an am-

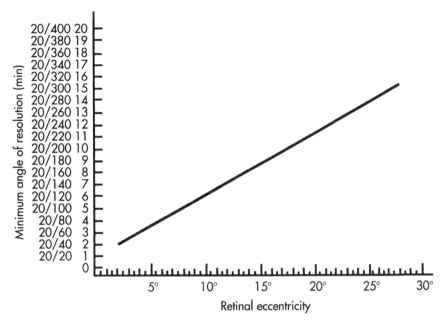

FIG. 2-16 Visual acuity as a function of retinal eccentricity.

blyopic eye with 3 degrees of eccentric fixation, the maximum visual acuity for that patient cannot exceed 20/60 and will probably be lower.

Theories

The reason some patients with amblyopia develop eccentric fixation and others maintain central fixation is essentially unknown. Various theories have been put forth to attempt to explain the development of eccentric fixation. Although none of these theories fully explains the development of eccentric fixation, all contribute somewhat to an explanation of the reason a nonfoveal area may be used for monocular fixation by a patient with amblyopia. Bangerter[198] explained eccentric fixation on the basis of depressed central or foveal vision that results in a suppression scotoma. According to Bangerter, the patient uses an eccentric area adjacent to the suppression scotoma that supposedly gives higher visual acuity. However, this cannot be the case because the area of eccentric fixation used by the patient is not always the highest area of sensitivity after the fovea. Furthermore, the visual acuity is not higher but lower in the eccentric area than at the fovea. Nevertheless, the stepwise improvement in the fixation pattern that is found with treatment in some patients gives some validity to Bangerter's theory.

Cüppers[199] proposes that with eccentric fixation the straight-ahead visual direction is shifted from the fovea to the eccentric area that the patient uses for fixation. This shift is supposedly related to a preexisting anomalous correspondence that exists under binocular viewing conditions. According to Cüppers, the same area in the amblyopic eye used under binocular conditions is also used for monocular fixation. Therefore the angle of eccentric fixation is identical to the angle of anomaly and the angle of strabismus, and no movement of the amblyopic eye occurs when covering the nonamblyopic eye during the unilateral cover test. Clinically, this is rarely the case; the magnitude of eccentric fixation does not usually correlate with the angle of strabismus. With the exception of microtropia of identity, the angle of strabismus is usually larger than the angle of eccentric fixation.[200] In addition, many cases of strabismic amblyopia exist without eccentric fixation. That eccentric fixation can develop in previously normal eyes of patients with amblyopia following occlusion therapy also opposes the theory of Cüppers.[201]

Schor[202] suggests that long-term constant strabismus leads to an "after-discharge" or potentiation of the agonist muscle in the strabismic eye when the dominant eye is covered. According to Schor, eccentric fixation develops not for best available acuity but because the habitual strabismic deviation causes an adaptive after-effect that modifies the subsequent monocular localization. This theory nicely predicts that patients with esotropia would have nasal eccentric fixation, and patients with exotropia would have temporal eccentric fixation. It does not, however, explain the rare occurrence of paradoxic eccentric fixation occurring spontaneously or after surgical overcorrection in some patients with strabismus.

ADDITIONAL FEATURES

ACCOMMODATION

A deficit of accommodation is a well-known characteristic of the amblyopic eye. Accommodation in amblyopia is imprecise and has been reported as being similar to organic scotomas.[203] It has been suggested that in some cases, abnormal accommodation is the cause of the amblyopia.[204] Accommodative defects in the amblyopic eye relative to the normal eye include decreased amplitude of accommodation, decreased accommodative facility, a flattened slope on the accommodative stimulus-response curve, and an increased depth of focus.[205-208] Improved visual acuity at near for some patients with amblyopia with plus lenses and blur in the presence of mild uncorrected hyperopia also suggests poor accommodation. The reduced accommodation most likely reflects a primary sensory loss over the central retinal region as a result of prolonged early abnormal visual responses, resulting in an overall reduced sensitivity of the eye.[208] Reduction of accommodation may also be attributed to the afferent pathway of the accommodation control system.[205] Other factors causing poor accommodation in amblyopia likely include the eccentric fixation and abnormal fixational movements associated with amblyopia. Low amplitudes of accommodation in children have been described mostly in connection with isoametropic amblyopia associated with high hyperopia.[99,101] These patients choose to remain blurred and do not fully accommodate at all times during early childhood, leading to accommodative insufficiency.

Some clinical tests are better discriminators between amblyopic and nonamblyopic eyes when measuring accommodation. Hokuda and Ciuffreda[209] found the minus-lens accommodative amplitude and the dynamic retinoscopy techniques to be the best discriminators between amblyopic and nonamblyopic eyes, when compared with the other tests of accommodation. All of their patients with amblyopia showed reduced accommodative amplitude in the amblyopic eye. The difference in accommodative amplitude between the amblyopic and nonamblyopic eye ranged from 0.5 D to 5 D, corresponding to an average interocular difference of about 25%. Reduced amplitudes, however, were not consistently found in the amblyopic eye with the subjective push-up technique. Following orthoptics/vision therapy, the amplitude of accommodation and other accommodative functions improved in some cases more rapidly than either visual acuity or fixation.[210,211]

OCULAR MOTILITY

The control and execution of eye movements is impaired in amblyopia.[212-217] The abnormal eye movements have been recorded electro-oculographically.[8] The unsteadiness in fixation in normal eyes (high-ve-locity microsaccades, slow drifts, tremors) is exaggerated in amblyopia. Fixation maintenance tends to be very unsteady. Amblyopic eyes have an increased tendency to drift while fixating a stationary target. In some cases, when reading is attempted monocularly with the amblyopic eye, there can be many losses of place and skipped words.[27,215]

The major abnormal fixational movements include increased drift amplitude, saccadic intrusions, and latent and manifest jerk nystagmus.[84] These tend to be larger in strabismic amblyopia than in anisometropic amblyopia. Increased drift refers to abnormally large and/or rapid smooth drift amplitudes (up to about 3 degrees) and velocities (up to about 3 degrees per second), respectively, during attempted monocular fixation. Increased drifts have been documented 75% of the time in patients with amblyopia but without strabismus, 50% of the time in patients with constant strabismic amblyopia, and 20% of the time in patients with intermittent strabismic amblyopia.[216] The large drift amplitudes are probably sufficient to carry the image to a retinal region with different acuity, thereby contributing to a temporal variability in visual acuity.[217] Saccadic intrusions refer to a pattern of movement in which there is a saccadic displacement of the visual axis away from the target, followed approximately 200 ms later by a return saccadic movement. Saccadic intrusions have rarely been found in anisometropic amblyopia. They do not significantly degrade vision because of their small amplitudes and velocities. Latent nystagmus is a disorder of the oculomotor system in which nystagmus is generally not present (or at least obvious) during binocular viewing, but upon occlusion of one eye a conjugate jerk nystagmus occurs, with the fast phase directed toward the viewing eye. In contrast to latent nystagmus, manifest jerk nystagmus is present during both monocular and binocular viewing conditions. Latent and manifest nystagmus are found predominantly in patients with amblyopia who have infantile esotropia or dissociated vertical deviations. Visual acuity deficits generally become greater with increased amplitude and velocity and tend to improve as foveation increases. The increased drift and nystagmus amplitude are also contributory to the reduced accommodation that accompanies amblyopia.[84]

Abnormalities of saccades (increased latency, reduced peak velocity, and dysmetria) produce overshoots and undershoots. Instead of a swift and accurate movement to the second target, the amblyopic eye may demonstrate a slowness of response and searching or corrective movements before finally assuming fixation of the target.[220] The abnormally long latency probably results from alterations in the neural pathways responsible for processing information used as input to the saccadic system.[218] The undershooting

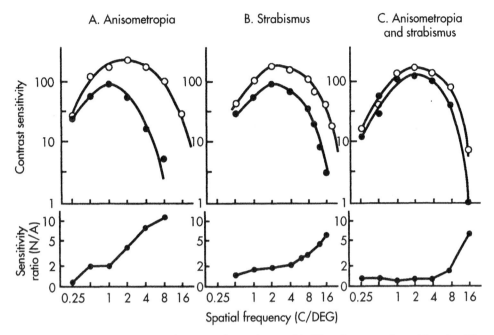

FIG. 2-17 Contrast sensitivity functions for patients with **(A)** anisometropic amblyopia, **(B)** strabismic amblyopia, and **(C)** combined anisometropic and strabismic amblyopia. The filled and open circles indicate the performance of the amblyopic and nonamblyopic eyes respectively. In all cases the high spatial frequencies are depressed for amblyopic eyes. (Modified from Bloch DA, Wick B: Differences between strabismic and anisometropic amblyopia: research findings and impact on management. In Rutstein RP: *Problems in optometry,* Philadelphia, 1991, JB Lippencott.)

and overshooting that amblyopic eyes make to displaced targets has been attributed to spatial distortion of strabismic amblyopic eyes.[11]

Instead of a smooth rotational movement at a speed and path corresponding to the target, abnormalities of pursuits (reduced gain, directional asymmetries, abnormal saccadic substitution) give an often jerky, irregular, nystagmoid, and lagging movement not corresponding to the path followed by the target.[8,84]

CONTRAST SENSITIVITY

The ability to detect contrast and brightness differences has long been recognized as abnormal in amblyopic eyes.[218,219] The loss of photopic contrast sensitivity appears to be one of the defining characteristics of amblyopia. Contrast sensitivity compares the ability of the patient to discriminate grating patterns or letters of a given spatial frequency as contrast is reduced. By determining the detection threshold of selected spatial frequency targets at different contrast levels, a function may be generated that can be compared with established norms. Targets in the form of charts with letters or gratings are available commercially.[220]

Patients with strabismic or anisometropic amblyopia show a decrease in intermediate and high spatial frequency detection when comparing the amblyopic and nonamblyopic eye.[221,222] The amblyopic eye consistently requires more contrast than the normal eye. This becomes more pronounced with increased severity of the amblyopia.[223] These reductions in contrast sensitivity of the amblyopic eye are not the result of optical factors, unsteady eye movements, or eccentric fixation.[222-224] The reduced contrast sensitivity function of the amblyopic eye represents a neural loss of foveal function.

Fig. 2-17 illustrates the contrast sensitivity function of three amblyopic eyes, one with anisometropia, one with strabismus, and one with both anisometropia and strabismus. The amblyopic eye of each patient shows reduced contrast sensitivity, particularly at high spatial frequencies. Contrast sensitivity deficits across the visual field of the patients differ greatly.[225] Patients with anisometropic amblyopia demonstrate a uniform and more extensive loss across the visual field, whereas patients with strabismic amblyopia exhibit an asymmetric and less extensive loss in contrast sensitivity across the visual field.[226,227] Milder forms of strabismic amblyopia show marked asymmetries, and more severe cases show more symmetric losses. In patients with anisometropic amblyopia, contrast sensitivity losses can extend as far as 50 to 55 degrees into the periphery, but in patients with strabismic amblyopia losses tend to stay within the central 30 degrees of the field.[226,227] A normalization of the visual function of patients with strabismic amblyopia occurs at low spatial frequencies. However, patients with anisometropic amblyopia tend to do poorly when viewing either high or low contrast. Of patients with strabismic amblyopia, those with exotropia tend to show their losses in the nasal field (temporal retina) and those with esotropia in the temporal field (nasal retina).[226]

Contrast sensitivity testing provides a more comprehensive measure of visual disability than is apparent from visual acuity testing alone. Some patients with amblyopia continue to report improvement in the function of their amblyopic eye, even though their Snellen or psychometric visual acuity has leveled off. This perceived improvement is likely the result of changes in contrast sensitivity. Also, following orthoptics/vision therapy the amblyopic eye's contrast sensitivity may normalize, even though little change occurs in visual acuity.[27,228-234] Losses in contrast sensitivity have been reported in the nonamblyopic eye, as well as the amblyopic eye, suggesting that the nonamblyopic eye is also abnormal.[235]

PATHOPHYSIOLOGY

Neurophysiologic research with kittens and monkeys has proved invaluable for studying the electrophysiologic and morphologic changes caused by stimulus deprivation in the visual system. Experimental amblyopia has been produced in these animals by unilateral and bilateral lid suturing, unilateral strabismus induced by surgery or prisms, and defocusing of the image by optical means or by the use of drugs.[88,236-239] Abnormal visual experience causes physiologic and histologic alterations in a nervous system that is normal at birth, with profound implications for vision. These changes have been induced when the animal is visually immature and the neural connections are not fixed. This is likely from 3 weeks to 3 months in kittens, extending to 4 months in monkeys. In man it is certainly longer. Changes in the visual systems of these kitten and monkeys have been documented in the retina, the lateral geniculate nucleus, and the visual cortex.

RETINA

Disagreement exists as to the degree of retinal involvement, if any, in amblyopia. Although most neurophysiologic and histopathologic abnormalities have been reported to occur in the lateral geniculate nucleus and striate cortex, there is some psychophysical and electrophysiologic evidence that the retina may also be abnormal in amblyopia. Visual information travels from the retina to cortical areas along at least two parallel pathways.[240,241] Each pathway appears to be supplied by a discrete type of retinal ganglion cell.[242,243] The X ganglion cells, or sustained cells, have a relatively high density in the fovea. These cells have

small receptive fields, respond best to high spatial frequencies, and are poor at discriminating quickly flickering images. The X ganglion cells are associated with central form vision and central visual acuity. The Y ganglion cells, or transient cells, are more evenly distributed across the retina, have large receptive fields, respond best to low spatial frequencies, and can detect high flicker frequencies. The Y cells are associated with the peripheral retina and are concerned with the location of objects in space. In kittens with strabismic amblyopia and in those given unilateral or bilateral atropine, a significant reduction in the spatial resolving power of the X cells has been reported.[244,245]

That the physiologic basis of strabismic amblyopia and possibly other forms of amblyopia is loss of cellular activity of foveal X cells is supported by studies that report abnormal patterns in the electroretinograms of patients with amblyopia.[246] Although not found by all investigators,[247] these abnormalities include a lowered amplitude of the "*b*" wave, a more rounded "*b*" wave, and a diminished potential of the "*a*" wave proportional to the degree of amblyopia. A reduction in electro-oculogram amplitudes in amblyopic eyes compared with normal eyes has also implicated the retinal pigment epithelium as being involved.[248]

The finding of an afferent pupillary defect in some patients with amblyopia also possibly suggests an abnormality at the retinal ganglion cell level; more specifically, failure of development of the X ganglion cells.[249-251] The more sensitive the examination, the higher the detection rate of this abnormality. Firth[250] recorded a relative afferent pupillary defect in 32% of patients with amblyopia, using a modification of the swinging flashlight test and the synoptophore. That there exists no relationship between the etiology or the degree of amblyopia and the magnitude of pupillary defect implies that any direct retinal contribution to acuity reduction must be minor.[252]

Additional evidence possibly supporting retinal involvement in amblyopia comes from measuring critical flicker frequency, color vision, differential and absolute light thresholds, and light and dark adaptation. Critical flicker frequency (CFF), the rate at which the flicker of an intermittent light stimulus disappears and becomes a continuous sensation, can be reduced in amblyopic eyes, but the losses are generally small.[253-255] The central CFF tends to approach the CFF of the peripheral retina or rod mechanism.[26]

Defects in color-vision have been observed only when the visual acuity is worse than 20/200.[256-259] The errors made by these patients are generally random and may be secondary to marked impairment of form vision rather than to an actual defect in color vision. Because these defects are similar to those found in normal peripheral vision, disturbances in color vision are more likely caused by eccentric fixation than a defect in the central retina.

Both patients with strabismic amblyopia and anisometropic amblyopia show elevated luminance increment thresholds for small targets.[218] The differential, or increment, threshold requires the patient to detect a target (ie., a bar, slit, or spot) that is superimposed on a homogeneous background. However, the ability for the amblyopic eye to perceive a simple light signal (the absolute visual threshold) is normal in both the light- and dark-adapted states.[260]

In summary, because patients with amblyopia have normal visual thresholds both foveally and peripherally, the consensus is that the basic retinal sensory mechanisms (rods, cones, photopigments) are probably intact in the amblyopic eye. Histopathologic reports of the retinas of monocularly deprived monkeys generally do not indicate significant differences in the size and density of retinal ganglion cells.[261] Any retinal changes are likely secondary to morphologic changes along the visual pathway.

LATERAL GENICULATE NUCLEUS

Changes from experimental amblyopia are well documented in the lateral geniculate nucleus (LGN), which serves as the relay station between the retina ganglion cells and the visual cortex. Cell sizes in the layers of the LGN receiving input from the normal and amblyopic eyes have been compared. The cells in those layers of the LGN receiving input from the amblyopic eye show a profound shrinkage.[262,263] Cells are decreased approximately 30% in size and contain shrunken nuclei and nucleoli.[241] In strabismic amblyopia the cell shrinkage is limited to the binocularly innervated portions of the LGN. After lid suture and induced anisometropia, all parts of the LGN are involved, including those that received visual input exclusively from the amblyopic eye. After suturing the sound eye, the cells in the LGN regain their normal size.[264] Deprivation for shorter periods (2 months vs. 3 months) produced similar but less severe changes, and no changes were seen when visual deprivation was carried out in adult animals. Cell shrinkage does not occur in strabismus induced by prisms, presumably because these animals alternately fixate and do not become amblyopic. Morphologic changes in the LGN similar to those described in kittens and monkeys have been reported in humans with anisometropic and strabismic amblyopia.[265,266]

VISUAL CORTEX

The most profound effects of amblyopia are found in the visual cortex. Microelectrode recordings from the visual cortex of kittens and infant monkeys with amblyopia differ from those without amblyopia. In the nonamblyopic animal with normal binocular vision, approximately 80% of the cells or neurons in the striate cortex are binocular and are driven or physiologically discharged by either eye (Fig. 2-18).[267] In uni-

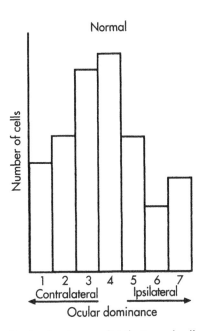

FIG. 2-18 Ocular dominance distribution of cells in cat striate cortex according to eye dominance (categories 1 and 7 contain neurons driven only through left or right eye, respectively. Remaining categories represent graded categories of binocular influence, with neurons in 4 being equally influenced by both eyes). No amblyopia.

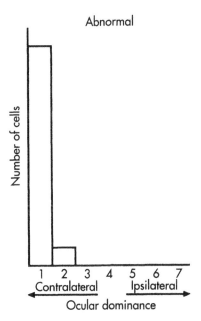

FIG. 2-19 Ocular dominance distribution of cells in cat striate cortex after eye ipsilateral to recorded cortex has been visually deprived, as in case of unilateral strabismus and other forms of deprivation. Amblyopia.

lateral strabismus and other forms of monocular visual deprivation, there is a shift of dominance and most cells are driven through the non-deprived eye (Fig. 2-19). The lack of responsiveness to the deprived eye results not only from loss of synaptic connections but also from a process of inhibition that is dependent

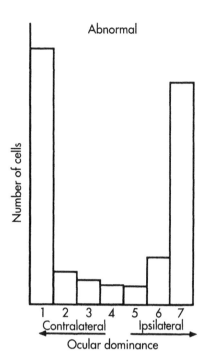

FIG. 2-20 Ocular dominance distribution of cells in cat striate cortex with alternating strabismus. No amblyopia.

on input from the normal eye and may be mediated through the neurotransmitter γ-aminobutyric acid (GABA). The number of cells responding to the amblyopic eye can be increased if the eye is used and the previously normal eye is deprived.[264] Treatment with the toxic compound bicuculline, a GABA antagonist, has also been shown to produce an increase in cortical responsiveness to the deprived eye (see Treatment). In the unilaterally deprived animal, there is also a reduction in the number of binocularly driven visual cortical cells. Depending on the degree of visual deprivation a reduction from the norm of 80% down to 10% to 20% or no binocular input at all can occur. The effects of monocular deprivation are more profound the earlier in life they occur. The reduction in binocularly driven cells also occurs in alternating strabismus without amblyopia (Fig. 2-20). The visual acuity of both eyes is maintained, but most cells are driven by either one eye or the other. This explains the loss of stereopsis in patients with strabismus but without amblyopia.

Positron emission tomography (PET) has been used to investigate changes in the metabolic activity of the visual cortex in humans with amblyopia. The local cerebral blood flow and glucose metabolism serve as the indicators of brain function. Deprivation, anisometropic, and strabismic amblyopia all show similar findings. A striking reduction exists in the amblyopic eye's ability to induce glucose metabolism in the visual cortex in response to visual stimulation.[268,269] This implies a lower level of activity, fewer cells responding, or both.

TREATMENT

The goal of amblyopia treatment is to normalize visual acuity and other functions of the amblyopic eye and, when this is not possible, improve the eye to optimal level. Amblyopia treatment is either passive or active. Passive treatment involves correction of refractive error, occlusion, and optical or pharmacologic penalization. There is little conscious effort on the part of the patient. Active treatment involves orthoptics/vision therapy to improve visual performance by the patient's conscious involvement in a sequence of specific controlled visual tasks that provide feedback to the patient.

Treating amblyopia involves prescribing the appropriate refractive correction and then deciding on the type of occlusion therapy. Orthoptics/vision therapy is given in conjunction to enhance the effect.

REFRACTIVE CORRECTION

As mentioned earlier, determination of the refractive error in amblyopia is best performed objectively with cycloplegic retinoscopy. The amblyopic eye should always have the most accurate optical correction. The clinician should not arbitrarily reduce the amount of cylindric correction or rotate the cylinder axis if it is not at 90 or 180 degrees. In some patients with isoametropia or anisometropia the glasses can be totally curative without additional treatment.[270,271]

The transient refractive errors common in infancy make it unclear when to prescribe.[106,107] Hopkisson and others[272] performed retinoscopy on 100 normal babies within 24 hours of delivery and at 6 weeks, 3 months, 6 months, and 1 year. Astigmatism of greater than 1 D increased from 10% at birth to 42% at 6 months but decreased to 15% at 1 year. Myopia was uncommon (4%) but 80% of eyes were hyperopic more than 2 D and 25% more than 4 D at birth, although these percentages decreased to 5% and 3% at 1 year. Anisometropia of more than 1 D was uncommon, but in two cases in which it persisted with high hyperopia, amblyopia occurred. Astigmatism and anisometropia probably must be persistent for 2 years or more from an early age to lead to amblyopia.[107,272]

For children with esotropia, the full amount of hyperopia is usually prescribed. In cases without esotropia and in which full correction may be impractical for the first correction, the amount of hyperopia can be reduced if done equally in each eye. Because each eye accommodates symmetrically and it is the less hyperopic eye that determines the amount of accommodation, any decrease in the plus must occur symmetrically or else the more hyperopic eye will continue to be blurred, even with glasses. Because amblyopic eyes tend to have reduced accommodation, we rarely cut the hyperopic correction in children by more than 1 D. The amount of astigmatism is fully corrected. Thus a child with amblyopia in the left eye with cycloplegic refraction of OD +1.50 − 1.00 × 90 and OS +5.00 − 1.50 × 95 can be treated with OD +0.75 − 1.00 × 90 and OS +4.25 − 1.50 × 95. In this way, when the nonamblyopic eye accommodates 0.75 D to see clearly at distance the amblyopic eye accommodates the same amount, and both eyes will have the correct amount of plus correction to see clearly. For children with myopia the full correction is always prescribed.

Glasses or Contact Lenses

A common concern is whether children with large amounts of anisometropia should be given contact lenses rather than glasses. Clinicians have reported success using contact lenses in treating anisometropic amblyopia.[273,274] For amounts of anisometropia exceeding 3 D, contact lenses have several advantages, including better cosmesis, reduction of induced prismatic imbalance when the child looks off the optical centers of the glasses, and elimination of the restricted visual field.[275]

Another concern with glasses is aniseikonia. According to Knapp's law, reduction in image size from normal is less in axial myopia and the increase in image size is less in axial hyperopia with glasses as compared with contact lenses.[276] There is similarly a more normal image size with contact lenses compared with glasses in patients with refractive myopia and hyperopia. Thus to minimize aniseikonia, contact lenses should be used in amblyopia related to refractive anisometropia and glasses should be used in amblyopia related to axial anisometropia. As discussed in Chapter 4, however, it has been shown that contact lenses for unilateral axial myopia actually reduce rather than increase aniseikonia.[273,277,278]

Nevertheless, we rarely use contact lenses initially in young children with anisometropic amblyopia. Glasses are the most practical means of dealing with the refractive error in these cases. Aniseikonia is not the most important issue in the beginning stage of amblyopia therapy, especially if the amblyopia is deep. A clear retinal image is the most important factor. Many of these children will also be occluded and will not be using binocular vision a portion of the time. It is only when the amblyopia is improved or eliminated entirely that aniseikonia possibly becomes a concern. Symptoms such as diplopia and closing of one eye should alert the clinician to aniseikonia. We recommend contact lenses be used following the successful treatment of anisometropic amblyopia. However, because of the large amount of anisometropia, contact lenses are used initially in aphakic children with deprivation amblyopia.

OCCLUSION

In spite of the new knowledge that has been added to our understanding of the underlying mechanisms of the various clinical manifestations of amblyopia, all the treatment modalities suggested in the last decades have not been able to replace occlusion. The use of occlusion or patching over the preferred eye to force visual function in the amblyopic eye was first described in the eighteenth century and remains the treatment of choice. Both convenient and economical, occlusion requires minimal office participation.

Occlusion therapy is prescribed according to the area of visual field occluded, wearing time, light transmission, and specific eye that is occluded.

Area of Visual Field Occluded

Occlusion can either be full and cover the entire visual field of one eye or be sector, or partial, and cover only a part of one or both eyes. An example of sector occlusion is binasal occlusion.

Wearing Time

Full-time, or constant, occlusion indicates that the patient wears the patch during all waking hours, removing it only during sleep. Periodic, or part-time, occlusion indicates that the patch is only worn a prescribed number of hours per day. Minimal occlusion indicates that the patch is generally worn 1 to 2 hours per day.

Light Transmission

Occlusion is either opaque (total) or attenuating (partial). Opaque is nontransmitting for light and form. The most common type of opaque occluders are the commercially available adhesive bandage patches. The Opticlude eye patch (Fig. 2-21) is semiporous and hypoallergenic and is available in junior and regular sizes. Other forms of opaque occlusion, such as tie-on patches, suction-cup occluders, and clip-on patches for glasses, are rarely used for young children because they are easily removed.[279] Peeking around a patch placed on glasses is frequent. This tendency usually lessens once vision has improved to 20/50 or better. Opaque contact lenses have been used on a limited basis.[276,280-282]

Attenuating, or partially transmitting, refers to nonopaque occlusion that permits the passage of diffuse light to the eye. Form vision is degraded but not completely eliminated by a scattering surface interposed before the eye. This generally takes the form of

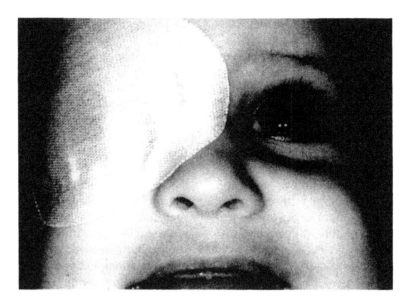

Fig. 2-21   Occlusion therapy used in an infant with amblyopia.

translucent tape applied to the entire lens of the non-amblyopic eye. Other forms of attenuating occlusion have included red filters, clear nail polish on the spectacle lens, blurring by optical means, and graded neutral-density filters.

Specific Eye to be Occluded

Occlusion is either direct, inverse, or alternating. With direct occlusion the nonamblyopic eye is patched, thereby forcing the amblyopic eye to fixate. With inverse or indirect occlusion the amblyopic eye is occluded and the nonamblyopic eye fixates. Alternating occlusion is when the patch is worn over the amblyopic eye sometimes and over the nonamblyopic eye at other times.

Constant, Total Direct (Conventional) Occlusion

Constant, total direct, or conventional, occlusion is total occlusion of the nonamblyopic eye that is used during all waking hours. It is the most common form of occlusion therapy.[283,284] Recovery of visual acuity with this form of occlusion occurs in most cases of strabismic and anisometropic amblyopia, provided treatment is begun early in life. The final level of acuity is rarely perfect, that is, 20/20. However, success rates greater than or equal to 20/40 visual acuity may occur for as many as 88% of all patients treated.[285] With eccentric fixation the figure falls to between 40% and 60%.[286]

Difficulties and Risks

Conventional occlusion is not without problems and risks. Approximately 10% to 25% of all patients treated may show little or no improvement.[287] Ineffectivity may be related to poor patient compliance, particularly with school-age children. Psychologic methods, such as ordering, pleading, threatening, or bribery, may be necessary on the part of the parents. Academic hardship may occur as the child is forced to participate in school and other activities with greatly reduced vision. Emotional and social problems may also develop. Some children do not show improvement because of poor parental compliance.

Constant, total direct occlusion must be used judiciously. The importance of regular follow-up is stressed. As a general rule, a child on full-time patching should be reevaluated at time intervals dependent on age. Children age 2 or younger should be seen every 2 weeks, whereas older children can be monitored on a monthly basis. As indicated earlier, indiscriminate or poorly supervised patching of the nonamblyopic eye can lead to occlusion (i.e., deprivation) amblyopia in young patients.[113,127]

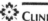 **Clinical Pearl**

A child on full-time patching should be reevaluated at time intervals dependent on age.

In attempting to prevent occlusion amblyopia, we use an alternating occlusion regimen for patients age 5 and younger. The schedule provided by Griffin[288] is most applicable, because it uses a ratio of 1 day of full-time direct occlusion per year of life, alternated with 1 day of inverse occlusion, repeating the procedure as necessary. For a 3 year old the occluder is worn over the nonamblyopic eye for 3 days and over the amblyopic eye for 1 day. This sequence is repeated until there is ideally no longer any difference in acuity between the two eyes. For a 4 year old the ratio is 4:1. Because occlusion amblyopia does not usually occur beyond the fifth year, we do not use alternate occlusion in children who are age 6 or older.

If improvement is slow or not progressing, the period of occlusion of the nonamblyopic eye can be increased (i.e., for a 3 year old, 5:1 instead of 3:1). The clinician should wait at least 5 minutes after removing the patch before checking visual acuity in that eye, so that the eye has time to adapt to light and recover from patching.

Because full-time occlusion discourages development of fusion, some clinicians prefer not to patch the amblyopic eye and instead allow binocular viewing for 1 or 2 days per week. For three reasons we prefer to occlude one eye or the other, rather than leaving both eyes open. First, occluding the amblyopic eye allows the fixating eye a brief period of the dominance it had been accustomed to before initiation of treatment. Second, occluding the amblyopic eye does not reinstate the same amblyopiagenic factors (i.e., form-vision deprivation and/or abnormal binocular interaction) that led to the amblyopia. The damage to binocularly driven cortical neurons is a consequence of strabismus and not occlusion. Using prisms to compensate for the angle of strabismus on the day of binocular viewing might eliminate this concern. Third, occluding one or the other eye adds to better compliance with therapy, both on the part of the child and the parents.

Skin irritation and allergies may occur during prolonged use, especially in the summer. Repeated removal of the adhesive patch tends to aggravate any skin condition. Applying tincture of benzoin or protective dressing wipes to the skin before applying the patch should eliminate this.[279] Benzoin also forms a protective layer on the skin that prevents the ulceration that occurs in some children. Allowing the patch to be placed on hypoallergenic tape rather than directly on the skin also reduces skin irritation (Fig. 2-22). When the patch is removed the adhesive on the patch is pulled from the underlying tape rather than the skin.

Conventional occlusion may be contraindicated for patients with amblyopia who have some form of binocular vision, such as anisometropia, microtropia, and intermittent strabismus. Swan[289] reports on heterophoric patients who developed esotropia following occlusion therapy for anisometropic amblyopia. All patients subsequently underwent extraocular muscle surgery for the strabismus. However, Swan's patients did not have their full hyperopic refractive error corrected before undergoing occlusion. However, we believe the risk of provoking strabismus by occluding a patient with anisometropic amblyopia is small. This occlusion-induced strabismus may be more likely for patients with ani-

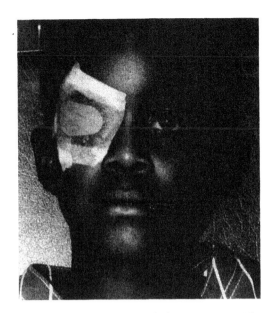

Fig. 2-22 Method used to avoid skin irritation with occlusion therapy.

sometropic amblyopia who wear only partial refractive corrections and have high AC/A ratios.[3]

Some patients with microtropia manifest a small-angle strabismus and an overlying heterophoria of variable and larger magnitude. The heterophoria is well controlled until the patient undergoes occlusion therapy for amblyopia. Occlusion can cause a breakdown of peripheral fusion, causing the small strabismic angle to change to a larger strabismus, although this is not always the case.[290-292] Changes may also develop when using occlusion with intermittent strabismus. The intermittent strabismus can become constant. For amblyopia associated with either anisometropia, microtropia, or intermittent strabismus, less aggressive occlusion therapy (i.e., part-time opaque or full-time attenuating) may be used initially, depending on the severity of the amblyopia.

Duration of Therapy

A question frequently asked by parents is how long occlusion therapy will last. Younger children tend to recover their acuity more quickly. With good compliance, however, the age of the child may not be the determining factor in strabismic and anisometropic amblyopia.[293-295] Oliver and others[295] treated 350 children with amblyopia exclusively with occlusion. Patients were categorized into 3 groups according to the age when treated. Most improvement occurred within 3 months after initiating treatment, regardless of the age of the patient (Fig. 2-23). Rutstein and Fuhr[293] report an average treatment period of 3.8 months to achieve maximum visual acuity for patients treated at age 7 or younger. For patients older than age 7 the av-

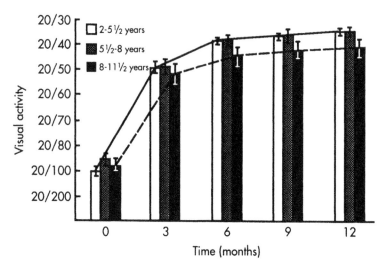

FIG. 2-23   Mean visual acuity achievement in three age groups of amblyopic patients. (Modified from Oliver and others: Compliance and results of treatment of amblyopia in children more that 8 years old, *Am J Ophthalmol,* 343:102, 1989.)

erage treatment period increased to 4.2 months. Thus we usually tell parents that most improvement in visual acuity should occur by 4 months of treatment. Using this information in another way, if after the same period no improvement occurs, we usually feel comfortable in terminating occlusion therapy, providing we are convinced that compliance was adequate. In the latter case, organic factors resulting in the visual loss should always be considered.[296]

Recurring Amblyopia

After improving visual acuity, strabismic patients may continue to show a strong fixation preference. If the original amblyopiagenic factors have not been eliminated and the patient is still visually immature, continuation of the abnormal visual experience may result in visual acuity regression. In these instances, amblyopia tends to recur until children reach ages 10 to 12. The average loss is nearly 50% of the visual acuity gain.[297] This is more likely if the amblyopia was deep. With children who have strabismus, we therefore also try to establish alternate fixation. Alternate fixation prevents a relapse of amblyopia, which may develop in as many as 40% to 70% of all cases.[293,298] The child with strabismus whose vision has improved but does not alternately fixate after amblyopia therapy and does not bifixate after strabismus therapy requires close observation so that relapses can be detected early. This can occur over a period of years, as illustrated by the following case example.[293]

CASE 4 (FIG. 2-24)

A 5-year-old girl presented in July, 1982 with a constant left esotropia of 40 PD at distance and near. Visual acuity was 20/40 right eye and 20/274 left eye, as measured with

the Psychometric cards. Cycloplegic refraction was +3.75 D OU and reduced the esotropia to 10 PD but did not improve the vision in the left eye. Treatment consisted of glasses with full correction and constant, total direct occlusion of the right eye. The left eye was patched every sixth day. Orthoptics/vision therapy was also done. In October, vision for the left eye improved to 20/38 and the patient still manifested a 10 PD, constant left esotropia. Because the patient demonstrated no potential for normal single binocular vision and the residual strabismus was not cosmetically displeasing, further treatment was not recommended.

The patient returned in May, 1983 with vision in the left eye of 20/222. Occlusion therapy of the right eye was performed on a part-time basis until April, 1984, when vision in the left eye was 20/25. Two years later, the vision for the left eye was essentially stable. However, at the patient's final visit in 1988, vision in the left eye had regressed to 20/190.

Some patients with strabismic amblyopia can achieve normal visual acuity but not alternate fixation. Campos and Gulli[299] treated 57 patients with strabismic amblyopia (ages 1 to 11), all of whom achieved 20/20 or better in each eye with occlusion. Only 29 (51%) could also alternately fixate after treatment (Fig. 2-25). Alternate fixation could not be achieved when treatment began after age 6. Establishing alternate fixation is also unlikely in strabismic children with high amounts of anisometropia. Such patients will usually not fixate with the more ametropic eye, even with equal visual acuity. Follow-up at least every 3 months, part-time occlusion, or attenuating occlusion can be used to maintain visual acuity (see Case 5).

OPAQUE CONTACT LENSES

Opaque contact lenses offer the advantages of requiring no contact with the skin and better cosme-

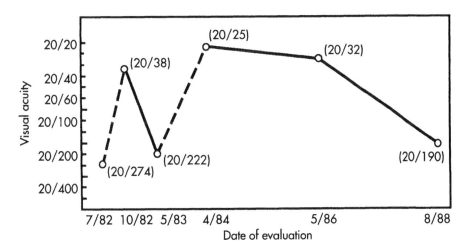

FIG. 2-24 Changes in visual acuity over time for patient with strabismic amblyopia (Case 4). Broken lines indicate periods of treatment; solid lines indicate periods without treatment. (Modified from Rutstein RP, Fuhr PD: *Optometry and vision science,* Baltimore, 1992, Williams & Wilkins.)

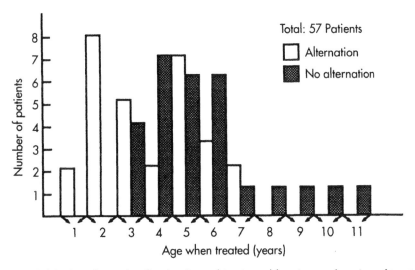

FIG. 2-25 Achieving alternating fixation in strabismic amblyopia as a function of treatment age. (Modified from Campos EC, Gulli R: Lack of alternation in patients treated for strabismic amblyopia, *Am J Ophthalmol,* 99:64, 1985.)

sis.[276,280-283] Moore[276] used opaque contact lenses over the preferred eye in children resistant to patching. For seven patients ranging in age from 1 to 8 years with amblyopia as a result of congenital cataracts, strabismus, or anisometropia, all patients showed improvement from 1 to 3 octaves, as measured by PL or by standard recognition acuity tests. Extended-wear occlusion soft contact lenses have also been used to treat amblyopia.[282]

Despite the reported success, opaque contact lenses are not our method of choice for treating amblyopia, especially in young children. Potential problems, such as corneal infection, difficulty in lens fit-

ting, parental difficulty in manipulating the lens, lens damage, lens displacement, frequent lens loss, low availability, and high cost, force us to use the more conventional methods of occlusion. Opaque contact lenses should be considered in cases in which physical or social problems with conventional patching are an obstacle. Older children and teenagers are usually the best candidates.

SECTOR OCCLUSION

Sector occlusion occurs when only a portion of the visual field or lens of one eye or both eyes is occluded. This method of selectively masking portions of

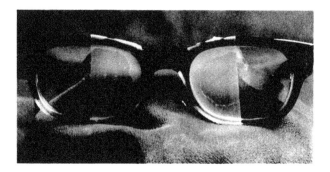

FIG. 2-26 Binasal occlusion.

the glasses was introduced in France. Binasal occlusion is the most common type of sector occlusion used to treat amblyopia.[300,301] It has been used also in treating esotropia and spasm of the near reflex.[302-303] Translucent adhesive tape or nail polish is used to occlude the nasal sector of the spectacle lens (Fig. 2-26). This allows only diffuse light to pass through, yielding a formless field. If opaque binasal occlusion is desired, black electrician's tape can be used.

To apply binasal occlusion, the patient, while wearing glasses, fixates a distant target in primary position with one eye while the other eye is occluded.[320] The pupil of the fixating eye is then bisected by the edge of the tape so that the nasal half of the monocular field of view is completely occluded. The procedure is repeated for the other eye. If deep amblyopia exists, a larger portion of the lens before the nonamblyopic eye can be taped. With binasal occlusion, alternate fixation is encouraged. Objects to the right can only be fixated by the right eye, and objects to the left can only be fixated by the left eye.

Although binasal occlusion has been used for many years, reports on its efficacy are scarce and controlled studies are lacking. We believe it should be restricted for patients who have improved following conventional occlusion therapy and manifest either a residual amblyopia or a nonalternating fixation pattern. Binasal occlusion may possibly establish alternate fixation and maintain the visual acuity gains for these patients. It should not be used as the initial therapy in children with strabismic amblyopia (see Chapter 13, Case 1).

ATTENUATING OCCLUSION

Attenuating, or partially transmitting, occlusion has the advantage that large forms still are visible to the occluded eye, and peripheral fusion is not disrupted. It is necessary that the visual acuity of the nonamblyopic eye be reduced to at least two lines lower than the amblyopic eye with the Snellen chart or else the patient will continue to favor the dominant eye. Attenuating occlusion is most commonly used

when the amblyopia is 20/60 or better and in cases with some fusion, as in anisometropic amblyopia, microtropia, or intermittent strabismus. It can also be used after constant, total direct occlusion when there is chance for visual acuity regression.

 CLINICAL PEARL

Attenuating occlusion is most commonly used when the amblyopia is 20/60 or better and in cases with some fusion, as in anisometropic amblyopia, microtropia, or intermittent strabismus.

Reports on the efficacy of attenuating occlusion are also scarce. Wesson[306] uses attenuating occlusion involving light-intensity reduction before the nonamblyopic eye to a level at which the amblyopic eye is still able to compete in a binocular manner with the nonamblyopic eye. He uses two pieces of polarized filters superimposed and rotated so that an angle is formed between their axes of polarization. As the angle approaches 90 degrees, the light transmitted through the Polaroid approaches extinction. The acuity of the nonamblyopic eye is reduced by slowly rotating the two polarized pieces in front of the nonamblyopic eye while the amblyopic eye is occluded. When an acuity level is reached that is two lines worse than the amblyopic eye, the Polaroid pieces are taped together and placed on the spectacle lens before the nonamblyopic eye. In one patient reported by Wesson,[306] the visual acuity improved from 20/100 to 20/26.

Cho and Norden[307] describe an attenuating occluder lens that can be used for amblyopia therapy. The steps for application include cutting and edging a plastic lens to the shape of the frame, sanding the entire back surface of the lens evenly with 600-grit sandpaper until the lens appears translucent, tinting both lenses with a light tint (the occluder lens will tint slightly darker than the regular lens because of the greater surface area on the back surface), and adjusting the tints so that the lenses are tinted approximately the same amount. The eye behind the occluder lens will be visible enough so that lid and eye movements are just visible; however, the visual acuity will be less than 20/400 for the occluded eye.

For attenuating occlusion, we prefer the Bangerter filters or foils (Fig. 2-27). These consist of a series of graded transparent filters (20/25 [0.8] to less than 20/300 [0.1]) that can be affixed directly to the patient's glasses, similar to Fresnel press-on prisms and lenses. The densest filter can be used in patients with deep amblyopia. In addition, rather than terminating occlusion therapy in children treated successfully for strabismic amblyopia, we taper it with Bangerter filters. With this technique, we have considerably reduced the incidence of recurring amblyopia. (See Case 5.)

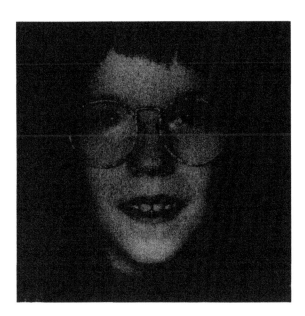

Fig. 2-27 Attenuating occlusion using Bangerter filters.

Case 5

A 6-year-old boy came to the clinic in September 1992 for a second opinion. He had been treated by an ophthalmologist for amblyopia. The treatment consisted of glasses and atropine ointment in the right eye over a 6-month period. The atropine had been discontinued 2 weeks earlier.

Our examination revealed corrected vision of OD 20/26 and OS 20/87, as measured with Psychometric cards. The patient manifested with the glasses a 5-PD constant left esotropia at distance and a 15-PD constant left esotropia at near. Without the glasses, the esotropia increased to 15 PD and 25 PD at distance and near, respectively. Suppression of the left eye occurred with the Worth four dot test at distance and near, and there was no appreciation of stereopsis. Cycloplegic refraction agreed with the current glasses (OD +4.00, OS +4.75). Visuoscopy revealed an unsteady 2-degree nasal, inferior eccentric fixation in the left eye. Ophthalmoscopic findings were normal.

The diagnosis was partly accommodative esotropia with amblyopia and eccentric fixation. Treatment consisted of total occlusion of the right eye during all waking hours and orthoptics/vision therapy.

One month later the visual acuity in the left eye had improved to 20/32 and visuoscopy showed central fixation. Another month of treatment improved the acuity to 20/20, but the patient still preferred to fixate with his right eye. At this point, occlusion was replaced with a Bangerter filter (0.2) on the right spectacle lens.

In February 1993, visual acuity remained stable. A Bangerter filter (0.3) was placed on the right lens. Two months later the filter was decreased even more. Over a period of 6 months the patient was weaned completely from occlusion.

At the last visit, 2 years later, visual acuities were 20/26 in each eye. Cover testing showed slight exophoria at distance and near. With the Worth four dot test the patient fused at near, but suppressed the left eye at distance. Stereopsis was 100 seconds of arc with the Randot stereotest.

PART-TIME OCCLUSION

Although constant, total direct occlusion is the most effective treatment, there may be certain instances when it is not appropriate. The age of the patient, the degree of amblyopia, and the fusion status all indicate whether constant or part-time occlusion will be used. Part-time occlusion can be used in patients with amblyopia with straight or almost straight eyes if there is concern about disrupting fusion. It can also be used to maintain the gain in visual acuity achieved with previous treatment. There is little or no risk of inducing occlusion amblyopia in the preferred eye with part-time occlusion.

With older children, we try not to occlude in school if at all possible. They experience a host of problems brought on by wearing the patch in school, the most frequent being taunting by other children. If the amblyopia is deep, these children may also experience serious academic impairment in their ability to perform well in school. In addition, the school may find that providing extra help to these children may be more than they are willing or able to do.

A 7-year-old patient we treated had 20/200 amblyopia secondary to a small-angle esotropia. Because of the severity of amblyopia and the lack of earlier treatment, we placed the youngster on conventional occlusion therapy. After only 2 weeks, the vision had improved to 20/70. However, during the progress evaluation the parents seemed quite upset. In their hands was a letter from the child's teacher stating how passive the child had become in school while wearing the patch. In the teacher's words, the child sat like a vegetable. Despite the large improvement, the type of occlusion therapy was switched to 3 hours per day after school and constantly on weekends and holidays. After 6 months the visual acuity had improved to 20/60. Constant, total direct occlusion was to be undertaken again in the summer.

Occlusion generally must be maintained at least 2 hours per day to be effective.[225] In the late 1970s and early 1980s numerous reports described a form of therapy known as *CAM treatment*.[308-314] The treatment consisted of patching the nonamblyopic eye for even shorter periods, usually 7 minutes and not exceeding 20 minutes per day. While wearing the patch the patient concentrated on some visually demanding near task, such as dot-to-dot pictures or mazes. These tasks were performed on a clear piece of plastic mounted directly above high-contrast square wave gratings of certain spatial frequencies, which were rotated at 1 rpm/min. The rationale of this treatment was the presentation of various spatial frequencies to the visual cortex connected with the amblyopic eye, to improve its function.

Earlier reports on this method were favorable. For example, in one study on 22 patients with amblyopia, the average near visual acuity improved from 20/133 to 20/57 after only six treatment sessions.[309] However, age-matched and controlled studies comparing this treatment with conventional occlusion found the former to be much less effective. Only 20% or less achieved significant improvement in visual acuity (more than 10% Snell-Sterling).[312] Any improvement likely resulted from the patient performing the visually demanding near tasks. These intense visual and eye-hand coordination tasks, as well as the general arousal of the patient during the exercises and possible practice effects, played more of a part than the minimal occlusion itself. In addition, most studies did not document improvement of acuity with tests that reduced or controlled memorization criteria shifts, or variability of acuity because of contour interaction and motor instability of amblyopic eyes. The use of CAM treatment is not popular in current practice.

INVERSE OCCLUSION

We have very little use for occluding the amblyopic eye for prolonged periods of time. Nevertheless, in children with strabismic amblyopia and steady eccentric fixation, some clinicians recommend inverse rather than direct occlusion.[315] According to these clinicians, occlusion of the fixating eye consolidates rather than eradicates the eccentric fixation in the amblyopic eye. It is hoped that the inverse occlusion will cause the eccentric fixation to disappear, because the amblyopic eye is not continuously reinforced by daily use. Daily therapy sessions emphasizing foveal fixation are performed when providing inverse occlusion.

The benefit of inverse occlusion has never been substantiated. The point or area that is used for eccentric fixation during monocular viewing is rarely the same point or area used during binocular viewing. To disrupt eccentric fixation, no occlusion at all should be just as effective. Several studies have indicated that direct occlusion is much more effective than inverse occlusion, regardless of the fixation status, especially in younger children.[316,317] We have used inverse occlusion only in extreme cases. For example, we recently examined a 9-year-old child who had undergone multiple surgical procedures for an esotropia and now was exotropic. Visual acuity was 20/400 in the strabismic eye, and visuoscopy showed fixation to be coincident with the optic nerve head. Inverse occlusion was attempted, with no change in the fixation status. Direct occlusion was also unsuccessful. We occasionally give inverse occlusion for a few days as a preliminary to direct occlusion, so the child can better adjust to occlusion.

OTHER TREATMENT MODALITIES
Penalization

Penalization is a method of amblyopia treatment that uses selective blurring rather than occlusion of the nonamblyopic eye.[318-327] The blurring is induced either pharmacologically or optically. The goal of penalization is to have the patient to use the amblyopic eye for a particular distance and the nonamblyopic eye for another distance or to have the patient use the amblyopic eye for all viewing distances. Supposedly, patients with esotropia with mild unilateral myopia use their myopic eye for near and their nonmyopic eye for distance fixation and are not amblyopic. If this condition could be simulated either optically or pharmacologically, this would be an effective method for treating and preventing amblyopia.

One of the earliest forms of penalization consisted of a combination of atropine in the nonamblyopic eye and isoflurophate in the amblyopic eye.[318] This caused the patient to use the amblyopic eye for near viewing and the nonamblyopic eye for distance viewing. The problem of instilling two medications, each with significant side effects, may have kept this from becoming a popular method of therapy.

Six types of penalization have been reported (Table 2-4). The most frequently used include near penalization, distance penalization, total penalization, and alternating penalization.

With near penalization, cycloplegia is induced in the nonamblyopic eye with atropine (0.5% or 1.0%) once or twice per day and fully corrected optically. The amblyopic eye is also optically corrected and given an additional plus lens ranging from 1.5 D to 3 D. The plus lens forces the amblyopic eye to be used for near fixation. Alternate fixation is encouraged as the nonamblyopic eye is used for distance fixation. Near penalization has been used mainly with deep amblyopia (20/100 or less).[319,320]

In distance penalization the nonamblyopic eye is cycloplegic and given a plus overcorrection of usually 3 D. The amblyopic eye is optically corrected for distance. This blurs the distance vision in the nonamblyopic eye, assuming it is hyperopic, but permits it to have clear near vision. The amblyopic eye is used for distance and has the option to use its recently improved vision also for near. Distance penalization has been used mostly with patients having mild amblyopia (20/60 or better) and in cases in which recurring amblyopia is likely.[320] Some children may remove the glasses to improve distance vision in their nonamblyopic eye.

Total penalization involves cycloplegia and either optically overcorrecting or undercorrecting the nonamblyopic eye. If the nonamblyopic eye is hyperopic, it is undercorrected by 3 to 4 D. If the eye is emmetropic or myopic, it is overminused by 4 to 5 D.

TABLE 2-4 TYPES OF PENALIZATION

Type	Nonamblyopic Eye	Amblyopic Eye	Aim	Indications
Near	Full correction; cycloplegia	Overcorrection of +1.50 to +3.00 D	Use of the amblyopic eye for near and the nonamblyopic eye for distance	Deep amblyopia with or without eccentric fixation
Distance	Overcorrection (+3.00 D); cycloplegia	Full correction	Use of the amblyopic eye for distance and the nonamblyopic eye for near	1. Mild amblyopia 2. Prevents recurring amblyopia
Total	Overminus (4.00-5.00 D) if emmetropic or myopic or optical undercorrection (3.00-4.00 D) if hyperopic; cycloplegia	Full correction	Use of the amblyopic eye for distance and near	1. High hyperopia 2. Mild amblyopia that has not responded to other treatment
Selective	Full correction; cycloplegia	Full correction; +2.00 D lower-segment bifocal	Use of the amblyopic eye for near and the nonamblyopic eye for distance	1. Following correction of strabismus if deviation remains only at near 2. To alternate or stabilize ocular dominance
Slight or mild	Overcorrection (+1.00 to +3.00 D)	Full correction	Use of the amblyopic eye for distance and the nonamblyopic eye for near	1. Prevents recurring amblyopia 2. Mild amblyopia
Alternating	Two pairs of glasses to be worn on alternate days. No. 1: RE +3.00 D overcorrection, No. 2: LE +3.00 D overcorrection		Right eye is used for near and left eye for distance on day 1. Reverses on day 2.	1. Used after vision is equalized and nonalternating strabismus remains. 2. Prevents recurring amblyopia

From Rutstein RP: Alternative treatment in amblyopia. In Rutstein RP, editor: *Problems in optometry,* Philadelphia, 1991, JB Lippincott.

The patient is forced to use the amblyopic eye both at distance and near. Total penalization has been used mostly for mild amblyopia (20/60 or better) and with hyperopia. Poor patient compliance is frequent with total penalization. Unless the nonamblyopic eye is highly hyperopic (6 D or greater), the patient usually gains better vision by removing the glasses and will do so. Treating children with hyperopia with cycloplegia combined with removal of the correcting lens before the nonamblyopic eye may be more effective.[320]

In selective penalization, cycloplegia is induced in the nonamblyopic eye, and it is given its full correction, whereas the amblyopic eye is fully corrected and given a +2.00-D lower segment bifocal. This can be recommended after treating amblyopia if the strabismic deviation remains only for near and also possibly to alternate or stabilize ocular dominance.

Slight and alternating forms of penalization rely on optical methods exclusively. Because no studies are available that suggest that pharmacologic penalization is superior to optical penalization and because adverse effects of prolonged cycloplegia can occur, the optical form is our method of choice. The nonamblyopic eye is overcorrected, allowing only the amblyopic eye to be used for distance. Fresnel press-on lenses can be used (Fig. 2-28).

Alternating penalization involves prescribing two pairs of glasses to be used on alternate days. One pair has a plus overcorrection incorporated in the lens of the right eye, and the other has the same overcorrection in the lens for the left eye. By varying these prescriptions, distance and near vision are blurred in each eye every other day. This can be effective in preventing recurring amblyopia in children with strabismus who do not alternately fixate.[322]

Often, fixed amounts of overcorrection are prescribed in optical penalization. We arbitrarily overcorrect the nonamblyopic eye by 2.50 to 3 D. Prescribing the minimal amount of blur necessary to ensure that the patient actually switches fixation to the amblyopic eye is probably better, especially if fusion potential exists. A polarized vectographic chart can be used for this purpose. Plus lenses are added to the nonamblyopic eye in 0.25-D increments, until the patient switches fixation to the amblyopic eye. The patient will begin to read the letters seen only by the ambly-

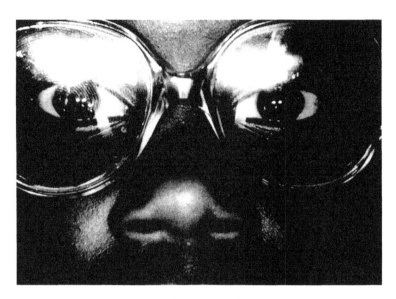

FIG. 2-28 Optical penalization with +3.00-D Fresnel press-on lens.

opic eye and omit the letters of the nonamblyopic eye. For 34 patients the average added power needed was only +1.25 D.[323]

Although investigators have reported on penalization therapy, few if any controlled studies verifying its efficacy appear in the literature.[324-327] The superiority of occlusion therapy not withstanding, optical penalization can be a useful alternative for amblyopia therapy, particularly when the visual acuity in the amblyopic eye is 20/60 or better and when occlusion has been unsuccessful. We have not found penalization useful when the amblyopia is deep. In these cases the child may still prefer the penalized eye for near vision, because visual acuity in that eye may remain slightly better despite the penalization.

The advantage of penalization is that it is inconspicuous and generally well tolerated. We have used penalization with children who cannot wear a patch because of skin allergy or severe behavioral problems. School children can use the nonamblyopic eye at least part-time and can therefore participate more easily in school activities. With penalization the peripheral binocular visual field is maintained, and peripheral fusion is not disrupted. Penalization can also be used to treat amblyopia with latent nystagmus, because there is no aggravation of the nystagmus with both eyes open. More frequently, we use penalization to prevent the loss of therapeutic gains made by previous occlusion therapy.

Another advantage of penalization is that it supposedly does not carry the risk of occlusion amblyopia in younger children. However, there have been documented cases of amblyopia induced by prolonged cycloplegia in children ages 3 to 5.[115,328] As with occlusion the susceptibility to visual deprivation with penalization declines with advancing age and likely ceases to exist after the fifth year of life. We are unaware of any reports of amblyopia following optical penalization being induced in children.

Orthoptics/Vision Therapy

Because amblyopia is a syndrome of vision disorders and not just reduced visual acuity, orthoptics/vision therapy attempts to train eye movements, fixation, spatial perception, accommodation, and binocular function, as well as to improve visual acuity. In conjunction with occlusion, it can lessen the total treatment time necessary to achieve the best visual acuity. With the young child, pointing, tracing, and coloring procedures while undergoing occlusion stimulates fixation and visual acuity of the amblyopic eye. Several case studies have documented improved vision function, particularly in older patients who had not responded to occlusion.[329] Improvements in accommodation, eye movements, and contrast sensitivity with orthoptics/vision therapy frequently occur more rapidly than visual acuity, suggesting residual neural plasticity for multiple sites in the visual pathway.[11,27,210,211,215]

The first formal orthoptics/vision therapy treatment for amblyopia was probably pleoptics. Bangerter[330] and Cüppers[199] introduced this technique in the mid-1950s. According to Bangerter and Cüppers, treatment of amblyopia works best when patients are provided with an external signal that enables them to monitor the accuracy of their performance. Pleoptics emphasizes awareness of eccentric fixation and feedback for correct localization. Pupillary dilation is required. According to Bangerter's method, pleoptics involves dazzling of the retina (including the area of eccentric fixation) by a bright flash of light that is followed by stimulation of the fovea with brief flashes of light. This process supposedly decreases the sensitivity of the peripheral retina to below that of the fovea. The flashing light on the fovea is thought to break through the foveal inhibition. According to Cüppers' method, nonfoveal retina is also bleached, but then the patient is also presented with visual and kinesthetic feedback regarding eccentric fixation in the amblyopic eye by the use of afterimages. A ring afterimage is created, and the patient monocularly aims, or localizes, the afterimage around targets and letters. Inverse occlusion is used full-time between pleoptics therapy sessions. When fixation becomes normalized, occlusion is switched to the nonamblyopic eye. Some patients were enrolled in "schools" and hospitals in Europe to allow daily attendance for high-intensity treatment.

Pleoptics involves an enormous commitment in terms of time, personnel, and costs. It requires substantial cooperation from the patient and is difficult to administer to children younger than ages 6 to 7. Nevertheless, in most cases, pleoptics was not as effective as conventional treatment and thus was never totally accepted.[331-333] Isolated reports do mention some success, especially with patients who failed with occlusion.[334-337] Presently, pleoptics may have its greatest value in adult patients with amblyopia who lose vision in their good eye either to an accident or ocular disease. Vereecken and Brabant[338] report on 203 such patients. Sixty-nine patients (34%) showed improved visual acuity in the amblyopic eye. Of these, 60% improved spontaneously over time without any treatment, and the remaining patients improved with orthoptics/vision therapy. Pleoptics was valuable for the patients with eccentric fixation.

Afterimage transfer techniques have been used to treat amblyopia.[339] This procedure does not require pupil dilation, and the patient uses conventional occlusion rather than inverse occlusion when not being treated. An afterimage is created, usually by means of a photographic flash unit in the nonamblyopic eye. That eye is then occluded, and the afterimage is transferred to the amblyopic eye. The location of the transferred afterimage represents the true straight-ahead position. For the eye to see correctly the patient should be able to align the afterimage with a small fixation target or letter. The increasing accuracy and speed in carrying out the alignment of the afterimage with a fixation object allows letters of decreasing size to be used, with an accompanying improvement in visual acuity. The afterimage can be replenished by switching the room lights off and on occasionally for at least 5 minutes. As mentioned earlier, the status of retinal correspondence must be known before using transferred afterimages. With anomalous correspondence the afterimage transfers to some nonfoveal area rather than the fovea and therefore makes afterimage treatment ineffective.

Although proponents[339] reported success in a single session in some cases and cite improvement from 20/200 to 20/40 or 20/20, this has not been our experience nor that of other investigators.[340,341] We find that many patients cannot perceive the transferred afterimage. Haidinger brushes can be used instead of transferred afterimages. As with afterimages the patient attempts to align the Haidinger brushes with the fixation target by using a subtle eye movement. This method, although never formally substantiated, may be useful for older and less easily occluded patients with amblyopia.

Auditory biofeedback and visual and kinesthetic biofeedback have been used to treat eccentric fixation and eye movement anomalies associated with amblyopia. Here the patient is supplied a signal that, by its pitch and position, informs the patient where he or she is fixating.[342,343] Auditory biofeedback does not require special conditions of visual stimulation and does not introduce extraneous visual stimuli that can interfere with foveal viewing on testing; can be used with patients who do not perceive Haidinger brushes or afterimages with the amblyopic eye; is not subject to fading or intermittent perception; and is more commanding perceptually than are low-contrast entoptic images such as afterimages and Haidinger brushes.[344-346] We have no experience with auditory feedback and realize it is in the experimental stage. Preliminary results for its use as a potential clinical treatment for amblyopia appear impressive.

Because abnormal binocular interaction is the major underlying mechanism in unilateral amblyopia, antisuppression procedures can be used to treat amblyopia under binocular viewing conditions.[359,360] Anaglypic and polarized TV trainers, cheiroscopic tracings, physiologic diplopia, stereoscopes, and bar reading are applicable for this purpose. These procedures are described in Chapter 5 and require the patient to maintain the amblyopic eye's perception under conditions involving stimulation of the nonamblyopic eye. By forcing the amblyopic eye to function in this manner the level of suppression or binocular inhibition is diminished and the amblyopia resolves. Peripheral fusion and binocular vision are encouraged. These procedures can be effective in preventing any amblyopia regression.[347] We use them almost exclusively in anisometropic amblyopia.

Pharmacologic Treatment

Chemical substances that might diminish or nullify amblyopia have been sought. Neurotransmitters such as GABA and catecholamines influence the visual-cortical plasticity in animals. Reversing certain ef-

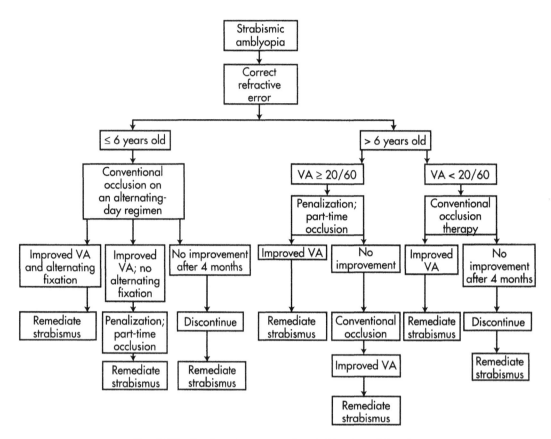

FIG. 2-29 Treatment sequence for strabismic amblyopia.

fects of visual deprivation in young animals with GABA-receptor blockers, catecholamine depletion, or the enhancing of neuronal plasticity by activating the central norepinephrine system has been reported. Duffy and others[349,350] show that bicuculline, a GABA-receptor blocker, if injected intracisternally in animals, could delay the central nervous system maturation time and eliminate the occurrence of amblyopia. Pettigrew and Kasumatsu[351] used activation of the central norepinephrine system for the purpose of enhancing neuronal plasticity.

Levodopa may have a similar effect on reversing human amblyopia. Following its administration, increases in contrast thresholds and decreases in size of fixation point scotomas occur.[352] Levodopa administered for as long as 1 week appears to provide positive results lasting for 1 to 3 weeks. Leguire and associates[353] investigated the efficacy of levodopa/carbidopa combined with part-time occlusion therapy on 10 children ages 6 to 14 with amblyopia. Ten other children received a placebo and part-time occlusion. The levodopa and carbidopa group improved significantly in mean visual acuity by 2.7 lines and in mean contrast sensitivity by 72% in the amblyopic eye. The placebo group improved in visual acuity by 1.6 lines. One month after ending treatment, the levodopa/car-

bidopa group maintained a 1.2-line improvement in visual acuity and 74% improvement in contrast sensitivity. The placebo group did not maintain their improvement. In a subsequent study on 15 children the average visual acuity improved from 20/170 to 20/107 after 5 weeks of treatment.[354] Although side effects such as emesis and nausea have been associated with its use, preliminary studies on levodopa are encouraging. Improvement in amblyopia has also been reported in over 90% of children treated with citicoline for 15 days, and results have been stable for at least 6 months.[355] This is a drug that is used to increase the level of consciousness in patients with head trauma and Parkinson's disease. Investigation of the use of such agents to influence visual performance in human amblyopia is in its very early stages. Perhaps in the future, amblyopia will be treated by taking a pill.

MANAGEMENT STRATEGIES
STRABISMIC AMBLYOPIA

The protocol for treating strabismic amblyopia is illustrated in Fig. 2-29. The initial step, as with all amblyopia, is correcting significant refractive errors. This alone seldom results in improvement of visual acuity. Constant, total direct occlusion therapy on an alternate-day regimen is the method of choice for younger children. Part-time occlusion is reserved for intermittent strabismus, school-age children, and mild amblyopia.

Treatment of the amblyopia should be completed before treatment of the strabismus. This yields a better chance for fusion. In cases of resistant amblyopia, however, treatment of the amblyopia also delays achieving ocular alignment and may hinder development of fusion at a later date. Lam, Repka, and Guyton[356] treated 47 children younger than age 8 who had esotropic amblyopia. Of these patients, 26 had their amblyopia fully treated before surgery and 21 underwent extraocular muscle surgery before completing the amblyopia therapy. Some patients required up to 5 years for reversal of their amblyopia. Interestingly, Lam, Repka, and Guyton[356] found no significant difference in the achieving of successful motor or sensory outcome, whether the amblyopia was fully or only partly treated before surgery. Motor success was defined as a posttreatment strabismic angle of 8 PD or less, and sensory success was the presence of any stereopsis with the Randot or Titmus stereotests.

 CLINICAL PEARL

Treatment of the amblyopia should be completed before treatment of the strabismus.

Treating the strabismus before treating the amblyopia has some disadvantages. The parents may gain a false sense of security after the eyes are straightened and may not continue with the amblyopia treatment after the strabismus has been treated. We occasionally see this following the treatment of accommodative esotropia. Furthermore, when correcting the strabismus before the amblyopia the fixation preference in younger children with residual small-angle strabismus will be difficult to judge, and significant amblyopia may be missed. Strabismus treatment should probably not be delayed any longer when the amblyopia has not improved following 4 months of treatment.

As mentioned earlier, patients with strabismic amblyopia and latent nystagmus are best treated with penalization rather than occlusion. Penalization appears to attenuate the amplitude and velocity and to a lesser degree the frequency of the latent nystagmus.[357] If this is not effective, occlusion therapy is given. Despite the possibility that occlusion therapy exacerbates the nystagmus, we, as well as others, have seen improvement of amblyopia in some cases.[358]

ANISOMETROPIC AMBLYOPIA

The protocol for treating amblyopia is illustrated in Fig. 2-30. Patients with anisometropic amblyopia present often as school-age children whose amblyopia has gone undetected because of lack of strabismus.[359,360] Refractive correction is always the first step; occlusion and orthoptics/vision therapy are added later, if necessary. We instruct the child to wear the glasses continuously for at least 1 month before we implement occlusion therapy. Unlike strabismic amblyopia, the refractive correction alone can be either partly or totally curative for some of these patients. Occlusion and orthoptics/vision therapy is not initiated until spontaneous visual acuity improvement with glasses ceases.

Predicting which patients will respond to glasses alone is difficult. Stereopsis is not a good indicator because many patients with anisometropic amblyopia possess high-grade stereoacuity even before treatment. Patients with smaller degrees of anisometropia (less than 2 D) may be more likely to improve with only the refractive correction.[270] Fusion of the Worth four dot test at distance, the presence of some astigmatism at a corresponding axis in the other eye, and steady improvement in visual acuity at each office visit may also be characteristic of the patients who will improve with glasses alone.[271]

When prescribing occlusion therapy for patients with anisometropic amblyopia, part-time occlusion is frequently given. The exception is the child with anisometropia who has deep amblyopia (20/100 or worse). In these situations, we treat aggressively with constant, total direct occlusion. As with strabismic amblyopia, if no improvement occurs after 4 months of conscientious treatment and patient compliance, the effort can be abandoned. This is more likely in unilateral high myopia associated with extensive myelinated nerve fibers.[50-54]

After reversing the amblyopia, some loss of visual acuity gain may occur in as many as 24% to 44% of all anisometropic patients.[293,361] Orthoptics/vision therapy has been shown to prevent this loss.[360] Because moderate amounts of central suppression exist in anisometropic amblyopia, binocular antisuppression therapy, such as cheiroscopic tracing and bar reading, can be given. This forces the amblyopic eye to function in a more natural and cooperative situation and reinforces the normal binocular interactions required for a complete cure.[358] Recurrent amblyopia with anisometropia is usually attributed to the patient's failure to continue wearing the glasses.

ISOAMETROPIC AMBLYOPIA

Because only one amblyopiagenic mechanism is in play and abnormal binocular interaction is not a factor, occlusion therapy is not necessary. Full correction of the symmetric and bilateral ametropia with either glasses or contact lenses is usually sufficient. Within 4 to 6 weeks after wearing the glasses, visual acuity and the refractive error are reevaluated. Thereafter, follow-up to monitor visual acuity changes may occur every 3 to 6 months.

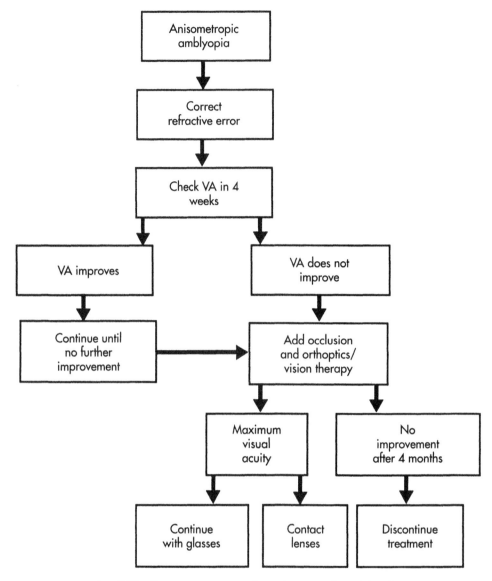

FIG. 2-30 Treatment sequence for anisometropic amblyopia.

Improvement of visual acuity may take a considerable amount of time, and some patients may never achieve normal visual acuity.[101] Maximum visual acuity improvement in isoametropic amblyopia usually occurs within 2 years following correction. Some patients' acuity improves rapidly after wearing the correction, after which the rate of improvement begins to level off but may continue for several years. With other patients a slow rate of improvement may continue for many years. Because many of these patients also have accommodative insufficiency, orthoptics/vision therapy to improve accommodative function can speed up the process.[100,101]

With hyperopic isoametropic amblyopia the likelihood of improving visual acuity to 20/30 or better is good. Fern[97] reported on 45 children (ages 7 months to 10 years 9 months) with 5 D or more isohyperopia.

Eighty-seven percent of the patients had amblyopia initially; 26% had amblyopia poorer than 20/40. After 1 year of wearing glasses, 43% had amblyopia and no patient had amblyopia poorer than 20/40. Patients corrected for more than 2 years exhibited significantly better aided visual acuity than those who were corrected for 1 year or less.

DEPRIVATION AMBLYOPIA

The intervention for children with congenital cataracts and other forms of deprivation amblyopia has changed dramatically during the last decade.[109] A total congenital cataract, with the classic "white pupil," can be routinely detected by anyone making a cursory examination of the child. With a total cataract or any visually significant cataract the condition is viewed as an emergency. Treatment includes surgery within the first weeks of life, short intervals between operations on the fellow eye in bilateral cases (48 hours or less), total bilateral occlusion between operations in bilateral cases, and immediate correction of the aphakia with extended-wear contact lenses.[126] Contact lens powers ranging from +20.00 D to +32.00 D are generally required.[362] The infant is prescribed greater plus power (2 to 3 D) than the measured refractive error to allow the child to participate in near-centered activities in the absence of accommodation. At approximately 12 to 18 months, because of the increased distance demands, bifocal glasses can be used over the contact lens. If the monocular cataract is felt to be consistent with development of good formed vision in the dilated state, long-term dilation and occlusion rather than lensectomy may be effective.[363]

Contact lens noncompliance is a particular problem for children with monocular aphakia; therefore intraocular lenses have been used instead of contact lenses.[364-367] There appears to be a greater reduction in the incidence of sensory strabismus with intraocular lenses than with contact lenses.[368] The concerns are long-term tolerance, biocompatibility of the intraocular lens material, safety, and efficacy. The large refractive error changes caused by rapid eye growth in infancy also discourages the use of intraocular lenses. Some have reported a mean decrease of 9 D in the contact lens correction of children during the first 4 years of life.[369] Because of the rapid change in refraction, especially during the first year or so, infants treated for unilateral congenital cataract are refracted frequently. The contact lens power for these infants is changed accordingly, to prevent inadequate optical correction, that may have an adverse influence on visual development and treatment outcome. Because most of the growth of the eyeball is complete by age 2, some surgeons use contact lenses initially and change to intraocular lenses beyond this age. [370,371]

With unilateral deprivation amblyopia the visual loss is potentially severe. Either constant, total direct occlusion on an alternate-day regimen or part-time occlusion (50% of the child's waking hours) is used to avoid inducing occlusion amblyopia. Most of these children will require maintenance therapy for several years to maintain the visual acuity gains achieved.

The earlier the treatment, the better the visual outcome. Whereas prompt treatment has provided results of 20/50 or better, delayed treatment is related to much poorer visual outcome. Robb, Mayer, and Moore[372] report on 12 infants with unilateral congenital cataracts. All infants had cataract extractions, aphakic contact lens correction, and occlusion of the unaffected eye by 6 months of age. At age 3½, five patients had 20/70 or better visual acuity, three patients had between 20/100 and 20/400 vision, and four patients had less than 20/400 in the aphakic eye. The

patients whose cataract surgery was done after 4 months of age had the poorest acuity outcomes. Difficulty in occlusion therapy and interruptions of contact lens wear also limited the development of better visual acuity.

Beller and others[373] report remarkably good results in eight patients with monocular congenital cataracts for which surgery, contact lenses, and occlusion were employed by 6 weeks of age. Five of the eight patients obtained visual acuities of 20/30 or better in the aphakic eye, and the other patients improved to 20/80 or better.

Drummond, Scott, and Keech[374] report a direct correlation for their patients between the median age at surgery and optical correction and the visual success. Those patients with 20/50 or better had a median age at surgery of only 17 days and a median age of optical correction and initiation of occlusion therapy of 24 days. Those patients with poorer results were progressively older. The oldest age at which visual acuity of 20/100 or better was achieved was noted when treatment began as late as 17 weeks of age.

High-grade stereopsis is rarely achieved in patients with monocular congenital cataracts.[375,376] However, operating within the first 24 hours of life and immediately applying a contact lens and judicious occlusion therapy allowed Gregg and Parks[377] to achieve 20/25 vision and 50 seconds of arc stereoacuity for one patient.

In the older child with deprivation amblyopia the prognosis for improvement in visual acuity is poor.

<u>CASE 6</u>
A 5-year-old girl presented with reduced vision in the right eye. From 3 months until 15 months of age, she had total right lid closure because of a plastic surgery procedure.

The examination showed visual acuity in the right eye of 10/200 and visual acuity in the left eye of 20/20. The patient was orthophoric. Cycloplegic refraction was +1.00 D in both eyes. Visuoscopy in the right eye showed eccentric fixation. Ophthalmoscopy was normal. Constant occlusion for the left eye and orthoptics/vision therapy for 1 year did not improve the acuity.[378]

CRITICAL PERIOD FOR TREATING AMBLYOPIA

All clinicians have an age beyond which they no longer treat amblyopia. Although the period for treating deprivation amblyopia is very restricted, this is not the case for strabismic and anisometropic amblyopia. The critical period for cure for these amblyopias lasts longer than the critical period for their creation. Numerous papers have shown that strabismic and anisometropic amblyopia can be treated in teenagers and even in some adults.[293,295,360,379-381] The rate and extent of improvement is less in older patients, however.

TABLE 2-5 **REGRESSION AND SUBSEQUENT RECOVERY OF VISUAL ACUITY FOR AMBLYOPIC PATIENTS**

Patient	Type	VA 1	VA 2	VA 3
1	S*	20/38	20/222	20/25
2	S	20/32	20/77	20/52
3	S	20/32	20/77	20/25
4	SA	20/30	20/90	20/60
5	SA	20/55	20/77	20/45
6	SA	20/40	20/100	20/40
7	S	20/32	20/45	20/32
8	A	20/30	20/60	20/30
9	S	20/45	20/137	20/32
10	SA	20/25	20/80	20/40
11	SA	20/25	20/80	20/40
12	A	20/20	20/38	20/25
13	S	20/50	20/200	20/48
14	S	20/30	20/68	20/30
15	S	20/52	20/104	20/68

Modified from Rutstein RP, Fuhr PD: Efficacy and stability of amblyopia therapy, *Optom Vis Sci,* 69:751, 1992.
*S, Strabismic amblyopia; A, Anisometropic amblyopia; SA, Strabismic/anisometropic amblyopia; VA 1, Visual acuity achieved with initial treatment; VA 2, Regression of visual acuity following termination of treatment; VA 3, Visual acuity achieved with second treatment.

 CLINICAL PEARL

Numerous papers have shown that strabismic and anisometropic amblyopia can be treated in teenagers and even in some adults.

Whether to treat amblyopia in the older patient presents an ethical and moral dilemma. For the young child it is the first step in establishing normal binocular vision. If visual acuity regresses after amblyopia treatment, there is also more likelihood of regaining at a later date most if not all of the visual acuity achieved with the earlier therapy (Table 2-5).

In the older patient the clinician must recognize that there are certain limitations with reduced vision in one eye, even when the fellow eye has 20/20 acuity. The better the visual acuity that is achieved in the amblyopic eye, the more potential obstacles are avoided in future employability. In an example case an adult patient lost his job in a local factory. He had been hired as a truck driver, pending the results of his eye examination. The truck company's vision screening had shown reduced vision in the left eye, and the patient suspected that glasses would solve the problem. Much to his dismay, best corrected visual acuity in the left eye was only 20/100 because of amblyopia secondary to a microtropia. The trucking company refused to hire him, despite the 20/20 vision in his right eye.

The clinician must also understand the additional risks involved in treating the older patient with strabismic amblyopia. Therapy in these patients can cause diplopia because of its weakening effect on suppression. On the other hand, the older patient with untreated amblyopia must live an entire lifetime with the risk of suffering serious disability to the normal eye. Patients with amblyopia have a much greater chance of loss of vision in the nonamblyopic eye than the overall population has of becoming blind (1.7/1000 vs. 0.79/1000).[25] In cases of unilateral amblyopia, diseases usually affecting both eyes affect first the eye whose functional integrity is less impaired.[25] However, some adults with untreated amblyopia, when losing the vision in their good eye through accident or disease, spontaneously recover part of the visual capabilities of their amblyopic eye.[336,380-384] In one case report, for example, visual acuity in the amblyopic eye in a 72-year-old patient improved from 20/400 to 20/50 after suffering anterior ischemic optic neuropathy in the nonamblyopic eye.[385] Similar findings have been documented in adult patients with age-related cataracts.[386] Although reports are mostly anecdotal, the vision of the amblyopic eyes of as many as 20% of patients may improve spontaneously after loss of the good eye.[338] However, the improvement in visual acuity may take from months to years and is rarely total.

 CLINICAL PEARL

Some adults with untreated amblyopia, when losing the vision in their good eye through accident or disease, spontaneously recover part of the visual capabilities of their amblyopic eye.

For the older patient presenting with deep amblyopia (20/100 or poorer), our policy is that if treatment has been attempted in the past and we believe that it was performed adequately, we do not treat. When treatment has never been given, we may recommend it. However, because of the poor compliance at an older age, we rarely see significant improvement and counsel the patient that if the amblyopic eye is ever needed, there is some chance that its vision will improve.

REFERENCES

1. Hillis A, Flynn JT, Hawkins BS: The evading concept of amblyopia: a challenge to epidemiologists, *Am J Epidemiol* 118:192, 1983.
2. Keech RV, Kutschke PJ: Upper age limit for the development of amblyopia, *J Pediatr Ophthalmol Strab* 32:89, 1995.
3. Kushner BJ: Functional amblyopia: a purely practical pediatric patching protocol. In Reinecke RD, editor: *Ophthalmology annual,* New York, 1988, Raven.
4. Dell W: The epidemiology of amblyopia. In Rutstein RP, editor: *Problems in optometry,* Philadelphia, 1991, JB Lippincott.
5. von Noorden GK: Amblyopia: a multidisciplinary approach, *Invest Opththalmol Vis Sci* 26:1704, 1985.

6. Srebo R: Fixation of normal and amblyopic eyes, *Arch Ophthalmol* 101:214, 1983.

7. Stark L, Ciuffreda KJ, Kenyon RV: Abnormal eye movements in strabismus and amblyopia. In Lennerstrad G, Zee D, Keller EL, editors: *Functional basis of ocular motility disorders,* New York, 1982, Pergamon.

8. von Noorden GK, Mackensen G: Pursuit movements of normal and amblyopic eyes: an electro-ophthalmographic study. II. Pursuit movements in amblyopic patients, *Am J Ophthalmol* 53:477, 1962.

9. Abraham SV: Accommodation in the amblyopic eye, *Am J Ophthalmol* 52:197, 1961.

10. Levi DM, Harwerth RS: Psychophysical mechanisms in humans with amblyopia, *Am J Optom Physiol Opt* 59:936, 1982.

11. Bedell HE, Flom MC: Normal and abnormal space perception, *Am J Optom Physiol Opt* 60:426, 1983.

12. Schor C, Levi D: Disturbances of small field horizontal and vertical optokinetic nystagmus in amblyopia, *Invest Ophthalmol Vis Sci* 19:668, 1980.

13. Flom MC, Bedell HE: Identifying amblyopia using associated conditions, acuity, and nonacuity factors, *Am J Optom Physiol Opt* 62:153, 1985.

14. Vinding T and others: Prevalence of amblyopia in old people without previous screening and treatment. An evaluation of the present prophylactic procedures among children in Denmark, *Acta Ophthalmol* 69:796, 1991.

15. Thompson JR and others: The incidence and prevalence of amblyopia detected in childhood, *Public Health* 105:455, 1991.

16. Casten J: The significance of prematurity on the eye, with reference to retrolental fibroplasia, *Acta Ophthalmol* 44(suppl):19, 1955.

17. Kitchen WH and others: A longitudinal study of very low birth weight infants. II. Results of controlled trial of intensive care and incidence of handicaps, *Dev Med Child Neurol* 21:582, 1979.

18. Kushner BJ: Strabismus and amblyopia associated with regressed retinopathy of prematurity, *Arch Ophthalmol* 100:256, 1982.

19. Pigassou-Albouy R, Fleming A: Amblyopia and strabismus in patients with cerebral palsy, *Ann Ophthalmol* 7:382, 1975.

20. Breaky AS: Ocular findings in cerebral palsy, *Arch Ophthalmol* 53:852, 1955.

21. Tuppuraninen K: Ocular findings among mentally retarded children in Finland, *Acta Ophthalmol (Copenh)* 61:634, 1983.

22. Rantakallio P, Krause V, Krause K: The use of the ophthalmological services during the preschool age, ocular findings and family background, *J Pediatr Ophthalmol Strab* 15:253, 1978.

23. Miller M, Israel J, Cuttone J: Fetal alcohol syndrome, *J Pediatr Ophthalmol Strab* 18:6, 1981.

24. National Eye Institute: *Visual acuity impairment survey pilot study,* Bethesda, Md, 1984, The Institutute.

25. Tommila V, Tarkkanen A: Incidence of loss of vision in the healthy eye in amblyopia, *Br J Ophthalmol* 65:575, 1981.

26. Schapero M: *Amblyopia,* Philadelphia, Pa, 1971, Chilton.

27. London R, Silver JL: Diagnosis of amblyopia: emphasis on nonacuity factors. In Rutstein RP, editor: *Problems in optometry,* Philadelphia, 1991, JB Lippincott.

28. Primo SA: Alcohol amblyopia, *J Am Optom Assoc* 59:392, 1988.

29. Cullom ME and others: Leber's heredity optic neuropathy masquerading as tobacco-alcohol amblyopia, *Arch Ophthalmol* 111:1482, 1993.

30. Rizzo JF: Adenosine: triphosphate deficiency a genre of optic neuropathy, *Neurology* 45:11, 1995.

31. Smiddy WE, Green WR: Nutritional amblyopia: a histopathological study with retrospective clinical correlation, *Graefes Arch Clin Exp Ophthalmol* 225:321, 1987.

32. Kellen RI, Schrank B, Burde RM: Yellow forelock: a new neuro-ophthalmological sign, *Br J Ophthalmol* 74:509, 1990.

33. Krumsiek J, Kruger C, Patzoid U: Tobacco-alcohol amblyopia: neuro-ophthalmological findings and clinical course, *Acta Neurol Scand* 72:180, 1985.

34. Iansek R, Edge CJ: Nutritional amblyopia in a patient with Crohn's disease, *J Neurol Neurosurg Psychiatry* 48:1307, 1985.

35. Rizzo JF, Lessell S: Tobacco amblyopia, *Am J Ophthalmol* 116:84, 1993.

36. Kermode AG and others: Tobacco-alcohol amblyopia: magnetic resonance image findings, *J Neurol Neurosurg Psychiatry* 52:1447, 1989.

37. Fields CR, Ozer G: Toxic amblyopia: literature review and case report, *South J Optom* 13:8, 1995.

38. Carrol FD: Nutritional amblyopia, *Arch Ophthalmol* 76:406, 1966.

39. Samples JR, Younge BR: Tobacco: alcohol amblyopia, *J Clin Neuro Ophthalmol* 1:213, 1981.

40. Quigley HA, Addicks EM, Green WR: Optic nerve damage in glaucoma. III. Quantitative correlation of nerve fiber layer loss and visual field defects in glaucoma, ischemic neuropathy, papilledema, and toxic neuropathy, *Arch Ophthalmol* 100:135, 1982.

41. Smilkstein MJ, Julig KW, Rumack RH: Acute toxic blindness: unrecognized quinine poisoning, *Ann Emerg Med* 16:98, 1987.

42. Moloney JB, Hillery M, Fenton M: Two-year electrophysiology follow-up in quinine amblyopia: a case report, *Acta Ophthalmol* 65:731, 1987.

43. Dyson EH, Proudfoot AT, Bateman DN: Quinine amblyopia: is current management appropriate? *Clin Toxicol* 23:571, 1986.

44. Boland ME and others: Complications of quinine poisoning, *Lancet* 1:384, 1985.

45. Brody SL, Slovis CM, Wrenn KD: Cocaine-related medical problems: consecutive series of 233 patients, *Am J Emerg Med* 88:352, 1990.

46. Hoffman RS, Reimer BI: "Crack" cocaine-induced bilateral amblyopia, *Am J Emerg Med* 11:35, 1993.

47. Enoch JM: The current status of receptor amblyopia, *Doc Ophthalmol* 23:130, 1967.

48. Henderson G, Clark J: "Shades of grey": a case study of achromatopsia, *Br Orthopt J* 52:16, 1995.

49. Romano PE: The cause of organic amblyopia in high myopia, *Ophthalmology* 95:288, 1988 (letter).

50. Ellis GS, Frey T, Gouterman RZ: Myelinated nerve fibers, axial myopia, refractory amblyopia: an organic disease, *J Pediatr Ophthalmol Strab* 24:111, 1987.

51. Ronen E, Biedner ER, Yassur Y: Anisometropic exotropic amblyopia associated with unilateral peripapillary myelinated nerve fibers, *Br Orthopt J* 49:46, 1992.

52. Hittner HM, Antoszyk JH: Unilateral peripapillary myelinated nerve fibers with myopia and/or amblyopia, *Arch Ophthalmol* 105:943, 1987.

53. Summers CG, Romig L, Lavoie JD: Unexpected good results after therapy for anisometropic amblyopia associated with unilateral peripapillary myelinated nerve fibers, *J Pediatr Ophthalmol Strab* 28:134, 1991.

54. Buys Y, Enzenauer R, Crawford JS: Myelinated nerve fibers and refractory amblyopia: a case report, *Ann Ophthalmol* 25:353, 1993.

55. Enoch JM: Amblyopia and the Stiles-Crawford effect, *Am J Optom* 34:298, 1957.

56. Green DG: Visual resolution when light enters the eye through different parts of the pupil, *J Physiol (London)* 190:583, 1967.

57. Yasuna ER: Hysterical amblyopia: its differentiation from malingering, *Am J Ophthalmol* 29:570, 1946.

58. Kathol RG and others: Functional visual loss: follow-up of 42 cases, *Arch Ophthalmol* 101:729, 1983.

59. Friesen H, Mann WA: Follow-up study of hysterical amblyopia, *Am J Ophthalmol* 62:1106, 1966.

60. Sletterberg O, Bertelsen T, Hovding G: The prognosis of patients with hysterical visual impairment, *Acta Ophthalmol* 67:159, 1989.

61. Miller BW: A review of practical tests for ocular malingering and hysteria, *Surv Ophthalmol* 17:241, 1973.

62. Kramer KK, LaPiana FG, Appleton B: Ocular malingering and hysteria: diagnosis and management, *Surv Ophthalmol* 24:89, 1979.

63. Hoffman DJ, Wilson R: Functional vision loss, *J Am Optom Assoc* 65:835, 1994.

64. Streff JW: Preliminary observations on a nonmalingering syndrome, *Optom Wkly* p 536, 1962.

65. Erickson GB, Griffin JR, Kurihara JI: Streff syndrome: a literature review, *J Optom Vis Dev* 25:64, 1994.

66. Behrman J, Levy R: Neurophysiological studies on patients with hysterical disturbances of vision, *J Psychosom Res* 14:187, 1970.

67. Rada RT and others: Visual conversion reaction in children. II. Follow-up. *Psychosomatics* 14:271, 1973.

68. Van Balen ATGM, Slyper FEM: Psychogenic amblyopia in children, *J Pediatr Ophthalmol Strab* 15:164, 1978.

69. Barsoum-Homsy M, Chevrette L: Incidence and prognosis of childhood glaucoma: a study of 63 cases, *Ophthalmology* 93:1323, 1986.

70. Kushner BJ: Successful treatment of functional amblyopia with juvenile glaucoma, *Graefes Arch Clin Exp Ophthalmol* 226:150, 1988.

71. Kushner BJ: Functional amblyopia associated with abnormalities of the optic nerve, *Arch Ophthalmol* 102:683, 1984.

72. Kushner JB: Functional amblyopia associated with organic ocular disease, *Am J Ophthalmol* 91:39, 1981.

73. Bradford GM, Kutschke PJ, Scott WJ: Results of amblyopia therapy in eyes with unilateral structural abnormalities, *Ophthalmology* 99:1616, 1992.

74. von Noorden GK, Frank JW: Relationship between amblyopia and the angle of strabismus, *Am Orthopt J* 26:31, 1976.

75. Smith K, Kaban TJ, Orton R: Incidence of amblyopia in intermittent exotropia, *Am Orthopt J* 45:90, 1995.

76. Flynn JT, Cassady JC: Current trends in amblyopia therapy, *Ophthalmology* 85:428, 1978.

77. Fahle M: Naso-temporal asymmetry of binocular inhibition, *Invest Ophthalmol Vis Sci* 28:1016, 1987.

78. Ellis FD, Helveston EM: Superior oblique palsy: diagnosis and classification, *Int Ophthalmol Clinic* 16:127, 1976.

79. Rutstein RP: Duane's retraction syndrome, *J Am Optom Assoc* 63:419, 1992.

80. Ikeda H, Wright MJ: A possible neurophysiological basis for amblyopia, *Br Orthopt J* 32:2, 1975.

81. Ikeda H, Wright MJ: Is amblyopia due to inappropriate stimulation of the "sustained" pathways during development? *Br J Ophthalmol* 58:165, 1971.

82. Guillery RW, Stelzner DJ: The differential effect of unilateral lid closure upon the monocular and binocular segments of the dorsal lateral geniculate nucleus of the cat, *J Comp Neurol* 139:413, 1970.

83. von Noorden GK, Crawford MLJ, Middleditch PR: The effects of monocular visual deprivation: disuse or binocular interaction? *Brain Res* 111:277, 1976.

84. Ciuffreda KJ, Levi DM, Selenow A: *Amblyopia: basic and clinical aspects,* Boston, 1991, Butterworth-Heinemann.

85. Chavasse B: *Worth's squint,* ed 7, Philadelphia, 1939, Blakiston & Son.

86. Dobson V, Teller DY: Visual acuity in human infants: a review and comparison of behavioral and electrophysiological studies, *Vision Res* 18:1469, 1978.

87. Hubel DH, Wiesel TN: Binocular interaction in striate cortex of kittens reared with artificial squint, *J Neurophysiol* 28:1041, 1965.

88. Woodruff G and others: The presentation of children with amblyopia, *Eye* 8:623, 1994.

89. Helveston EM: The incidence of amblyopia exanopsia in young adult males in Minnesota in 1962-1963, *Am J Ophthalmol* 60:75, 1965.

90. Hardman LSJ and others: Microtropia versus bifoveal fixation in anisometropic amblyopia, *Eye* 5:576, 1991.

91. France TD: Amblyopia. In Isenberg SJ, editor: *The eye in infancy,* Chicago, 1989, Mosby.

92. Helveston EM: The relationship between the degree of anisometropia and the depth of amblyopia, *Am J Ophthalmol* 62:757, 1966.

93. Malik SRK, Gupta AK, Choudry S: Anisometropia: its relation to amblyopia and eccentric fixation, *Br J Ophthalmol* 52:773, 1968.

94. Sen DK: Anisometropic amblyopia, *J Pediatr Ophthalmol Strab* 17:180, 1980.

95. Townshend AM, Holmes JM, Evans LS: Depth of anisometropic amblyopia and difference in refraction, *Am J Ophthalmol* 116:431, 1993.

96. Kutschke PJ, Scott WE, Keech RV: Depth of anisometropic amblyopia and difference in refraction, *Am J Ophthalmol* 117:681, 1994 (letter).

97. Fern KD: Visual acuity outcome in isometropic hyperopia, *Optom Vis Sci* 66:649, 1989.

98. Ingram RM and others: Prediction of amblyopia and squint by means of refraction at age 1 year, *Br J Ophthalmol* 70:12, 1986.

99. Werner DB, Scott WE: Amblyopia case reports: bilateral hypermetropic ametropic amblyopia, *J Pediatr Ophthalmol Strab* 22:203, 1985.

100. Friedman Z, Neumann E, Abel-Peleg B: Outcome of treatment of marked ametropia without strabismus following screening and diagnosis before the age of three, *J Pediatr Ophthalmol Strab* 22:54, 1985.

101. Schoenleber DB, Crouch ER: Bilateral hypermetropic amblyopia, *J Pediatr Ophthalmol Strabismus* 24:75, 1987.

102. von Noorden GK, Avilla CW: Accommodative convergence in hypermetropia, *Am J Ophthalmol* 110:287, 1990.

103. Mitchell DE and others: Meridional amblyopia: evidence of modification of the visual system by early visual experience, *Vision Res* 13:535, 1973.

104. Freeman RD: Contrast sensitivity in meridional amblyopia, *Invest Ophthalmol* 14:78, 1975.

105. Charman WN, Voisin L: Astigmatism, accommodation, the oblique effect, and meridional amblyopia, *Ophthalmic Physiol Opt* 13:73, 1993.

106. Mohinda I and others: Astigmatism in infants, *Science* 202:329, 1978.

107. Gwiazda J and others: Infant astigmatism and meridional amblyopia, *Vision Res* 25:1269, 1985.

108. Garzia RP, Nicholson SB: Deprivation amblyopia. In Rutstein RP, editor: *Problems in optometry,* Philadelphia, 1991, JB Lippincott.

109. Scott WE and others: Management and visual acuity results of monocular congenital cataracts and persistent hyperplastic primary vitreous, *Aust N Z J Ophthalmol* 17:143, 1989.

110. Anderson RL, Baumgartner SA: Amblyopia in ptosis, *Arch Ophthalmol* 98:1068, 1980.

111. Harrad RA, Graham CM, Collin JRO: Amblyopia and strabismus in congenital ptosis, *Eye* 2:625, 1988.

112. Schanzlin DI, Goldberg DB, Brown SI: Transplantation of congenitally opaque corneas, *Ophthalmology* 97:1253, 1980.

113. Levi DM: Occlusion amblyopia, *Am J Optom Phys Opt* 53:16, 1976.

114. Simon JW, Parks MM, Price EL: Severe visual loss resulting from occlusion therapy, *J Pediatr Ophthalmol Strab* 24:244, 1987.

115. von Noorden GK: Amblyopia caused by unilateral atropinization, *Ophthalmology* 88:131, 1981.

116. North RV, Kelly ME: Atropine occlusion in the treatment of strabismic amblyopia and its effect upon the non-amblyopic eye, *Ophthalmicl Physiol Opt* 11:113, 1991.

117. Flom MC, Neumaier RW: Prevalence of amblyopia, *Public Health Rep* 81:329, 1966.

118. Fraser GR, Friedman AL: *The causes of blindness in childhood: a study of 776 children with severe visual handicaps,* Baltimore, 1967, Johns Hopkins.

119. Francois J: *Congenital cataracts,* Springfield, Ill, 1965, Charles C. Thomas

120. Bouzas AG: Anterior polar congenital cataract and corneal astigmatism, *J Pediatr Ophthalmol Strab* 29:210, 1992.

121. Parks MM: Visual results in aphakic children, *Am J Ophthalmol* 94:441, 1982.

122. Nelson LB, Ullman S: Congenital and developmental cataracts. In Tasman W, Jaeger EA, editors: *Duane's clinical ophthalmology,* vol 1, Philadelphia, 1989, JB Lippincott.

123. Urema Y, Katsumi O: Form-vision deprivation amblyopia and strabismic amblyopia, *Graefes Arch Clin Exp Ophthalmol* 226:193, 1988.

124. Wright KW, Christensen LE, Noguchi BA: Results of late surgery for presumed congenital cataracts, *Am J Ophthalmol* 114:409, 1992.

125. Catalano RA and others: Preferential looking as a guide for amblyopia in monocular infantile cataracts, *J Pediatr Ophthalmol Strab* 24:56, 1987.

126. Kushner BJ: Visual results after surgery for monocular juvenile cataracts of undetermined onset, *Am J Ophthalmol* 102:468, 1986.

127. Awaya S, Sugawara M, Miyake S: Observations in patients with occlusion amblyopia: results of treatment, *Trans Ophthalmol Soc U K* 99:447, 1979.

128. Assaf AA: The sensitive period: transfer of fixation for strabismic amblyopia, *Br J Ophthalmol* 66:64, 1982.

129. von Norden GK: New clinical aspects of stimulus deprivation amblyopia, *Am J Ophthalmol* 92:416, 1981.

130. Thomas J, Mohindra I, Held R: Strabismic amblyopia in infants, *Am J Optom Physiol Opt* 56:197, 1979.

131. von Noorden GK: Idiopathic amblyopia, *Am J Ophthalmol* 100:214, 1985.

132. Firth AY, Davis H: Idiopathic amblyopia: the role of anisometropia in etiology—a case report, *Binoc Vis Eye Muscle Surg* 9:129, 1994.

133. Cantolino SJ, von Noorden GK: Heredity in microtropia, *Arch Ophthalmol* 81:753, 1969.

134. Zipf RF: Binocular fixation pattern, *Arch Ophthalmol* 94:401, 1976.

135. Wright KW and others: Reliability of fixation preference in diagnosing amblyopia, *Arch Ophthalmol* 104:549, 1986.

136. Wright KW, Walonker F, Edelman PM: 10-diopter fixation test for amblyopia, *Arch Ophthalmol* 99:1242, 1981.

137. Kiorpes L, Boothe RG: The time course for the development of strabismic amblyopia in infant monkeys, *Invest Ophthalmol Vis Sci* 19:841, 1980.

138. Kiorpes L, Boothe RG, Carlson MR: Acuity development in surgically strabismic monkeys, *Invest Ophthalmol Vis Sci* 25(suppl):216, 1984.

139. Thomas J, Mohindra I: Amblyopia in esotropic infants, *Invest Ophthalmol Vis Sci* 20(suppl):201, 1979.

140. Jacobson SG, Mohindra I, Held R: Age of onset of amblyopia in infants with esotropia, *Doc Ophthalmol Proc Ser* 30:210, 1981.

141. Birch EE, Steger DR: Monocular acuity and stereopsis in infantile esotropia, *Invest Ophalmol Vis Sci* 26:1624, 1985.

142. Simon JW and others: The time course of development of amblyopia in human infants as detected by preferential looking and fixation assessment, *Invest Ophthalmol Vis Sci* 27:2, 1986.

143. Calcutt C: Is fixation preference assessment an effective method of detecting strabismic amblyopia? *Br Orthopt J* 52:29, 1995.

144. Marsh-Tootle WL: Clinical methods of testing visual acuity in amblyopia. In Rutstein RP, editor: *Problems in optometry,* Philadelphia, 1991, JB Lippincott.

145. Mayer DL, Fulton AB, Hansen RM: Preferential looking acuity obtained with a staircase procedure in pediatric patients, *Invest Ophthalmol Vis Sci* 23:538, 1982.

146. Birch EE, Stager DR: Prevalence of good visual acuity following surgery for congenital unilateral cataract, *Arch Ophthalmol* 106:40, 1988.

147. Catalano RA and others: Preferential looking as a guide for amblyopia therapy in monocular infantile cataracts, *J Pediatr Ophthalmol Strab* 24:56, 1987.

148. Birch EE, Stager DR, Wright WW: Grating acuity development after early surgery for congenital unilateral cataract, *Arch Ophthalmol* 104:1783, 1986.

149. Mayer DL, Moore B, Robb RM: Assessment of vision and amblyopia by preferential looking tests after early surgery for unilateral congenital cataracts, *J Pediatr Ophthalmol Strab* 26:61, 1989.

150. Stager DR, Birch EE: Preferential looking acuity and stereopsis in infantile esotropia, *J Pediatr Ophthalmol Strab* 23:160, 1986.

151. Ellis GS and others: Teller acuity card versus clinical judgment in the diagnosis of amblyopia with strabismus, *Ophthalmology* 95:788, 1988.

152. Brovarone FV and others: Preferential looking techniques yield important information in strabismic follow-up, *Doc Ophthalmol* 83:307, 1993.

153. Dobson V, Sebris SL: Longitudinal study of acuity and stereopsis development in infants with or at risk of esotropia, *Invest Ophthalmol Vis Sci* 30:1146, 1989.

154. Kushner BJ, Lucchese NJ, Morton GV: Grating visual acuity with Teller cards compared with Snellen visual acuity in literate patients, *Arch Ophthalmol* 113:485, 1995.

155. Friendly DS, Jaafar MS, Morillo DL: A comparative study of grating and recognition visual acuity testing in children with anisometropia without strabismus, *Am J Ophthalmol* 110:293, 1990.

156. Mandava N, Simon JW, Jenkins PL: Preferential looking and recognition acuities in clinical amblyopia, *J Pediatr Ophthalmol Strab* 28:323, 1991.

157. Reinecke RD: Objective and subjective testing of visual acuity in amblyopic patients, *Am Orthopt J* 9:93, 1959.

158. Enoch JM, Rabinowicz IM: Early surgery and visual correction of a infant born with unilateral lens opacity, *Doc Ophthalmol* 41:371, 1976.

159. Westfall CA, Shute RH: OKN asymmetries in orthoptic patients: contributing factors and effect of treatment, *Behav Brain Res* 49:77, 1992.

160. London R: Optokinetic nystagmus: a review of pathways, techniques, and selected diagnostic applications, *J Am Optom Assoc* 53:791, 1982.

161. Skarf B and others: A new VEP system for studying binocular vision in human infants, *J Pediatr Ophthalmol Strabismus* 30:237, 1993.

162. Davis ET, Bass SJ, Sherman J: Flash visual evoked potential (VEP) in amblyopia and optic nerve disease, *Optom Vis Sci* 72:612, 1995.

163. Wright KW, Eriksen KJ, Shors TJ: Detection of amblyopia with P-VEP during chloral hydrate sedation, *J Pediatr Ophthalmol Strab* 24:107, 1987.

164. Friendly DS and others: Pattern-reversal visual evoked potentials in the diagnosis of amblyopia in children, *Am J Ophthalmol* 102:329, 1986.

165. Henc-Petrinovic L and others: Prognostic value of visual evoked responses in childhood amblyopia, *Eur J Ophthalmol* 3:114, 1993.

166. Fern KD, Manny RE: Visual acuity of the preschool child: a review, *Am J Optom Physiol Opt* 63:319, 1986.

167. Richman JE, Petito GT, Cron MT: Broken wheel acuity test: a new and valid test for preschool and exceptional children, *J Am Optom Assoc* 55:561, 1984.

168. Giaschi DE and others: Crowding and contrast in amblyopia, *Optom Vis Sci* 70:192, 1993.

169. Stager DR, Everett ME, Birch EE: Comparison of crowding bar and linear optotype acuity in amblyopia, *Am Orthopt J* 40:51, 1990.

170. Bailey IL, Lovie JE: New design principles for visual acuity letter charts, *Am J Optom Physiol Opt* 53:740, 1976.

171. Lovie-Kitchin JE: Validity and reliability of visual acuity measurements, *Ophthalmic Physiol Opt* 9:458, 1989.

172. Flom MC, Weymouth FW, Kahneman D: Visual resolution and contour interaction, *J Opt Soc Am* 53:1026, 1963.

173. Davidson DW, Eskridge JB: Reliability of visual acuity measures of amblyopic eyes, *Am J Optom Physiol Opt* 54:756, 1977.

174. Griffin JR: Visual acuity testing in amblyopia using Flom psychometric analysis, *Optom Mthly* 73:460, 1973.

175. von Noorden GK, Burian HM: Visual acuity in normal and amblyopic patients under reduced illumination. I. Behavior of visual acuity with and without neutral density filter, *Arch Ophthalmol* 61:533, 1959.

176. Caloroso E, Flom MC: Influence of luminance on visual acuity in amblyopia, *Am J Optom* 46:189, 1969.

177. Duckman R: Using photorefraction to evaluate refractive error, ocular alignment, and accommodation in infants, toddlers, and multiply handicapped children. In Scheiman MM, editor: *Problems in optometry*, Philadelphia, 1990, JB Lippincott.

178. Molteno AC and others: Reliability of the Otago photoscreener: a study of a thousand cases, *Aust N Z J Ophthalmol* 21:257, 1993.

179. Angi MR and others: Results of photorefraction screening for amblyogenic defects in children aged 20 months, *Behav Brain Res* 49:91, 1992.

180. Freedman HL, Preston KL: Polaroid photoscreening for amblyogenic factors: an improved methodology, *Ophthalmology* 99:1785, 1992.

181. Dortmans RJ, McKenny BS, Gole GA: Eccentric photorefraction: improving the predictive value and yield in detection of refractive errors, *Aust N Z J Ophthalmol* 17:417, 1989.

182. Hope C and others: Community photoscreening of six-to-nine-month-old infants for amblyopiogenic risk factors, *Aust N Z J Ophthalmol* 22:193, 1994.

183. Bischoff P, Althaus K: How exact is photorefraction in infants when compared to retinoscopy and how much do the values change within a period of six months? *Klin Monatsbl Augenheilkd* 205:128, 1994.

184. Lepard CW: Comparative changes in the error of refraction between fixing and amblyopic eyes during growth and development, *Am J Ophthalmol* 80:485, 1975.

185. Nastri G and others: The evolution of refraction in the fixing and the amblyopic eye, *Doc Ophthalmol* 56:265, 1984.

186. Leffertstra LJ: A comparative study of the difference in the evolution of refraction in the two eyes in patients with convergent strabismus, *Klin Monatsbl Augenheilkd* 170:74, 1977.

187. von Noorden GK: *Binocular vision and ocular motility: theory and management of strabismus*, ed 5, St Louis, 1996, Mosby.

188. Sherman A: Eccentric fixation in functional amblyopic patients, *J Am Optom Assoc* 41:174, 1970.

189. Hermann JS, Priestly BS: Bifoveal instability: the relationship to amblyopia, *Am J Ophthalmol* 60:452, 1965.

190. Kirschen DG, Rosenbaum AL, Weiss S: Strabismus measurement errors on (prism) alternate cover test in amblyopes with eccentric fixation, *Binoc Vis Eye Muscle Surg* 7:155, 1992.

191. Griffin JR: *Binocular anomalies: procedures for vision therapy*, ed 2, Chicago, 1982, Professional.

192. Gording EJ: A report on Haidinger brushes, *Am J Optom Arch Am Acad Optom* 27:604, 1950.

193. Brock F, Givner I: Fixation anomalies in amblyopia, *Arch Ophthalmol* 47:1465, 1952.

194. Jones R, Eskridge JB: The Hirschberg test: a re-evaluation, *Am J Optom Arch Am Acad Optom* 47:105, 1970.

195. Wick B, London R: The Hirschberg test: analysis from birth to age five, *J Am Optom Assoc* 51:1009, 1980, erratum 52:55, 1981.

196. Flom MC, Weymouth FW: Centricity of Maxwell's spot in strabismus and amblyopia, *Arch Ophthalmol* 66:260, 1961.

197. Flom MC: Personal communication. In: Schapero M, editor: *Amblyopia*, Philadelphia, Pa, 1971, Chilton.

198. Bangerter A: Uber Pleoptik, *Wiener Klin Wochenschr* 65:966, 1953.

199. Cüppers C: Moderne Schiebehandlung, *Klin Monatsbl Augenheilkd* 5:579, 1956.

200. Helveston EM, von Noorden GK: Microtropia: a newly defined entity, *Arch Ophthalmol* 78:272, 1968.

201. Burian HM: Occlusion amblyopia and the development of eccentric fixation in occluded eyes, *Am J Ophthalmol* 62:853, 1966.

202. Schor CM: A motor theory for monocular eccentric fixation of amblyopic eyes, *Am J Optom Physiol Opt* 55:183, 1978.

203. Otto J, Safra D: Methods and results of quantitative determination of accommodation in amblyopia and strabismus. In Moore S, Mein J, Stockbridge L, editors: *Orthoptics past, present, future*, New York, 1976, Stratton.

204. Okai K, Ishii M, Ishikawa S: A quasi-static study of accommodation in amblyopia, *Ophthalmic Physiol Opt* 6:287, 1986.

205. Hatsukawa Y, Otori T: A study of accommodation of amblyopic eye by simultaneous measurement of refraction of both eyes. In Campos E, editor: *Proceedings of the Fifth International Strabismological Association Congress*, Rome, 1986, ETA.

206. Wood ICJ, Tomlinson A: The accommodative response in amblyopia, *Am J Optom Physiol Opt* 52:243, 1975.

207. Kirschen DG, Kendall JH, Riesen KS: An evaluation of the accommodative response in amblyopic eyes, *Am J Optom Physiol Opt* 58:597, 1981.

208. Ciuffreda KJ and others: Static aspects of accommodation in human amblyopia, *Am J Optom Physiol Opt* 60:436, 1983.

209. Hokoda SC, Ciuffreda KJ: Measurement of accommodative amplitude in amblyopia, *Ophthalmic Physiol Opt* 2:205, 1982.

210. Selenow A, Ciuffreda KJ: Vision function recovery during orthoptic therapy in an exotropic amblyope with high unilateral myopia, *Am J Optom Physiol Opt* 60:659, 1983.

211. Hokoda SC, Ciuffreda KJ: Different rates and amounts of vision function recovery during orthoptic therapy in an older strabismic amblyope, *Ophthalmic Physiol Opt* 6:213, 1986.

212. Schor CM, Flom MC: Eye position control and visual acuity in strabismus amblyopia. In Lennerstrand G, Bach-y-rita P, editors: *Basic mechanisms of ocular motility and their clinical implications*, New York, 1975, Pergamon.

213. Schor CM, Hallmark W: Slow control of eye position in strabismic amblyopia, *Invest Ophthalmol Vis Sci* 17:577, 1978.

214. Ciuffreda KJ, Kenyon RV, Stark L: Increased drift in amblyopic eyes, *Br J Ophthalmol* 64:7, 1980.

215. Ciuffreda KJ, Kenyon RV, Stark L: Saccadic intrusions contributing to reading disability: a case report, *Am J Optom Physiol Opt* 60:242, 1983.

216. Ciuffreda KJ, Kenyon RV, Stark L: Fixational eye movements in amblyopia and strabismus, *J Am Optom Assoc* 50:1251, 1979.

217. Westheimer G, McKee SP: Visual acuity in the presence of retinal image motion, *J Opt Soc Am* 65:847, 1975.

218. Grovesnor T: The effects of duration and background luminance upon brightness discrimination of an amblyope, *Am J Optom Arch Am Acad Optom* 34:634, 1957.

219. Flynn JT: Spatial summation in amblyopia, *Arch Ophthalmol* 78:470, 1967.

220. Glover H, Bird S, Yap M: Performance of amblyopic children on printed contrast sensitivity charts, *Am J Optom Physiol Opt* 64:361, 1987.

221. Levi DM, Harwerth RS: Spatial-temporal interactions in anisometropic and strabismic amblyopia, *Invest Ophthalmol Vis Sci* 16:90, 1977.

222. Hess RF, Howell ER: The threshold contrast sensitivity function in strabismic amblyopia: evidence for a two-type classification, *Vision Res* 17:1049, 1977.

223. Levi DM: The Glenn A Fry Award Lecture: the "spatial grain" of the amblyopic visual system, *Am J Optom Physiol Opt* 65:767, 1985.

224. Higgens KE, Daugamann JG, Mansfield RSW: Amblyopic contrast sensitivity: insensitivity to unsteady fixation, *Invest Ophthalmol Vis Sci* 23:113, 1982.

225. Bloch DA, Wick B: Differences between strabismic and anisometropic amblyopia. Research findings and impact on management. In Rutstein RP, editor: *Problems in optometry*, Philadelphia, 1991, JB Lippincott.

226. Hess RF, Pointer JS: Differences in the neural basis of human amblyopias: the distribution of the anomaly across the visual field, *Vision Res* 25:1577, 1985.

227. Levi DM, Klein SA: The role of local contrast in the visual deficits of humans with naturally occurring amblyopia, *Neurosci Lett* 136:63, 1992.

228. Wali N and others: CSF interocular interactions in childhood amblyopia, *Optom Vis Sci* 68:81, 1991.

229. Gottlob I, Stangler-Zuschrott E: Effect of levodopa on contrast sensitivity and scotomas in human amblyopia, *Invest Ophthalmol Vis Sci* 31:776, 1990.

230. Abrahamsson M, Sjostrand J: Contrast sensitivity and acuity relationship in strabismic and anisometropic amblyopia, *Br J Ophthalmol* 72:44, 1988.

231. Koskela PU: Contrast sensitivity in amblyopia. II. Changes during pleoptic treatment, *Acta Ophthalmol* 64:563, 1986.

232. Tsuchiya S: Changes in the contrast sensitivity of an amblyopic eye after losing the other normal eye, *Tokai J Exp Clin Med* 11:145, 1986.

233. Koskela PU: Contrast sensitivity in amblyopia. I. Changes during CAM treatment, *Acta Ophthalmol* 64:344, 1986.

234. Koskela PU, Hyvarinen L: Contrast sensitivity in amblyopia. III. Effect of occlusion, *Acta Ophthalmol* 64:386, 1986.

235. Leguire LE, Rogers GL, Bremer DL: Amblyopia: the normal eye is not normal, *J Pediatr Ophthalmol Strab* 27:32, 1990.

236. Wiesel TN, Hubel DH: Single-cell responses in striate cortex of kittens deprived of vision in one eye, *J Neurophysiol* 26:1003, 1963.

237. Crawford MLJ, von Noorden GK: The effects of short-term experimental strabismus on the visual system in Macaca mulatta, *Invest Ophthalmol Vis Sci* 18:496, 1979.

238. von Noorden GK: Histological studies of the visual system in monkeys with experimental amblyopia, *Invest Ophthalmol Vis Sci* 12:727, 1973.

239. Headon MP, Powell TPS: Cellular changes in lateral geniculate nucleus of infant monkeys after suture of the eyelids, *J Anat* 16:135, 1973.

240. Enroth-Cugell C, Robson JG: The contrast sensitivity of retinal ganglion cells of the cat, *J Physiol (London)* 187:517, 1966.

241. Cleland BG, Dubin MW, Levick WR: Sustained and transient neurons in the cat's retina and lateral geniculate nucleus, *J Physiol (London)* 217:473, 1971.

242. Ikeda H: Is amblyopia a peripheral defect? *Trans Ophthalmol Soc U K* 99:347, 1979.

243. Navon SE, McKeown CA: Amblyopia, *Int Ophthalmol Clin* 32:35, 1992 (review).

244. Ikeda H, Tremain KE: Amblyopia resulting from penalization: neurophysiological studies of kittens reared with atropinization one or both eyes, *Br J Ophthalmol* 62:21, 1978.

245. Ikeda H, Tremain KE: Amblyopia occurs in retinal ganglion cells in cats reared with convergent squint without alternating fixation, *Exp Brain Res* 35:559, 1979.

246. Arden GB, Vaegan ?, Hogg CR: Pattern ERGs are abnormal in many amblyopes, *Trans Ophthalmol Soc U K* 100:453, 1980.

247. Gottlob I, Welge-Lussen L: Normal pattern electroretinograms in amblyopia, *Invest Ophthalmol Vis Sci* 28:187, 1987.

248. Williams C, Papakostopoulos D: Electro-oculographic abnormalities in amblyopia, *Br J Ophthalmol* 79:218, 1995.

249. Barbur JL, Hess RF, Pinney HD: Pupillary function in human amblyopia, *Ophthalmol Physiol Opt* 14:139, 1994.

250. Firth AY: Pupillary responses in amblyopia, *Br J Ophthalmol* 74:676, 1990.

251. Greenwald MJ, Folk ER: Afferent pupillary defects in amblyopia, *J Pediatr Ophthalmol Strab* 20:63, 1983.

252. Portnoy JZ and others: Pupillary defects in amblyopia, *Am J Ophthalmol* 96:609, 1983.

253. Feinberg I: Critical flicker frequency in amblyopia ex anopsia, *Am J Ophthalmol* 42:473, 1956.

254. Alpern M, Flitman DB, Joseph RH: Central fixed flicker thresholds in amblyopia, *Am J Ophthalmol* 49:1194, 1960.

255. Miles WP: Flicker fusion frequency in amblyopia ex anopsia, *Am J Ophthalmol* 32:225, 1949.

256. Francois J, Verriest G: La discrimination chromatique dans l'amblyopie strabique, *Doc Ophthalmol* 23:318, 1967.

257. Winn B and others: Amblyopia, accommodation, and colour, *Ophthalmol Physiol Opt* 7:365, 1987.

258. Bradley A and others: A comparison of color and luminance discrimination in amblyopia, *Invest Ophthalmol Vis Sci* 27:1404, 1986.

259. Mtanda AT and others: Evaluation of color vision, mesopic vision, visual evoked potentials, and lightness discrimination in adult amblyopes, *Doc Ophthalmol* 62:247,1986.

260. Wald G, Burian HM: The dissociation of form vision and light perception in strabismic amblyopia, *Am J Ophthalmol* 27:950, 1944.

261. von Noorden GK, Crawford MLJ, Middleditch PR: Effect of lid suture on retinal ganglion cells in Macaca mulatta, *Brain Res* 122:437, 1977.

262. Crawford MLJ: Visual deprivation syndrome, *Ophthalmology* 85:465, 1978.

263. Garey L, Blakemore C: Monocular deprivation: morphological effects on different classes of neurons in the lateral geniculate nucleus, *Science* 195:414, 1977.

264. von Noorden GK, Crawford MLJ: Morphological and physiological changes in the monkey visual system after short-term lid suture, *Invest Ophthalmol Vis Sci* 17:762, 1978.

265. von Noorden GK, Crawford MLJ, Levacy RA: The lateral geniculate nucleus in human anisometropic amblyopia, *Invest Ophthalmol Vis Sci* 24:788, 1983.

266. von Noorden GK, Crawford MLJ: The lateral geniculate nucleus in human strabismic amblyopia, *Invest Ophthalmol Vis Sci* 33:2729, 1992.

267. Hubel DH, Wiesel TN: Receptive fields binocular interaction and functional architecture in the cat's visual cortex, *J Physiol* 160:106, 1962.

268. Demer JL and others: Imaging of cerebral blood flow and metabolism in amblyopia by positron emission tomography, *Am J Ophthalmol* 105:337, 1988.

269. Demer JL: Positron emission tomographic studies of cortical function in human amblyopia, *Neurosci Biobehav Rev* 17:469,1993 (review).

270. Kivlin JD, Flynn JT: Therapy of anisometropic amblyopia, *J Pediatr Ophthalmol Strab* 18:47, 1981.

271. Clarke WN, Noel LP: Prognostic indicators for avoiding occlusion therapy in anisometropic amblyopia, *Am Orthopt J* 40:57, 1990.

272. Hopkisson B and others: Can retinoscopy be used to screen infants for amblyopia? A longitudinal study of refraction in the first year of life, *Eye* 6:607, 1992.

273. Mets M, Price RL: Contact lenses in the management of myopic anisometropic amblyopia, *Am J Ophthalmol* 91:484, 1981.

274. Levinson A, Ticho V: The use of contact lenses in children and infants, *Am J Optom* 49:59, 1972.

275. Cotter S: Conventional therapy for amblyopia. In Rutstein RP, editor: *Problems in optometry,* Philadelphia, 1991, JB Lippincott.

276. Moore B: Contact lens therapy for amblyopia. In Rutstein RP, editor: *Problems in optometry,* Philadelphia, 1991, JB Lippincott.

277. Winn B and others: Reduced aniseikonia in axial anisometropia with contact lens correction, *Ophthalmol Physiol Opt* 8:341, 1988.

278. Romano PE: An exception to Knapp's Law: unilateral axial high myopia, *Binoc Vis Eye Muscle Surg* 1:166, 1985.

279. von Noorden GK: *Binocular vision and ocular motility: theory and management of strabismus,* ed 5, St Louis, 1990, Mosby.

280. Fierreri G, Squeri CA: Occlusion by means of soft contact lenses for treatment of amblyopia, *Klin Monatsbl Augenheilkd* 169:362, 1976.

281. Blassman K, Neuhann T: Treatment of amblyopia with soft contact lenses, *Klin Monatsbl Augenheilkd* 172:766, 1978.

282. Tsubota K, Yamada M: Treatment of amblyopia by extended-wear occlusion soft contact lenses, *Ophthalmologica* 208:214, 1994.

283. Garzia RP: Efficacy of vision therapy in amblyopia: a literature review, *Am J Optom Physiol Opt* 64:393, 1987.

284. Ham O: Strabismic amblyopia: final results of occlusion treatment in 205 cases, *Binoc Vision* 1:195, 1985.

285. Catford GV: Amblyopic occlusion: the results of treatment, *Trans Ophthalmol Soc U K* 87:179, 1967.

286. Pope LG: Treatment of eccentric fixation without occlusion, *Br Orthopt J* 28:77, 1971.

287. Jenkins TC: Some aspects of amblyopia, *Ophthalmic Physiol Opt* 3:331, 1983.

288. Griffin JR: *Binocular anomalies: procedures for vision therapy,* ed 2, Chicago, 1982, Professional.

289. Swan KC: Esotropia following occlusion, *Arch Ophthalmol* 37:444, 1947.

290. Charney K, Morris JE: Decomposition of pre-existing esotropia during occlusion therapy, *Am Orthopt J* 34:83, 1984.

291. Pine L, Shippman S: The influence of occlusion therapy on esodeviations, *Am Orthopt J* 32:61, 1982.

292. Holbach H, von Noorden GK, Avilla GW: Changes in esotropia after occlusion therapy in patients with strabismic amblyopia, *J Pediatr Ophthalmol Strab* 28:6, 1991.

293. Rutstein RP, Fuhr PD: Efficacy and stability of amblyopia therapy, *Optom Vis Sci* 69:747, 1992.

294. Nucci P and others: Compliance in antiamblyopia occlusion therapy, *Acta Ophthalmol* 70:128, 1992.

295. Oliver M and others: Compliance and results of treatment of amblyopia in children more than 8 years old, *Am J Ophthalmol* 102:340, 1986.

296. Yang LLH, Lambert SR: Reappraisal of occlusion therapy for severe structural abnormalities of the optic disc and macula, *J Pediatr Ophthalmol Strab* 32:37, 1995.

297. Gregersen E, Rindziunski E: Conventional occlusion in the treatment of squint amblyopia, *Acta Ophthalmol (Kbh)* 43:462, 1965.

298. Sparrow JC, Flynn JT: Amblyopia: a long-term follow-up, *J Pediatr Ophthalmol Strab* 14:333, 1977.

299. Campos EC, Gulli R: Lack of alternation in patients treated for strabismic amblyopia, *Am J Ophthalmol* 99:63, 1985.

300. Tassinari JD: Binasal occlusion, *J Behav Optom* 1:16, 1990.

301. Sarniguet-Badoche J: Early medical treatment of strabismus before the age of 18 months. In Reinecke RD, editor: *Strabismus II,* New York, 1984, Grune and Stratton.

302. Vereecken E: Conservative treatment. In Evens L, editor: *Convergent strabismus,* Boston, 1982, W Junk.

303. Manor R: Use of special glasses in spasm of the near reflex, *Am Ophthalmol* 11:903, 1979.

304. Rutstein RP: Alternative treatment for amblyopia. In Rutstein RP, editor: *Problems in optometry,* Philadelphia, 1991, JB Lippincott.

305. Classe JG, Rutstein RP: Binocular vision anomalies: an emerging cause of malpractice claims, *J Am Optom Assoc* 66:305, 1995.

306. Wesson MD: Use of light intensity reduction treatment for amblyopia, *Am J Optom Physiol Opt* 60:112, 1983.

307. Cho MH, Norden LC: A cosmetic spectacle occluder lens, *South J Optom* 6:10, 1988.

308. Banks RV and others: A new treatment for amblyopia, *Br Orthopt J* 35:1, 1978.

309. Watson RG and others: Clinical assessment of a new treatment for amblyopia, *Trans Ophthalmol Soc U K* 93:201, 1978.

310. Daiziel CC: Amblyopia therapy by the Campbell-Hess technique, *Am J Optom Physiol Opt* 57:280, 1980.

311. Nyman KG and others: Controlled study comparing CAM treatment with occlusion therapy, *Br J Ophthalmol* 67:178, 1983.

312. Lennerstrand G, Samuelsson B: Amblyopia in 4-year-old children treated with grating stimulation and full-time occlusion: a comparative study, *Br J Ophthalmol* 67:181,1983.

313. Terrell A: Cambridge stimulator treatment for amblyopia: an evaluation of 80 consecutive cases treated by this method, *Aust J Ophthalmol* 9:121, 1981.

314. Schor C, Wick B: Rotation grating treatment of amblyopia with and without eccentric fixation, *J Am Optom Assoc* 54:545, 1983.

315. Duke-Elder S: *System of ophthalmology: ocular motility and strabismus,* vol 6, St Louis, 1973, Mosby.

316. von Noorden GK: Occlusion therapy in amblyopia with eccentric fixation, *Arch Ophthalmol* 73:776, 1965.

317. Urist MJ: Eccentric fixation amblyopia ex anopsia, *Arch Ophthalmol* 54:345, 1955.

318. Knapp P: Capobianco N: Use of miotics in esotropia, *Am Orthopt J* 6:40, 1956.

319. Cibis L: Penalization treatment of ARC and amblyopia, *Am Orthopt J* 25:79, 1975.

320. von Noorden GK, Milam JB: Penalization in the treatment of amblyopia, *Am J Ophthalmol* 88:511, 1979.

321. Gregerson E, Pontoppidan M, Ridziunski E: Optic and drug penalization and favoring in the treatment of squint amblyopia, *Acta Ophthalmol* 52:60, 1974.

322. von Noorden GK, Attiah F: Alternating penalization in the prevention of amblyopia recurrence, *Am J Ophthalmol* 102:473, 1986.

323. Repka MX and others: Determination of optical penalization by vectographic fixation reversal, *Ophthalmology* 92:1584, 1985.

324. Timmerman GJ: The results of penalization therapy, *Doc Ophthalmol* 42:385, 1977.

325. McKenney S, Beyers M: Aspects and results of penalization treatment, *Am Orthopt J* 25:85, 1975.

326. Ron A, Nawratzki I: Penalization treatment of amblyopic: a follow-up study of two years in older children, *J Pediatr Ophthalmol Strab* 19:137, 1982.

327. Repka MX, Ray JM: The efficacy of optical and pharmacological penalization, *Ophthalmology* 100:769, 1993.

328. Kubota N, Usui C: The development of occlusion amblyopia following atropine therapy for strabismic amblyopia, *Acta Soc Ophthalmol Jpn* 97:763, 1993.

329. Selenow A, Ciuffreda KJ: Vision recovery during orthoptic therapy in an adult esotropic amblyope, *J Am Optom Assoc* 57:132, 1986.

330. Bangerter A: *Amblyopiedbehandlung*, Aufl 2, Basel, 1955, Karger.

331. Girard LJ and others: Results of pleoptic treatment of suppression amblyopia, *Am Orthopt J* 12:12, 1962.

332. Nordman E: Results of pleoptic treatment, *Acta Ophthalmol Suppl* 114:1, 1972.

333. von Noorden GK, Lipsius RML: Experiences with pleoptics in 58 patients with strabismic amblyopia, *Am J Ophthalmol* 58:41, 1964.

334. Koskela PU, Mikkola T, Laatikainen L: Permanent results of pleoptic treatment, *Acta Ophthalmol* 69:39, 1991.

335. Sen DK: Results of treatment of anisohypermetropic amblyopia without strabismus, *Br J Ophthalmol* 66:680, 1982.

336. Sen DK: Results of treatment in amblyopia associated with unilateral high myopia without strabismus, *Br J Ophthalmol* 68:681, 1984.

337. Wanter BS: Pleoptic therapy in amblyopia, *Am Orthopt J* 30:77, 1980.

338. Vereecken EP, Brabant P: Prognosis for vision in amblyopia after the loss of the good eye, *Arch Ophthalmol* 102:220, 1984.

339. Colaroso E: After-image transfer: a therapeutic procedure for amblyopia, *J Am Optom Assoc* 49:65, 1972.

340. McCormick BJ: After-image transfer therapy in non-strabismic amblyopia, *Ophthalmic Optician* 18:641, 1976.

341. Jenkins TCA, Pickwell LD, Sheridan M: After-image transfer: evaluation of short-term treatmen, *Br J Physiol Opt* 33:33, 1979.

342. Halpern E, Yolton RL: Ophthalmic applications of biofeedback, *Am J Optom Physiol Opt* 63:985, 1986.

343. Schor C, Hallmark W: Slow control of eye position in strabismic amblyopia, *Invest Opthalmol Vis Sci* 17:577, 1978.

344. Kirschen DG, Flom MC: Visual acuity at different retinal loci of eccentrically fixating functional amblyopes, *Am J Optom Physiol Opt* 55:144, 1978.

345. Flom MC, Kirschen DG, Bedell HE: Control of unsteady eccentric fixating in amblyopic eyes by auditory feedback of eye position, *Invest Ophthalmol Vis Sci* 19:1371, 1980.

346. Kirschen DG: Biofeedback therapy for amblyopia. In Rutstein RP, editor: *Problems in optometry.* Philadelphia, 1991, JB Lippincott.

347. Cohen AH: Monocular fixation in a binocular field, *J Am Optom Assoc* 52:801, 1981.

348. Pickwell LD: The management of amblyopia without occlusion, *Br J Physiol Opt* 31:115, 1976.

349. Duffy FH and others: Bicuculline reversal of deprivation amblyopia in the cat, *Nature* 260:256, 1976.

350. Burchfiel JL, Duffy FH: Role of intracortical inhibition in deprivation amblyopia: reversal by microiontophoretic bicuculline, *Brain Res* 206:479, 1981.

351. Pettigrew JD, Kasamatsu T: Local perfusion of noradrenaline maintains cortical plasticity, *Nature* 271:761, 1978.

352. Gottlob I, Stangler-Zuschrott E: Effect of levodopa on human amblyopia: a cross-over double-masked study, *Invest Ophthalmol Vis Sci* 30(suppl):302, 1989 (ARVO abstract).

353. Leguire LE and others: Longitudinal study of levodopa/carbidopa for childhood amblyopia, *J Pediatr Ophthalmol Strab* 30:354, 1993.

354. Leguire LE and others: Levodopa/carbidopa treatment for amblyopia in older children, *J Pediatr Ophthalmol Strab* 32:143, 1995.

355. Campos EC and others: Effect of citicoline on visual acuity in amblyopia: preliminary results, *Graefes Arch Clin Exp Ophthalmol* 233:307, 1995.

356. Lam GC, Repka MX, Guyton DL: Timing of amblyopia therapy relative to strabismus surgery, *Ophthalmology* 100:1751, 1993.

357. Simonsz HJ: The effect of prolonged monocular occlusion on latent nystagmus in the treatment of amblyopia, *Doc Ophthalmol* 72:375, 1989.

358. von Noorden GK and others: Latent nystagmus and strabismic amblyopia, *Am J Ophthalmol* 103:87, 1987.

359. Noda S, Hayasaka S, Setogawa T: Occlusion therapy of Japanese children with anisometropic amblyopia without strabismus, *Ann Ophthalmol* 25:145, 1993.

360. Wick B and others: Anisometropic amblyopia: is the patient ever to old to treat? *Optom Vis Sci* 69:866, 1992.

361. Kutschke PJ, Scott WE, Keech RV: Anisometropic amblyopia, *Ophthalmology* 98:258, 1991.

362. Moore BD: Optometric management of congenital cataracts, *J Am Optom Assoc* 65:719, 1994 (review).

363. Drummond GT, Hinz BJ: Management of monocular cataract with long-term dilation in children, *Can J Ophthalmol* 29:227, 1994.

364. Hiles DA: Intraocular lens implantation in children with monocular cataracts:1974-1983, *Ophthalmology* 91:1231, 1984.

365. BenEzra D, Paez JH: Congenital cataract and intraocular lenses, *Am J Ophthalmol* 96:311, 1983.

366. Burke JP, Willshaw HE, Young JDH: Intraocular lens implants for unilateral cataracts in childhood, *Br J Ophthalmol* 73:860, 1989.

367. Sinskey RM, Amin PA, Lingua R: Cataract extraction and intraocular lens implantation in an infant with a monocular congenital cataract, *J Cataract Refract Surg* 20:647, 1994.

368. BenEzra D: Cataract surgery and intraocular lens implantation in children, *Am J Ophthalmol* 121:224, 1996 (letter to the editor).

369. Moore BD: Changes in the aphakic refraction of children with unilateral congenital cataracts, *J Pediatr Ophthalmol Strab* 19:290, 1989.

370. Gordon RA, Donzis PB: Refractive development of the human eye, *Arch Ophthalmol* 103:785, 1985.

371. Basti S, Ravishankar U, Gupta S: Results of prospective evaluation of the three methods of management of pediatric cataracts, *Ophthalmology* 103:713, 1996.

372. Robb RM, Mayer DL, Moore BD: Results of early treatment of unilateral congenital cataracts, *J Pediatr Ophthalmol Strab* 24:178, 1987.

373. Beller R and others: Good visual function after neonatal surgery for congenital monocular cataracts, *Am J Ophthalmol* 91:559, 1981.

374. Drummond GT, Scott WE, Keech RV: Management of monocular congenital cataracts, *Arch Ophthalmol* 107:45, 1989.

375. Wright KW, Matsumoto E, Edelman PM: Binocular fusion and stereopsis associated with early surgery for monocular congenital cataracts, *Arch Ophthalmol* 110:1607, 1992.

376. Tytla ME and others: Stereopsis after congenital cataract, *Invest Ophthalmol Vis Sci* 34:1767, 1993.

377. Gregg FM, Parks MM: Stereopsis after congenital monocular cataract extraction, *Am J Ophthalmol* 114:314, 1992.

378. von Noorden GK: Classification of amblyopia, *Am J Ophthalmol* 63:238, 1967.

379. Pritchard C: Why won't you treat my 10-year-old's lazy eye, *Am Orthopt J* 40:15, 1990.

380. Birnbaum MH, Koslowe K, Sanet R: Success in amblyopia therapy as a function of age: a literature survey, *Am J Optom Physiol Opt* 54:269, 1977.

381. Saulles H: Treatment of refractive amblyopia in adults, *J Am Optom Assoc* 58:959, 1987.

382. Rabin J: Visual improvement in amblyopia after visual loss in the dominant eye, *Am J Optom Physiol Opt* 61:334, 1974.

383. Klaeger-Manzanell C, Hoyt CS, Good WV: 2-step recovery of vision in the amblyopic eye after visual loss and enucleation of the fixing eye, *Br J Ophthalmol* 78:506, 1994.

384. Tierney DW: Vision recovery in amblyopia after contralateral subretinal hemorrhage, *J Am Optom Assoc* 60:281, 1989.

385. Hamed LM, Glaser JS, Schatz NJ: Improvement of vision in amblyopia eye following visual loss in the contralateral normal eye: a report of three cases, *Binoc Vis Eye Muscle Surg* 6:97, 1991.

386. Wilson ME: Adult amblyopia reversed by contralateral cataract formation, *J Pediatr Ophthalmol Strab* 29:100, 1992.

Anomalies of Accommodation

Accommodation alters the dioptric power of the eye and, in so doing, enables objects from the punctum remotum (far point) to the punctum proximum (near point) to be viewed clearly.[1-9] Without accommodation, all objects closer than the far point would be blurred, and near task performance would drastically decrease.

Although the normal accommodative system is quite flexible and resistant to fatigue, accommodative dysfunction is common.[10-15] Precise data regarding its prevalence is not available.[16] The prevalence of accommodative dysfunction not associated with the process of presbyopia probably affects at least 2% to 3% of the population (Table 3-1), although estimates vary. A review of 119 patients in an urban clinic suggests that accommodative dysfunction was the most frequently encountered binocular anomaly in the group, affecting 16.8% of the cases.[17] Another study of a screening of 200 school children found apparent accommodative dysfunction to be very common (as high as 25%).[18] The criteria used to define accommodative dysfunction and the setting in which it is evaluated affect the apparent prevalence.

Accommodative dysfunction has been recognized since the time of Donders.[19] Although sometimes elusive, accommodation deficiency causes significant symptoms, such as blur, headaches, asthenopia (eyestrain), and decreased performance.

TESTING ACCOMMODATIVE FUNCTION

A complete evaluation of a patient's accommodative system includes an examination of the amplitude, facility, and accuracy of the response of accommodation in each eye. Because the vergence and accommodative systems mutually interact in binocular viewing, accommodative function should be isolated from the vergence system by testing monocularly. Problems in one system may be attributed to the other.[20-24]

ACCOMMODATIVE AMPLITUDE

The accommodative amplitude is the maximum dioptric increase that the accommodative system can provide the eye.[25-27] Measured in diopters, the accommodative amplitude is the inverse of the distance (in meters) from the spectacle plane to the closest point (punctum proximum) that can be made clear for a properly corrected eye.[18] Accommodative amplitude can be determined using the push-up method, dynamic

TABLE 3-1   A SURVEY OF MAJOR DIAGNOSES IN A RANDOMLY DRAWN SAMPLE OF 330 CLINIC PATIENTS

Diagnosis	Number	Percentage (%)	Rank
Refractive error requiring correction	121	36.7	1
Routine vision examination	100	30.3	2
Presbyopia related anomalies	43	13	3
Miscellaneous	24	7.3	4
Binocularity problems	20	6.1	5
Accommodative dysfunction	8	2.4	6
Pathology	7	2.1	7
Amblyopia	5	1.6	8
Aniseikonia	2	0.6	9
Total	330	100	—

retinoscopy, or the minus lens technique. The push-up method is most commonly used.

Push-Up Technique

To measure accommodative amplitude, one eye of a properly corrected patient is occluded. The patient views a small target (20/20 to 20/40 for eyes with normal acuity) with the uncovered eye, and, as the target is slowly brought closer to the eye the patient is instructed to signal the point of first sustained blur. Movement of the target too slowly or quickly can create a bias in the patient that the blur has occurred too soon or too late, respectively. The ability to see blur is enhanced by the small target and bright illumination. Dim illumination may cause the amplitude to appear erratically larger or smaller. Binocular amplitudes of accommodation appear slightly higher than monocular amplitudes because of the effect of vergence and the fact that the distance is measured along the perpendicular to the face rather than along the hypotenuse.[25]

Dynamic Retinoscopy Technique

The amplitude, accuracy, and sustaining ability of a patient's accommodation can be objectively determined using dynamic retinoscopy and near-point targets, even on infants. To determine the amplitude, the patient occludes one eye.[28-29] The clinician affixes a near-point target to a retinoscope and instructs the patient to keep the target clear as long as possible as it is moved closer. The clinician moves toward the patient while viewing the retinoscopic reflex, usually a small amount of "with" movement. As the patient's amplitude of accommodation is reached the reflex will suddenly extend, indicating that the target is too close and accommodation is relaxed. The amplitude determined using this method is highly correlated with the push-up method (r = 0.92), although the push-up method is generally preferred by clinicians.[30] Double-masked studies have shown that the objective technique commonly suggests amplitudes approximately 2 to 3 D higher than the usual subjective push-up technique in normal patients and patients with amblyopia.[31] This objective technique produces more accurate results of accommodative amplitude on patients with amblyopia than the subjective technique.

Minus Lens Technique

To measure accommodative amplitude, minus lenses are progressively introduced in 0.25-D steps before a monocularly viewed target (letter size 20/20 to 20/40 for eyes with normal acuity) at a known distance (usually 40 cm). To keep the target clear the patient must use progressively greater accommodation as the lens power is increased. The endpoint is the strongest minus lens with which the subject can maintain clarity

of the target. The target being viewed also usually requires accommodation because of its distance; therefore the accommodative amplitude is the sum of the endpoint minus lens and the accommodation necessary because of the distance of the target (i.e., 40 cm, 2.50 D). The minus lens technique frequently produces a smaller result (approximately 0.5 D) than the push up technique, probably because of proximal effects.[31]

Expected Levels of Accommodative Amplitude

The expected accommodative amplitude as a function of age has been well described (Fig. 3-1).[25,32] Generally, past approximately age 55, apparent accommodation is a function of the depth of focus of the eye.[25] The expected maximum and minimum amplitudes of accommodation for a corrected patient of a given age can be determined using Hofstetter's formulas.[32]

Expected amplitude (D) = 18.5 − 0.3 (age in yrs)
Maximum amplitude (D) = 25 − 0.4 (age in yrs)
Minimum amplitude (D) = 15 − 0.25 (age in yrs)

Hofstetter's formulas should not be used for children younger than age 8, because subjects of that age or younger were not included in the study.

Factors Affecting Accommodative Amplitude

Accommodative function in infants approaches normal by age 6 months.[33] Evaluating the accommodative ability of infants requires special techniques; however, it is infrequently evaluated and not usually clinically important.[33-34]

A decrease in amplitude with repeated measurement is evidence of fatigue of accommodation, because accommodative function normally is quite stable over an extended period.[35,36] Repeatedly assessing accommodative amplitude is the most efficient method of eliciting accommodative fatigue.[35]

The amplitude of accommodation is susceptible to adaptation associated with prolonged viewing at either near or far.[37] For example, individuals who sustained focus at far point before an assessment of amplitude had an amplitude of accommodation 0.37 D less than after an 8-minute near task. Viewing a target at the near point for 8 minutes before amplitude was assessed caused an average increase of accommodative amplitude of 0.62 D. Although both of these changes are statistically significant, they are not often clinically relevant.

A decreased amplitude of accommodation is associated with amblyopia, although the method of evaluation has a considerable affect on the assessment.[38-39] The decrease in amplitude apparently is the result of a lower accommodative controller output and may remain, even if orthoptics/vision therapy successfully normalizes visual acuity.[38]

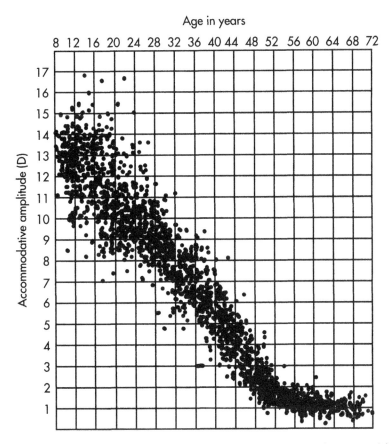

Age in years

FIG. **3-1**   The expected amplitude of accommodation as a function of age. (Modified from Hofstetter HW: A comparison of Duane's and Donders' tables of the amplitude of accommodation, *Am J Optom Arch Am Acad Optom* 21:345, 1944.)

The accommodative amplitude of patients with corrected myopia and hyperopia is identical, although lens effectivity may be important if the correction is relatively high.[40] That is, a patient with very high myopia may appear to have less spectacle accommodation, and a patient with high hyperopia may appear to have more spectacle accommodation than when corrected with contact lenses. Lens effectivity causes about a 0.25-D difference when the correction in question is +5.00 D or −5.00 D. At +10.00 D or −10.00 D, effectivity can cause a difference in accommodation of about 0.5 D.

Apparent accommodation (of up to 3 D or more) that is an inverse function of pupil size can occur in pseudophakic eyes and is related to minimizing the size of retinal blur circles as in a pinhole camera.[41]

ACCOMMODATIVE FACILITY

Accommodative facility is the ability of the accommodative system to change from one level to another.[18] Accommodative facility is most commonly assessed as the number of cycles of plus and minus lenses (+/−

2.00 D) that can be cleared within a given time (1 minute) while viewing a near-point target (20/30 at 40 cm).[42] Other techniques used to assess accommodative facility include far-near subjective assessment, computerized techniques, and dynamic retinoscopy.[43-45]

Flip Lens Technique

As with other measures of accommodation, accommodative facility should be assessed with the patient properly corrected. To measure accommodative facility, testing should be completed monocularly. The near-point target should be small letters (approximately 20/30) held at 40 cm.[42] The patient is instructed to say "clear" as soon as the letters are clear. Plus and minus 2.00-D lenses are most commonly used to measure accommodative facility.[18] The clinician rotates the lenses from one side to the other as soon as the patient indicates that clear vision is obtained. The patient is tested for 1 minute for each eye (typically, first the right eye, then the left). Binocular accommodative facility testing can also be completed to obtain a combined measure of accommodative and vergence ability.

For binocular testing, suppression checks have been recommended.[42,46] Suppression can be monitored with physiologic diplopia.[47]

Accommodative facility testing should be completed only for individuals age 40 or younger. Older prepresbyopic individuals have a marked reduction in accommodative facility, as assessed by the flip lens test.[48-49] Over half of 45 adults (ages 30 to 42) could not complete a single cycle of +/−2.00-D binocular flip lenses (mean 1.2 cpm [cycles per minute]).[49] For this group, the average facility value with +/−1.00-D flip lenses was 8.9 cpm. The flip lens test for these older ages also is not sensitive in identifying symptomatic individuals.[49]

 CLINICAL PEARL

Accommodative facility testing should be completed only for individuals 40 years of age or younger.

Measurements of accommodative facility are affected by the power of the lenses used (increased power causes decreased facility) and the size of the target (larger letters cause better facility) but not by the trial (facility measurements tend to stay the same with repeated measures).[48,50] If a patient's failure is close to the criterion value, extended testing time (1 minute additional) for monocular facility may allow the patient to improve and pass the test.[51] With an additional minute to evaluate accommodative facility, patients tend to increase their facility rate approximately 1 cpm. The test-retest reliability (r = 0.45, 0.40) is poorest for individuals in the "high" fail group (those closest to passing).[51] Reliability of the test is significantly better for those more clearly failing the test (the "low" fail group, r = 0.67, 0.72).

Far-Near Subjective Technique

In a subjective judgment of the facility of accommodation the patient is first given targets requiring good focus at both distance and near and is then asked to alternate fixation between the two targets as quickly as the targets can be cleared.[10,43,52] The patient is cautioned to completely clear each target and is observed by the clinician for 1 minute. The clinician makes a subjective assessment of accommodative facility, based on clinical experience (as either good, fair, or poor). This technique is limited by its qualitative nature but is useful as a screening technique.

Dynamic Retinoscopy Technique

Dynamic retinoscopy (MEM) has been used to objectively evaluate the facility of accommodation.[45] The dynamic retinoscopy technique and a flip lens subjective technique for testing accommodative facility gave similar results in 86% of patients; however, there was a relatively low level of agreement between the two techniques (r = 0.21). This technique could be useful for evaluating the accommodative facility of children when subjective results are questionable.

Expected Levels of Accommodative Facility

The appropriate criterion for accommodative facility is challenging to determine because the patient's age and the technique affect the assessment. For adolescents (older than age 13), monocular facility that is less than 12 cpm with +/−2.00-D lenses is suspect.[18] For adults (20 years or older), we consider binocular accommodative facility that is less than 10 cpm with +/−2.00-D lenses abnormal. Binocular values in adults that are less than 12 cpm with +/−1.00-D lenses are also abnormal. Suppression checks also cause lower values for binocular facility. A monocular facility rate of 6 cpm is one standard deviation below the mean and also has been suggested as appropriate for a criterion value.[51]

 CLINICAL PEARL

For adolescents (older than age 13), monocular facility that is less than 12 cpm with +/−2.00-D lenses is suspect. For adults 20 years or older, we consider binocular accommodative facility that is less than 10 cpm with +/−2.00-D lenses abnormal.

For monocular accommodative facility in adolescents using +/−2.00-D lenses, averages have ranged from 11.6 to 17 cpm.[14,42,46,50,52] For binocular facility (also adolescents using +/−2.00-D lenses), averages have ranged from 6 to 10.6 cpm.[14,42,46,50,53a] Standard errors of measurement (monocular or binocular assessment) range from 0.5 to 1.68 cpm.[42,46]

Average accommodative facility values for children (age 12 or younger) are lower than for adolescents. Mean monocular facility values (+/−2.00 D) for children ages 6, 7, and 8 to 12 were 5.5, 6.5 and 7 cpm, respectively.[53b] Appropriate pass rates may be 3, 4.5, and 5 cpm (monocular, +/−2.00 D cpm).[14] Binocular facility using +/−2.00 D in children is so low that the value of such testing is uncertain (mean 3, 3.5, and 5 cpm for ages 6, 7, and 8 to 12 years, respectively). With stringent criteria (7 cpm, binocular facility, +/−2.00 D), very high numbers of school children fail, 53% in one study.[18] Even so, young children frequently have difficulty completing the accommodative facility test; approximately 30% of 6 and 7 year olds cannot complete even one cycle with +/−2.00 D flip lenses.[45]

Individuals with accommodative facility 1 standard deviation lower than the mean often show symptoms such as asthenopia when reading (less than 6 cpm monocularly with +/−2.00 D).[53a] In one study, no difference was found between males and females with respect to accommodative facility values, and a mean was determined of 12.8 cpm with +/−2.00-D flippers and 15.1 cpm with +/−1.00-D flip lenses.[1]

Various studies have examined the expected change in accommodative speed as a function of age.[44,54] The best of these used a psychophysical technique to measure the speed of accommodation for subjects of different ages who were changing accommodation from near to far and far to near.[54] Far-to-near accommodative ability decreased slowly with age, and the mean time for the change increased from 0.5 seconds to about 0.75 seconds between ages 25 and 35. The mean time for changing from near to far did not slow significantly over the ages included in the study (ages 24 to 44).

ACCOMMODATIVE RESPONSE

When viewing an object closer than optical infinity the accommodative response is typically less than the stimulus (Fig. 3-2). The difference between the accommodative stimulus and the accommodative response is called the lag of accommodation. If the accommodative response is greater than the accommodative stimulus, a lead of accommodation exists. The accommodative response is typically determined objectively using dynamic retinoscopy, which was developed by Cross around 1900.[28,55,56] Objective testing of the accommodative response often can help confirm that an accommodative anomaly exists.[28,57] The lag of accommodation at the 40-cm range assessed in the clinic averages +0.50 to 0.75 D.[56,58] If the stimulus is brought closer the lag of accommodation increases precipitously and may trail off markedly if the target is brought inside the amplitude of accommodation.[59,60]

The lag of accommodation is the steady-state error for the accommodative system.[22] Letter size has little effect on the accommodative lag.[61,62] Accommodation is more stable with binocular viewing.[63]

Dynamic retinoscopy is critical to understanding accommodative and binocular function because the test shows the results of many factors acting on the visual system.[55,64] Generally, these are related to accommodation, vergence, refractive status, or the level of cooperation of the patient (Table 3-2). Poor accommodative function can cause an extended lag (insufficiency or presbyopia) or a lead (spasm). A patient bothered by esophoria and poor negative vergences usually will have an extended lag. Similarly, one afflicted with exophoria and poor positive vergences can have a lead of accommodation.[56,65-67] The lead of accommodation in the latter case (exophoria) is not as consistently present as the extended lag that occurs with esophoria.

The AC/A (accommodative-convergence accommodation) ratio (Δ/D) is a measure of the relationship between changes in vergence that occur for a particular change in accommodation. Because the AC/A value is usually moderate to high in patients with esophoria, extending the lag of accommodation can significantly

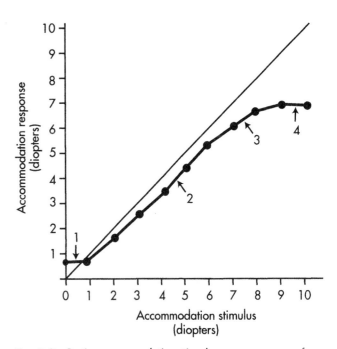

FIG. 3-2 Static accommodative stimulus-response curve for a normal subject. 1= initial nonlinear region, 2= linear region, 3= transitional soft saturation region, and 4= hard saturation presbyopic region. (Modified from Ciuffreda KJ and others: Static aspects of accommodation in human amblyopia, *Am J Optom Physiol Opt* 60(6):436, 1983.)

reduce the esophoria and therefore whatever symptoms are present. On the other hand, patients with exophoria often have low AC/A ratios. Any changes in the accommodative response consequently produces less of an effect on an exophoria and the symptoms that go with it.[68]

A patient with uncorrected hyperopia frequently has an extended lag, whereas uncorrected myopia may result in a lead. Evaluation of the near response for an extended accommodative lag is a good screening test for children suspected of latent hyperopia.[69] The accommodative response can be challenging to assess in children because their fixation tends to vary. In one study of school children, 26% had a lag outside of a range of 0.25 to 0.75 D.[18]

Prolonged reading causes a shift of the accommodative response in the myopic direction, that is, toward a smaller lag or lead.[70] Twenty-eight college students who read for an hour with material at a distance of 20 cm had an increase in their accommodative response of 0.3 D at every stimulus distance. In addition, their mean far point shifted 0.43 D in the myopic direction, and similar changes occurred in the dark focus of accommodation.[70,71] These changes were correlated with increased levels of visual fatigue and suggest a tendency toward spasm of the accommodative system with prolonged reading.

TABLE 3-2 **POSSIBLE INTERPRETATIONS FOR THE RESULTS OF DYNAMIC RETINOSCOPY AT 40 CM**

Qualitative Results of Dynamic Retinoscopy	Quantitative Results of Dynamic Retinoscopy (D)	Possible Interpretation	Other Data Consistent with This Interpretation*
Normal	+0.25 to 0.75	Normal	v, a, Rx: WNL
Extended or high lag	+1.00 or greater	Normal	v, a, Rx: WNL
		Presbyopia or prepresbyopia	a: decreased
		Accommodative dysfunction (insufficiency, fatigue, paresis, or infacility)	v, Rx: WNL
		Hyperopia or latent hyperopia†	Rx: uncorrected hyperopia (cycloplegia may be required to detect)
			v: esophoria when uncorrected
			a: decreased when uncorrected
		Vergence dysfunction (esophoria, poor negative vergences)	Rx: WNL
			v: esophoria, decreased negative vergences
			a: decreased binocularly, OK monocularly
		Overminused†	Rx: too much minus
			a: decreased through Rx
			v: esophoria, decreased negative vergences through Rx
		Malingering	Rx, a, v: normal but variable
Decreased or minus lag or lead	Less than +0.25	Normal	v, a, Rx: WNL
		Accommodative dysfunction (spasm or spasm of near reflex)	a: impaired
			v: esophoria, decreased negative vergences
			Rx: normal to more myopic
		Vergence dysfunction: exophoria and decreased positive vergences	Rx, a: WNL
			v: exophoria, decreased positive vergences
		Overplused correction	Rx: overplused, poor distance visual acuity
			a: larger than normal
			v: exophoria
		Malingering	Rx, a, v: normal but variable

Modified from Daum KM: Accommodative response. In Eskridge JB, Amos JF, Bartlett JD, eds: *Clinical procedures in optometry*, Philadelphia, 1991, JB Lippincott.
v, vergences; *a*, accommodation; *Rx*, correction; *WNL*, within normal limits.
†These are the only factors that could account for a lag greater than +2.50 D if the target is at 40 cm.

The accommodative response to minus lenses is reduced in myopia.[72-73] With an accommodative demand of 3.0 D, children with myopia accommodated 0.91 D less (total accommodation, 0.75 D; lag, 2.25 D) than the typical 1.66 D of children with emmetropia (lag, 1.34 D). No such difference occurred with plus lenses. This differential sensitivity to blur has been suggested as a possible etiologic factor in myopia.[74,75] Poor accommodative response (a large lag) has also been hypothesized to precede the onset of juvenile myopia.[76]

The accommodative system also manifests the after-effects of stimulation with lenses and/or prisms.[20] Convergence (demanded by BO prisms and minus lenses) tends to cause an increase in the accommodative response. In the same fashion a reduction in the accommodative response tends to occur with divergence (demanded by BI prisms or plus lenses). With time the accommodative response tends to increase to nearly match the stimulus. These effects appear to be primarily related to the patient's awareness of nearness.[77] When the stimuli are removed, the response tends to return to baseline level in a fashion that is dependent on the environment (the decay of the response to its original level occurs more quickly in darkness).[20]

The response of accommodation to any stimulus further depends on the spatial frequency makeup of the stimulus, because accommodation is most efficient with spatial frequencies in the 3 to 5 c/degree range.[78] The lag of accommodation increases as the spatial frequency makeup of the stimulus departs from that optimal range. The accommodative response also depends on other aspects of the stimulus.[79] Stimuli with higher contrast and greater detail elicit the greatest response. A field without detail opens the accommodative loop, resulting in accommodation returning to its resting level.

The accommodative response is reduced in amblyopia.[38,39] As vision is improved with orthoptics/vision

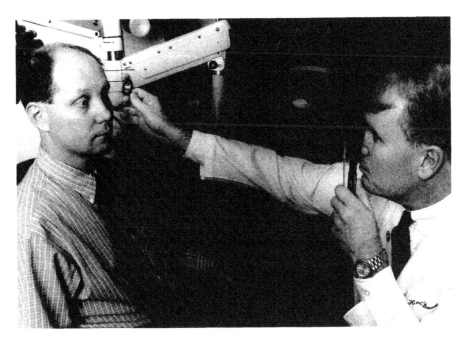

FIG. 3-3   Set-up of clinician, patient, stimulus, and lenses for MEM retinoscopy.

therapy the accommodative response tends to normalize. The accommodative response often is unstable in multiple sclerosis, increasing over viewing time.[80] The eye's accommodative response can also be effected by the direction of gaze, tending to increase in downward gaze.[81]

The MEM (monocular estimation method) and Nott dynamic retinoscopy techniques are the most common techniques for measuring accommodative response, providing essentially identical results.[82] The selection of one technique over the other should be a function of the examiner's preference, the particular nature of the lag (larger lags or larger leads are easier to see using MEM), or equipment available (MEM requires trial lenses). Dynamic retinoscopy can be used to determine a near-point correction.[64,83,84] As the accommodative response is being observed on a patient reading near-point material, sets of plus lenses are introduced until a normal lag is determined. The near-point addition is chosen to be that set of lenses that provide clear and comfortable reading and a lag that is in the normal range.

Monocular Estimation Method (MEM) Technique

The Monocular Estimation Method (MEM) technique is the most common technique for dynamic retinoscopy. A patient views a target located at the plane of the examiner's retinoscope.[55] The reading material should be suitable for the patient's reading ability and should be in the 20/25 to 20/40 range. The lighting should be arranged so that the patient can easily see the printed material at the same time that the clini-

cian can see the retinoscopic reflex. Usually, slightly dimmed room lights, as is the case when measuring distance visual acuity, and a stand light directly illuminating the printed material being observed by the patient is sufficient. The accommodative status is determined by neutralizing the retinoscopic reflex motion with lenses briefly interposed into the line of vision of the eye being examined with the retinoscope (Fig. 3-3).[55] Plus lenses neutralize "with" motion (a lag of accommodation), and minus lenses neutralize "against" motion (a lead of accommodation).[85] To minimize any effect of the lenses on accommodation, they should not be in the patient's line of sight more than about half of a second (the latency of accommodation). The neutralizing lenses should be placed before the eye for which the lag is being measured.

The MEM technique provides results that closely correspond to measures of accommodation using a vernier optometer (r = 0.9754, p<0.001).[86] A modified MEM technique of only estimating the lag is sometimes used by experienced clinicians (similar to estimating the magnitude of a phoria when performing the alternate cover test, rather than measuring it with prisms). The MEM technique can also be used to assess accommodative facility in children or others in whom communication or cooperation is suspect.[45] The reflex is examined with each change of the flip lenses, and the speed of accommodation is judged.

Nott Technique

The Nott technique of dynamic retinoscopy does not involve added lenses and is therefore superior theoretically to the MEM technique in that the chance of altering accommodation is less.[58,87,88] As in the MEM technique a properly corrected patient views a good accommodative stimulus (approximately 20/25 to 20/40 and at a reading level suitable for the patient) located at a known distance in front of the patient. The lighting is arranged so that the patient can clearly see the target and the clinician can see the retinoscopic reflex. The clinician initially holds the retinoscope in the same plane as the target while viewing the movement of the reflex. If the reflex is "with" motion, the clinician leaves the target in place and moves away from it (and the patient) until neutrality is achieved. If the movement seen initially is "against," the clinician moves in front of the target, toward the patient, until neutrality is achieved.

The lag or lead of accommodation with the Nott technique is the dioptric difference between the stimulus and the endpoint for neutrality (Fig. 3-4). For example, if the target is at 40 cm and "with" motion is seen initially, the clinician moves away from the patient until neutrality is achieved. If neutrality is gained at 50 cm, the lag is 0.5 D (stimulus = 1/0.4 M or 2.5 D and neutrality = 1/0.5 M or 2 D; 2.5 D (stimulus) − 2 D (neutrality) = 0.5-D lag). Note that the lag is *not* the linear distance between the stimulus and neutrality, that is, it is *not* 50 cm − 40 cm = 10 cm or 1/0.10 = 10 D).

There are certain practical problems with the Nott technique. If the lag is large, the retinoscopic reflex is hard to see from a long distance away from the patient. If there is a lead, the clinician's head tends to get in the way of the target as he or she moves between the target and the patient. Despite these difficulties, the Nott technique is a quick and accurate way to determine the lag because it does not require additional lenses.

Cross-Cylinder Technique

Although it is not a preferred technique, the cross-cylinder test is another method of assessing accommodative response. The cross-cylinder technique is performed by presenting a cross-lined target at a known distance (usually 40 cm) while the lines are viewed through a cross-cylinder lens (+/−0.5 D) set with the minus axis vertical. The cross-cylinder lens creates a blurred interval of Sturm. The target is viewed with slightly dim illumination and, if there is a lag of accommodation as is typical, the horizontal lines will appear clearest. Plus lenses are added until the vertical lines are just clearest and the lens that equalizes the appearance of the lines is a measure of the lag of accommodation. This technique can be completed monocularly to assess accommodation in isolation, if desired. If completed binocularly, the technique assesses the accommodative response as affected by accommodation and vergence.

Although the monocular cross-cylinder technique is less commonly used to assess the accommodative response and is affected by other factors, it can provide a comparable estimate of the lag to the MEM or Nott techniques.[82] The patient often attempts to maintain clarity of the set of lines that is initially clearer. In addition, when a negative cylinder is introduced before a previously fully corrected eye, patients tend to accommodate to clear the anterior focal point, in contrast to the expected accommodation to the circle of least confusion.[89]

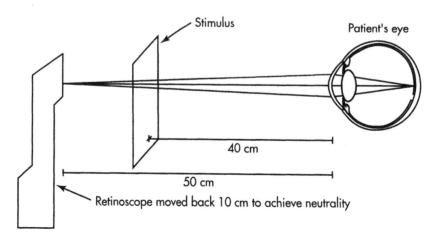

FIG. 3-4 Diagram of position of retinoscope when neutrality is achieved for eye with +0.50-D lag using Nott technique. The lag is dioptric difference (0.5 D) between stimulus located at 40 cm (2.50 D) and retinoscope when neutrality is achieved (2 D).

DIVISION OF ACCOMMODATIVE ANOMALIES

When an individual presents with an accommodative anomaly the clinician must first determine whether the etiology is functional or organic. This functional/organic distinction is important because the management of these two classes is very different.

 CLINICAL PEARL

> When an individual presents with an accommodative anomaly the clinician must first determine whether the etiology is functional or organic.

Patients with organic anomalies of accommodation, such as paresis of accommodation, are much less common than those with functional anomalies and have a distinctive set of signs and symptoms.[10] People with accommodative anomalies of organic etiology often suddenly lose accommodation in one eye and have a severely diminished amplitude. Ordinarily, other neurologic findings, such as pupillary signs (mydriasis) and/or incomitant strabismus, also are present. A loss of accommodation and a mydriatic pupil in a patient with incomitant exotropia usually indicates paresis of the oculomotor nerve. In addition, there is a relatively unique constellation of symptoms in an organic dysfunction. Micropsia or macropsia (i.e., changes in apparent size), sharp headaches, vertigo, or dizziness may be reported, along with a stiff neck and/or diplopia. (See Case 1.)

CASE 1

A 21-year-old woman reported by phone that she had diplopia for about the past 3 weeks when looking to the right. On examination, she had 20/20 visual acuity in each eye through her disposable soft contact lenses. Her accommodative ability was reduced on the right side, 6 D, vs. 12 D on the left. Anisocoria was present (5 mm OD vs. 3 mm OS) and was more apparent in dim illumination, suggesting a parasympathetic defect. There was an obvious incomitancy with versions. Other signs were unremarkable.

The patient was referred for neuroimaging, which revealed a large intracranial tumor that was subsequently removed surgically. The acute onset, presence of diplopia in a particular gaze, and the asymmetric accommodation all pointed to an organic accommodative anomaly. Cases such as this must be handled correctly because the patient's life may be at stake.

In contrast, a functional loss of accommodation typically only involves accommodation, although it may be associated with other conditions, such as convergence insufficiency.[43] The pupil is not involved, and associated oculomotor deviations if present are comitant in nature. Symptomology stemming from functional losses of accommodation includes headaches (often dull), eyestrain, and blurred vision. Functional conditions also do not usually have a precise onset, are bilateral, and most conditions have existed for months.

CLASSIFICATION OF ACCOMMODATIVE ANOMALIES

Although the boundaries are often blurred the anomalies of accommodation are frequently classified as one of the following five syndromes: (1) insufficiency of accommodation (premature presbyopia), (2) fatigue of accommodation (ill-sustained accommodation), (3) infacility of accommodation (inertia of or tonic accommodation), (4) spasm of accommodation (accommodative excess, excess accommodation, pseudomyopia), and (5) paresis of accommodation (palsy of accomodation or paralysis of accommodation).[9,10,12,15] Although unlikely, multiple anomalies of accommodative function sometimes occur in the same patient.[18]

Data suggesting the relative prevalences of these conditions is anecdotal. Insufficiency of accommodation is the most prevalent syndrome, followed by infacility, spasm, and fatigue (Table 3-3).[90] Fatigue of accommodation probably occurs more often than has been reported by either patients or clinicians because it is not reported until it is a more severe problem. People with accommodative dysfunction are usually young, and accommodative dysfunction usually does not occur past age 40.[10]

DESCRIPTION OF ACCOMMODATIVE ANOMALIES

INSUFFICIENCY OF ACCOMMODATION
Definition

Insufficiency of accommodation is a condition in which the amplitude of accommodation is chronically below the lower limits of the expected amplitude for a patient's age.[12-13] This condition, sometimes called premature presbyopia, is one of the most frequently diagnosed binocular visual anomalies.[43,90,91] Although the diagnosis often is straightforward, many problems can determine whether a patient has a chronically low am-

TABLE 3-3 DISTRIBUTION OF ACCOMMODATIVE DYSFUNCTION SYNDROMES

Type	Frequency	Percentage
Insufficiency	96	84
Infacility	14	12
Spasm	3	3
Fatigue	1	1
Total	114	100

Modified from Daum KM: Accommodative dysfunction, *Doc Ophthalmol* 55:177, 1983.

TABLE 3-4 SYMPTOMS IN ACCOMMODATIVE
INSUFFICIENCY (N = 96)

Description	Frequency	Percentage (%)
Blur	57	59
Headaches	54	56
Asthenopia	43	45
Diplopia	29	30
Reading problems	13	14
Fatigue	9	9
Poor facility	7	7
Photophobia	3	3
None	2	2
Suppression	1	1
Dizziness	1	1

Modified from Daum KM: Accommodative insufficiency, *Am J Optom Physiol Opt* 60(5):352, 1983.

plitude of accommodation, because the ability to accommodate sometimes varies from day to day.[92]

Symptoms

Patients with accommodative insufficiency usually suffer from blur, headaches, and asthenopia associated with near work (Table 3-4).[43,92-95] Burning, irritated vision, photophobia, and nausea are also occasionally reported.[93] These symptoms have been recognized since the time of Donders and often begin within a few minutes of beginning a near-work task.[10,12,13,19,96] Although the symptoms are bothersome, often young adult patients are able to continue working at their task but with reduced comfort and performance. Frequently, children with accommodative insufficiency avoid near tasks such as reading. The presence (or absence) of symptoms is not reliable for diagnosis because of this avoidance of near-work tasks.

The symptoms of accommodative insufficiency are similar to those reported with convergence insufficiency and are also akin to those reported at the onset of presbyopia, although patients do not report that "my arms are not long enough" as do patients with presbyopia. Because of the prevalence of accommodative insufficiency, when a young patient reports headaches, eyestrain, and discomfort that commences after 10 to 15 minutes of work at the near point, accommodative insufficiency should be suspected. Only refractive error problems (e.g., astigmatism or hyperopia) are more common.

 CLINICAL PEARL

> Because of the prevalence of accommodative insufficiency, when a young patient reports headaches, eyestrain, and discomfort that commences after 10 to 15 minutes of work at the near point, accommodative insufficiency should be suspected.

Signs

Table 3-5 shows a clinical profile of 96 patients diagnosed with accommodative insufficiency.[43] The most striking feature of patients afflicted with accommodative insufficiency is a decreased amplitude of accommodation. These patients also tend toward convergence insufficiency, and most are exophoric and have unimpressive positive vergences.

Amplitude of Accommodation

A decreased amplitude of accommodation is the most significant and most common feature of accommodative insufficiency.[43,95] The mean amplitude of accommodation is often approximately 5 D to 6 D less than the expected level for the patient's age.[43,95] The average amplitude often is approximately 2 D below the minimum age level, using Hofstetter's formulas.[13]

A complicating factor for diagnosis of accommodative insufficiency is that a patient's amplitude of accommodation can vary substantially, moving from a normal level to insufficient.[93] In addition, the variability can occur over a rather short period.[93] Patients who clearly have insufficient accommodation during the late afternoon may have better accommodative ability during the morning.

Age and Sex

Patients with accommodative insufficiency usually are school age, often from age 10 to the mid-to-late twenties.[43,97] After the age of approximately 35 to 40, accommodative insufficiency is simply called presbyopia.[92] There have not been any well-constructed epidemiologic studies examining the prevalence by age or sex in the general population. Accommodative insufficiency is predominantly seen in women, about twice as often as in men (e.g., one series contained 60 females and 36 males).[43,98] The condition may actually be found about equally in the two sexes, but women may be more likely to seek care than men and therefore make up a larger proportion of patients in clinical series.

Other Clinical Features

Clinical features other than a reduced amplitude identifying accommodative insufficiency are often absent.[43] Patients with this condition tend to have a slightly reduced facility of accommodation (poorer than normal in 35 of 70 patients in one series).[43] A tendency of patients with accommodative insufficiency toward convergence insufficiency (exophoria, reduced vergences, remote NPC, and so on) has frequently been described.[43,92] These types of patients accounted for 65% of one series of 96 patients[43] and 44% of another series.[92] This is a higher prevalence of convergence insufficiency than in other types of accommodative dysfunction.

TABLE 3-5 CLINICAL PROFILE, ACCOMMODATIVE INSUFFICIENCY

Parameter	N	Before Treatment		After Treatment		Statistical Significance of Change*	
		Mean	Standard Deviation (SD)	Mean	Standard Deviation (SD)	t	p > t
Amplitude of accommodation	74	7.98 D	2.57 C	11.46 D	3.42 D	9.43	0.0001
Lag of accommodation 40 cm	10	0.15 D	0.47 D	0.39 D	0.33 D	1.30	NS
Phoria 6 m	55	0.75△ exophoria	4.17△	1.21△ exophoria	3.77△	1.38	NS
40 cm	70	3.68△ exophoria	8.80△	3.75△ exophoria	7.88△	0.17	NS
AC/A	54	4.76△/1.0 D	2.15△/1.0 D	4.83△/1.0 D	1.75△/1.0 D	1.14	NS
Stereopsis 40 cm	26	44.62 sec	37.97 sec	29.23 sec	16.95 sec	−2.02 3.86	0.054 0.0005
Vergences (negative) 40 cm	33	8△/14△/10△	4△/5△/6△	12△/15△/12△	5△/5△/5△	1.59 1.84	0.121 0.0755
Vergences (positive) 40 cm	53	12△/18△/13△	7△/8△/6△	20△/29△/24△	10△/10△/11△	5.68 7.44	0.0001
Nearpoint of convergence (NPC)	78	8.24 cm	6.67 cm			6.90	

Modified from Daum KM: Accommodative insufficiency, *Am J Optom Physiol Opt* 60(5):352, 1983.
*Paired t-test: *t* computed for those subjects who had data recorded before and after treatment using same technique.

Strabismus and Weakness of Accommodation. Accommodative insufficiency often has been associated with exodeviations.[97,99-106] Von Noorden, Brown, and Parks[104] describe several adolescent and young adults with intermittent exotropia and severe accommodative insufficiency. Stark and others[106] and Rutstein and Daum[107] also describe individuals with exotropia associated with defective accommodation that is often severely reduced. Exotropia and accommodative insufficiency in skin divers suffering from decompression sickness has also been described.[105] In this condition, it may be impossible to differentiate which system is primary.

A patient presenting with exotropia and severely reduced accommodative function complicates the clinical picture and suggests a much poorer prognosis.[97,101,104,108] If the exotropia is primary and the accommodative disorder secondary, the accommodative system may produce additional accommodative convergence to compensate for the exodeviation and achieve fusion. If this is the case, accommodative function may become chronically fatigued. The main emphasis in these cases should be to treat the primary exodeviation.[107]

Accommodation weakness may be primary and has been suggested as the cause of exotropia.[97] In these cases the lag of accommodation is high. With poor focus of the target and a low accommodative vergence level, the vergence system may become chronically fa-

tigued, leading to exotropia. Emphasis in these patients should be on treating the accommodative problem and its cause, if discoverable.[107]

We have reported on a number of patients with intermittent exotropia and accommodative dysfunction (see Chapter 9).[107] Because the lag of accommodation was large when the exotropia occurred, accommodation was considered to be the primary etiologic factor. If accommodation was functioning properly, the lag would remain stable whether the patient was fusing or exotropic. Weak accommodation was suspected because the lag increased as if accommodation had given out when the exotropia occurred.

Accommodative insufficiency may also exist in esotropia. This esotropia is characterized by a small refractive error, a small deviation at distance, a larger esotropia at near, and a remote near point of accommodation. Because of the reduced accommodative ability, these patients may exert excessive accommodative effort and thus exhibit increased convergence with esotropia.

Prevalence

The prevalence of accommodative insufficiency is unknown, and anecdotal information varies. An evaluation of 119 patients suggests that 16.8% of patients were symptomatic because of accommodative dysfunction.[17] Others have suggested prevalence rates ranging from 14.4%, 10%, and 9.5% of 1615 consecutive cases to 44% abnormal function in a special population of children with learning disabilities.[96,109-111] We believe that a 3% to 5% rate is most likely.[93]

Associated Conditions

Most cases of accommodative insufficiency are associated with either convergence insufficiency or some type of emotional distress or fatigue.[43,108,111-112] Other factors associated with the condition (listed below) are less frequently seen, and the nature of the association is probably indirect. Any condition that causes an overall debilitation may also cause accommodative insufficiency.

 CLINICAL PEARL

Any condition that causes an overall debilitation may also cause accommodative insufficiency.

A variety of factors have been suggested to be associated with insufficient accommodation. Among these are the following: (1) convergence insufficiency*; (2) neurasthenia or emotional factors, often as a result of fatigue and/or overwork†; (3) toxic conditions as a result of tuberculosis, influenza, whooping cough, or measles[92-94,110,116,118]; (4) severe dental caries or infections[92-94,116,119]; (5) endocrinal disturbances, such as diabetes[92,94,110,120]; (6) anemia[92,93,112,121]; (7) vascular hypertension[92,93]; (8) anoxia, altitude[118,122]; (9) eyestrain[92]; (10) decompression sickness[105]; (11) sclerosis of the crystalline lens[92,93]; (12) inability of the ciliary body to contract‡ (13) menopause[27]; (14) arteriosclerosis[26]; (15) Down syndrome[30]; (16) cerebral palsy[124-127]; (17) trauma[100,128,129]; (18) toxoplasmosis[95,130]; (19) hereditary factors; (20) various systemic medications[18,112,131]; (21) asthma or medications associated with it, such as albuterol[132]; (22) toxemia of pregnancy[133]; (23) perceptual dysfunction[134]; (24) amblyopia[31,39]; (25) nasal obstruction[92,93]; (26) encephalitis[112,135]; (27) concussion[105,112]; (28) mesencephalic disease (pineal tumor, multiple sclerosis, infectious polyneuropathy, and other vascular lesions [e.g., middle cerebral artery embolism])[105,136]; (29) cataract or glaucoma[118]; (30) suspected chronic fatigue and immune dysfunction syndrome[14]; (31) diphtheria, meningitis, hepatitis[112]; (32) dysthyroid conditions[112]; (33) alcoholism[112]; (34) malnutrition[112]; (35) multiple sclerosis[112]; and (36) idiopathic occurrences.[95]

Individuals with diabetes are on the average deficient by approximately 2 D in accommodative amplitude for any particular age.[120] Individuals who have a longer duration of the condition, are more poorly controlled, or have retinopathy show significantly lower amplitudes.

Etiology

Although accommodative insufficiency is relatively commonly seen in the clinic the precise etiology of this condition is rarely known.* Fatigue is a very common factor in the development of accommodative insufficiency. In most patients it is not possible to establish a definite etiology, however exceptions exist.† These are typically accommodative insufficiency and convergence insufficiency related to trauma, anemia, or decompression sickness or anoxia because of altitude or vascular insufficiency.‡ Improper or delayed development may also be an etiologic factor.

A study of 12 professional divers with severe accommodative deficiency and convergence insufficiency suggests that the etiology of accommodative insufficiency is central in origin.[105,115] The accommodative amplitude of these individuals increased by 2 to 3 D when parasympathomimetic agents such as physostigmine (0.1%) and carbachol (3%) were applied, suggesting that the peripheral accommodative apparatus was still intact.

A psychogenic component of accommodative insufficiency is sometimes present and is frequently associated with visual field defects (e.g., constricted and tubular fields as assessed on the tangent screen).[93] Most patients with accommodative insufficiency consistently exhibit certain additional signs, such as convergence insufficiency; cannot accommodate through minus lenses of which they are not aware; lack additional signs of psychogenic distress, such as constricted and tubular visual fields; and do not respond to placebo devices.

Uncorrected refractive error, such as against-the-rule astigmatism or anisometropia, can cause accommodative insufficiency.[142] Blur leads to a decreased output from the disparity detectors in the vergence controller loop of the oculomotor control system (i.e., decreased sensitivity).[142] Over time, this lack of sensitivity can lead to a larger fixation disparity in an effort to stimulate convergence. If the fixation disparity becomes too large, suppression and a simultaneous decrease in the blur detector output of the accommodative loop can occur, and the patient may develop voluntary accommodative vergence to avoid the blur and diplopia.[142] Voluntary convergence leads to suppressed sensitivity of the blur detectors because the information they supply is no longer used.[142-144] Uncorrected refractive errors are important in effectively treating accommodative insufficiency as indicated by the following case example.

---

*References 25, 92-94, 97, 99, 104, 105, 108, 113-115.
†References 35, 92-94, 105, 111, 112, 116, 117.
‡References 25, 92, 93, 96, 98, 113, 123.

*References 12, 13, 14, 15, 92, 95, 139.
†References 12, 100, 103, 105, 122, 136, 140, 141.
‡References 100, 105, 122, 135, 140, 141.

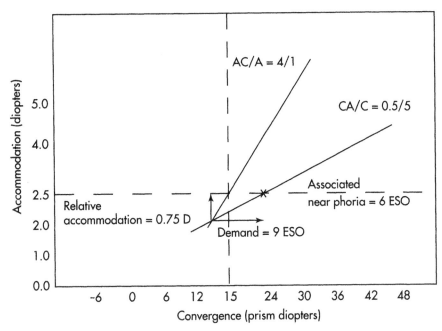

FIG. 3-5 CA/C line is drawn through associated phoria *(X)*, and AC/A line is drawn through convergence accommodation reference representing near test distance. AC/A and CA/C lines intersect at a point indicating the demand upon accommodation (1.5 D) and convergence (18PD) necessary to correct or overcome an associated phoria of 6PD esophoria for person with normal (0.50/6) CA/C ratio and high AC/A ratio. The demand on accommodation and convergence controllers will become very large as slopes of AC/A and CA/C become parallel. Note that reciprocal of AC/A is plotted. (Modified from Schor CM, Narayan V: Graphical analysis of prism adaptation, convergence accommodation, and accommodative convergence, *Am J Optom Physiol Opt* 59:774, 1982.)

<u>CASE 2</u>

A 27-year-old woman presented with severe symptoms and a very poor amplitude of accommodation (2 D). She had a refraction of +0.75 −0.50 × 092 and +1.00 −1.00 × 070, which was prescribed. After wearing the glasses for a few weeks, accommodation improved and the symptoms were alleviated.

Etiology of Symptoms in Accommodative
Insufficiency with Slightly
Reduced Accommodation

Patients with accommodative insufficiency frequently complain of problems with near-point vision, even though this reduced amplitude of accommodation is enough to produce comfortable near vision for other, older individuals. Although the presence of symptoms is correlated with the amplitude being below the expected level, stresses on the binocular visual system that are present with monocular measurements are not necessarily those that are present under binocular conditions.[93] The criteria that are commonly used to predict the requirements on the accommodative and fusional systems (Sheard's[144] or Percival's criteria, as

described in Chapter 6) use data derived from the dissociated state. Schor[21,22] and others have shown that the accommodative and fusional systems (AC/A, CA/C, and associated phoria) (Fig. 3-5) interact under binocular conditions in ways that are not revealed with dissociated testing, so that accommodative effort can be more than the demand indicates.[20-24,145,146]

Diagnosis

The diagnosis of accommodative insufficiency is appropriate in the following instances: (1) when there are visually related symptoms at the near point and a depressed amplitude of accommodation in the absence of other possible problems or (2) with only a diminished amplitude and missing symptoms because of the avoidance of near work or insensitivity of the patient. The diagnosis is complicated by the variability that occurs in accommodative amplitude; however, a reduced amplitude of accommodation is the single necessary finding for the diagnosis.[93]

Assessing the true amplitude of accommodation is sometimes difficult because of poor patient understanding or cooperation. If necessary, the test should be redone with the patient holding the push-up stick,

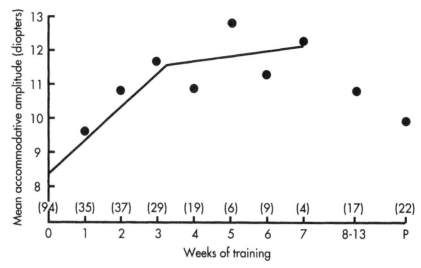

FIG. 3-6 Mean accommodative amplitude during treatment period. Numbers in parentheses above abscissa indicate number of points making up mean. Solid lines represent best-fitting lines (least squares method) for weeks 0 to 3 and 3 to 7. Mean accommodative amplitude indicated at *P* is mean value at progress checks, which were an average of 12.3 months after dismissal (range 3 to 60 months). (Modified from Daum KM: Accommodative insufficiency, *Am J Optom Physiol Opt* 60(5):352, 1983.)

to try and obtain accurate results. Symptoms also may not be reported accurately. If the condition is long-standing, the patient may not be aware of eyestrain.

When a child with a low accommodative amplitude presents, we suggest a tentative diagnosis of accommodative insufficiency, even in the absence of significant symptoms. We believe that this is appropriate in view of the importance of clear, comfortable near vision. Subsequently, if the amplitude can be demonstrated at an expected level, the diagnosis should be revised.

Treatment

Any clinically significant refractive error that may be causative should be corrected initially, including small amounts of astigmatism (see Case 2). The treatment should address the cause of the insufficiency of accommodation if it is apparent.[92-94,98,110] The removal, reduction, or control of any source of fatigue or debility is important.[93] The two most important treatments for accommodative insufficiency are plus lens additions for nearwork or orthoptics/vision therapy exercises.* Progressive addition lenses may be useful for these patients and remove some of the stigma of wearing bifocals.[147] Bifocal contact lens corrections also have been tried with limited success.[148] Orthoptics/vision therapy exercises are frequently used to strengthen the accommodative and vergence mechanism.† We do not recom-

---

*References 25, 92-98, 104, 114, 118, 130, 147.
†References 11, 25, 92-94, 98, 104, 114, 118.

Box 3-1 **TREATING ACCOMMODATIVE INSUFFICIENCY**

- Correct all clinically significant refractive error.
- Treat the cause of debility or fatigue, if apparent.
- Use either plus lenses at the near point for convenience, or
- Use orthoptics/vision therapy exercises to achieve remediation.

mend pharmacologic remedies that have been used with poor success.[93,94]

The prognosis is generally good, although recurrences are common.[12,43] Significantly and severely reduced accommodative ability carries a substantially poorer prognosis.[105] When accommodative ability is severely reduced, we generally suggest that plus lenses be used initially, possibly with base-in prisms if there is a significant exodeviation present.[104] (Box 3-1.)

Results of Treatment

Orthoptics/vision therapy has a significant effect on accommodative ability.[2-8,149] If orthoptics/vision therapy is instituted, the accommodative amplitude can increase approximately 1 D per week (Fig. 3-6), until it reaches approximately the normal level.[43] Concurrently, over the period of treatment the amplitude and facility of accommodation, stereopsis, and fusional vergence ranges also may change significantly (Table 3-5). Training will necessitate at least 4 weeks of treatment.[43] With orthoptics/vision therapy, most cases can be successfully treated.

 CLINICAL PEARL

> If orthoptics/vision therapy is instituted, the accommodative amplitude can increase approximately 1 D per week, until it reaches approximately the normal level.

In some cases, particularly when accommodative dysfunction is combined with vergence dysfunction, a more extensive treatment period may be necessary and useful. For example, the treatment of 129 patients with combined accommodative-vergence dysfunction consisted of two 45-minute office sessions per week, with an average of 25 visits necessary to complete the treatment.[91] With this extended therapy, successful treatment occurred in 87% of the cases. Similar results with varied methods of treatment have been reported in other studies.[150,151] In one study, 24 of 26 patients with significant accommodative insufficiency and an associated convergence insufficiency improved with treatment.[108] Seventeen of the 26 became asymptomatic, although three quarters of the patients continued to exhibit deficiencies in objective criteria. Another group of patients reached normal accommodative function in an average of 4.5 sessions of training.[152]

The effective treatment of accommodative insufficiency improves not only the clinical data (e.g., accommodative amplitude) and symptoms but can also improve performance. Treated patients achieved a significant decrease in the number of errors on a pencil-and-paper task.[152] Improvements in school performance occurred as a result of a program of carefully applied orthoptics/vision therapy and other training in children with accommodative defects related to cerebral palsy.[126]

Objective assessment of improvement in accommodative amplitude also has been provided.[129] In one study a group of children with accommodative deficiencies was divided into control and treatment groups.[134] The treatment group showed improvement in accommodative ability and in visual perceptual ability, whereas the control group remained stable.

INFACILITY OF ACCOMMODATION
Definition

Infacility of accommodation is the condition in which difficulty or sluggishness occurs in the change from one level of accommodation to another.[92] Also known as *tonic accommodation* or *inertia of accommodation*, this condition is a common anomaly of accommodation.[52,90,91] When the time taken to alter focus from one distance to another consumes one second or more, an abnormal condition is present.[52] The ability to change focus is separate from the ability to eventually achieve a given level of accommodation.[153]

TABLE 3-6 SYMPTOMS IN TONIC ACCOMMODATION

Description	Frequency	Percentage (%)
Blur	9	64
Poor facility	6	43
Headaches	5	36
Asthenopia	5	36
Diplopia	4	29
Fatigue	3	21
Reading problems	2	14
Other	1	7

Modified from Daum KM: Orthoptic treatment in patients with inertia of accommodation, *Am J Optom Physiol Opt* 66(2):68, 1983.

Symptoms

Individuals with infacility of accommodation most often complain of intermittent blur when they look up from near work and poor facility in using their accommodative system (Table 3-6).[12,13,154] In some patients there are no subjective complaints, in spite of an obvious deficiency in altering focus.[12,13,15,134] Several studies have shown that low facility of accommodation tends to be correlated with asthenopia (Fig. 3-7).[53a,155]

Signs

The most significant (and sometimes the only) sign of infacility of accommodation is a poor facility of accommodation.[52] The measurement of accommodative facility is a crucial aspect of the assessment of these patients. The amplitude of accommodation is generally within the normal range.[52]

Patients with accommodative infacility not only have poor facility but also have prolonged latencies and time constants using objective means (Fig. 3-8).[153,156] This objective data, particularly the prolonged time constants, suggests that this condition is not the result of a psychogenic etiology.

Prevalence

There is a relative lack of data about the prevalence of accommodative infacility in the general population. One study found 23.3% of 60 randomly selected children who had passed a vision screening had accommodative infacility.[53a] Another study found 8.6% of controls and 22.8% of learning disabled demonstrated accommodative infacility.[157]

Etiology and Associated Conditions

The etiology of accommodative infacility is generally unknown.[139] Often, it occurs as an isolated entity. The condition has been associated with advancing scle-

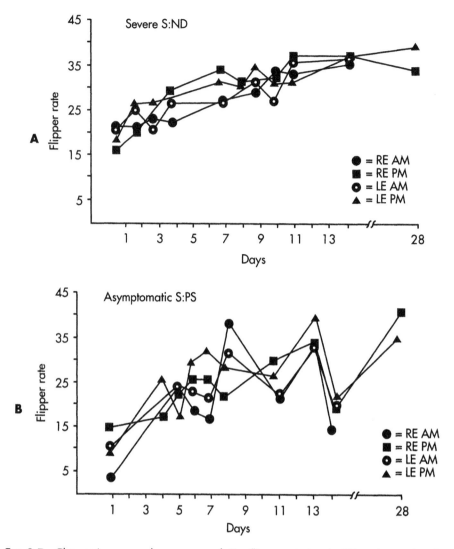

FIG. 3-7   Change in monocular accommodative flipper rate (cycles/80 sec) over time in representative asymptomatic and severely symptomatic subject for each eye and for morning and afternoon measurements. (Modified from Levine S, Ciuffreda KJ, Selenow A, Flax N: Clinical assessment of accommodative facility in symptomatic and asymptomatic individuals, *J Am Optom Assoc* 56:286, 1985.)

rosis of the lens and with some of the same factors associated with insufficiency of accommodation, such as measles, diabetes, Graves' disease, and chronic alcoholism,* migraine,[160] disturbances of the autonomic nervous system,[160] learning disability,[157] and cerebral palsy.[124-127] It has also been associated with the tonic pupil syndrome and appears to be a late phenomenon of Adie's syndrome.[12,13,15,154,158,159] One study found that 43% of individuals with infacility of accommodation also had an associated convergence insufficiency.[52] The level of accommodative facility has been shown to be equal in a matched population of normals and dyslexics.[161]

*References 12, 13, 15, 92, 153-154, 158, 159.

Diagnosis

Infacility of accommodation is frequently diagnosed on the basis of symptoms and a single test, the lens flipper test of accommodative facility. If a reliable patient reports difficulty changing focus from one level to another and the test is positive, the diagnosis is direct. If the patient is reliable and not reporting symptoms although the accommodative facility test reveals low facility, the patient should be questioned anew about ability to alter focus. If the patient is unreliable or is a child, questions about visual performance may be helpful (if performance is poor without complaints, assume that the dysfunction is present). Borderline cases generally should be monitored. Infacility of accommodation tests should be completed monocularly;

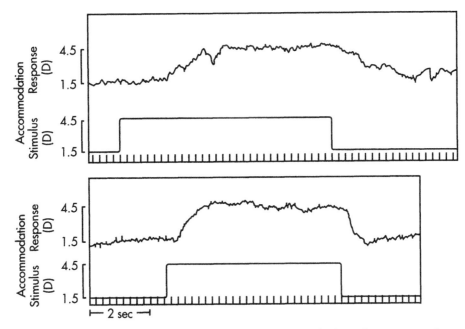

FIG. 3-8 Accommodation response of subject 2. Upper records show slow response dynamics for positive accommodation and slow, multiphasic response dynamics for relaxation of accommodation before orthoptics training. Bottom records show patient's improvement after training with faster velocities in both directions of accommodation. Note two discontinuous spikes in upper record when patient blinked; stimuli for each eye are unpredictable step changes, between targets set at 1.5 and 4.5 D. (Modified from Liu J and others: Objective assessment of accommodation orthoptics. I. Dynamic insufficiency, *Am J Optom Physiol Opt* 56:285, 1979.)

however a low binocular facility test indicates a possible vergence dysfunction. If the accommodative facility test reveals a borderline value and the symptoms are equivocal, we recommend a second evaluation on another date. If the result is again uncertain, we recommend monitoring the condition, unless the patient is a child. In these cases we typically make a tentative diagnosis and initiate treatment.

Treatment

Assuming that the underlying problem has been addressed, treatment of accommodative infacility is usually either orthoptics/vision therapy and/or a plus lens addition.[51] Initially, we recommend orthoptics/vision therapy. This consists of training directed at facility of accommodation, typically flip lens training. A training lens combination (often +/− 1.00-D lenses) is selected that can be completed at least for 4 to 5 cpm. The training is designed to repeatedly fatigue the system in a controlled fashion. Several training sessions per day (up to five) work well if the training is to be completed at home. In-office training has the advantage that compliance problems can be more easily overcome. The patient's goal is to exceed normal levels on the flipper lenses. We usually recommend training to reach 15 to 20 cpm with +/− 2.00-D lenses. In an ef-

fort to overcome boredom with the flip lens technique, we also recommend that the patient read while randomly altering the flip lenses. Alterations at sentences, paragraphs, pages, and so on stimulate the accommodative system while the patient is otherwise engaged in reading. (See Case 3.)

CASE 3

A 20-year old woman reported difficulty when attempting to change focus from distance to near. She had good visual acuities in each eye. Her phorias were orthophoria and 3PD exophoria at distance and near, respectively. Her refraction was low myopia (−0.50 DS and −0.25 −0.50 × 090, right and left). Near point of convergence was 7 cm, and vergences were within normal ranges. Accommodative amplitude was 9 D in each eye. Accommodative facility with the +/− 2-D flipper was only 5 cpm (monocular).

The refraction was prescribed for distance wear, which improved vision. Accommodative infacility was diagnosed, and accommodative flip lens training was prescribed. Over approximately 6 weeks the symptoms gradually disappeared and accommodative facility improved to 12 cpm with +/− 2-D lenses.

In situations in which the patient is older, does not wish to complete training, or is unable to comply with the requirements of training, we provide plus lens addi-

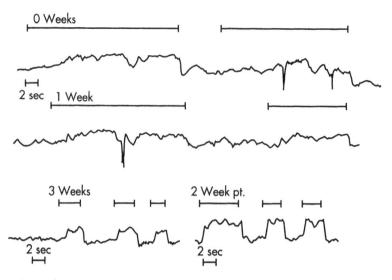

FIG. 3-9 Photorefractive records of subject JJ. Accommodative responses shown were taken at 0 (no training), 1, and 3 weeks of training and 3 weeks posttraining *(PT)*. Stimulus bars represent illumination of near target. Significant improvement of accommodative response occurred at 3 weeks and was maintained during the posttraining interval. (Modified from Bobier WR, Sivak JG: Orthoptic treatment of subjects showing slow accommodative responses, *Am J Optom Physiol Opt* 60(8):678, 1983.)

tions. Typically, a bifocal prescription, often a progressive addition lens, is most successful. The magnitude of the lenses should be the smallest possible providing immediately clear and comfortable vision when changing from distance to near. The patient should be examined while wearing the tentative add. If the add is correct, dynamic retinoscopy when completed through the add should range from +0.25 to +0.75 D (Box 3-2.)

 CLINICAL PEARL

In situations in which the patient is older, does not wish to complete training, or is unable to comply with the requirements of training, we provide plus lens additions.

Results of Treatment

Many studies have demonstrated that accommodative infacility is treatable using orthoptics/vision therapy. Over the course of treatment the facility of accommodation in one group of 14 patients being treated with flip lens training was significantly improved.[52] Liu and others[156] objectively demonstrate decreases in the latencies and time constants of accommodation and an improvement in facility with orthoptics/vision therapy (Fig. 3-8). Bobier and Sivak[162] also have shown improvements in the latency, movement time, and response time in a study of five patients with poor facility of accommodation, as a result of orthoptics/vision therapy (Fig. 3-9). These investigators used a dynamic photorefractive technique and concluded that orthop-

---

BOX 3-2 TREATING ACCOMMODATIVE INFACILITY

- Correct any significant refractive error.
- Address any discoverable underlying problem causing fatigue or stress.
- Use orthoptics/vision therapy to treat the problem.
- Consider plus lens additions if training is not desired or is unsuccessful.

---

tics/vision therapy is a useful and valid technique for solving the problems of patients with infacility of accommodation. The changes in the dynamic aspects of accommodation were independent of changes in the amplitude of accommodation, suggesting that the changes were unlikely to be peripheral in nature.

Improvements in the dynamic components of accommodation with training over a 7-day period have been documented.[149] Others have shown that patients could learn to accommodate while wearing −9.00-D contact lens, suggesting that they could learn to control essentially their entire accommodative ability and alter the level with voluntary control.[3] Another study reviewed records of 129 patients who had undergone orthoptics/vision therapy treatment of accommodative insufficiency or infacility problems, 87% of whom had

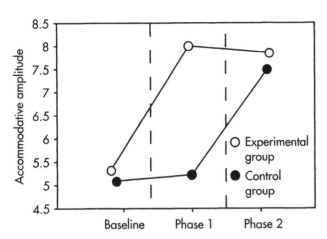

FIG. 3-10 Abscissa depicts three phases of testing, that is, baseline, phase 1, and phase 2. Mean accommodative amplitude for all patients in each phase (determined by minus lens to blur) is plotted on ordinate. Open circles ○ represent patients who received experimental, accommodative training during phase 1 and placebo training during phase 2. Closed circles ● represent patients who received the opposite condition, that is, phase 1, control (placebo); and phase 2, experimental. (Modified from Cooper J and others: Reduction of asthenopia after accommodative facility training, *Am J Optom Physiol Opt* 64(6):430, 1987.)

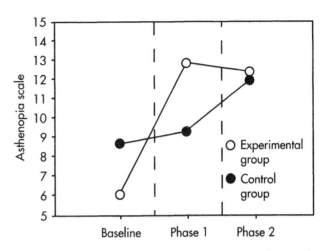

FIG. 3-11 Mean asthenopia scores are presented on ordinate, whereas phases of testing are presented on the abscissa. Open circles ○ represent patients who received experimental therapy first; closed circles ● represent those patients who received placebo therapy first. (Modified from Cooper J and others: Reduction of asthenopia after accommodative facility training, *Am J Optom Physiol Opt* 64(6):430, 1987.)

a successful outcome.[91] Others have reported similar results.[43,163]

Successful treatment of infacility of accommodation using orthoptics/vision therapy in a population of children with cerebral palsy has also been reported.[124-127] Before treatment, 100% failed the +/− 2.00-D lenses flip test; after treatment, 57% could complete the same flip lenses test. The treatment was associated with improved performance and attention of the children to near tasks.

Cooper and others[131] completed a matched-subjects, cross-over design study testing the effect of accommodative facility training on five subjects with accommodative infacility. To control for the placebo effect, the subjects were divided into control and experimental groups (Fig. 3-10).[131] Statistical changes for accommodative amplitude and asthenopia occurred for the groups who underwent training using the test lenses but did not occur for the groups using the plano lenses (Fig. 3-11).[131] This significant study was not contaminated by many of the methodologic problems of studies of the treatment of accommodative infacility, most significantly the lack of a control group. Orthoptics/vision therapy was confirmed as the source of the changes in accommodative ability. Other data show plasticity in the accommodative (and vergence) system in response to prolonged near work and to changes in the optical relationship of vergence and accommodation.[164 166]

FATIGUE OF ACCOMMODATION
Definition

Fatigue of accommodation is the condition in which the accommodative amplitude is within the normal range but is sustained only with effort and soon (or eventually) gives out.[92] It is akin to insufficiency of accommodation and is relatively infrequently diagnosed, probably because the symptomology is not severe and objective findings can be elusive.[90] Fatigue of accommodation is a harbinger of impending difficulties with the accommodative system.

Symptoms

The symptoms reported are those reported in virtually all accommodative dysfunction, that is, blur and/or asthenopia, usually commencing after a period of near work.[110,167-169] These symptoms are not usually severe.

Signs

Frequently, the only sign of fatigue of accommodation is a reduced amplitude of accommodation with repetition.[35,170] The repeated measurement of accommodative amplitude with the push-up technique is the best method of detecting the problem.[35]

Associated Conditions

Many of the same factors associated with insufficiency of accommodation have also been linked with fatigue of accommodation.[92] Overall debilitation and fatigue, myasthenia gravis, poor lighting, and low oxygen tension in the air because of high altitude or a rebreathing apparatus have been shown to produce fatigue in the accommodative system.[122,170-172] Fatigue of accommodation may be an additional feature of insufficiency of accommodation.[93] Nursing women are particularly susceptible, as are any other individuals who are chronically fatigued.[133]

Etiology

The normal accommodative system is quite flexible and resistant to fatigue.[35,36,172-174] Lancaster and Williams[36] have shown that with prolonged accommodation the punctum proximum (near point) moves nearer to the eye (1 to 4 D), rather than fatigues and moves away.[35] Only after 30 minutes or longer of accommodation did the near point recede even slightly in most cases. Lancaster and Williams attributed these changes to the viscosity of the crystalline lens.

Several early investigators studied the fatigue of accommodation using ophthalmic ergographs, which are still being marketed.*[170,174,175] Of a group of asthenopic subjects, 69% showed no evidence of fatigue of accommodation over a 15-minute period.[172] A correlation exists between objective evidence of fatigue (recession of the near point) and the report of blur by the subject (r = 0.69). There is a lower correlation coefficient (r = 0.46) between a normal near point of accommodation for the individual's age and the presence of fatigue, suggesting that fatigue of accommodation is a separate entity from accommodative insufficiency.

Each of 19 subjects using an ergographic device showed an initial increase in accommodative amplitude over a period of up to 10 minutes.[35] Following the increase the amplitude remained at a constant level over a test period of 20 minutes. Of a variety of test procedures, repeated alternation of fixation from far point to near point and vice versa most often produced fatigue in the accommodative system. Fatigue was only rarely found, and a single recording of fatigue often could not be repeated. If an individual showed fatigue on two or more successive tests, the phenomenon was consistently present.

The site of accommodative fatigue is not likely to be at the accommodative apparatus in the eye or at the extraocular muscles because no change in the AC/A ratio occurred with fatigue.[24,35] The fatigue process likely is a central nervous system condition, in as much as peripheral changes would produce a changed AC/A.

Diagnosis

A diagnosis of fatigue of accommodation is generally a result of the patient's description of symptoms beginning after a period of near work in concert with a finding of diminished amplitude of accommodation upon repeated measurement. The diagnosis is often difficult because the symptoms are not severe.

Treatment

There have been few studies of the results of treating fatigue of accommodation.[43] The prognosis and treatment plan are similar to those for insufficiency of accommodation.[43] If the etiology is discovered, it should be treated directly. Orthoptics/vision therapy is the method of choice and is usually effective in dealing with the condition, although plus lenses at the nearpoint can also be effectively applied.[35]

SPASM OF ACCOMMODATION
Definition

Spasm of accommodation is the habitual condition in which there is an involuntary tendency to maintain accommodation in the absence of a dioptric stimulus.[92,177,178] Accommodative spasm (AS) is a greater-than-normal accommodative response for a given stimulus or demand.[179] With AS, a patient with hyperopia may appear less hyperopic, a patient with emmetropia may appear myopic, and a patient with myopia may appear more myopic.[12] AS has also been called *accommodative excess,*[14] *hyperaccommodation,*[14] *pseudomyopia,*[9,180-182] and *ciliary* spasm[178,183] and includes spasm of the near reflex. True spasm of accommodation is an unusual accommodative anomaly.[90] To date only five studies have reported case series containing 17 or more patients.[177,184-186]

✿ CLINICAL PEARL

Accommodative spasm (AS) is a greater-than-normal accommodative response for a given stimulus or demand.

AS may begin suddenly, may occur unilaterally or bilaterally (the usual case), may be constant or intermittent, and in most cases disappears with cycloplegia.[187,188] A lead of accommodation ("against" movement) is seen with dynamic retinoscopy.[14] A "physiologic" spasm of accommodation occurs after prolonged near work, which amounts to about 1.5 D or less and diminishes after about 10 minutes.[36] These temporary biases occur with a variety of conditions and produce a variety of response magnitudes.[188-190]

Symptoms

A wide variety of symptoms has been associated with spasm of accommodation.* Individuals with this condition may manifest any or all of the symptoms found in Box 3-3. Patients report variably blurred vision, uncomfortable vision with asthenopia, pain and

---

*NP Accommodation Meter, Kowa Instruments; Accommotrac vision trainer, Biofeedtrac, Inc., Brooklyn Heights, NY.

*References 10, 92, 177, 178, 180, 187, 192-196.

Box 3-3 SYMPTOMS ASSOCIATED WITH SPASM OF ACCOMMODATION

Blurred vision (sometimes variable, often worse near the end of the day)
Asthenopia
Ocular pain
Headaches
Subjective difficulties in relaxing accommodation
History of frequent changes of spectacles
History of ineffective spectacles
Micropsia/macropsia
Diplopia
Systemic problems (gastric disturbances, vomiting)

Modified from Rutstein RP, Daum KM, Amos JF: Accommodative spasm: a study of 17 cases, *J Am Optom Assoc* 59(7):527, 1988.

Box 3-4 SIGNS ASSOCIATED WITH SPASM OF ACCOMMODATION

Esophoria or esotropia (variable)
Hyperopia or anisohyperopia
Poor facility of accommodation; variable accommodation
Frequent decreases in plus power in spectacles
Variable responses
Variable suppression

Modified from Rutstein RP, Daum KM, Amos JF: Accommodative spasm: a study of 17 cases, *J Am Optom Assoc* 59(7):527, 1988.

headaches, and a sense of difficulty relaxing accommodation. These patients often experience difficulties with spectacles, such as blurred or uncomfortable vision. On occasion, diplopia or other symptoms, such as micropsia, occur. Patients in one study complained primarily of blurred vision (71%), ocular pain and fatigue (47%), and diplopia (29%).[186] The onset of the symptoms was within a year of the clinical presentation. Some cited an exact time that the symptoms began, others did not. Four patients reported symptoms lasting longer than a year, in one case up to 14 years. Seven of the patients (41%) had emotional disturbances of some type (nervous stomach, recent divorce, harassment associated with obesity, change of employment, hysterical neuroses, poor school performance, death in family).

Signs

The clinical presentation of accommodative spasm varies, making it difficult to diagnose (Box 3-4).[186] In some cases the spasm occurs for both distance and near fixation, in other cases for near only or distance only.[177] In some patients the spasm may become manifest only after prolonged testing.

Spasm of accommodation may be accompanied by heterophoria, orthophoria, or heterotropia, but usually is accompanied by esophoria or esotropia.[10,178] An accommodative spasm may occur in patients secondary to large exodeviations.[197] These patients, because of deficient fusional convergence, activate excessive accommodation and accommodative convergence in the interest of fusion (see Chapter 9, Case 6). The accommodative spasm is not present when the patient is not binocular.

Long-standing shifts in accommodative level occur with as little as 8 minutes of work.[22,164,189] The precise

relationship of such shifts in the resting focus of accommodation to the clinical picture of spasm of accommodation has not been demonstrated.

A profile of 17 patients with AS has been compiled.[186] The visual acuity of these patients was generally 20/30 or better. The mean spheric refraction with cycloplegia was 0.45 D hyperopia, almost exactly the mean of the population. The noncycloplegic spheric refraction was 0.16 D hyperopia. The difference between cycloplegic and noncycloplegic refractions exceeded 0.50 D in only two patients. No patient had astigmatism exceeding 1.0 D or anisometropia exceeding 0.50 D. Spasm of the near reflex (SNR), as discussed below, occurred in 10 of these patients (59%). Some of the patients also experienced marked blepharospasm.

The spasm of accommodation was intermittent and variable. Measuring the precise degree of spasm with dynamic retinoscopy was difficult because of the variability of the response. The magnitude of the "against" movement ranged from 0.75 to 5 D (mean, 2.4 D).[186] Patients with SNR overaccommodated to a greater degree (mean, 3.2 D) than those not manifesting SNR (mean, 1.4 D).[186]

Many patients demonstrated constricted and tubular visual fields and had a probable psychogenic component to the etiology. In tubular fields the linear size of the visual field is identical and reduced at both 1- and 2-m testing distances using the tangent screen. Similar visual fields occur with psychogenic amblyopia (see Chapter 2). Patients with abnormal visual fields tended to overaccommodate more than those with normal fields (2.6 vs. 1.7 D).[186]

Prevalence

AS is an uncommon clinical entity. Some early investigators doubted its existence.[198] One report of 114 patients with accommodative disorders included only 3 (2.6%) diagnosed with AS.[10] An examination using dynamic retinoscopy of the accommodative status of 721 school-age children demonstrated only eight children (1%) with an overaccommodation of 0.5 D or greater.[199] Several reports about AS have occurred in the Russian literature.[196,200-207] AS seems to occur most frequently in young, serious, and conscientious individuals.[186] Over age 40, AS is nonexistent or rare. Studies have consistently reported AS more frequently in females than males, the proportion of females ranging from 65% to 82% of the patients.[177,184-186]

Etiology

The etiology of spasm of accommodation is nearly always speculative.[139] Most of the studies have concluded that the condition is functional in origin.[186] Some have emphasized causes associated with overstimulation of the ciliary apparatus as a result of uncorrected or improperly corrected refractive errors.[194,208,209] Many clinicians have reported differences between the subjective and objective refraction, as well as differences between cycloplegic and noncycloplegic refraction.[12,193,194]

A review of 30 patients with AS concluded that eyes not affected with refractive error or anisometropia were unlikely to develop AS.[177] This series was discovered in the examination of 20,289 patients (prevalence 0.15%). Patients with hyperopia and/or mixed astigmatism who rejected their true correction and rejected minus lenses were at risk for spasm of accommodation. Compound hyperopic astigmatism occurred in 76% of the AS patients, 45% having more than 2 D of hyperopia. In addition, 76% had anisometropia, and 50% had more than 1.5 D of astigmatism. Prangen[177] concludes that AS could not occur without an underlying refractive error, often with a reinforcement from some secondary cause, usually a psychogenic disorder or focal infection. Most of these patients probably had latent hyperopia. Fenton[185] found an average cycloplegic refraction of 4 D of hyperopia in 17 patients with AS. Accordingly, the condition should be suspected when the amplitude of accommodation is abnormally low.[12] Prescribing 0.5 D less than the cycloplegic findings eliminated the symptoms for these patients.

Alexander[194] claimed that improperly corrected astigmatism led to AS as a result of the constant variation of accommodation in the desire to see different meridional aspects of objects clearly. Smith[209] also reported that AS has a refractive substrate, especially astigmatism causing the patient to actively accommodate.

Rutstein, Daum, and Amos[186] and Cogan and Freese[184] did not report significant hyperopia in their series of 17 and 16 patients, respectively. This contradicts earlier reports that suggested uncorrected or improperly corrected refractive errors are frequently associated with AS or at least suggests that AS can occur without significant refractive error.

Other suspected causes have included extensive near work*; imbalances, such as convergence insufficiency[12,19,193-195,197]; convergence excess[10,12,210]; latent hyperphoria[195]; underlying emotional factors[10,177,187,211]; or disorders of visual perception.[206] Accommodative spasm may be induced in some patients by an intense, glaring light, such as the light during retinoscopy.[12,194] Viewing through an improperly set lens for long periods when performing fundus photography can induce AS.[212] Extensive near work alters the resting focus of accommodation, and accommodative adaptation takes longer than vergence adaptation.[72,213]

A wide variety of ocular and systemic drugs may induce AS. Ocular pharmaceutic agents such as carbachol, isoflurophate, neostigmine, physostigmine, and pilocarpine, along with systemic drugs such as guanethidine, morphine, opium, isosorbide dinitrate, and methylene blue have all been associated with AS.[214-218]

Associated Conditions

Several conditions have been associated with accommodative spasm, including emotional disturbances, inadequate or variable fusional vergences, overwork, fatigue, disorders of visual perception, and hyperopia (latent, uncorrected).[180,186,194,195] Organic anomalies, such as dental, nasal, and meningeal inflammations, irritative lesions of the brain stem, migraine, head injury, pupillotonia, ciliary muscle inflammation, diabetes mellitus, measles, and myasthenia gravis have also been associated with spasm of accommodation.†

Accommodative Spasm in Conjunction with Convergence Spasm

Definition

Intermittent esotropia (overconvergence), miosis, and accommodative spasm comprise spasm of the near reflex (SNR).[184,223-227] Esotropia occurs when the accommodative spasm is large enough to also give an excess of convergence. Limited abduction mimicking lateral rectus paresis has been associated with SNR.[211,224,227-231] A patient with SNR is discussed in Chapter 7 (see Fig. 7-16 and Case 6).

The condition is relatively infrequently diagnosed and, as mentioned earlier, is often misdiagnosed.[223] Five patients with SNR were diagnosed with bilateral lateral rectus paresis, and some had undergone unnecessary surgery.[224] Two patients were treated for ocular myasthenia.[233] The most significant clue in distinguishing myasthenic weakness from SNR is pupillary weakness.[233] SNR always manifests a strong pupillary miosis, whereas ocular myasthenia does not.[233]

---

*References 10, 12, 92, 177, 178, 194.
†References 10, 12, 168, 177, 192, 193, 219, 220.

TABLE 3-7 **CLINICAL CHARACTERISTICS OF LATENT HYPEROPIA AND ACCOMMODATIVE SPASM**

Characteristic	Latent Hyperopia	Spasm of Accommodation Accommodative Excess (Pseudomyopia)	Spasm of Near Reflex (SNR)
Refractive error	Hyperopia (often high)	Varies (frequently emmetropia)	Varies (frequently emmetropia)
Visual acuity	Good to fair (depends on the degree of hyperopia)	Varies (may be somewhat reduced)	Varies (markedly reduced during spasm)
Diplopia	Rare	No	Yes
Dynamic retinoscopy	Usually an extended lag (large "with" movement)	A lead ("against" movement)	Lead (large "against" movement)
Action or effect of accommodation	Equals or is less than the hyperopia	Exceeds the basic refractive error	Exceeds the basic refractive error
Amplitude of accommodation	Often reduced	Normal	Normal
Pupils	Normal	Normal	Miotic
Convergence spasm	No	No	Yes
Motility	Normal	Normal	Usually limited abduction simulating lateral rectus paresis
Etiology	Undercorrected refractive error	Typically psychogenic; rarely organic	Typically psychogenic; rarely organic

Modified from Rutstein RP, Daum KM, Amos JF: Accommodative spasm: a study of 17 cases, *J Am Optom Assoc* 59(7):527, 1988.

Symptoms

Patients with SNR report symptoms, including intermittent blurred vision, intermittent diplopia, pain, dizziness, and nausea, that are identical to those reported with AS, although the intensity may be greater.[186,223]

Signs

SNR is characterized by an intermittent and variable esotropia, primarily at the near point. It is provoked by near work and manifests an intermittent spasm of accommodation of a substantial amount. There is also deficient and variable abduction during the spasm, along with miotic pupils.[186,223]

Etiology

A strong psychogenic factor is generally accepted in the etiology of SNR.[186] The presence of constricted and tubular visual fields confirms a psychogenic factor that may not be obvious to the clinician.[184,186,224] Organic causes are very rare but should be considered.[168,186,212] Etiologies such as cerebellar tumor or Arnold-Chiari malformation (both posterior fossa abnormalities), pituitary adenoma, vestibulopathy, and head trauma have been reported.[225,226] Some of these patients showed papilledema and/or nystagmus that are not seen in psychogenic etiologies. None of the seven patients in the series with organic etiologies had signs of emotional disturbance or complained of significant visual disability.[186,225,226] Most clinicians emphasize the psychogenic nature of SNR and have concluded that a neurologic examination is not necessary for patients with SNR.[186,227-229]

Associated Conditions

Many conditions have been reported in conjunction with SNR, including hysteria or neurosis, cerebral palsy, labyrinth pathology, head trauma, encephalitis, tumors, mesencephalic lesions, tabes dorsalis, and myotonic dystrophy.[186,223]

Diagnosis

Confirming the variable nature of the syndrome is important. Dynamic retinoscopy is critical to establishing overaccommodation. Any time an esotropia (or any significant esodeviation) is detected, dynamic retinoscopy is critical to an accurate diagnosis. A close examination of the pupils during the spasm reveals the pupillary involvement. The cover test can be confusing because the spasm and the resulting esotropia occur irregularly, producing inconsistent information. In addition, retinoscopy and refraction may be difficult because of the intermittent nature of the spasm and apparent variation in refractive error.

Treatment

The treatment of SNR is similar in nature to that of accommodative spasm (see below). Because it is an end-stage form of accommodative spasm the treatment often is prolonged and difficult.

Differential Diagnosis

Latent hyperopia, AS, and SNR are sometimes confused. Table 3-7 presents a classification system for these anomalies.[186] Historically, many clinicians have classified latent hyperopia as a form of AS. This concept may have its roots in Donders' original description.[19] With respect to a zero level of accommodation, patients with latent hyperopia have a chronically elevated level of accommodation, but the response is a compensatory action that serves to correct the hyperopia and improve visual acuity, rather than a spastic action. The time necessary for the ciliary body to relax is related to its chronic use. Latent hyperopia is the condition in which the patient's true refractive error is greater than is manifested by noncycloplegic techniques.[230] These individuals are usually significantly hyperopic and may show an extended lag of accommodation as measured by dynamic retinoscopy.[233] The accommodative response in these cases appears to be a compensatory adaptation in the interest of clear vision.[198] In contrast, spasm of accommodation patients have a lead of accommodation, generally of 0.75 D or greater.[186] Cases of AS can be further classified as either *accommodative excess (pseudomyopia)* or *SNR* (Table 3-7). Unlike latent hyperopia the accommodative response in these cases is not useful to the patient because the overaccommodation blurs vision. Some have suggested that any AS involves the near triad, and that the difference between AS and SNR is only one of degree.[142] From this perspective, pupillary miosis and convergence occur to a noticeable extent in SNR and not in spasm.

Measuring accommodative response is critical in the diagnosis of AS.[142] If a lead of accommodation is clearly present, AS is a relatively straightforward diagnosis, assuming proper correction of the patient. Recognition of the variable esodeviation of these patients is also useful in making a diagnosis. Intermittent esotropia without accommodative involvement does not manifest the accommodative lead. The deviation in intermittent esotropias also is less variable. The cover test can be difficult to interpret until the anomaly is recognized, because the deviation occurs unpredictably.

Treatment

The treatment of spasm of accommodation varies considerably. Most authorities concur that removing the underlying cause is essential.[186] The specific therapy for alleviating the spasm has included removing the cause of the fatigue of the patient*; short-acting cycloplegic agents[12,193]; long-acting cycloplegic agents[12,177,181,182]; miotics and plus lenses[10,12,192,234,235]; minus lenses[184,193]; orthoptic/vision therapy training;† placebo therapy[238]; occlusion[239]; hypnosis[186]; electrical shock therapy[205]; blurring[202]; and ultrasound.[240]

The most efficacious form of treatment is removal of the cause of the patient's fatigue and prescription of the maximum plus (least minus) correction. The cautious application of orthoptics/vision therapy aimed at

strengthening the accommodative system in concert with plus lenses at near to minimize the necessity for accommodation is also useful. Orthoptics/vision therapy training for this condition is aimed at increasing the flexibility of the accommodative system, using alternate plus and minus lenses and plus acceptance.[206] Push-up training is contraindicated for these patients.

Gradually reducing the strength of the minus lenses and prescribing plus reading glasses or bifocals to prevent accommodation has been used to treat the condition.[181] We do not recommend the use of added minus lenses because these induce rather than inhibit accommodation.[184,193]

Generally, we do not recommend the use of pharmacologic agents to treat AS, although they have long been used.[12,177,181,182,193] This is an uncomfortable solution for patients because of the pain and discomfort associated with the instillation of the drops and the photophobia from the resultant mydriasis. The administration of cycloplegic agents may be useful in difficult cases.

Results of Treatment

In one study, 12 patients were treated with plus reading lenses to inhibit the excessive accommodation.[186] Four of these also underwent orthoptics/vision therapy training using flipper lenses.[14,202] One patient had been treated with atropine by his referring physician. Four were treated with psychologic counseling. Two others were not treated.

Fourteen of these patients were followed for periods ranging from 2 to 30 months. Total resolution of the anomaly (an alleviation of symptoms, no overaccommodation with dynamic retinoscopy, and normal visual fields) occurred in four patients (29%). The remaining patients continued to experience a spasm of some degree, with various degrees of alleviation of symptoms and fields.

The modest success of such a variety of forms of treatment is probably related to the common psychogenic etiology of the condition. An important portion of the treatment is to reassure the patient during the course of treatment.

Summary

Spasm of accommodation does not have to be associated with refractive error, most patients have emmetropia. Diagnosis should be based on dynamic retinoscopy (an "against" reflex). Most cases have a psychogenic etiology indicated by the case history and visual fields. In these cases a significant portion of therapy may be counseling. We recommend treating most patients with the most plus (least minus) correction of refraction, a plus lens addition at the near point, and, in some cases, orthoptics/vision therapy.

---

*References 177, 178, 180, 187, 194, 195.
†References 12, 14, 178, 180, 187, 195, 202, 206, 236, 237.

PARESIS OF ACCOMMODATION

Definition

Paresis (or paralysis) of accommodation is an accommodative dysfunction with a direct organic etiology. The pupil is usually involved.[93]

> There is no hard and fast line between paralysis and insufficiency of accommodation. Any insufficiency of considerable amount may be called paresis and one that is complete or nearly so a paralysis. The terms paresis and paralysis, are especially applied to marked insufficiencies of sudden development and either of toxic or due to organic lesions of the nervous system. But this is a distinction hard to draw and maintain.[92]

 CLINICAL PEARL

Paresis (or paralysis) of accommodation is an accommodative dysfunction with a direct organic etiology.

Symptoms

Patients with paresis of accommodation report some or all of the following: near blur, photophobia (because of the dilated pupil), diplopia (because of the frequently associated incomitant strabismus), micropsia, and headaches.[10,12] The onset is generally sudden and often is unilateral, with the pupil and extraocular musculature involved, in relation to lesions affecting the ipsilateral oculomotor nerve.[243] The diplopia may be restricted to a particular gaze, depending on the associated incomitant strabismus.

Signs

Although the initial picture may mimic a functional anomaly the signs of paresis of accommodation are markedly different. The signs are ipsilateral decreased amplitude of accommodation; ipsilateral mydriatic, possibly nonreactive pupil; and incomitant strabismus.[243] The involvement of the pupil and the incomitant strabismus set this condition apart from functional losses of accommodation. Accommodative ability is consistently poor, even with rest.[110]

Etiology

Many factors may be involved in the etiology of paresis of accommodation. These include the following (1) dental infections or caries[92-94,116,119,243]; (2) tonsillar infections[243-247]; (3) grippe[32]; (4) infectious mononucleosis[247]; (5) encephalitis[248,249]; (6) cerebral disease[32]; (7) diphtheria[92,133,153]; (8) malaria[133]; (9) syphilis[32,92,94]; (10) hysteria[94,247,248]; (11) toxic systemic conditions[32]; (12) mumps[247,248]; (13) childbirth[247,248]; (14) lactation[32]; (15) infectious hepatitis[247,248]; (16) pharmacologic agents (particularly parasympatholytic agents)[92]; (17) trauma[92,100,128,248]; (18) psychotherapeutic drugs (phenothiazine derivatives)[250]; (19) lesions of the parasympathetic nuclei in the midbrain[247,248]; (20) ciliary ganglionitis[248]; (21) anoxia[32,122]; (22) excessive near work[32]; (23) poor lighting[32]; (24) a variety of toxins[12,92,153]; (25) food poisoning[12]; (26) Guillain-Barré syndrome and Wilson's disease[252]; (27) exhaustion[32]; (28) distocia[32]; (29) scarlet fever, malaria, and typhoid fever[133,247,248]; (30) viral diseases, such as measles, zoster, and influenza[133,153,247,248]; (31) botulism[247]; (32) Adie's syndrome[154,158,159]; (33) diabetes mellitus[12,32,248]; and (34) idiopathic factors.[153]

The loss of accommodation associated with ciliary muscle dysfunction in Adie's tonic pupil syndrome is more likely to present within the first 2 years of developing the condition.[154] Patients who had Adie's tonic pupil syndrome for longer than 2 years had a decreased accommodative amplitude of 0.7 D, compared with the fellow normal eye.[154]

Guillain-Barré syndrome, also known as *acute idiopathic polyneuritis,* does not usually present with paresis of accommodation. Only 1 of 40 patients with the syndrome had a paralysis of accommodation. The loss of accommodation in Wilson's disease can be severe and seems to be supranuclear in origin.[251]

Diagnosis

Paresis of accommodation of peripheral etiology is often unilateral; cases with a central etiology are nearly always bilateral.[93] As mentioned before, an organic loss of accommodation is accompanied by other signs involving the pupil and the extraocular musculature. A loss of accommodation and a mydriatic pupil in a patient with incomitant exotropia usually indicates paresis of the oculomotor nerve. Depending on the location of the lesion the particular features vary. Generally, the incomitant deviation and the associated diplopia are more obvious than the accommodative dysfunction (see Case 1). Because unraveling the type of incomitancy can be confusing and pupillary findings can sometimes be overlooked, the accommodative deficit can be helpful in suggesting that there is an organic etiology. The presence of a larger pupil on the same side as the accommodative dysfunction is an important confirmatory sign.

Treatment

Foremost in dealing with paresis of accommodation is to deal with the etiology.[10] Often this should include imaging of the head, because tumors are a possible cause of the problem. In this regard the possibility of a paretic (organic) etiology should be considered for every accommodative problem.

Once appropriate care for the etiology has been rendered, relief of the symptoms can be accomplished using additional plus lenses (possibly combined with base-in prism) at near.[12,95] On occasion, patients are more comfortable with a unilateral addition. Orthoptics/vision therapy may be useful in the recovery stages.[12,98]

The prognosis for recovery is generally considered good.[12] Recovery, if it occurs, usually occurs within 3 to 4 weeks.[12] The condition may be considered permanent after that time.[12]

UNEQUAL ACCOMMODATION
Definition

Unequal accommodation is the condition in which the accommodative ability is unequal between the two eyes. Differences in either accommodative amplitude or facility can occur. Spasm of accommodation in only one eye has been reported.[187] Unequal accommodation is a very unusual anomaly but occasionally occurs.[92,93] Accommodative ability is usually equal within 0.25 D between the eyes (which is the accuracy of the measurement technique).[163,252]

Apparently unequal accommodative ability should not be classified in this category. For example, the accommodative amplitude is sometimes measured lower (or higher) for the right eye as a result of factors related to the measurement technique or the motivation of the patient. Patients may give more (or less) of an effort to perform the test after one eye is measured. Proper measurement technique includes a reassessment of the amplitudes of accommodation whenever a difference is determined. Other factors related to the measurement technique can cause differences, such as parallax errors, in measuring the endpoint of accommodation, suggesting in error a difference in amplitude. Similar errors can occur in the measurement of accommodative facility.

Differential anisoaccommodation is possible.[253] The magnitude is generally limited to approximately 0.75 D or less and is nearly always accompanied by eyestrain and headache. Anisoaccommodation may occur during near viewing, when the balance between the refractive correction of the eyes is improper.

Symptoms

Symptoms associated with unequal accommodation are blurred vision (at distance and/or near); discomfort and asthenopia, especially with near work; poor depth perception; photophobia; and headache.[154] Diplopia can occur secondary to an associated strabismus. Occasionally, patients report a sensitivity to differences in accommodation between the eyes.[154]

Signs

The signs of unequal accommodation include unequal accommodative amplitude, possibly along with other signs of third cranial nerve dysfunction, such as mydriasis and exotropia. Frequently, a loss of accommodative facility is also present.[154] The accommodative amplitude in the affected eye ranges from slight to an essential absence of accommodation on one side.

With Adie's syndrome, a frequent cause of unequal accommodation, patients also sometimes report fluctuating accommodation.[154] Pupillary dysfunction is the rule with Adie's syndrome.[154] The average pupil changes size over the course of the syndrome, being at first mydriatic and moving toward miosis with time. The pupil reacts very poorly if at all to light and reacts to accommodation in a tonic fashion, hence the tonic pupil syndrome. Hypersensitivity to direct-acting parasympathomimetic agents (e.g., pilocarpine, 0.25%) may be present. Adie's tonic syndrome that spares the pupil but affects the accommodative system has been reported.[154]

Accommodation is profoundly affected with the onset of Adie's syndrome. The amplitude tends to drop very low with the onset of the condition and then recovers over a period of several years. The condition tends to become bilateral, although frequently years pass between one eye and the other being affected. With Adie's syndrome an induced astigmatism upon attempted accommodation may be present.[154]

Etiology

Normally, the accommodative function between the two eyes is identical, suggesting the reception of innervational information from a common neural center.[190,254] Associated pupillary dysfunction, such as in Adie's syndrome, suggests a neurologic etiology.[92,158,159] Unilateral cataract also may cause unequal accommodation.[92] Other factors associated with unequal accommodation are unilateral peripheral involvements, such as glaucoma and trauma; contusions of the eyeball; mydriatics; and inability of the eyes to respond to a stimulus to accommodation (e.g., amblyopia).[32,39,128] Frequently the etiology is unknown.[93]

Diagnosis

Unequal accommodation is infrequently diagnosed. Most often the condition is related to either paresis of accommodation or, as in our clinic, to Adie's tonic pupil syndrome. Other causes are frequently obscure or overlooked. For example, unequal accommodation secondary to a poor refractive balance is rarely discovered. Poor balances seldom miss by even as much as a diopter, a difference that is often overlooked in measuring accommodative amplitude. A major responsibility of the clinician is to make sure any organic etiology is appropriately handled with neuroimaging or otherwise.

Treatment

As with other anomalies, if the cause is treatable, it should be addressed first. In cases such as Adie's syndrome, for example, no direct treatment is available.

Unequal adds may be useful. Orthoptics/vision therapy may be useful in the recovery stage.

SECONDARY ANOMALIES OF ACCOMMODATION
Definition

Secondary anomalies of accommodation are not true anomalies of accommodation. They are only apparent anomalies of accommodation resulting from interaction of the accommodative system with some other binocular or refractive anomaly. Secondary anomalies of accommodation are most obvious when binocular testing is undertaken for accommodation rather than testing of each eye individually. Conditions affecting the vergence system, such as convergence insufficiency or convergence excess, can cause significant binocular dysfunction of accommodation. The apparent accommodative dysfunction only is present when accommodation is active under the binocular situation and is actually the response of the accommodative system to vergence problems. In some cases the accommodative system responds to assist the convergence system to alleviate symptoms and/or diplopia via the accommodative-convergence linkage.

 CLINICAL PEARL

The apparent accommodative dysfunction only is present when accommodation is active under the binocular situation and is actually the response of the accommodative system to vergence problems.

Symptoms

Symptoms described by patients with secondary anomalies of accommodation are those associated with the primary binocular anomaly. These are typically nonspecific and may include any or all of the following: blur (often intermittent and variable), asthenopia, headaches, and diplopia. Most often, difficulties are reported associated with a period of near work. Symptoms also can be a result of binocular visual stress at distance or some intermediate distance.

Signs

The sign of a secondary anomaly of accommodation is reduced accommodation when testing is completed binocularly. Usually with monocular testing, accommodation is normal. Other accommodative signs of a primary binocularity problem for exodeviations include a low negative relative accommodation (NRA) value and a high positive relative accommodation (PRA) value, a low lag or a lead of accommodation, and inadequate positive fusional vergences. Esodeviation types of problems often show a high NRA value and a low PRA value, a high lag of accommodation, and inadequate negative fusional vergence. Deviations secondary to an exodeviation or an esodeviation may manifest an apparently decreased binocular amplitude and/or facility of accommodation. However, the monocular amplitude and facility are not decreased.

 CLINICAL PEARL

The sign of a secondary anomaly of accommodation is reduced accommodation when testing is completed binocularly. Usually with monocular testing, accommodation is normal.

Etiology

Dynamic retinoscopy is critical to discovering the true etiology of a binocular visual problem.[57] The etiology of the secondary pseudoanomaly of accommodation is always the primary binocular dysfunction.

Associated (Primary) Conditions

Conditions that can result in an apparent or secondary anomaly of accommodation are convergence insufficiency, convergence excess, basic or equal esodeviation, or basic or equal exodeviation, as well as intermittent strabismic deviations in all of these.

Diagnosis

Proper assessment technique prevents confusion that accommodative deficiency is primary in nature. Accommodative function should be tested monocularly.

Treatment

The appropriate treatment is to deal with the primary binocular anomaly.

TREATMENT OF ACCOMMODATIVE ANOMALIES

The two basic choices in the treatment of accommodative defects are plus lens additions and orthoptics/vision therapy.[10,95,186] Accommodative defects are often related to great demands on the system that can be minimized with sufficient rest.

 CLINICAL PEARL

The two basic choices in the treatment of accommodative defects are plus lens additions and orthoptics/vision therapy.

The following are key factors in successfully treating accommodative dysfunction: (1) successfully diagnosing the problem, particularly with respect to differentiating accommodative dysfunction from vergence dysfunction; (2) clearly communicating the nature of the problem to the patient, especially the link between fatigue, stress, and overwork and accommodation problems; and (3) determining and applying the most effective treatment.

Objective

The aim of any treatment of accommodative dysfunction is to provide visual comfort, especially for near tasks; to enhance if possible the ability to alter accommodation quickly and efficiently; to ensure the ability to maintain accommodation for extended periods; and to obtain values expected for the age of the patient for amplitude, facility, and response of accommodation.

Do's and Don'ts in the Treatment of Accommodative Defects

Clinicians should consider and apply the following do's and dont's in treating patients with accomodative defects.

- *Do make a diagnosis before beginning treatment.* Because treatment options are limited, treatment is sometimes initiated without the proper formulation of the nature of the problem and an examination of possible etiologies.
- *Do let the patient choose the treatment.* Traditionally, orthoptics/vision therapy has been viewed as fixing the problem, whereas plus lenses often have been seen as a sort of a crutch. These are different options, and patients should be assisted in making an educated choice that is best suited to their needs.
- *Do explain* that orthoptics/vision therapy avoids the use of an add with its limitations and possibly the use of glasses altogether for patients with clinical emmetropia. On the other hand, note that an add can be an immediate solution and does not require the investment of time and effort that is necessary in orthoptics/vision therapy.
- *Do not consider accommodative problems insignificant.* Eyestrain and blur while reading and so on can be very disturbing and can cause significant decreases in performance.

Orthoptics/Vision Therapy vs. Plus Lenses

Several factors should be considered when determining whether to recommend orthoptic/vision therapy training or plus lenses.[103] The most significant of these factors is the patient's preference for one type of treatment or the other. A study of 114 patients with various types of accommodative dysfunction treated with orthoptics/vision therapy suggested that the age of the patient and the patient's AC/A ratio are the most significant predictors of success with orthoptics/vision therapy.[103] Patients that are closest to normal are most likely to be successful using either treatment modality.

Generally, orthoptics/vision therapy is better for young patients who are able to cooperate. As patients get older, an add is increasingly better, particularly for patients in their thirties. The prognosis for results with training at these ages is not nearly as good as for younger patients. Some data have suggested that adds are better than training, although not enough evidence has been amassed to answer the question satisfactorily.[130,150] Other data suggests approximately equal efficacy with orthoptics and lens additions.[10]

Orthoptics/Vision Therapy for Accommodation

As a result of the training process, orthoptics/vision therapy will probably make things slightly worse before it makes things better over the long term. This is an unfortunate by-product of training because it necessarily causes a certain amount of eyestrain. Effort is an important part of the training process. Patients should understand that they will get out of training what they put into it.

Because compliance with home training can be a major problem, in-office training should be undertaken if possible. Practical considerations are important in any training program. Most patients are not able to complete large amounts of training each day; 20 to 30 minutes of training a day is the maximum for most people.

Training Efficacy

Changing the ability of the accommodative system has been well documented. Objective assessment of modifications of the interactions between accommodation and vergence have been documented by several investigators.[24,156,162,255] Learning voluntary control of accommodation has been documented.[1-8,149]

Flip Lens Training

Accommodative training using flip lenses, that is, accommodative rock, is the most common type of training for accommodative dysfunction (Fig. 3-12).[10]

 CLINICAL PEARL

Accommodative training using flip lenses, that is, accommodative rock, is the most common type of training for accommodative dysfunction.

The following are important considerations when implementing flip lens training:

- The patient should be properly corrected.
- There should be adequate lighting of the near-point material and comfortable seating for the patient.
- Clear, written instructions should explain the training and reinforce the clinician's instructions.
- A log should be kept of orthoptics/vision therapy.
- Several short, intense training sessions are preferable to one long session; however, the clinician should be willing to compromise.
- Consistency in performing the training is very important. For this reason, in-office training is probably superior to in-home training.

The initial training lenses should be selected so that the patient uses a lens set that is challenging but possible.

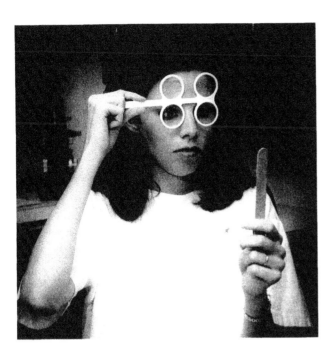

FIG. 3-12 Accommodative facility training is the most common training for accommodative dysfunction.

The patient should be able to complete at least 5 cpm with the training lenses. The lens choices are typically +/− 1.00-, +/− 1.50-, and +/− 2.00-D lens flippers.

The lenses should be changed when the patient is able to comfortably complete the goal for that set of lenses. Goals for flip lens training should be relatively high; we recommend 15 to 20 cpm with +/− 2.00-D lenses.[143] For at-home training the clinician should set a goal for the patient to reach in the first week and in the second week, until the patient is seen again; for in-office training the clinician should set a goal for the patient to reach for each session.

There are several techniques that can be used in training with the flip lenses. A push-up stick or the block of letters from a near chart should be used for a target. If a block-of-letters chart is used, the patient should read in sequence the next letter each time the lenses are alternated. The patient's task is to alternately clear the print as quickly as possible as the lenses are changed from plus to minus and vice versa. Generally, the lenses should be switched from 15 to 25 times with each eye so that the time spent training is 5 to 10 minutes per session. If in-home training is completed, the patient should keep a log book of training so that the consistency and the amount of effort that the patient is putting into the training can be evaluated. Exceptionally motivated patients should be encouraged to do more if they like, spending 30 to 45 minutes per session. For example, the patient can use a magazine, book, or other reading material for a target. The patient should alternate the lenses intermittently, such as

at every word for a while, then every sentence, then every paragraph. With each alternation of the lenses the patient should clear the reading material as quickly as possible.

Far-Near Alternating Fixation Training

Far-near alternating fixation training can be used to supplement or replace flip lens training. As before, the patient should be corrected with adequate lighting. The best method is to affix in the distance a block-letter chart (a chart containing 10 rows of 10 letters) on a wall, where the letters can be seen if in good focus. The patient holds a near block-letter chart. The patient's task is to read all of the letters on both charts, beginning with the first one at near then the first one at distance, the second one at near and the second at distance, and so on until finished. Other techniques, such as a distance chart and intermittent minus lenses or a near target and intermittent plus lenses, also can be used to stimulate accommodation.

Push-Up Training

Push-up training is a very common, easy, convenient, and effective technique.[43] The patient should be corrected with good lighting. The target can be a push-up stick with small letters attached or, alternatively, a pencil or some other material containing small lettering. The patient should hold the target at arm's length, look at the smallest row that can be seen clearly, and then bring the target in toward the face until the row of letters slightly blurs. At that point the patient should hold the material stable for a bit while attempting to clear it up; if the material clears, the patient should continue moving the target in. When the patient reaches a point at which the target cannot be cleared, the process is repeated. The whole process should be completed 5 times a day, with approximately 25 repetitions per session. Push-up training should be monitored in a log, with the patient recording the date, time, number of repetitions, and closest distance at which the target can be kept clear.

Considerations in Training

An initial decision in treatment is whether training should be monocular or binocular. If an associated vergence problem is severe, accommodation training should commence monocularly, to lessen the strain on the system. If the accommodative problem is severe and the vergence problem is not, initially the accommodative training should be binocular, to allow the vergence system to assist accommodation. Accommodative rock (flip lens) training is effective for both facility and amplitude problems; push-up is primarily for amplitude problems. Push-up training should not be selected for spasm problems.

Accommodation training is simple and easy. Patients become bored with the exact same training. Over time, the training should be altered so that various techniques are used in different ways. There are few problems in explaining to the patient how to do the training. Training of accommodation is relatively inexpensive and improvement is usually noticeable after only a short period. Improvement, of course, enhances the motivation of the patient to continue. On the other hand, the training sometimes appears unsophisticated because it is so simple and easy, which frequently interferes with the patient's motivation. Also, working hard at training causes eyestrain and fatigue that can interfere with other visual activities.

Using Plus Lenses

The minimum amount of plus lenses that will provide relief should be selected for a patient with accommodative dysfunction. The most consistent method to choose plus lenses is for the clinician to select an add and adjust its power, based on dynamic retinoscopy. If the add is of the proper strength, the lag of accommodation through the add while viewing a near-point target should be +0.25 to +0.75 D. Too much of a lag suggests that the add should be increased, too little (or a lead) suggests that the add can be decreased. The patient's comments about the magnitude of the add should also be taken into account.

 CLINICAL PEARL

The most consistent method to choose plus lenses is for the clinician to select an add and adjust its power, based on dynamic retinoscopy. If the add is of the proper strength, the lag of accommodation through the add while viewing a near-point target should be +0.25 to +0.75 D.

REFERENCES

1. Tucker J, Charman WN, Ward PA: Modulation dependence of the accommodative response to sinusoidal gratings, *Vision Res* 26:1693, 1986.
2. Roscoe SN, Couchman DH: Improving visual performance through volitional focus control, *Hum Factors* 29:311, 1987.
3. Provine RR, Enoch JM: On voluntary ocular accommodation, *Percept Psychophys* 17:209, 1975.
4. Carr H, Allen JB: A study of certain relations of accommodation and convergence to the judgment of the third dimension, *Psychol Rev* 13:258, 1906.
5. Sisson ED: A case of voluntary accommodation, *J Gen Psychol* 17:170, 1937.
6. Sisson ED: Voluntary control of accommodation, *J Gen Psychol* 18:195, 1938.
7. Marg E: An investigation of voluntary as distinguished from reflex accommodation, *Am J Optom Arch Am Acad Optom* 28:347, 1951.
8. Cornsweet TN, Crane HD: Training the visual accommodative system, *Vision Res* 13:713, 1973.
9. Brooke B: Anomalies of accommodation, *Br Orthopt J* 19:113, 1962.
10. Daum KM: Accommodative dysfunction, *Doc Ophthalmol* 55:177, 1983.
11. Theobald S: Some typical cases of "subnormal accommodative power," *Trans Am Ophthalmol Soc* 7:138, 1894.
12. Borish IM: *Clinical refraction,* ed 3, Chicago, 1970, Professional.
13. Duke-Elder S: System of ophthalmology. In Abrams D, Duke-Elder S, editors: *Ophthalmic optics and refraction,* St Louis, 1970, Mosby.
14. Griffin Jr: *Binocular anomalies: procedures for vision therapy,* ed 2, Chicago, 1982, Professional.
15. Walsh FB, Hoyt WF: *Clinical neuro-ophthalmology,* ed 3, Baltimore, 1969, Williams & Wilkins.
16. Bennett GR, Blondin M, Ruskiewicz J: Incidence and prevalence of selected visual conditions, *J Am Optom Assoc* 53:647, 1982.
17. Hokoda SC: General binocular dysfunctions in an urban optometry clinic, *J Am Optom Assoc* 56:560, 1982.
18. Wick B, Hall P: Relation among accommodative facility, lag, and amplitude in elementary school children, *Am J Optom Physiol Opt* 64:593, 1987.
19. Donders FC: *On the anomalies of accommodation and refraction of the eye,* London, 1864, Hatton.
20. Schor CM, Kotulak JC, Tseutaki T: Adaptation of tonic accommodation reduces accommodative lag and is masked in darkness, *Invest Ophthalmol Vis Sci* 27:820, 1986.
21. Schor CM: Analysis of tonic and accommodative vergence disorders of binocular vision, *Am J Optom Physiol Opt* 60:1, 1983.
22. Schor CM: The Glenn A Fry Award Lecture: adaptive regulation of accommodative vergence and vergence accommodation, *Am J Optom Physiol Opt* 63:587, 1986.
23. Schor CM, Kotulak JC: The dissociability of accommodation from vergence in the dark, *Invest Ophthalmol Vis Sci* 27:544, 1986.
24. Schor CM, Tseutaki TK: Fatigue of accommodation and vergence modifies their mutual interaction, *Invest Ophthalmol Vis Sci* 28:1250, 1987.
25. Duane A: Studies in monocular and binocular accommodation with their clinical applications, *Am J Ophthalmol* 5:865, 1922.
26. Bernstein F, Bernstein M: Law of physiologic aging as derived from long-range data on refraction of the human eye, *Arch Ophthalmol* 34:378, 1945.
27. Slataper FJ: Age norms of refraction and vision, *Arch Ophthalmol* 43:466, 1950.
28. Sheard C: Dynamic skiametry, *Am J Optom* 6:609, 1929.
29. Eskridge JD: Clinical objective assessment of the accommodative response, *J Am Optom Assoc* 60:272, 1989.
30. Woodhouse JM and others: Reduced accommodation in children with Down syndrome, *Invest Ophthalmol Vis Sci* 34:2382, 1993.
31. Rutstein RP, Fuhr PD, Swiatocha J: Comparing the amplitude of accommodation determined objectively and subjectively, *Optom Vis Sci* 70:496, 1993.
32. Hofstetter HW: A comparison of Duane's and Donders' tables of the amplitude of accommodation, *Am J Optom Arch Am Acad Optom* 21:345, 1944.
33. Braddick O, Atkinson J, French J: A photorefractive study of infant accommodation, *Vision Res* 19:1319, 1979.
34. Banks MS: The development of visual accommodation during early infancy, *Child Dev* 51:646, 1980.
35. Hofstetter HW: An ergographic analysis of fatigue of accommodation, *Am J Optom Arch Am Acad Optom* 20:115, 1943.
36. Lancaster W, Williams E: New light on the theory of accommodation, with practical applications, *Trans Am Acad Ophthalmol Otolaryngol* 19:170, 1914.
37. Ebenholtz SM, Zander PA: Accommodative hysteresis: influence on closed loop measures of far point and near point, *Invest Ophthalmol Vis Sci* 28:1246, 1987.

38. Ciuffreda KJ and others: Static aspects of accommodation in human amblyopia, *Am J Optom Physiol Opt* 60:436, 1983.

39. Ciuffreda KJ, Rumpf D: Contrast and accommodation in amblyopia, *Vision Res* 25:1445, 1985.

40. Mantyjarvi MI: Accommodation in hyperopic and myopic school children, *J Pediatr Ophthalmol Strab* 24:37, 1987.

41. Nakazawa M, Ohtsuki K: Apparent accommodation in pseudophakic eyes after implantation of posterior chamber intraocular lenses, *Am J Ophthalmol* 96:435, 1983.

42. Zellers JA, Alpert TL, Rouse MW: A review of the literature and a normative study of accommodative facility, *J Am Optom Assoc* 55:31, 1984.

43. Daum KM: Accommodative insufficiency, *Am J Optom Physiol Opt* 60:352, 1983.

44. Allen MJ: Accommodative rock via computer, *J Am Optom Assoc* 59:610, 1988.

45. Gallaway M, Scheiman M: Assessment of accommodative facility using MEM retinoscopy, *J Am Optom Assoc* 61:36, 1990.

46. Burge S: Suppression during binocular accommodative rock, *Optom Monthly* 70:867, 1979.

47. Garzia RP, Richmond JE: Accommodative facility: a study of young adults, *J Am Optom Assoc* 10:821, 1982.

48. Siderov J, Johnston AW: The importance of the test parameters in the clinical assessment of accommodative facility, *Optom Vision Sci* 67:551, 1990.

49. Siderov J, DiGuglielmo L: Binocular accommodative facility in pre-presbyopic adults and its relation to symptoms, *Optom Vision Sci* 68:49, 1991.

50. McKenzie KM and others: Study of accommodative facility testing reliability, *Am J Optom Physiol Opt* 64:186, 1987.

51. Rouse MW and others: Monocular accommodative facility testing reliability, *Optom Vis Sci* 66:72, 1989.

52. Daum KM: Orthoptic treatment in patients with inertia of accommodation, *Aust J Optom* 66:68, 1983.

53a. Hennessey D, Iosue RA, Rouse MW: Relation of symptoms to accommodative infacility of school-aged children, *Am J Optom Physiol Opt* 61:177, 1984.

53b. Scheiman M and others: Normative study of accommodative facility in elementary schoolchildren, *Am J Optom Physiol Opt* 65:127, 1988.

54. Temme LA, Morris A: Speed of accommodation and age, *Optom Vision Sci* 66:106, 1989.

55. Sheard C: The comparative value of various methods and practices of skiametry, *Am J Physiol Opt* 3:177, 1922.

56. Tait EF: A quantitative system of dynamic retinoscopy, *Am J Optom* 6:669, 1929.

57. Romano PE: Objective accommodometry: isn't it time? (from infrared optometers to dynamic retinoscopy), *Binoc Vis Eye Muscle Surg Qtrly* 8:229, 1993 (editorial).

58. Nott, IS: Dynamic retinoscopy, accommodation, and convergence, *Am J Physiol Opt* 6:490, 1925.

59. Rosenfield M, Ciuffreda KJ, Rosen J: Accommodation response during distance optometric test procedures, *J Am Optom Assoc* 63:614, 1992.

60. Ciuffreda KJ, Kenyon RV: Accommodative vergence and accommodation in normals, amblyopes, and strabismics. In Schor CM, Ciuffreda KJ, editors: *Vergence eye movements: basic and clinical aspects,* Boston, 1983, Butterworth-Heinemann.

61. Lovasik JV, Kergeat H, Kothe AC: The influence of letter size on the focusing response of the eye, *J Am Optom Assoc* 58:631, 1987.

62. Tan RK, O'Leary DJ: Steady-state accommodation response to different Snellen letter sizes, *Am J Optom Physiol Opt* 62:751, 1985.

63. Kreuger H: Fluctuations in the accommodation of the human eye to mono- and binocular fixation, *Graefes Arch Clin Exp Ophthalmol* 205:129, 1978.

64. Pomeranz RB: The use of bell retinoscopy to determine the near-point Rx, *Optic J* 1964.

65. Tait EF: A quantitative system of dynamic retinoscopy, *Am J Optom Arch Am Acad Optom* 30:113, 1953.

66. Whitaker AC: The Tait dynamic system of retinoscopy, *Am J Optom* 6:497, 1929.

67. Daum KM: Accommodative response. In Eskridge JB, Amos JF, Bartlett JD, editors: *Clinical procedures in optometry,* Philadelphia, 1991, JB Lippincott.

68. Semmlow JL, Heerema D: The role of accommodative convergence at the limits of fusional convergence, *Invest Ophthalmol Vis Sci* 18:970, 1979.

69. Velasco e Cruz AA, Sampaio NMV, Vargas JA: Near retinoscopy in accommodative esotropia, *J Pediatr Ophthalmol Strab* 27:245, 1990.

70. Owens DA, Wolf-Kelly K: Near work, visual fatigue, and variations of oculomotor tonus, *Invest Ophthalmol Vis Sci* 28:743, 1987.

71. Tan RK, O'Leary DJ: Stability of the accommodative dark focus after periods of maintained accommodation, *Invest Ophthalmol Vis Sci* 27:1414, 1986.

72. McBrien NA, Millodot M: The effect of refractive error on the accommodative response gradient, *Ophthalmic Physiol Opt* 6:145, 1986.

73. McBrien NA, Millodot M: Differences in adaptation of tonic accommodation with refractive state, *Invest Ophthalmol Vis Sci* 29:460, 1988.

74. Gwiazda J and others: Myopic children show insufficient accommodative response to blur, *Invest Ophthalmol Vis Sci* 34:690, 1993.

75. Chung KM: Critical review: effects of optical defocus on refractive development and ocular growth and relation to accommodation, *Optom Vis Sci* 70:228, 1993.

76. Goss DA: Clinical accommodation and heterophoria findings preceding juvenile myopia, *Optom Vision Sci* 68:110, 1991.

77. Rosenfield M, Ciuffreda KJ, Hung GK: The linearity of proximally induced accommodation and vergence, *Invest Ophthalmol Vis Sci* 32:2985, 1991.

78. Owens DA: A comparison of accommodative responsiveness and contrast sensitivity for sinusoidal gratings, *Vision Res* 20:159, 1980.

79. Fisher SK, Ciuffreda KJ: Accommodation and apparent distance, *Perception* 17:609, 1988.

80. Ogden NA, Raymond JE, Seland TP: Visual accommodation and sustained visual resolution in multiple sclerosis, *Invest Ophthalmol Vis Sci* 33:2744, 1992.

81. Takeda T, Neveu C, Stark L: Accommodation on downward gaze, *Optom Vis Sci* 69:556, 1992.

82. Locke LC, Sommers W: A comparison study of dynamic retinoscopy techniques, *Optom Vis Sci* 66:72, 1989.

83. Owens DA, Mohindra I, Held R: The effectiveness of a retinoscope beam as an accommodative stimulus, *Invest Ophthalmol Vis Sci* 19:942, 1980.

84. Morgan MW, Peters HB: Accommodative-convergence in presbyopia, *Am J Optom Arch Am Acad Optom* 28:3, 1951.

85. Bester HM: The interpretation of dynamic skiametric findings, *Am J Physiol Opt* 1:223, 1920.

86. Rouse MW, London R, Allen DC: An evaluation of the monocular estimate method of dynamic retinoscopy, *Am J Optom Physiol Opt* 59:234, 1982.

87. Nott IS: Convergence, accommodation, and fusion, *Am J Optom* 6:19, 1929.

88. Fry GA: Skiametric determination of the near-point Rx, *Optom Wkly* 41: 1469, 1950.

89. Freeman RD: Asymmetries in human accommodation and visual experience, *Vision Res* 15:483, 1975.

90. Rouse MW: Management of binocular anomalies: efficacy of vision therapy in the treatment of accommodative deficiencies, *Am J Optom Physiol Opt* 64:415, 1987.

91. Hoffman L, Cohen AH, Feurer G: Effectiveness of nonstrabismus optometric vision training in a private practice, *Am J Optom Arch Am Acad Optom* 50:813, 1973.

92. Duane A: Anomalies of accommodation clinically considered, *Arch Ophthalmol* 45:124, 1916.

93. Duane A: Subnormal accommodation, *Arch Ophthalmol* 54:566, 1925.

94. Prangen AD: Subnormal accommodation, *Arch Ophthalmol* 6:906, 1931.

95. Chrousos GA and others: Accommodation deficiency in healthy young individuals, *J Pediatr Ophthalmol Strab* 25:176, 1988.

96. Theobald S: Subnormal accommodative power in young persons a not infrequent cause of asthenopia, *Trans Am Ophthalmol Soc* 6:127, 1893.

97. Prakash P, Agarwal LP, Nag SG: Accommodation weakness and convergence insufficiency, *Orient Arch Ophthalmol* 10:261, 1972.

98. Gould G: Premature presbyopia, *Am Med* 9:103, 1905.

99. Hammerberg E, Norn MS: Defective dissociation of accommodation and convergence in dyslectic children, *Acta Ophthalmol (Kbh)* 50:651, 1972.

100. Anderson M: Orthoptic treatment of loss of convergence and accommodation caused by road accidents ("whiplash" injury), *Br Orthopt J* 18:117, 1961.

101. Bugola J: Hypoaccommodation and convergence insufficiency, *Am Orthopt J* 27:85, 1977.

102. Cooper J, Duckman R: Convergence insufficiency: incidence, diagnosis, and treatment, *J Am Optom Assoc* 49:673, 1978.

103. Daum KM: Predicting the results in the orthoptic treatment of accommodative dysfunction, *Am J Optom Physiol Opt* 61:184, 1984.

104. von Noorden GK, Brown DJ, Parks M: Associated convergence and accommodative insufficiency, *Doc Ophthalmol* 34:393, 1973.

105. Lieppman ME: Accommodative and convergence insufficiency after decompression sickness, *Arch Ophthalmol* 99:453, 1981.

106. Stark L and others: Accommodative disfacility presenting as intermittent exotropia, *Ophthalmol Physiol Opt* 4:233, 1984.

107. Rutstein RP, Daum KM: Exotropia associated with defective accommodation, *J Am Optom Assoc* 58:548, 1987.

108. Mazow ML and others: Acute accommodative and convergence insufficiency, *Trans Am Ophthal Soc* 87:158, 1989.

109. Robinson BN: A study of institutionalized juveniles who are demonstrated underachieving readers, *Am J Optom Arch Am Acad Optom* 50:113, 1973.

110. Blatt N: Weakness of accommodation, *Arch Ophthalmol* 5:362, 1931.

111. Hoffman LG: Incidence of visual difficulties in children with learning disabilities, *J Am Optom Assoc* 51:447, 1980.

112. Raskind RH: Problems at the reading distance, *Am Orthopt J* 26:53, 1976.

113. Duane A: A new classification of the motor anomalies of the eyes based on physiological principles, together with their symptoms, diagnosis, and treatment, *Ann Ophthalmol Otolaryngol* 6:84, 1897.

114. Berens C, Connolly PT, Kern D: Certain motor anomalies of the eye in relation to prescribing lenses, *Am J Ophthalmol* 16:199, 1933.

115. Sasaki JD: Exophoria and accommodative convergence insufficiency, *Optom Wkly* 47:811, 1956.

116. Prangen AD: Some problems and procedures in refraction, *Arch Ophthalmol* 18:432, 1937.

117. Morris CW: A theory concerning adaptation to accommodative impairment, *Optom Wkly* 50:255, 1959.

118. Hofstetter HW: Factors involved in low amplitude cases, *Am J Optom Arch Am Acad Optom* 19:279, 1942.

119. Brownell ME: Paresis of accommodation due to dental caries, *Arch Ophthalmol* 26:1057, 1941.

120. Moss SE, Klein R, Klein BEK: Accommodative ability in younger-onset diabetes, *Arch Ophthalmol* 105:508, 1987.

121. Mathur JS, Vaithilinham E: Accommodative insufficiency and anemia, *Optician* 160:396, 1970.

122. Wilmer WH, Berens C: The effect of altitude on ocular functions, *JAMA* 71:1394, 1918.

123. Duane A: Accommodation, *Arch Ophthalmol* 5:1, 1931.

124. Duckman RH: The incidence of visual anomalies in a population of cerebral palsied children, *J Am Optom Assoc* 50:1013, 1979.

125. Duckman RH: Effectiveness of vision training in a population of cerebral palsied children, *J Am Optom Assoc* 51:607, 1980.

126. Duckman RH: Accommodation in cerebral palsy: function and remediation, *J Am Optom Assoc* 55:281, 1984.

127. Duckman RH: Vision therapy for the child with cerebral palsy, *J Am Optom Assoc* 58:28, 1987.

128. Westcott V: Concerning the accommodation before and after head injury, *Illinois Med J* 83:170, 1943.

129. Lovasik JV, Wiggins R: Cortical indices of impaired ocular accommodation and associated convergence mechanisms, *Am J Optom Physiol Opt* 61:15, 1984.

130. Russell G, Wick B: A prospective study of treatment of accommodative insufficiency, *Optom Vis Sci* 70:131, 1993.

131. Cooper J and others: Reduction of asthenopia after accommodative facility training, *Am J Optom Physiol Opt* 64:430, 1987.

132. Almgill VT: Case notes: reduced accommodation in asthmatic young adults, *Brit Orthopt J* 46:123, 1989.

133. Wood DJ: Accommodative failure in malaria and influenza, *Brit J Ophthalmol* 4:415, 1920.

134. Hoffman LG: The effect of accommodative deficiencies on the developmental level of perceptual skills, *Am J Optom Physiol Opt* 59:254, 1982.

135. Walsh TJ: *Neurophthalmology,* Philadelphia, 1972, Lea & Febiger.

136. Ohtsuka K and others: Accommodation and convergence insufficiency with middle cerebral artery occlusion, *Am J Ophthalmol* 106:60, 1988.

137. Potaznick W, Kozol N: Ocular manifestations of chronic fatigue and immune dysfunction syndrome, *Optom Vis Sci* 69:811, 1992.

138. Deleted in proof.

139. Heath GG: Representative important questions in clinical optometry, *Am J Optom Physiol Opt* 58:289, 1981.

140. Carroll R, Seaber JH: Acute loss of fusional convergence following head trauma, *Am Orthopt J* 24:57, 1974.

141. Krohel GB and others: Post-traumatic convergence insufficiency, *Ann Ophthalmol* 18:101, 1986.

142. Jampolsky A: Ocular divergence mechanisms, *Trans Am Ophthalmol Soc* 68:730, 1970.

143. Saladin JJ: Convergence insufficiency, fixation disparity, and control systems analysis: *Am J Optom Physiol Opt* 63:645, 1986.

144. Sheard C: Zones of ocular comfort, *Am J Optom Arch Am Acad Optom* 7:9, 1930.

145. Wick B, London R: Analysis of binocular visual function using tests made under binocular conditions, *Am J Optom Physiol Opt* 64:227, 1987.

146. Semmlow JL, Hung GK: The near response: theories of contro. In Schor CM, Ciuffreda KJ, editors: *Vergence eye movements: basic and clinical aspects,* Boston, 1984, Butterworth-Heinemann.

147. Valentino JA: Clinical use of progressive addition lenses on non-presbyopic patients, *Optom Mthly* 73:1, 1982.

148. Libassi DP, Barron CL, London R: Soft bifocal contact lenses for patients with nearpoint asthenopia, *J Am Optom Assoc* 56:866, 1985.

149. Randle RJ, Murphy MR: The dynamic response of visual accommodation over a seven-day period, *Am J Optom Physiol Opt* 51:530, 1974.

150. Russell G, Wick B: A prospective study of treatment of accommodative insufficiency, *Optom Vis Sci* 68(12s):197, 1991.

151. Wold RM, Pierce JR, Keddington J: Effectiveness of optometric vision therapy, *J Am Optom Assoc* 49:1047, 1978.

152. Weisz CL: Clinical therapy for accommodative responses: transfer effects upon performance, *J Am Optom Assoc* 50:209, 1979.

153. Tucker J, Tomlinson A: An investigation of persistent paresis of accommodation, *Am J Optom Physiol Opt* 51:3, 1974.

154. Bell RA, Thompson HS: Ciliary muscle dysfunction in Adie's syndrome, *Arch Ophthalmol* 96:638, 1978.

155. Levine S and others: Clinical assessment of accommodative facility in symptomatic and asymptomatic individuals, *J Am Optom Assoc* 56:286, 1985.

156. Liu J and others: Objective assessment of accommodation orthoptics. I. Dynamic insufficiency, *Am J Optom Physiol Opt* 56:285, 1979.

157. Sucher DF, Stewart J: Vertical fixation disparity in learning disabled, *Optom Vis Sci* 70:1038, 1993.

158. Graveson GS: The tonic pupil, *J Neurol Neurosurg Psychiatry* 12:219, 1949.

159. Russell GFM: Accommodation in the Holmes-Adie syndrome, *J Neurol Neurosurg Psychiatry* 21:290, 1958.

160. Cogan DG: Accommodation and the autonomic nervous system, *Arch Ophthalmol* 18:739, 1937.

161. Buzzelli AR: Stereopsis, accommodative, and vergence facility: do they relate to dyslexia? *Optom Vis Sci* 68:842, 1991.

162. Bobier WR, Sivak JG: Orthoptic treatment of subjects showing slow accommodative responses, *Am J Optom Physiol Opt* 60:678, 1983.

163. Wold RM: The spectacle amplitude of accommodation of children aged six to ten, *Am J Optom Physiol Opt* 44:642, 1967.

164. Ebenholtz SM: Accommodative hysteresis: a precursor for induced myopia? *Invest Ophthalmol* 24:513, 1983.

165. Ebenholtz SM: Accommodative hysteresis: relation to resting focus, *Am J Optom Physiol Opt* 62:755, 1985.

166. Miles FA, Judge SJ, Optican LM: Optically induced changes in the couplings between vergence and accommodation, *J Neurosci* 7:2576, 1987.

167. Brown B: The convergence insufficiency masquerade, *Am Orthopt J* 40:94, 1990.

168. Herman P: Convergence spasm, *Mt. Sinai J Med* 44:501, 1977.

169. Haldi BA: Surgical management of convergence insufficiency, *Am Orthopt J* 28:106, 1978.

170. Howe L: The fatigue of accommodation as registered by the ergograph, *JAMA* 67:100, 1916.

171. Ferree CE: The efficiency of the eye under different systems of lighting, *Ophthalmol (Seattle)* 10:622, 1914.

172. Berens C, Stark EK: Studies in ocular fatigue. IV. Fatigue of accommodation: experimental and clinical observations, *Am J Ophthalmol* 15:527, 1932.

173. Berens C, Sells S: Experimental studies on fatigue of accommodation. *Arch Ophthalmol* 31:148, 1944.

174. Berens C, Stark EK: Studies in ocular fatigue. III. Fatigue of accommodation: history, apparatus, and methods of graphic study, *Am J Ophthalmol* 15:216, 1932.

175. Berens C: An accommodation ergograph, *Trans Am Acad Ophthalmol Otolaryng* 24:472, 1929.

176. Pigion RG, Miller RJ: Fatigue of accommodation: changes in accommodation after visual work, *Am J Optom Physiol Opt* 62:853, 1985.

177. Prangen AD: Spasm of accommodation with report of thirty cases. In: *Transactions of the Section on Ophthalmology of AMA of 82nd Annual Session,* Chicago, 1922, AMA.

178. Irvine G: A survey of esophoria and ciliary spasm, *Br J Ophthalmol* 31:289, 1947.

179. Suchoff IB, Petito GT: The efficacy of visual therapy: accommodative disorders and nonstrabismic anomalies of binocular vision, *J Am Optom Assoc* 57:119, 1986.

180. Walker J: Myopia and pseudo-myopia, *Br J Ophthalmol* 30:735, 1946.

181. Hein PA: Pseudomyopia, *Ann Ophthalmol* 6:1197, 1974.

182. Stenson SM, Raskind RH: Pseudomyopia: etiology, mechanisms, and therapy, *J Pediatr Ophthalmol Strab* 7:110, 1970.

183. Lupica VP, Hypnosis therapy for ciliary spasm, *J Am Optom Assoc* 47:102, 1976.

184. Cogan DG, Freese CG: Spasm of the near reflex, *Arch Ophthalmol* 54:752, 1955.

185. Fenton P: Accommodative spasm. In Koichi and others, editors: Ophthalmology: Proceedings of the XXIII International Congress, Series 450, *Excerpta Medica* 2:1217, 1979.

186. Rutstein RP, Daum KM, Amos JF: Accommodative spasm: a study of 17 cases, *J Am Optom Assoc* 59:527, 1988.

187. Sollom AW: Unilateral spasm of accommodation and transient convergent squint due to an anxiety neurosis, *Br Orthopt J* 23:118, 1966.

188. Murrah WF: Recurrent unilateral accommodative spasms and miosis, *South Med J* 58:1135, 1965.

189. Fisher SK, Ciuffreda KJ, Bird JE: The effect of monocular versus binocular fixation on accommodative hysteresis, *Ophthalmic Physiol Opt* 8:438, 1988.

190. Fisher SK, Ciuffreda KJ, Hammer S: Interocular equality of tonic accommodation and consensuality of accommodative hysteresis, *Ophthalmic Physiol Opt* 7:17, 1987.

191. Miwa T, Tokoro T: Accommodative hysteresis of refractive errors in light and dark fields, *Optom Vis Sci* 70:323, 1993.

192. Press LJ: Management of Adie's syndrome, *Am J Optom Physiol Opt* 58:235, 1981.

193. Sloane AE, Kraut JA: Spasm of accommodation, *Doc Ophthalmol* 34:365, 1973.

194. Alexander GF: Spasm of accommodation, *Trans Ophthalmol Soc U K* 60:207, 1940.

195. Marlow FW: Persistent accommodative spasm due to latent hyperphoria, *Arch Ophthalmol* 51:223, 1922.

196. Sokolovsky A: Asthenopias and accommodation spasms and their treatment, *Oftalmol Zh* 30:348, 1975.

197. Seaber JH: Pseudomyopia in exodeviations, *Am Orthopt J* 16:67, 1966.

198. Paton L: Functional spasm of accommodation, *Trans Ophthalmol Soc U K* 37:370, 1917.

199. Rouse MW, Hutter RF, Shiflett R: A normative study of the accommodative lag in elementary school children, *Am J Optom Physiol Opt* 61:693, 1984.

200. Adigazalova-Polchaeva KA, Zeynalov VZ: Vision dimming by cylindrical lenses and use of this method for treating accommodation spasm, *Vestn Oftalmol* 1:25, 1980.

201. Adigezalova-Polchaeva KA, Zeynalov VZ: Treatment of spasm accommodative by blurring with cylindrical glasses, *Oftalmol Zh* 34:213, 1970.

202. Adigezalova-Polchaeva KA, Khanlarova NA: Effectivity of orthoptic treatment of pseudomyopia in remote terms of observation, *Oftalmol Zh* 36:454, 1981.

203. Smereka LG: Remote results of treatment of fresh accommodation spasms in country school children, *Oftalmol Zh* 36:467, 1981.

204. Grushko SG: Results of treatment of accommodative spasm, *Oftalmol Zh* 36:462, 1981.
205. Cherikchi LE: Electrostimulation of the ciliary muscle in treatment of accommodation spasm, *Oftalmol Zh* 39:83, 1984.
206. Volksou VV, Kolesnikova LN: Treatment of an accommodation spasm with an immediate association with the weakness of the ciliary muscles, *Vestn Oftalmol* 1:50, 1972.
207. Oligina AM: Detection and treatment of accommodation spasm in school children, *Oftalmol Zh* 21:423, 1966.
208. Dashevsky AI, Andreeva NA: Elimination of accommodation prespasm by methods of microblurring and divergent deaccommodation after, *Oftalmol Zh* 36:164, 1981.
209. Smith JL: Letter to editor, *J Clin Neuro Ophthalmol* 4:71, 1984.
210. Moore S: The accommodative effort syndrome, *Am Orthopt J* 17:5, 1967.
211. Schwartze GM, McHenry LC, Proctor RC: Convergence spasm: treatment by amytal interview, *J Clin Neuro Ophthalmol* 3:123, 1983.
212. Panisett A, Pop M: The Panisett-Pop syndrome, *Can J Ophthalmol* 14:55, 1979.
213. Schor CM, Johnson CA, Post RB: Adaptation of tonic accommodation, *Ophthalmic Physiol Opt* 4:133, 1984.
214. Dangel ME, Weber PA, Leier CB: Transient myopia following isosorbide dinitrate, *Ann Ophthalmol* 15:7156, 1983.
215. Fraunfelder FT: *Drug-induced ocular side-effects and drug interactions,* ed 2, Philadelphia, 1982, Lea & Febiger.
216. Jaanus SD, Pagano VT, Bartlett JD: Drugs affecting the autonomic nervous system. In Bartlett JD, Jaanus SD, editors: *Clinical ocular pharmacology,* Boston, 1984, Butterworth-Heinemann.
217. Jaanus SD, Bartlett JD: Adverse ocular side effects of systemic drug therapy. In Bartlett JD, Jaanus SD, editors: *Clinical ocular pharmacology,* Boston, 1984, Butterworth-Heinemann.
218. Rengstorff R, Royston M: Miotic drugs: a review of ocular, visual, and systemic complications, *Am J Optom Physiol Opt* 53:70, 1976.
219. Guiloff RJ, Whiteley A, Kelly RE: Organic convergence spasm, *Acta Neurol Scand* 61:252, 1980.
220. Romano PE, Stark WJ: Pseudomyopia as a presenting sign in ocular myasthenia gravis, *Am J Ophthalmol* 75:872, 1973.
221. Baker R, Brown B, Garner L: Time course and variability of dark focus, *Invest Ophthalmol Vis Sci* 24:1528, 1983.
222. Wolfe JM, O'Connell KM: Adaptation of the resting state of accommodation, *Invest Ophthalmol Vis Sci* 28:992, 1987.
223. Rutstein RP, Galkin KA: Convergence spasm, *J Am Optom Assoc* 55:495, 1984.
224. Griffin JF, Wray SH, Anderson DP: Misdiagnosis of spasm of the near reflex, *Neurology* 26:1018, 1976.
225. Dagi LR, Chrousos GA, Cogan DC: Spasm of the near reflex associated with organic disease, *Am J Ophthalmol* 103:582, 1987.
226. Tijessen CC, Goor C, Van Woerkom TC: Spasm of the near reflex: functional or organic disorder? *J Clin Neuro Ophthalmol* 3:59, 1983.
227. Nirankari VS, Hameroff SB: Spasm of the near reflex, *Ann Ophthalmol* 12:1050, 1980.
228. Keane JR: Convergence spasm, *Neurology* 33:1637, 1983 (reply from author).
229. Sarkies NJC, Sanders MD: Convergence spasm, *Trans Ophthalmol Soc U K* 104:782, 1985.
230. Keane JR: Neuro-ophthalmic sign and symptoms of hysteria, *Neurology (NY)* 32:757, 1982.
231. Silbert JA, Alexander A: Cyclotherapy in the treatment of symptomatic latent hyperopia, *J Am Optom Assoc* 58:40, 1987.
232. Hutter RF, Rouse MW: Visually related headache in a preschooler, *Am J Optom Physiol Opt* 61:711, 1984.
233. Rosenberg ML: Spasm of the near reflex mimicking myasthenia gravis, *J Clin Neuro Ophthalmol* 6:106, 1986.
234. Viikari K: The prophylactic fogging method of revealing spasm of accommodation, *Acta Ophthalmol* 125(suppl):17, 1975.
235. Viikari K: Minus or plus lenses in the therapy of the convergence spasm? *J Clin Neuro Ophthalmol* 4:71, 1984.
236. Koslowe KC and others: Evaluation of Accommotrac biofeedback training for myopia control, *Optom Vis Sci* 68: 338, 1991.
237. Gallaway M and others: Biofeedback training of visual acuity and myopia: a pilot study, *Am J Optom Physiol Opt* 64:62, 1987.
238. Catalano RA and others: Functional visual loss in children, *Ophthalmology* 93:385, 1986.
239. Manor RS: Use of special glasses in treatment of spasm of near reflex, *Ann Ophthalmol* 11:903, 1979.
240. Kubareva NS: The usage of ultrasonic therapy for treatment of patients with accommodative spasm and myopia of mild degree, *Oftalmol Zh* 36:162, 1981.
241. Trachtman JN: Biofeedback of accommodation to reduce myopia: a review, *Am J Optom Physiol Opt* 64:639, 1987.
242. Trachtman JN, Giambalvo V, Feldman J: Biofeedback of accommodation to reduce functional myopia, *Biofeedback Self Regul* 6:547, 1981.
243. Zorn M, Sajban T: Convergence insufficiency masks a growing tumor, *Rev Optom* October, 1986, p 96.
244. Sumner P: Subnormal accommodation: the result of focal infection, *Am J Ophthalmol* 4:356, 1921.
245. Veasey: Paralysis of accommodation, *Trans Am Ophthalmol Soc* 17:440, 1919.
246. White JW: Paralysis of accommodation following a peritonsillar abscess, *Am J Ophthalmol* 4:276, 1921.
247. Thal LS, Phillips SR, Stark L: Paralysis of accommodation in infectious mononucleosis, *Am J Optom Physiol Opt* 54:19, 1977.
248. Cogan DG: *Neurology of the ocular muscles,* ed 2, Springfield, Ill, 1956, Charles C Thomas.
249. Alpers BJ, Palmer HD: The cerebral and spinal complications occurring during pregnancy and the puerperium: a critical review with illustrative cases, *J Nerv Ment Dis* 70:465, 1929.
250. Hollister LE: Complications from psychotherapeutic drugs: 1964, *Clin Pharm Therapeutics* 5:322, 1964.
251. Klingele TG, Newman SA, Burde RM: Accommodation defect in Wilson's disease, *Am J Ophthalmol* 90:22, 1980.
252. Turner MJ: Observations on the normal subjective amplitude of accommodation, *Br J Physiol Opt* 15:70, 1958.
253. Murran L: How the visual system might respond to design flaws of head mounted displays that result in aniso-accommodative stimuli, *Optom Vis Sci* 72(suppl 12):169, 1995.
254. Campbell FW: Correlation of accommodation between the two eyes, *J Opt Soc Am* 50:738, 1960.
255. Tseutaki TK, Schor CM: Clinical method for measuring adaptation of tonic accommodation and vergence accommodation, *Am J Optom Physiol Opt* 64:437, 1987.
256. Schor CM, Narayan V: Graphical analysis of prism adaptation, convergence accommodation and accommodative convergence, *Am J Optom Physiol Opt* 59:774, 1982.

Aniseikonia (unequal images) is the condition stemming from relative differences in the size and/or shape of the ocular images seen by the two eyes at the cortex.[1-5] The image difference may or may not be the same as the difference in the retinal images of the eyes.[6] Aniseikonia can cause subjective distortions of space, discomfort, suppression, amblyopia, diplopia, and difficulties with stereopsis and other visual functions.[7-9]

HISTORICAL BACKGROUND

Even before the turn of the century, Donders (and others) understood that spectacle lenses of unequal powers could cause differences in image size.[1,10] Many clinicians, however, have not taken aniseikonia seriously, apparently because much of the evidence is subjective. The symptoms reported in aniseikonia are similar to those reported with other binocular vision problems, and the symptoms do not consistently correlate with the magnitude of the image size difference. Aniseikonia also is sometimes doubted because correcting the image size difference does not always provide relief.[11]

SIGNIFICANCE

As early as 1939, Berens noted that, "Opinions vary in regard to the importance of aniseikonia and as to what the correction of this condition may accomplish;" a similar statement could be made today.[12] To sort out this dilemma, it is important to recognize that aniseikonia of 0.1% to 0.2% can be detected with the proper equipment, and it is especially important to specify the level of aniseikonia in question.[13] Most clinicians suggest that a 1% to 2% difference in image size should be corrected.[1,5,8] Opinions vary somewhat; for example, Burian[5] felt 1% was significant, whereas Hawkswell[14] held with 2% because this difference may cause considerable discomfort.[1,8,9] Substantially larger amounts may or may not cause symptoms, although they generally have a profound effect on performance. The significance of a given patient's aniseikonia depends largely on the patient's ability to adapt to the image size difference, much as a person adapts to a new pair of glasses.[5] Aniseikonia typically causes symptoms when there is a moderate image size difference (approximately 1% to 5%). It also generally causes symptoms only when the anisometropia is corrected; suppression occurs otherwise.

✿ CLINICAL PEARL

Aniseikonia typically causes symptoms when there is a moderate image size difference (approximately 1% to 5%).

Large image size differences may or may not cause discomfort, although they will interfere with other visual function. In fact, significant image size differences may prevent binocularity entirely; aniseikonia larger than about 5% is incompatible with fine binocular vision and fusion.[13,15,16] Aniseikonia significant enough to prevent fusion can cause strabismus, suppression, and/or amblyopia, particularly if the individual is very young when the image size difference occurs.[15,17,18]

CLASSIFICATION

Aniseikonia can be classified as either physiologic, neurologic, or optical in nature (or some combination). Physiologic aniseikonia is produced either by eccentrically viewing an object or as a result of differing binocular perspectives of an object. Optical aniseikonia is usually further classified as overall, meridional, or asymmetric magnification differences.

Although not usually of direct concern to clinicians or patients, physiologic aniseikonia occurs to a surprising extent. Eccentric viewing of a particular object causes different viewing distances because of the separation of the eyes in the head. These differing relative-distance magnification effects easily produce image size differences of 10% to 20% that are managed by the visual system in an extremely sophisticated and complex manner. Binocular perspective also causes a difference in the image size and orientation seen by the eyes. These differences provide disparity that is interpreted by the visual system in the judgment of depth, that is, stereopsis. Physiologic aniseikonia will not be considered further in this discussion.

In transmitting a retinal image to the cortex, the neurologic apparatus produces a certain image magnification. The retinal mosaic superimposes a magnification factor on any retinal image.[19,20] Neurologic aniseikonia can occur in the absence of other anomalies (e.g., anisometropia or astigmatism) that cause aniseikonia. Neurologic aniseikonia may be as important as optical aniseikonia, particularly if the patient is highly anisometropic because of differences in axial lengths of the eyes.

Optical aniseikonia is a difference in the image size of retinal images brought about by the power and location of the refractive lens correction in combination with the ametropia of the eye. Much of the classical work on aniseikonia concerns optical aniseikonia.

TESTING

Most of the procedures for testing aniseikonia are either direct comparison or stereoscopic techniques. The direct comparison techniques are usually easy to administer but are not always very accurate because they require difficult judgments by the patient. Stereoscopic techniques are sometimes more difficult for patients to perceive; however, if the patient sees the target and understands the task, the techniques are usually accurate. Of course, all procedures for aniseikonia require that the patient understand and respond appropriately to the test. Problems such as suppression, reduced binocularity, or amblyopia can complicate or prevent the assessment.[21]

TRIAL LENSES

Any measurement of aniseikonia using a correction or trial lenses of the image size difference is affected by the lenses used in the measurement.[22] Therefore the trial lenses should have the same base curve and center thickness, so that the shape factor is constant.[23]

Afocal Magnifiers for Testing

A series of afocal magnifiers is valuable for testing purposes. To create such a set the formula for overall spectacle magnification should be solved for a back vertex power of zero. In solving for the power of the front surface, F_1, the clinician can specify both the thickness and the index (i.e., choose the material) and determine the base curve.

TABLE 4-1 PARAMETERS OF AFOCAL MAGNIFIERS MADE OF GLASS

M	Magnification (%)	F1 (D)	F2 (D)	CT (mm)
1.005	0.5	+2.50	−2.51	3.0
1.010	1	+3.37	−3.40	4.5
1.020	2	+6.00	−6.12	5.0
1.030	3	+8.00	−8.24	5.5
1.040	4	+10.12	−10.40	5.8
1.050	5	+12.12	−12.73	6.0

Modified from Remole A: Anisophoria and aniseikonia. II. The management of optical anisophoria, *Optom Vis Sci* 66:736, 1989.

$$\text{Spectacle magnification} = (1/1 - [t/n]F_1)(1/1 - hF_v)$$

where t = center thickness, n = index of refraction, F_1 = front surface power, h = vertex distance, and F_v = back vertex power, and

$$F_t = F_1 + F_2 - t/n\ (F_1F_2)$$

where F_t = true power of the lens, F_1 = front surface power, F_2 = back vertex power, t = center thickness, and n = refractive index.

A minimum set of size lenses for testing purposes would probably be six lenses ranging from 0.5% to 5% magnification. Table 4-1 shows possible diagnostic afocal magnifiers for glass lenses.[1]

An afocal magnifier actually can have zero vertex power for only one distance.[23] Fortunately the power at other distances is small and can be ignored. Most laboratories will make such a set of magnifiers easily and inexpensively.

DIRECT COMPARISON TESTS

One class of aniseikonia tests, direct comparison, involves a comparison of the image sizes seen by the eyes. Patients often experience difficulties making the appropriate judgments for tests in this class.[24,25] Frequently the targets are displaced in the same direction, and the result is that fixation disparity, heterophoria, or anisophoria is judged, rather than aniseikonia.[25]

Direct Comparison of Objects

A very simple but gross method of testing for aniseikonia is to cause diplopia with a vertical prism while the patient observes an object, such as an acuity chart.[26,27] Apparent differences in size suggest aniseiko-

FIG. 4-1 Brecher test for aniseikonia. **A,** Patient observes two penlights with one eye and images of two penlights through a Maddox rod with other eye. **B,** No aniseikonia is present, and images seen by each eye are equal. **C,** With aniseikonia, image seen by left eye is larger than that seen by right eye. **D,** Image size again equalized with an afocal magnifier before right eye.

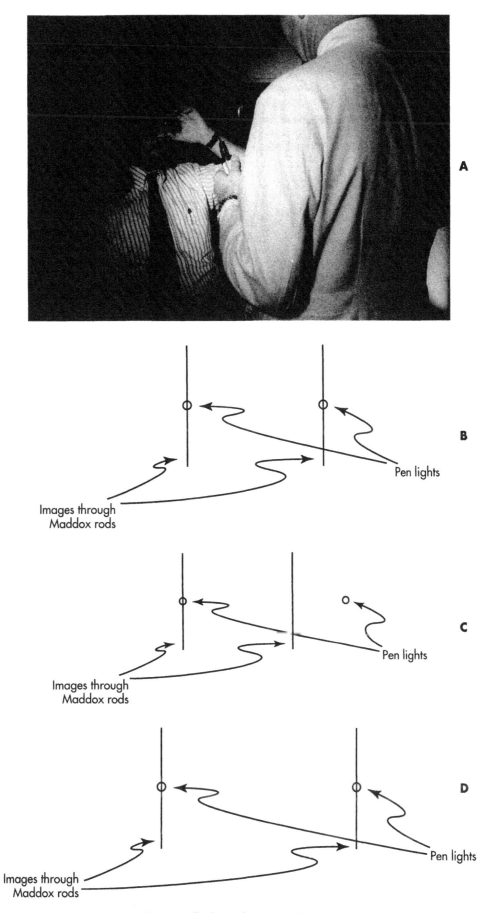

FIG. 4-1   For legend see opposite page.

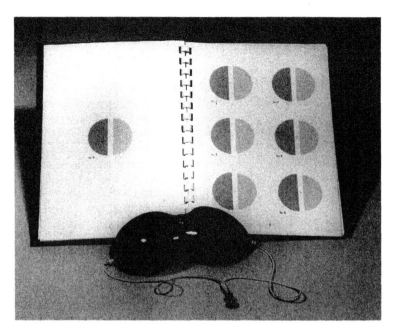

FIG. 4-2   Awaya test for aniseikonia. Patient wears red and green filters and observes whether circles are same size.

nia. Some patients may be able to detect as little as a 2% image size difference between the eyes.

Brecher Test

The Brecher[24] test for aniseikonia is very simple. Two small lights separated by several centimeters are presented in front of the patient. The patient holds a Maddox rod in front of one eye, so that one eye sees the lights while the other eye sees two streaks of light that depend on the orientation of the Maddox rods (Fig. 4-1).[24] The Maddox rod is oriented according to the meridian that is to be tested for image size differences.

The patient's task is to decide whether the separation between the lights is the same as the separation between the streaks. Iseikonia (equal image sizes) causes an equal separation, even if one set is displaced because of a deviation (phoria or strabismus).[24] The magnitude of the image size difference is measured with hand-held afocal magnifiers that are placed into the line of sight until the separation between the lights and the streaks is equal. Both the difference in image size between the eyes and the sensitivity (i.e., variability) of the observer to the task should be assessed. The sensitivity is the amount of magnification difference that just makes a difference. It has been reported to be as accurate as 0.5%; however, a more realistic figure is 1% to 2%.

Awaya "New" Aniseikonia Test

Katsumi and others[28] describe the use of a test for aniseikonia consisting of a book of red and green figures and spectacles containing red and green filters

(Fig. 4-2).* Vision is dissociated using the colored filters as the subject views sets of red and green half circles in the book. There are two series of circles in which the image size difference ranges from 0% to 24%. While wearing the filters the patient first examines the two half circles that are the same size to see whether they appear equal or not. If a difference is perceived, then the patient looks at the 24% difference circles and sequentially views smaller and smaller differences to determine a pair in which the red is just bigger than the green, a pair in which they are the same size, and a pair in which the red circle is just smaller than the green. Although the Awaya test is easy to administer and interpret, the amount of aniseikonia is significantly underestimated.[29,30] Therefore we do not recommend this test.

STEREOSCOPIC TECHNIQUES
Space Eikonometer

The space eikonometer is the gold-standard test for aniseikonia (Fig. 4-3) because of its high level of accuracy (0.1% to 0.2% differences detectable).†[30] This device is unique in that a differentiation between the geometric, induced, and declination effects can be made with minimal difficulty.[31] The geometric effect is caused by image size differences in the horizontal meridian (axis 90-degree magnifier) and is so called because the image differences are geometrically predictable. The induced effect is caused by image size differences in the vertical meridian (axis 180-degree

*Handaya, Tokyo, Japan.
†American Optical Corporation, Southbridge, Mass.

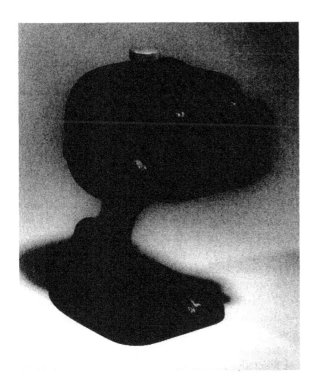

FIG. 4-3 The American Optical space eikonometer is the gold standard test for aniseikonia.

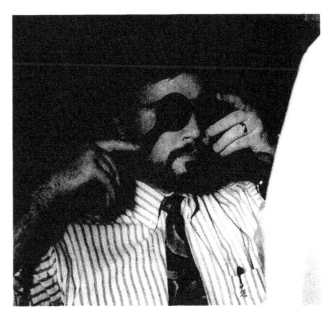

FIG. 4-4 Miles test for aniseikonia. Patient observes two penlights with each eye covered by a Maddox rod oriented to produce vertical streaks.

magnifier). The induced effect is not geometrically predictable unless the clinician assumes that the magnification in the vertical meridian also induces changes on the horizontal meridian. Declination effects are a result of oblique magnification differences usually related to oblique cylinder correction. Usually, a patient with aniseikonia has an overall difference, along with a meridional effect (that may or may not be at an oblique meridian). To complete the measurement sequence for a given patient a measurement of the horizontal magnification difference (axis 90 degrees), the vertical magnification difference (axis 180 degrees), and the declination effect (oblique axes) is made in order. Although the space eikonometer is no longer being manufactured, extensive descriptions of its use are available.[32]

 CLINICAL PEARL

The space eikonometer is the gold-standard test for aniseikonia because of its high level of accuracy (0.1% to 0.2% differences detectable).

Miles Test

The Miles test for aniseikonia uses two small lights observed through two Maddox rods (one over each eye) oriented to produce vertical images (Fig. 4-4).[33] The patient sees two vertically oriented lines that are the result of the fusion of the two sets of two lines seen through the Maddox rod before each eye. The patient's

task is to observe which line is closer, because the eye requiring additional magnification to equalize the images will see a closer image. Afocal magnifiers should be added before the eye seeing the closer image, until the images are in the same plane. Bracketing the magnitude allows an estimation of the sensitivity of the test. The Miles test is often difficult for patients to perform and can only be used for horizontal image size differences because of the use of horizontal disparities.

ESTIMATION

Frequently, 1% per diopter of anisometropia image size difference is assumed. This is less than the actual image difference.[22] This estimation technique is used when aniseikonia is strongly suspected but is difficult to measure.

 CLINICAL PEARL

Frequently, 1% per diopter of anisometropia image size difference is assumed.

SYMPTOMS

Patients with image size differences commonly report long-standing ocular discomfort, such as burning, itching, ocular fatigue when performing particular tasks, various types of headaches, photophobia, poor depth perception, vertigo, and general physical disturbances, such as irritability, dizziness, nausea, or nervousness.[5,7,34-37] Patients with aniseikonia resulting from radial keratotomy (RK) frequently complain of dull headaches in the back of the head, fluctuating vision, poor image quality, monocular diplopia, dull pain, glare, and blurred vision at distance or near or both.[38] The asthenopia associated with aniseikonia is much the same as that reported with vergence and refractive problems.[9] Some patients with asthenopia complain of binocular eyestrain and blur in which images before one eye are seen at a different distance and are of a different size.[9] Eye strain includes any of a large variety of symptoms, including redness, itching, blur, discomfort, and fatigue associated with use of the eyes. Surprisingly, patients with aniseikonia only infrequently report spatial distortion. The etiology of symptoms caused by aniseikonia is unknown, although they are not likely of muscular origin.[3]

 CLINICAL PEARL

> Patients with image size differences commonly report long-standing ocular discomfort, such as burning, itching, ocular fatigue when performing particular tasks, various types of headaches, photophobia, poor depth perception, vertigo, and general physical disturbances, such as irritability, dizziness, nausea, or nervousness.

The production of asthenopia is probably what causes impaired reading skill associated with aniseikonia.[39] Patients most often report symptoms as a result of aniseikonia with moderate amounts of image size difference.[40,41] Symptoms most likely arise when the visual system's adaptation ability for image size differences is overwhelmed.[42] Lancaster[3] speculates that the symptoms arise because of the additional burden on the visual system (much as symptoms arise when reading in very dim light). Frequently, the symptoms reported by the patient do not correlate with the degree of aniseikonia.[12] That is, small degrees of aniseikonia may produce severe symptoms, whereas larger degrees may not be troublesome. This varies according to the patient.

Personality Traits

The ability to perceive aniseikonia is sometimes suggested to be related to a patient's personality.[43] The typical aniseikonic patient often has been described as hypercritical and neurotic. Few well-designed studies verify these assertions.

SIGNS

The most significant signs of aniseikonia are anisometropia, occurring naturally or as oblique astigmatism, aphakia, and pseudophakia.

 CLINICAL PEARL

> The most significant signs of aniseikonia are anisometropia, occurring naturally or as oblique astigmatism, aphakia, and pseudophakia.

Anisometropia

Anisometropia, a condition of unequal refraction of 1 D or more between the eyes, is strongly associated with overall aniseikonia.[2,44] Many studies have examined the prevalence of anisometropia in various populations (Table 4-2). Depending on the population the prevalence of anisometropia (greater than 1 D) is approximately 5% to 10%.

Dynamic Aniseikonia

Anisometropia can cause problems with overall optical aniseikonia (which is present without any eye movement) and also can cause "dynamic" aniseikonia, a result of the optical anisophoria.[1,8] Dynamic aniseikonia is a problem whenever the eyes are moved away from the optical center of the spectacle lenses but is not a problem with contact lens corrections. Frequently, the visual system eliminates the swimming sensation of dynamic aniseikonia within days by reprogramming each eye's directional values.

Oblique Astigmatism

Significant amounts of oblique astigmatism can cause declination errors and a consequent distortion of space and/or symptoms.[45] A declination error is a tilt of the image, which causes disparities and stereoscopic distortion. To be considered oblique, an astigmatic axis must be at least 15 degrees away from the vertical or horizontal.[45] The amount of distortion seen is partly a function of the lack of cyclorotation of the eyes.[46] Larger, more complex stimuli elicit more eye movement and therefore cause less distortion. Oblique astigmatism can occur naturally or as a result of radial keratotomy (RK).[38,47]

Aphakia

A patient with unilateral aphakia corrected with a contact lens usually has aniseikonia of about 8% to 9%.[6,18,48,49] Fine fusion and high-grade stereopsis are not possible with image size differences greater than about 5%.[14-16] These size differences can make many patients with aphakia unhappy with only a contact lens correction of their aphakia. Often a spectacle-contact lens reverse telescopic arrangement may be helpful.

Pseudophakia

Most of the more than one million patients who have cataract surgery each year in the United States are corrected with intraocular lenses.[30] Approximately

TABLE 4-2 PREVALENCE OF ANISOMETROPIA IN VARIOUS POPULATIONS

Study	Population	Remarks and Percentage (%)
Blum, Peters, and Bettman, 1959, (Orinda study)	School children, ages 5 to 15	Mean approximately 0.25 D, std. dev. approximately 0.52 D; Smooth change from 2% at age 5 to approximately 4% at age 15 exceed 1.0-D anisometropia
Rayner, 1966	Laboratory orders for spectacles	79.8% less than 0.50 D anisometropia
Kehoe, 1942		65.0% less than 0.50 D anisometropia; 23.1% between 0.50 and 1.00 D; 7.4% between 1.00 and 1.50 D; 2.9% between 1.50 and 2.00 D; 1.6% more than 2.00 D
Hirsch, 1967	Ojai children ages 5 to 14	0.9% in ages 5 to 6 increasing to 2.4% in ages 13 to 14
Brock, 1962	1500 consecutive patients	27.8% of patients with myopia anisometropic greater than 1.00 D; 9.0% of patients without myopia anisometropic by the same amount
Hamilton (Bezan, 1990)	Children	1.37% females and 0.74% males have anisometropia greater than 1.00 D among Native American children; 7.2% Caucasian children have same amount or more
Jones, 1908 (Bezan, 1990)	100 Indian children	28% anisometropia less than 0.25 D; 65% between 0.25 and 1.00 D; 7% greater than 1.00 D
Woodruff and Samek, 1977	7660 Ontario Indians	52.2% less than 0.25 D; 40.56% between 0.25 and 1.00 D; 7.24% greater than 1.00 D
Woodruff, 1977	168 children	13.1% prevalence of anisometropia of 1 D or more
Garber, 1985	Navajo children with at least 1.50-D astigmatism in either eye	49% have 0.75 D or greater anisometropia
Bezan, 1990	1000 Native Americans ages 8 to 89 receiving vision examinations at the W.W. Hastings Indian Health Service Hospital Optometry Clinic	21.7% no anisometropia; 68.5% anisometropia between 0.25 and 1.00 D; 9.8% anisometropia greater than 1.00 D

40% of these patients have symptoms associated with aniseikonia.[30,50] Disturbing the internal optical elements of the eye and a small amount of anisometropia are responsible for the image size difference between the eyes.

Stereopsis

Image size differences greater than about 5% greatly hinder binocular performance; therefore, stereopsis often is reduced in aniseikonia.[16] Although binocular performance is reduced significantly in the presence of aniseikonia (a 14% reduction in the binocular VEP with 2% aniseikonia), stereopsis is still likely to be present, even with large amounts of aniseikonia. Stereoacuity decreases linearly with small amounts of induced aniseikonia, and, for the full range of aniseikonia and stereopsis, there is a curvilinear relationship.[51-54] Approximately 82% of individuals can detect some stereopsis while wearing a correction causing between 13% and 22% aniseikonia.[53] Only 34% of subjects can perceive stereopsis while wearing afocal magnifiers causing image size differences greater than 22%.[53] Random-dot stereopsis is still possible with aniseikonia of up to 15%.[55,56]

 CLINICAL PEARL

Image size differences greater than about 5% greatly hinder binocular performance; therefore, stereopsis often is reduced in aniseikonia.

Space Perception

Aniseikonia can cause several types of spatial distortion, although the distortion is most likely to occur in situations with few clues to rectilinearity.[36,52,57,58] The ability to see such distortion varies considerably from subject to subject and is not likely to be reported.[52,59] Spatial distortion as a result of aniseikonia can be detected if the image size difference is as little as 0.1% to 0.2%, and a standard deviation (an index of the consistency of measurement) of as little as 0.06% can occur.[52] Unsurprisingly, the larger the aniseikonia, the easier it is to see a distortion of space.[52]

Spatial perception of aniseikonic effects depends markedly on the target. A tilting plane device will clearly show aniseikonic distortions if the pattern is random; if a regular pattern is on the plane, the subject typically will perceive it correctly.[57] A meridional mag-

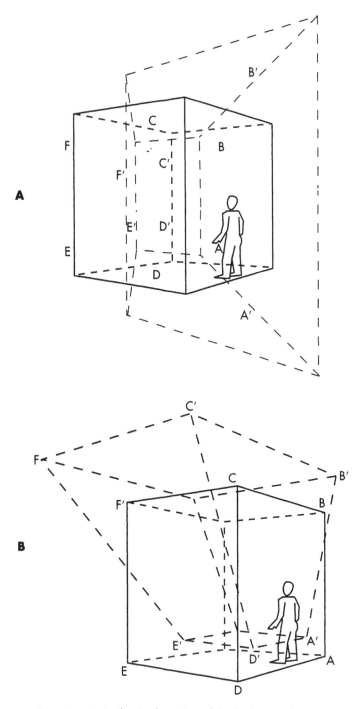

FIG. 4-5 Aniseikonic distortion of the leaf room. **A,** Geometric effect; axis 090-degree magnifier before right eye. This distortion is the same when an axis 180-degree magnifier is placed before left eye (induced effect). **B,** Effect of declination; axis 135-degree magnifier before right eye and axis 045-degree magnifier before left eye. (Modified from Ogle KN: *Researches in binocular vision,* New York, 1972, Hafner.)

nifier (axis 90 degrees) in front of one eye effectively moves the horopter toward that eye, which moves images back on that side. Therefore points that are equidistant from the eyes will appear equidistant, and the side with the larger magnified image will appear farther away. If the patient is looking at pairs of vertical cords and the magnifier (axis 90 degrees) is in front of the right eye, the cords on the right will appear farther away. If the patient is looking at a leaf room, for example, the right side of the room will look larger and farther away. This is called the geometric effect (Fig. 4-5).

When a leaf room is viewed through an overall magnifier held before one eye, the expected view would be that the right side of the room would appear larger and farther away. In fact, very little distortion occurs. This puzzle begins to make sense with the understanding that a meridional magnifier positioned before the right eye (axis 180 degrees) makes the leaf room appear larger and further away on the left (see Fig. 4-5). This is not expected on the basis of geometry, because only horizontal disparities are used in the generation of stereopsis, whereas the axis 180-degree magnifier creates only vertical disparities. It is as if the vertical magnification to the right eye's image has caused the left eye's vertical image to be enlarged to equal it and, in the process, has created a horizontal disparity before the left eye. This effect with the axis 180-degree magnifier is called the induced effect.

It is interesting, however, that an axis 180-degree magnifier does not affect the appearance of a pair of vertical cords. Apparently, some detail in meridians other than the vertical must be present for the induced effect to become operative.

Meridional magnifiers cause the monocular images to be distorted (Fig. 4-6).[60] A +1.00 DC at axis 135 before the right eye and +1.00 DC at axis 45 before the left eye could cause a tilt of a vertical rod (which is 3 m away) of 35 degrees.[60] Usually, these distortions are not seen because of strong perceptual biases toward seeing things straight up and down.

Oblique meridional magnifiers also cause a distortion of the leaf room. If magnifiers are placed axis 135 degrees before the right eye and axis 45 degrees before the left, the magnification is in meridians 45 degrees and 135 degrees in a V pattern. In this case the leaf room will appear bigger and farther away at the bottom (see Fig. 4-5). Because the geometric and induced effects cancel each other, this distortion of space is a result of the declination errors, the rotation or torsional effect of the magnifiers. These types of magnification errors also do not effect the appearance of a pair of vertical cords.

These distortions of space can be predicted on a mathematic basis or measured otherwise.[61-63] An exception is the induced effect (magnification in the vertical meridian), which cannot be easily computed.[62] All of these changes in the perception of space occur because aniseikonia effects the location of the horopter.[64,65] Alterations in image size also produce effects on the contrast sensitivity curve.[66] Magnification shifts the contrast sensitivity curve to the right, producing increased sensitivity to high spatial frequencies.

Because the distortions from opposite magnifications before the eyes can cause space to be magnified either the same or differently depending on what is being looked at, specially designed instruments have been constructed to allow a correct diagnosis of the aniseikonia (i.e., the space eikonometer).

Strabismus, Amblyopia, and Suppression

Aniseikonia can be a significant factor in the etiology of strabismus, especially if unilateral cataracts are removed early in the life of an infant.[16,40,67,68] As with strabismus, substantial aniseikonia also can cause amblyopia and/or suppression.[14,69] Without correcting image size differences, relatively good visual acuity may be obtained, but binocular vision is usually lost.[16] Failure to adequately treat image size differences in an infant with aphakia and anisometropia who also has deprivation amblyopia and strabismus can drastically diminish the prognosis for the continued cure of any of these conditions.[6]

 CLINICAL PEARL

Aniseikonia can be a significant factor in the etiology of strabismus, especially if unilateral cataracts are removed early in the life of an infant.

Reduced Vergence Amplitudes

Unequal image sizes can cause reduced vertical vergence amplitudes and other binocular findings.[70]

PREVALENCE

The exact prevalence of aniseikonia is unknown.[7] Estimates of its prevalence do not include image size differences that occur as a result of eccentric viewing or binocular vision (physiologic aniseikonia). The question of the prevalence of clinically significant amounts of aniseikonia is very difficult to answer because of the nature of the studies that have been completed. Common weaknesses of these studies are that they have (1) not made a determination of whether suspected individuals have symptoms, (2) failed to fully describe the characteristics of the sample, (3) not clearly identified the criteria used to diagnose the condition, and/or (4) not specified how aniseikonia was measured. Many have simply measured image size differences between the eyes, assuming that any difference of 1% or more was significant. The best studies are

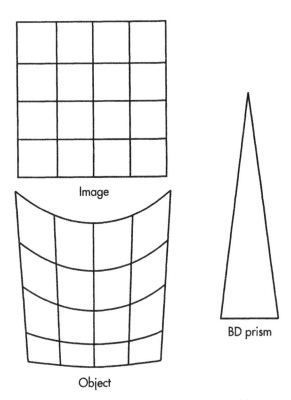

FIG. 4-6 Distortion of monocular images by oblique astigmatism. (Modified from Brown WL: Optical principles of prism. In Cotter SA, London R, editors: *Clinical uses of prism: a spectrum of applications,* St Louis, 1995, Mosby.)

probably those reported by Burian[5] and others that suggest that significant image size differences (2% or more) occur approximately 1% to 3.5% of the time in the general population.[15,71,73]

Aniseikonia clearly has a higher prevalence in the subpopulations of people with pseudophakia and significant oblique astigmatism.[15,50,74] Patients with these conditions should have aniseikonia ruled out if they have symptoms.

ETIOLOGY

The etiology of aniseikonia is very complex; however, the nature of the condition revolves around differences in the size of images arriving at the cortex. Many factors are associated with differences of image sizes. With a spectacle lens the base curve, thickness, vertex distance, and refractive power of the lens all have a significant effect on the size of an image. Likewise, the position and design of an intraocular lens (IOL) have a great effect on image size.[37]

DIAGNOSIS

Anisometropia is the best clue suggesting that aniseikonia will occur, with the larger image occurring in the eye with the most plus or least minus.[7] The presence of symptoms is helpful in the diagnosis, particularly if they are long-standing and are binocular in nature (i.e., relieved by monocular occlusion). However, symptoms alone could be a result of binocular dysfunction (e.g., vergence problems). A fit-over magnifier on each eye can be used to determine whether the symptoms are relieved with the suspected image size difference corrected and aggravated when the magnifier is reversed and the image size difference is increased.[22] Aniseikonia is not likely to be a problem unless the patient has reasonably good visual acuity (about 20/40 or better) and binocular vision.[41]

Although not important for the diagnosis of aniseikonia, keratometry readings are a useful method of suggesting whether a given refractive error is likely axial or refractive in origin.[7] Keratometry values have relatively little impact on the diagnosis or treatment of aniseikonia, because contact lenses should be prescribed initially for anisometropia of either refractive or axial etiology.

TREATMENT

Contact Lenses

The first alternative in the treatment of problems related to aniseikonia should be the application of contact lenses. Contact lenses are the best choice whether the etiology of the image size difference is axial or refractive. Contact lenses are also the best choice for oblique astigmatism correction. Contact lenses minimize image size difference and eliminate dynamic aniseikonia and other induced prismatic effects.[19,20] They have other optical advantages that argue for use even when aniseikonia remains.[75] They minimize aberrations associated with spectacle lenses; visual field defects, such as the Jack-in-the-box phenomenon; and prismatic imbalance caused by eccentric viewing.

 CLINICAL PEARL

The first alternative in the treatment of problems related to aniseikonia should be the application of contact lenses.

A contact lens is far superior to glasses in correcting aniseikonia in patients who have had cataract surgery who do not receive intraocular lenses.[28] Those with contact lenses averaged a 4.6% image size difference, whereas those with spectacles averaged 17.8%.

Spectacle Lenses
Small Eye Sizes
Smaller eye sizes allow thicker and steeper lenses to be used without excessive penalties of weight. Aniseikonic patients should always choose the smallest acceptable eye size.

Short Vertex Distance
For patients with aniseikonia who wear glasses, fitting the lenses as close to the eyes as possible is important because short vertex distances always minimize image size differences between the eyes.[26] Theoretically, vertex distance should be of more benefit with refractive than with axial errors of refraction and should be unnecessary in cases of axial anisometropia. However, changes in vertex distance remain helpful as a result of factors in addition to the optical system, such as neurologic magnification (e.g., magnification as a result of different receptor packing).[20,76]

 CLINICAL PEARL

For patients with aniseikonia who wear glasses, fitting the lenses as close to the eyes as possible is important because short vertex distances always minimize image size differences between the eyes.

Vertex distance can be modified within certain limits.[77] Changing vertex distance, of course, not only has an effect on magnification but also alters the effective power of the lens. If the lens is plus, decreasing the vertex distance decreases the magnification provided by the lens, thus minimizing any difference between the lenses. Therefore patients with anisohyperopia should have their spectacle lenses fitted as closely as possible to minimize any differences. If the lens is minus, decreasing the vertex distance increases the magnification provided by the lens. Likewise, patients with anisomyopia should wear their lenses as close as possible. The vertex distance also can be changed by specifying the location of the bevel.[78] A bevel toward the front of the lens moves the lens back; conversely, a bevel toward the back of the lens effectively moves the lens forward. For a high correction, this can move the lens 2 or 3 mm closer or farther away from the eyes.

Changing the vertex distance of a spectacle lens affects the magnification as a function of the power of the lens (Table 4-3).[78,79] For a lens with a vertex power of 10 D a change of vertex distance of 1 mm changes the magnification by 1% in a linear relationship. Therefore for a +10.00-D right eye and a +5.00-D left eye a change in the vertex distance of 4 mm (closer to the eyes) would substantially effect an assumed 5% image size difference between the eyes. In this case the +10.00-D eye will have its magnification decreased by 4% while the +5.00-D lens will have a decreased magnification of 2%. The difference between the eyes would then be reduced by 2%. Because the clinician is almost always trying to increase the magnification of minus lenses and decrease that of plus lenses, spectacles with which size differences are potentially a problem should always be moved as close as possible to the eyes.

TABLE 4-3 **APPROXIMATE MAGNIFICATION (%) CHANGES FOR EYEWIRE DISTANCE CHANGES OF VARIOUS LENS POWERS**

Change in Eyewire distance (h, mm)	Power (D)					
	1	2	4	6	8	10
1	0.1	0.2	0.4	0.6	0.8	1.0
2	0.2	0.4	0.8	1.2	1.6	2.0
3	0.3	0.6	1.2	1.8	2.4	3.0
4	0.4	0.8	1.6	2.4	3.2	4.0
5	0.5	1.0	2.0	3.0	4.0	5.0

Modified from Wick B: Iseikonic considerations for today's eyewear, *Am J Optom Arch Am Acad Optom* 50:952, 1973.

Equal Base Curve and Center Thickness

Anisohyperopic patients with aniseikonia benefit from lenses with equal base curves and center thickness. Patients with myopia will benefit from correcting the anisometropia with stock lenses, because these patients naturally tend to minimize size differences.

Antireflection Coatings and Aspheric Lenses

An antireflection coating makes thicker, steeper lenses much less noticeable and should be liberally used in aniseikonic design.[79] Aspheric lenses are another good method to minimize center thickness for a particular base curve.

High-Index Spectacle Lenses

High-index lenses should be used if base curves and center thicknesses are manipulated to minimize image differences, because greater changes in magnification can be achieved.[80] These lenses are also lighter and thinner.

Partial Correction, Cutting Cylinder, and Sphere

Partial correction is a very common method of dealing with aniseikonic complaints, particularly those resulting from oblique astigmatism.[22,60,81] Because this method decreases visual function, it should not be used for young people who are given the full cylindric correction. The correction for an adult is rotated toward the horizontal and vertical axes and/or the cylinder power is decreased while keeping the circle of least confusion on the retina.[60] The monovision technique of fitting one eye for distance and one for near may eliminate aniseikonic symptoms in certain situations.[82]

Manipulating Parameters of Spectacle Lenses

In some cases the manipulation of the parameters of spectacle lenses to minimize image size differences is necessary. There are several aspects of this process.

Knapp's Law

Traditionally, Knapp's law has been used to justify using spectacle lenses to correct patients with axial anisometropia, although this is not currently accepted.[20] Knapp's law states that the focal power of an eye-spectacle system is the same as without the spectacle lens when a spectacle lens is placed at the anterior focal plane of the eye.[77,83] If the refractive error is produced by axial length differences, the power of the system with or without the spectacle lens is the same and the image size produced is also the same, regardless of the refractive error.

This relationship occurs because of the special relationship between the thickness of the system, the lens power formula (below), and the focal length of the eye.

$$F_{\text{eye-spectacle system}} = F_{\text{eye}} + F_{\text{spectacle lens}} - t/n \, (F_{\text{eye}} \, F_{\text{spectacle lens}})$$

Substituting $f_{\text{eye}}/1$ for t/n because t is the distance between the principal planes of the system (equal to the anterior focal length of the eye) and 1 for n (the index common to the eye-spectacle lens system is air) and the equivalent $1/f_{\text{eye}}$ for F_{eye}, the formula for the power of the system becomes:

$$F_{\text{eye-spectacle system}} = F_{\text{eye}} + F_{\text{spectacle lens}} - (f_{\text{eye}}/1)(1/f_{\text{eye}})(F_{\text{spectacle lens}})$$

which reduces to:

$$F_{\text{eye-spectacle system}} = F_{\text{eye}} + F_{\text{spectacle lens}} - F_{\text{spectacle lens}}$$

which in turn reduces to:

$$F_{\text{eye-spectacle system}} = F_{\text{eye}}$$

Because the power of the eye-spectacle system is the same with the addition of the spectacle lens, the image size is also the same size as before the spectacle lens was added. The addition of the spectacle lens to the eye simply moves the principle planes of the system.

Not long ago, clinicians were careful to correct refractive errors caused by improper axial lengths with spectacle lenses and to correct refractive errors caused by improper coordination of refractive components with contact lenses. However, now this convention is no longer appropriate because it is now known that the ocular (cortical) images are affected also by neurologic aniseikonia.[7,20] The first and best choice in dealing with any image size problem is contact lenses. Knapp's law is a true description of the geometrically determined *retinal* image size. Knapp's law does not accurately describe the size of *ocular* images arriving at the cortex because it does not incorporate neurologic factors, such as the packing of retinal receptors, that affect aniseikonia.[7,20] Knapp's law perhaps should be considered Knapp's *suggestion* because the relationship does not hold true when the transmission to the cortex is considered.

Magnification Properties of Ophthalmic Lenses

Spectacle magnification is usually defined as:

$$\text{Spectacle magnification} = \{1/[1 - (t/n)F_1]\} \times [1/(1 - hF_v)]$$

in which t = spectacle lens center thickness (in meters), n = index of refraction of the spectacle lens, F_1 = front surface power of the lens (D), h = distance from the back surface of the spectacle lens to the entrance pupil of the eye (also in meters), and F_v = back vertex power of the lens (D).[80]

The first portion of the equation involves the lens front surface power (i.e., the base curve), the thickness of the lens, and the lens refractive index, which together make up the shape factor. The second portion is a function of the eye-lens vertex distance and the back vertex power of the lens, which is the power factor. Spectacle magnification can be reduced to these two factors:

$$\text{Spectacle magnification} = \text{shape factor} \times \text{power factor}$$

Ordinarily, a clinician does not wish to alter the power of the lens to be prescribed, in-as-much as it reduces visual acuity and binocular visual capability. The power factor can be altered by changing the vertex distance and, for this reason, lenses are often fit as close as possible. The components of the shape factor can be readily changed in most cases. Often, the image size difference can be altered by 2% (or more) by altering the index, the thickness, and the base curve of the lenses.

Spectacle Lens Factors and Image Sizes

The index of refraction, base curve, and center thickness are commonly used to change the magnification associated with the shape factor. Increasing the base curve (i.e., making it steeper) tends to increase the shape factor and the magnification of the lens. Likewise, increasing the center thickness increases the magnification of the lens. Selecting a different material to increase the refractive index makes changes to either the base curve or the center thickness more dramatic.[80] A minus lens moved nearer the eye increases magnification; a plus lens moved farther from the eye increases the magnification.[22] In sensitive patients, care should be taken to match the dimensions of the previous correction to avoid creating an adaptation problem.[59]

The base curve of a lens can alter magnification, although the interaction of base curve changes with vertex distance must be understood. For example, increasing the base curve of a minus lens does not necessarily increase the magnification.[26,59,78,84,85] Increasing the base curve also moves the lens farther away from the eye, thus negating a portion of the increase. For a plus lens, increasing the front curve increases the shape factor as expected and also produces a concomitant change in the power factor. For a minus lens, however, the increase in the shape factor is effected to a greater

or lesser extent, according to the power of the lens and the eye size. For very small eye sizes (48 mm) and glass lenses (Masterpiece II) the decrease in the power factor more than offsets the increase, because of the shape factor for all lenses -5.50 D or more. For eye sizes of 56 mm the crossover point drops to -3.87 D.

The center thickness of minus lenses of significant refractive power and/or eye size must be altered to significantly change the shape magnification. A change in center thickness will increase both the shape and power magnification. The position of the bevel is important.[85] Placing it far to the front reduces the vertex distance and increases the magnification (actually minifies the image less).

All of these changes to spectacle lenses should be considered in the context of practicality. Patients typically will reject a lens thicker than about 4 or 5 mm. The clinician should prescribe a correction that is thinner and corrects only a portion of the image size difference rather than one that fully eliminates image size differences but is thicker. Likewise, vertex distance and base curves also have practical limits. Changes in the base curve depend on the power of the lens and the eye size of the frame. When there is no anisometropia the necessary changes in lens configuration must be greater.

CASE 1

A 38-year-old man experienced a breakdown in fusion secondary to a central serous macular lesion in the left eye. After several months a laser photocoagulation procedure was used to seal the lesion. When examined in our clinic, he reported that image sizes were smaller with the OS than with the OD. His refraction was +0.75 −0.25 × 045 (20/20, right eye) and +0.75 −0.25 × 180 (20/20, left eye). His current glasses had base curves of 6.25 D and were 3.2 mm thick. A steeper and thicker lens was prescribed for the left eye (12-D base curve and 4-mm thickness). The patient reported that the images appeared equal between the two eyes and that vision was more comfortable.

Nomographs

A nomograph is a convenient way to see the relationships between several variables.[78] In dealing with aniseikonia, nomographs are commonly used to determine the relationship between magnification and the base curve and center thickness of a spectacle lens.[80] The magnification provided by a particular base curve and center thickness also can be calculated using an equation, but a nomograph does not require an equation or a calculator to work out the answer. In addition, the nomograph allows the user to visualize the results of several combinations of two of the variables on the third. Therefore nomographs are quicker and easier than working magnification formulas.

Nomographs have been created for both shape and power factors. The shape factor nomograph is used to select base curves and center thicknesses for the spectacles lenses in question (Fig. 4-7). Because the clinician does not typically wish to alter the power being prescribed, the power factor nomograph shows magnification as a function of power and distance. The accompanying nomograph can be used to give combinations of base curves and center thicknesses of lenses that could be prescribed to eliminate aniseikonia. In the absence of any other information, generally the clinician should assume an image size difference of about 1% per diopter.[80]

If a patient has a correction of OD +4.00 DS and OS +2.25 −0.25 × 090, assuming an image size difference of 1% per diopter, the clinician should magnify the image before the left eye about 2% to equalize the images. To do this using the nomograph requires a stepwise approach. First, select a high-index material, such as polycarbonate, to maximize the effect of changes in parameters and select base curves and center thicknesses that will minimize the shape factor of the right eye while being practical.

Second, use the nomograph to find pairs of base curves and center thicknesses that will give a shape factor that is 2% greater than that of the right eye. In this case the shape factor for the right lens is 1% (2.3 mm thick, 6-D base curve). The goal for the design of the left lens is to make the shape factor 2% + 1%, which is 3%. On a theoretic basis, many combinations provide the appropriate magnification. The critical concern is to find practically useable parameters. Eliminating the entire difference is impractical because the resulting lens for the left eye will be too steep and too thick (e.g., 3.4 mm thick, 12-D base curve). We recommend compromising and correcting only 1.3% of the difference (shape factor, 2.3%; center thickness, 3.5 mm; base curve, 9 D).

Finding practically useable parameters is a very important part of prescribing for aniseikonia. Several things can help, such as calling the laboratory and asking if the proposed lens design is practical. Manufacturers sometimes provide base curve tables showing which base curves are used for which powers, along with center thickness. In selecting iseikonic lenses the usual parameters should be altered as little as possible.

The center thickness must be kept practical because changing it can dramatically alter the weight of the lens. A set of lenses that cannot be worn because they are too heavy will not do the patient much good, even if they correct image size differences perfectly. Bitoric lenses are difficult and expensive for the laboratory to make, and we do not recommend their use.

Computerized Methods

Various computerized interactive methods of selecting proper lenses to correct size differences are available.[86]

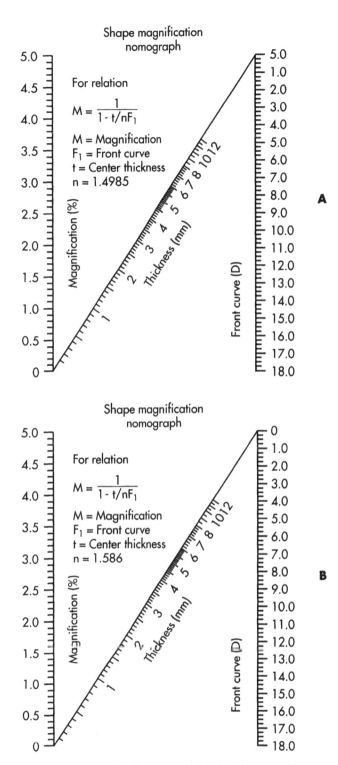

FIG. 4-7 Nomographs showing relationship between base curve, center thickness, and shape factor for lenses of various materials. **A,** CR-39 plastic (n = 1.4985). **B,** Polycarbonate plastic (n = 1.586). (Modified from Stephens GL, Polasky M: New options for aniseikonia correction: the use of high index materials, *Optom Vis Sci* 68:899, 1991.)

Spectacle-Contact Lens Combination: Aniseikonia in Neonatal or Infantile Unilateral Aphakia

Spectacle correction of monocular aphakia causes image size differences of from 22% to 35% (magnified in the aphakic eye). Correction with a contact lens still causes differences of 7% to 12%.[18,74,87,88] A concern for aniseikonia in cases of neonatal or infantile unilateral aphakia should occur only when the patient has good visual acuity in both eyes and the potential for excellent binocularity.[18] To correct greater than about a 4% image size difference, a Galilean telescope arrangement must be used. Patients using a Galilean system will have induced prism whenever they look away from the center of the optical system.[74] Therefore because patients with aphakia are always prescribed an add, slab-off prism may be necessary. A frame with adjustable pads will allow the vertex distance to be altered. In addition, induced vertical prism is possible if the contact lens decenters.

Binocular function in unilateral aphakia is unlikely in an infant, unless the resultant aniseikonia is corrected.[68] A Galilean telescope arrangement can be constructed by adding plus power to a contact lens and partially compensating for it in a spectacle lens. Using this arrangement, 5% to 8% reductions in image size can be rather easily accomplished (Table 4-4). For infants a +3.00-D overcorrection is also appropriate, because their effective visual world is near.

A contact lens fitted to an infant must be frequently and carefully evaluated because the child may cause difficulties by rubbing the eye and/or lens.[68] For the optics, as well as the physiology, it is important that the contact lens remain centered, except for movement with a blink.

Intraocular Lenses and Aniseikonia

The use of intraocular lenses (IOLs) does not eliminate aniseikonia. Studies show an average aniseikonia of about 2% with a unilateral IOL, 20 times greater than the calculated aniseikonia.[88,89] An examination after cataract surgery of 57 patients with unilateral IOLs measured an average of 2.8% aniseikonia, with a range of 0% to 8.5%.[28] The position of an IOL has an effect on the amount of aniseikonia present.[90] An average of 2.5% image size difference existed in 41 posterior-chamber IOL wearers, and a 3.1% difference in 10 anterior-chamber IOL wearers was determined.[90] Although the tendency holds true, anterior-chamber lenses do not always produce larger image sizes.[37] Even patients with two IOLs can have significant aniseikonia of at least 3.4%.[37]

Adaptation and Aniseikonia

The visual system has a substantial amplitude for adjustment for image size differences in aniseikonia, although disagreement exists.[36,42,59] The ability to adapt

TABLE 4-4 RELATIONSHIP BETWEEN VERTEX DISTANCE, SPECTACLE POWER, AND PERCENT SIZE REDUCTION FOR IMAGE SIZE IF A +7.00-D OVERCORRECTION IS PRESCRIBED IN A CONTACT LENS

Vertex Distance (mm)	Power in Spectacle Plane (D)	Percent Size Reduction (%)
7	−7.36	4.9
8	−7.42	5.7
9	−7.47	6.3
10	−7.53	7.0
11	−7.58	7.7

Modified from Enoch JM, Campos EC: Helping the aphakic neonate to see, *Int Ophthalmol* 8:237, 1985.

to magnification differences before the eyes is one of the most significant factors in determining whether a patient will be comfortable with a given image size difference. Unfortunately, it is difficult to evaluate the ability of any given patient to adapt to an image size difference. To date, no tests have been developed that reliably provide an estimate of a patient's adaptability. For this reason the most common method of determining a patient's adaptation ability is simply to have the patient wear the proposed correction and see if improvement occurs.

Several investigations of adaptation to size differences before the eyes have been performed. Burian[5] studied three subjects who wore meridional magnifiers for a 1- to 2-week period. Over that time, these subjects experienced a significant degree of adaptation to the size difference. The decreases ranged from 20% to 67% of the original aniseikonia. After a period the spatial distortion tended to go away in familiar places with lots of vertical and horizontal lines, such as the city. When the subjects went into unfamiliar places (such as the countryside) that were relatively devoid of known verticals and horizontals, the symptoms returned.

Miles[33] described the effects of wearing size lenses of various types for periods of 25, 37, 23, and 28 days by two individuals. Immediately upon wearing the lenses of axis 180 degrees on one eye or the other (either 3% or 4%), there was substantial distortion of both familiar and unfamiliar space, and considerable eyestrain occurred. After about 5 days of wear the distortion largely disappeared in familiar surroundings. After that, in surroundings that were unfamiliar and without many clues to rectilinearity the distortion of space reappeared. The eyestrain largely disappeared after a few days of wear. The measured amount of aniseikonia remained fairly constant. Glasses with oblique meridional effects caused a large constant degree of eyestrain, headaches, and spatial distortion over the entire time that they were worn.

These studies in which adults have worn lenses producing aniseikonia for extended periods (up to 2 weeks) suggest that the adaptation is primarily one of interpretation rather than physiologic adaptation, although it is likely that some physiologic adaptation takes place, probably about 20% to 60% of the total adaptation.[60] The physiologic component of adaptation to aniseikonia is larger if the correction has been worn since childhood because it appears to be age-dependent.[60] Katsumi and others[28] also assume that aniseikonic adaptation ability is age-dependent and works well up to about 3% differences between the eyes.

Adapting to image size differences produced by RK is a special challenge. RK is usually performed in adulthood, when adaptation ability is less. In addition, RK occurs at a specific point in time, so that adaptation is necessary within a short period. Duling and Wick[38] report on four patients with RK-related aniseikonia, noting that the primary objective of RK is to provide good monocular vision (uncorrected if possible), whereas binocular visual problems are frequently ignored. RK causes aniseikonic problems as a result of the unequal correction of the eyes or distortion of the cornea, causing astigmatic and therefore meridional image size errors.[38]

Success in the Treatment of Aniseikonia

There is little literature regarding the treatment of aniseikonia. For most patients at least some relief is likely when the condition is treated. Bannon and others,[36] in a review of the subject, found that approximately 70% of those patients given aniseikonic corrections report beneficial results. Of 18 patients with unilateral aphakia that were corrected with spectacle-contact lens combinations (Galilean telescopes), 14 were successful.[18] The patients ranged in age from 12 and 60 years. Newcomb's patient[82] with 16 D of anisometropia and aniseikonia was successfully helped using the monovision technique with contact lenses. The purposeful prevention of binocular vision eliminated any aniseikonic problems. In addition, there are anecdotal cases of patients with treated aniseikonia who experienced relief after years of discomfort.[7]

REFERENCES

1. Remole A: Anisophoria and aniseikonia. I. The relation between optical anisophoria and aniseikonia, *Optom Vis Sci* 66:659, 1989.
2. Schapero M, Cline D, Hofstetter HW: *Dictionary of visual science,* ed 2, Philadelphia, 1968, Chilton.
3. Lancaster WB: Nature, scope, and significance of aniseikonia, *Arch Ophthalmol* 28:767, 1942.
4. Bannon RE: On the technique of measuring and correcting aniseikonia, *Am J Optom Arch Am Acad Optom* 18:145, 1941.
5. Burian HM: Clinical significance of aniseikonia, *Arch Ophthalmol* 29:116, 1943.
6. Winn B and others: Reduced aniseikonia in axial anisometropia with contact lens correction, *Ophthalmic Physiol Opt* 8:341, 1988.
7. Rabin JC, Bailey IL: Treatment of an unusual case of aniseikonia, *J Am Optom Assoc* 54:153, 1983.
8. Remole A: Anisophoria and aniseikonia. II. The management of optical anisophoria, *Optom Vis Sci* 66:736, 1989.
9. Wick B: Aniseikonia following unilateral intraocular lens implant, *J Am Optom Assoc* 54:423, 1983.
10. Bannon RE: *Clinical manual on aniseikonia,* Buffalo, 1974, American Optical.
11. Hicks AH: A review of 200 consecutive cases examined on the eikonometer, *Arch Ophthalmol* 30:298, 1943.
12. Moskowitz W: Meridional size disparity as a function of compressed inferior visual space: a case in point, *Percept Mot Skills* 51:1255, 1980.
13. Ogle KN: *Researches in binocular vision,* New York, 1972, Hafner.
14. Hawkswell A: Routine aniseikonic screening, *Brit J Physiol Opt* 29:126, 1974.
15. Davis RJ: Empirical corrections for aniseikonia in preschool anisometropes, *Am J Optom Arch Am Acad Optom* 36:351, 1959.
16. Campos EC, Enoch JM: Amount of aniseikonia compatible with fine binocular vision: some old and new concepts, *J Pediatr Ophthalmol Strab* 17:44, 1980.
17. Roper KL, Bannon RE: Diagnostic value of monocular occlusion, *Arch Ophthalmol* 31:316, 1944.
18. Enoch JM: Use of inverted telescope corrections incorporating soft contact lenses in the (partial) correction of aniseikonia in cases of unilateral aphakia, *Adv Ophthalmol* 32:54, 1976.
19. Rabin J, Bradley A, Freeman RD: On the relation between aniseikonia and axial anisometropia, *Am J Optom Physiol Opt* 60:553, 1983.
20. Bradley A, Rabin J, Freeman RD: Non-optical determinants of aniseikonia, *Invest Ophthalmol Vis Sci* 24:507, 1983.
21. Stoddard KB: Aniseikonia, *Am J Optom Arch Am Acad Optom* 17:253, 1940.
22. Berens C, Bannon RE: Aniseikonia: a present appraisal and some practical considerations, *Arch Ophthalmol* 70:181, 1963.
23. Ogle KN: The correction of aniseikonia with ophthalmic lenses, *J Opt Soc Am* 26:323, 1936.
24. Brecher GA: A new method of measuring aniseikonia, *Am J Ophthalmol* 34:1016, 1951.
25. Bannon RE: Space eikonometry in aniseikonia, *Am J Optom Arch Am Acad Optom* 30:86, 1953.
26. Ryan VI: Predicting aniseikonia in anisometropia, *Am J Optom Physiol Opt* 52:96, 1975.
27. Pratt-Johnson JA, Tillson G: Intractable diplopia after vision restoration in unilateral cataract, *Am J Ophthalmol* 107:23, 1989.
28. Katsumi O and others: Binocular function in unilateral aphakia, *Ophthalmology* 95:1088, 1988.
29. Cohen HL, Forman MZ, Milan RH: A qualitative and quantitative method of screening aniseikonia, *Am J Optom Arch Am Acad Optom* 34:184, 1957.
30. McCormack G, Peli E, Stone P: Differences in tests of aniseikonia, *Invest Ophthalmol Vis Sci* 33:2063, 1992.
31. Ogle KN: Theory of the space eikonometer, *J Opt Soc Am* 36:20, 1946.
32. Scheiman M, Wick B: *Clinical management of binocular vision,* Philadelphia, 1994, JB Lippincott.
33. Miles PW: A comparison of aniseikonic test instruments and prolonged induction of artificial aniseikonia, *Am J Ophthalmol* 36:687, 1948.
34. Hughes WL: Aniseikonia: some clinical observations, *Am J Ophthalmol* 18:607, 1935.

35. Bannon RE: Headaches and aniseikonia, *Am J Optom Arch Am Acad Optom* 17:448, 1940.

36. Bannon RE and others: Aniseikonia and space perception: after 50 years, *Am J Optom Arch Am Acad Optom* 47:423, 1970.

37. Snead MP and others: Aniseikonia: a method of objective assessment in pseudophakia using geometric optics, *Ophthalmic Physiol Opt* 11:109, 1991.

38. Duling K, Wick B: Binocular vision complications after radial keratotomy, *Am J Optom Physiol Opt* 65:215, 1988.

39. Simmons HD, Gassler PA: Vision anomalies and reading skill: a meta-analysis of the literature, *Am J Optom Physiol Opt* 65:893, 1988.

40. Madigan LF: Examination and correction of aniseikonia, *Arch Ophthalmol* 13:696, 1934.

41. Berens C, Loutfallah M: Aniseikonia: a study of 836 patients examined with the ophthalmo-eikonometer, *Am J Ophthalmol* 22:625, 1939.

42. Lancaster WB: Aniseikonia, *Arch Ophthalmol* 20:907, 1938.

43. Schaninger CM: *Percept Mot Skills* 43:915, 1976.

44. Blum HL, Peters HB, Bettman JW: *Vision for elementary schools: the Orinda study,* Berkeley, Calif, 1959, University of California.

45. Burian HM, Ogle KN: Meridional aniseikonia at oblique axes, *Arch Ophthalmol* 33:293, 1945.

46. Hampton DR, Kertesz AE: Human response to cyclofusional stimuli containing depth cues, *Am J Optom Physiol Opt* 59:21, 1982.

47. Binder PS: Radial keratotomy in the United States, *Arch Ophthalmol* 105:37, 1987.

48. Christman EH: Correction of aniseikonia in monocular aphakia: *Arch Ophthalmol* 85:148, 1971.

49. Krefman RA: Reverse Galilean telescopic spectacles in unilateral aphakia, *Am J Optom Physiol Opt* 58:772, 1981.

50. Lubkin V and others: Aniseikonia in unilateral and bilateral pseudophakia, *Invest Ophthalmol Vis Sci* 31(suppl): 94, 1990.

51. Lovasik JV, Robertson KM: Electrophysiological detection of aniseikonia, *J Am Optom Assoc* 55:499, 1984.

52. Ogle KN: Association between aniseikonia and anomalous binocular spatial perception, *Arch Ophthalmol* 30:54, 1943.

53. Lovasik JV, Szymkiw M: Effects of aniseikonia, anisometropia, accommodation, retinal illuminance, and pupil size on stereopsis, *Invest Ophthalmol Vis Sci* 26:741, 1985.

54. Reading RW, Tanlamai T: The threshold of stereopsis in the presence of differences in magnification of the ocular images, *J Am Optom Assoc* 51:593, 1980.

55. Julesz B: *Foundations of cyclopean perception,* Chicago, 1971, University of Chicago.

56. Ogle KN, Wakefield JM: Stereoscopic depth and binocular rivalry, *Vision Res* 7:89, 1967.

57. Ames A: Aniseikonia: a factor in the functioning of vision, *Am J Ophthalmol* 18:1014, 1935.

58. Ames A: The space eikonometer test for aniseikonia, *Am J Ophthalmol* 28:246, 1945.

59. Linksz A: The diagnosis and correction of aniseikonia, *Trans Am Acad Ophthalmol Otolaryngol* 70:340, 1966.

60. Guyton DL: Prescribing cylinders: the problem of distortion, *Surv Ophthalmol* 22:177, 1977.

61. Ogle KN: Meridional magnifying lens systems in the measurement and correction of aniseikonia, *J Opt Soc Am* 34:302, 1944.

62. Ogle KN, Boeder P: Distortion of stereoscopic spatial localization, *J Opt Soc Am* 38:723, 1948.

63. Shipley AT, Rawlings SC: The nonius horopter: an experimental report, *Vision Res* 10:1263, 1970.

64. Reading RW: Vergence instabilities and the longitudinal horopter, *Ophthalmic Physiol Opt* 6:63, 1986.

65. Reading RW: Horopter shifts due to a magnification change, *Am J Optom Physiol Opt* 61:310, 1984.

66. Bradley A, Freeman RD: Contrast sensitivity in anisometropic amblyopia, *Invest Ophthalmol Vis Sci* 21:467, 1981.

67. Saloman E: An aniseikonic alternating esotrope, *Am J Optom Arch Am Acad Optom* 48:859, 1971.

68. Enoch JM, Campos EC: Helping the aphakic neonate to see, *Int Ophthalmol* 8:237, 1985.

69. Lancaster WB: Aniseikonia, *Arch Ophthalmol* 20:907, 1938.

70. Ellerbrock VJ: The effect of aniseikonia on the amplitude of vertical divergence, *Am J Optom Arch Am Acad Optom* 29:403, 1952.

71. Burian HM: The history of the Dartmouth Eye Institute, *Arch Ophthalmol* 40:163, 1948.

72. Burian HM: The Dartmouth Eye Institute, *Surv Ophthalmol* 19:101, 1974.

73. Burian HM, Walsh R, Bannon RE: Note on the incidence of clinically significant aniseikonia, *Am J Ophthalmol* 29:201, 1946.

74. Enoch JM: A spectacle-contact lens combination used as a reverse Galilean telescope in unilateral aphakia, *Am J Optom Arch Am Acad Optom* 45:231, 1968.

75. Levinson A, Ticho U: The use of contact lenses in children and infants, *Am J Optom Arch Am Acad Optom* 49:60, 1972.

76. Mills PV: Aniseikonia in corrected aniseikonia, *Brit Orthopt J* 36:36, 1979.

77. von Bahr G: An analysis of the change in perceptual size of the retinal image at correction of ametropia, *Doc Ophthalmol* 20:530, 1966.

78. Rayner AW: Aniseikonia and magnification in ophthalmic lenses: problems and solutions, *Am J Optom Arch Am Acad Optom* 43:617, 1966.

79. Wick B: Iseikonic considerations for today's eyewear, *Am J Optom Arch Am Acad Optom* 50:952, 1973.

80. Stephens GL, Polasky M: New options for aniseikonia correction: the use of high index materials, *Optom Vis Sci* 68:899, 1991.

81. Linksz A: Aniseikonia with notes on the Jackson-Lancaster controversy, *Trans Am Acad Ophthalmol Otolaryngol* 63:117, 1959.

82. Newcomb RD: Dissimilar contact lenses for a 16-D anisometrope: a case study, *Am J Optom Physiol Opt* 54:114, 1977.

83. Knapp H: The influence of spectacles on the optical constants and visual acuteness of the eye, *Arch Ophthalmol Otolaryngol* 1:377, 1869.

84. Brown RM, Enoch JM: Combined rules of thumb in aniseikonic prescriptions, *Am J Ophthalmol* 1970; 69:1128.

85. Good GW, Polasky M: Eikonic lens design for minus prescriptions, *Am J Optom Physiol Opt* 56:345, 1979.

86. Alexander JA: Computer assisted optometry: a tutorial with examples, *Am J Optom Arch Am Acad Optom* 50:730, 1973.

87. Cohen A: Calculating magnification differences in monocular aphakia, *Am J Optom Physiol Opt* 53:294, 1976.

88. Schechter RJ: Elimination of aniseikonia in monocular aphakia with a contact lens-spectacle combination, *Surv Ophthalmol* 23:57, 1978.

89. Lightholder PA, Phillips LJ: Evaluation of the binocularity of 147 unilateral and bilateral pseudophakic patients, *Am J Optom Physiol Opt* 56:451, 1979.

90. Boissonnot M, Risse JF, Ingrand P: Aniseiconie, *Ophtalmologie* 4:213, 1990.

91. Brown WL: Optical principles of prism. In Cotter SA, London R, editors: *Clinical uses of prism: a spectrum of applications,* St Louis, 1995, Mosby.

Suppression and Anomalous Correspondence

The evaluation of a patient with a binocular vision disorder includes an evaluation of the patient's sensory fusion status, as well as the evaluation of patient's motor fusion status. The sensory status greatly affects the prognosis for normal binocular vision. Patients with strabismus, for example, vary in the ability they exhibit to suppress diplopia, state of retinal correspondence, and quality of sensory fusion. Generally, the younger patient is more able to cope with strabismus, because the visual system is more pliable. The longer the strabismus is present, the more likely that the sensory adaptations have developed. Sensory fusion testing determines the following conditions:

- Whether visual confusion and/or diplopia exists
- Whether there is suppression and its extent
- Whether amblyopia exists (see Chapter 2)
- The type of retinal correspondence
- The patient's responsiveness to disparate retinal stimulation, or stereopsis

SUPPRESSION: PHYSIOLOGIC AND PATHOLOGIC

Suppression is an active inhibition resulting in the loss of awareness of visual impression for one eye in binocular vision. It can be either physiologic or pathologic. Physiologic suppression, or suspension, occurs in all patients and is part of normal single binocular vision. It is in play when looking through a monocular microscope or using a direct ophthalmoscope. The brain sees only what interests it and suppresses all other images.

 CLINICAL PEARL

Suppression is an active inhibition resulting in the loss of awareness of visual impression for one eye in binocular vision.

Whenever binocular fixation is maintained at a fixed distance, objects that are closer or that are farther away are imaged on noncorresponding retinal regions (Fig. 5-1). These images are potential stimuli for physiologic diplopia when they are not located within Panum's area. Under ordinary circumstances, the individual is not aware of physiologic diplopia because the images strike nonfoveal retinal elements of poorer acuity and of much less interest than the object of regard. The perceptual avoidance of the images of objects that are not located within Panum's area is the result of physiologic suppression. Occasionally, the awareness of physiologic diplopia will occur; we have examined patients with "acute-onset diplopia" in whom this situation was found to be the case. The phenomenon can be readily explained to the patient.

Physiologic suppression is also functioning in retinal or binocular rivalry. When two dissimilarly patterned images are simultaneously presented to the two foveae, the brain suppresses one or the other of the images. The image from one eye competes with the image from the other eye for conscious regard. A state of rapid alternation of parts of the stimuli takes place, and at no time are the dissimilarly patterned images seen in the same

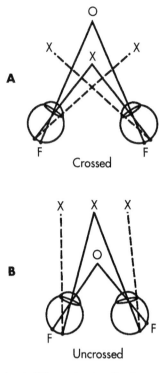

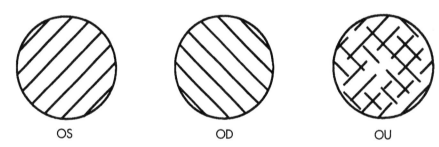

FIG. 5-1 Physiologic diplopia. **A,** When viewing fixation target *O,* point *X* is seen in crossed diplopia when it is closer than target *O* and is seen in **(B)** uncrossed diplopia when it is farther than target *O.*

FIG. 5-2 Retinal rivalry. Diagonal lines are not fused but seen in a mosaic-like pattern.

place at the same time. The patient is therefore alternately aware of the image of one eye and the image of the other eye. Examples of rivalrous stimuli are red and green versions of the same object, each seen by only one eye, or lines seen vertically by one eye and horizontally by the other. Retinal rivalry can be demonstrated by a simple experiment. If two dissimilar images, each consisting of thin diagonal lines but differing in orientation, are viewed by each eye separately and simultaneously using a stereoscope, rapid and varying regional suppression results, without fusion. The binocular impression is one of a constantly changing mosaic (Fig 5-2).

Pathologic suppression is present in constant and intermittent strabismus and in patients with anisometropic amblyopia who maintain binocular vision and have achieved their optimum visual acuity. It can also occur in aniseikonia and in heterophoria that is not well compensated. It rarely produces symptoms of asthenopia. The following discussion pertains to the suppression that occurs in strabismus.

VISUAL CONFUSION AND DIPLOPIA

In a patient with manifest strabismus, corresponding retinal points in the two eyes are no longer similarly directed. The immediate consequences are visual confusion and diplopia. Visual confusion arises when the images of two objects (e.g., a circle and a square) that are physically separated in space and dissimilar in size, shape, and orientation are suddenly placed on the cor-

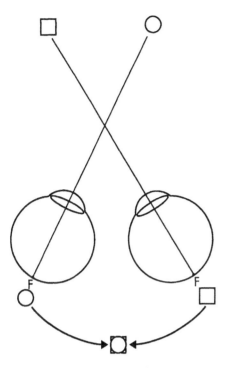

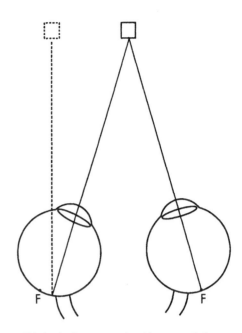

FIG. 5-3 Visual confusion. The two foveae are stimulated by different objects and will localize them in same position in space.

FIG. 5-4 Diplopia in esotropia. Uncrossed (homonymous) diplopia.

responding foveae. Subjective localization of different foveal images in a common visual direction occurs. The two dissimilar images are seen as being superimposed and projected to the same point in space (Fig. 5-3).

Visual confusion is rarely reported by the patient, probably because of the binocular rivalry that exists between the foveae. As previously mentioned, superimposition of dissimilar images on the two foveae is eliminated by physiologic suppression, and the existence of visual confusion as a symptom, even transiently, is doubtful. There is good evidence that the moment the eyes deviate, regardless of the patient's age, an intense physiologic foveal suppression develops in the strabismic eye that obviates the simultaneous imaging of different objects onto the foveae. Such a suppression would be present only when both eyes are being used. Whereas in normal binocular vision the dissimilarly contoured images on the two foveae compete with each other for conscious regard (see Fig. 5-2), in strabismus, retinal rivalry is lost and is replaced by foveal suppression of the deviating eye.[1,2] Only the images received by one fovea enter consciousness.

 CLINICAL PEARL

Visual confusion is rarely reported by the patient, probably because of the binocular rivalry that exists between the foveae.

Unlike visual confusion, diplopia is usually quite disturbing to the patient. It results when the images from a single object fall on noncorresponding points that are too disparate for the visual system to fuse and thus the images are seen in two different visual directions. The image falling on the fovea of the fixating eye will always be clearer than the image seen with the noncorresponding, nonfoveal retinal element of the other eye. In esotropia the image falls on the fixating eye's fovea and is projected straight ahead. The same image falls on nasal retina in the esotropic eye (Fig. 5-4) and is projected temporally, giving uncrossed, or homonymous, diplopia (the image of the left eye will be seen in the left side of the visual field). In exotropia the image from a single object falls on the fixating eye and is projected straight ahead. The same image falls on temporal retina of the exotropic eye (Fig. 5-5) and is projected nasally, giving crossed, or heteronymous, diplopia (the image of the left eye will be seen in the right side of the visual field). In hypertropia the image in the deviating eye is displaced superiorly and localized inferiorly, whereas in hypotropia the image of the deviating eye is displaced inferiorly and localized superiorly.

 CLINICAL PEARL

Diplopia is usually quite disturbing to the patient.

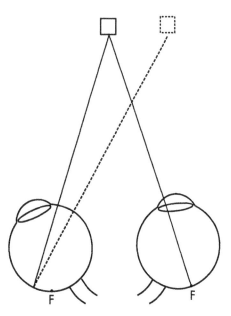

FIG. 5-5 Diplopia in exotropia. Crossed (heteronymous) diplopia.

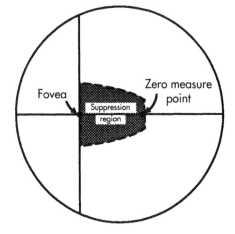

FIG. 5-6 Suppression zone in esotropia. A region of nasal hemiretina is suppressed. (From Jampolsky A: A simplified approach to strabismus diagnosis. In: *The first international congress of orthoptists,* St Louis, 1968, Mosby.)

SUPPRESSION IN STRABISMUS

Many patients with strabismus develop suppression and do not have diplopia. Strabismic suppression is regional, is facultative, exists only with similar contours, has a latent period, and is age-dependent.

Regional

Patients with strabismus rarely suppress the entire retina of the deviating eye. Only a portion or zone of the deviating eye's visual field is suppressed. The exception is the patient with large-angle alternating strabismus who appears to have two seemingly independent visual systems. To eliminate diplopia, suppression must exist in the periphery of the deviated eye in which the object of attention is imaged. This is referred to as the *diplopia point, zero measure point,* or *point "z".*[3]

The shape and size of the suppression zone in esotropia and exotropia differ. In esotropia the two localized suppression regions in the deviating eye, the foveal suppression, which is physiologic and eliminates visual confusion, and the peripheral suppression at the zero measure point in the nasal hemiretina, which is pathologic and eliminates diplopia, merge into one to form an elliptic D-shaped zone, with its long axis horizontal (Fig. 5-6). The suppression zone is positioned on one hemiretina. Targets imaged on the temporal hemiretina of the deviating eye are not suppressed. The depth of suppression is not uniform across the zone and is most intense at the zero measure point and at the fovea. The size of the zone is generally proportional to the size of the deviation. Some investigators,

however, have indicated that the size of the suppression zone in the nasal retina is small and constant, measuring approximately 5 degrees, regardless of the size of the esotropia.[4] The regionality of suppression can be demonstrated by placing prisms of increasing power before the strabismic eye (see Clinical Diagnosis). The prisms move the image out of the suppression zone, and the patient begins to notice diplopia. Regional suppression is further confirmed by the finding that some patients with small-angle esotropia maintain some binocular cooperation. Knowledge of a regional suppression can be helpful in adults with childhood-onset strabismus who begin to experience diplopia (see the following case and Chapter 10, Case 9).

CASE 1

A 50-year-old man presented with complaints of diplopia that began approximately 20 months earlier. The diplopia was only present when he looked up. Previous ocular history had indicated long-standing esotropia for which treatment had not been given. He denied any recent trauma or illnesses.

Our examination showed corrected vision of 20/20 for each eye. The patient manifested a constant 5-PD right esotropia at distance and near. He fused the Worth four dot test at near and suppressed with the right eye at distance. Harmonious anomalous correspondence with central suppression was shown with the Bagolini striated lenses. Stereopsis with the Titmus test was 400 seconds of arc.

Despite having normal versions the patient had a V-pattern deviation and became 10-PD exotropic and diplopic in upgaze. Base-in prisms placed the diplopic image within the nasal hemiretina suppression zone and eliminated the diplopia in upgaze.

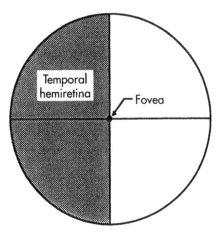

FIG. 5-7 Suppression zone in exotropia. Entire temporal hemiretinal is suppressed. (From Jampolsky A: A simplified approach to strabismus diagnosis. In: *The first international congress of orthoptists,* St Louis, 1968, Mosby.)

Suppression in exotropia is supposedly more extensive and involves most if not all of the temporal hemiretina, from the fovea to the temporal periphery, regardless of the size of the deviation (Fig. 5-7). No suppression exists on the nasal hemiretina. The suppression zone is larger than in esotropia, supposedly because of the higher incidence of intermittency that exists in exotropia. The continuous changing of the deviation from exophoria to exotropia requires a larger zone of suppression than in the case of constant strabismus, as is more likely in esotropia. Differences in the size of nasal and temporal hemiretinal suppression zones are also attributed to differences in the phylogenetic development of the two hemiretinas. The crossed and phylogenetically older nasal retinal-cortical projections are more resistant to suppression than are the newer uncrossed temporal retinal-cortical projections.[3]

The area and size of suppression zones differ, depending on the method of examination and may not be as stereotypical as indicated.[5-13] The hemiretinal suppression zones described above have been found mostly with the more dissociative testing techniques.[14] For example, using Polaroid filters rather than haploscopic instruments has shown that suppression does not exclusively involve the nasal hemiretina in esotropia and the temporal retina in exotropia. Instead, it extends nasally and temporally from the fixation point, regardless of the direction of the deviation.[7] Color complexity of the stimulus and similarity of targets presented to the two eyes also change suppression zone characteristics. The concept of hemiretinal suppression, according to some authorities, may actually be based on measurement artifact because it frequently cannot be duplicated with less dissociating tests.[11,13] Pratt-Johnson and others,[9,10] using an Airmark perimeter, found that there was actually no difference between suppression in esotropia and in exotropia and that suppression was not confined to one half of the retina in either type of strabismus. The exception was patients with microtropia, in whom the deviation is small enough for peripheral fusion to occur in the presence of a foveal/parafoveal suppression area in the deviating eye. Pratt-Johnson and others[9,10] found that strabismic patients without fusion suppress the whole area of the deviating eye that would have correspondence with the dominant eye. They proposed the existence of a "trigger mechanism" that operates on a hemiretinal basis rather than a suppression zone mechanism. The hemiretinal "trigger mechanism" deter-

mines whether suppression or diplopia occurs and is activated by the image of the fixation object crossing the vertical hemiretinal midline from one side of the retina to the other.

Facultative

Strabismic suppression is present only when it is needed. It exists when both eyes are open, with the normally fixating eye viewing an object, and disappears when one eye is closed. In unilateral strabismus the suppression is monocular and is always in the deviating eye. In alternating strabismus in which either eye in turn can be used to fixate, the suppression also occurs only in the deviating eye but changes from eye to eye as the patient alternately fixates. Some patients with large-angle exotropia acquire a habit of alternately suppressing each eye so rapidly that a kind of panoramic vision is achieved, such as that in animals with wide eye separation. In intermittent strabismus, suppression occurs when the eyes are misaligned and is absent when the eyes are straight. In incomitant strabismus, suppression occurs in the position of gaze in which the strabismus is manifest, and normal binocular vision without suppression occurs in the other positions.

Similar Contours

The most effective stimuli to elicit strabismic suppression are contours of similar shape, color, and orientation. Testing situations that alter the exact similarity of each retinal image that exists under conditions of usual, everyday situations may be sufficient to alter the characteristics of suppression found in the patient. The more dissimilar the images on noncorresponding retinal points (the zero measure point of deviating eye and the fovea of fixating eye), the less likely the strabismic patient will be able to suppress. This is seen clinically when using colored filters. A patient with strabismus who denies diplopia frequently becomes aware of diplopia when viewing a fixation light with one eye through a red filter before one eye. Using increasingly darker filters makes the differences of the images more likely to be noticed. This is the principle of the Bagolini filter bar.

Latent Period

There is a latent period associated with strabismic suppression. If an object is presented to a deviating eye so that the image falls on a normally suppressed area and the time of exposure is relatively short, the suppression may not be present. The onset of suppression has a 75- to 150-ms latency following binocular stimulation.[15] Quickly flashing each eye alternately with instruments such as the synoptophore may be sufficient to disrupt the suppression momentarily and cause diplopia.

Diplopia can sometimes be elicited while the strabismic patient is fixating a light source. If an occluder is placed before the deviating eye and removed abruptly for a brief exposure of the deviating eye, diplopia may be elicited. This transient diplopia quickly fades.

Age of Onset

Strabismic suppression develops only in visually immature patients. Nearly 100% of children who have strabismus suppress. A young child who becomes strabismic will have diplopia and may close one eye for a while but will quickly develop suppression. However, an adult who acquires strabismus will not likely develop suppression, and the diplopia persists. The second image may be ignored but can be consciously recognized and accurately localized if desired. This is not true with childhood-onset strabismus, in which an actual functional suppression zone can usually be plotted under binocular viewing conditions.

 CLINICAL PEARL

> Nearly 100% of children who have strabismus suppress. However, an adult who acquires strabismus will not likely develop suppression.

The youngest age at which suppression is unlikely to develop is unclear. Most authorities believe it to be age 5, but there are many exceptions.[16] A 2-year-old with intermittent exotropia with equal vision and high-grade stereopsis potential whose condition is converted to esotropia following extraocular muscle surgery would likely acquire sensory changes to this new situation, with suppression on the nasal hemiretina. Similar treatment in an adult in whom suppression can no longer develop would likely result in continuous diplopia.

PATHOPHYSIOLOGIC MECHANISM

Although some work suggests a retinal cause, the majority of findings point to suppression as being an active cortical inhibition.[17,18] This has been confirmed electrophysiologically. The pattern visual evoked potential (VEP) is greatly diminished when the stimulus is presented within the area of suppression.[19,20] Suppression completely abolishes P-1 amplitudes in patients with large suppression zones and greatly reduces them in patients with small suppression zones. In patients with alternating esotropia, larger amplitude responses in the VEP have been found when the fixating eye is stimulated than when the deviating eye is stimulated.[18] In addition, simultaneous recordings of the electroretinogram (ERG) have indicated that when the VEP is reduced with suppression, the ERG is not.[21]

CLINICAL DIAGNOSIS OF SUPPRESSION

Clinical tests for suppression determine the area encompassed by the suppression, the presence of alternating or unilateral suppression, the frequency of the suppression, and the depth of the suppression. The tests are designed to create a different stimulation to each eye. A target with binocular and monocular details is presented to the two eyes under binocular viewing conditions. A portion of the binocular image presented to each eye is coded so that the ability of each eye to see under the binocular viewing conditions can be tested. This way the suppressed eye can be identified.

A variety of tests have been used to evaluate suppression with varying degrees of contrasting stimulation to each eye. The more common tests include the Worth four dot test, binocular perimetry, the synoptophore, the Bagolini striated lens test, prisms, stereopsis tests, and the Bagolini filter bar. The Worth four dot test, the synoptophore, and the Bagolini striated lens test are also used to determine the retinal correspondence status.

Worth Four Dot Test

The Worth four dot test is the traditional test for suppression and has remained one of the most frequently used tests for over 75 years. It can be effective with young children. The patient looks through a pair of red and green glasses at a target consisting of four illuminated colored dots or lights (Fig. 5-8). The red lens is usually placed before the right eye and the green lens is placed before the left eye. The dots are arranged as a diamond on a special hand-held flashlight: two green dots are opposite one another on the right and left, a red dot is on the top, and a white dot is on the bottom. The patient sees the green dots only with the eye looking through the green lens and the red dot only with the other eye. The white dot can be seen through either lens.

The clinician asks the patient how many dots he or she sees and what color they are. Results of this testing

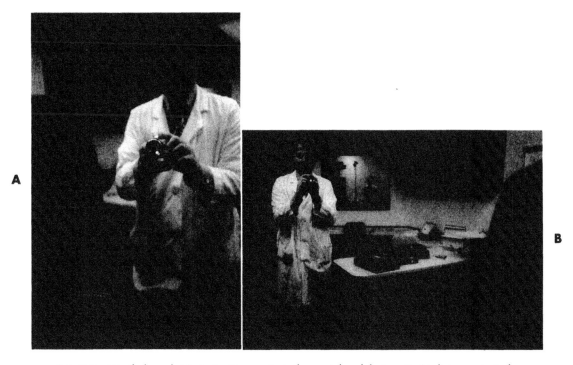

FIG. 5-8 Worth four dot test. **A,** At near, tests for peripheral fusion. **B,** At distance, tests for bifoveal fusion.

are recorded as either fusion, diplopia, alternating suppression, or unilateral suppression (Fig. 5-9). If the patient sees only three green lights, suppression exists in the right eye. If the patient sees only two red lights, there is suppression in the left eye. If the patient sees five lights, there is no suppression; instead, the patient is diplopic. If the red lights are seen to the patient's right and the green lights to the patient's left, the lights are homonymously (uncrossed) localized, as occurs in esotropia. If the green lights are seen to the right and the red lights to the left, the lights are heteronymously (crossed) localized, as occurs in exotropia. With vertical diplopia the higher eye will always see the image displaced lower and the lower eye always higher. If the patient is fusing, he or she will see four dots, with the white dot alternately seen as a mixture of red or green as a result of retinal rivalry. As discussed later, a response of four dots may also indicate that the patient is fusing on the basis of anomalous correspondence if the unilateral cover test reveals a strabismus.

A patient who is suppressing may at times report seeing five lights. This is caused by very rapid alternating fixation in which the patient first sees two lights with one eye, then changes fixation and sees three lights with the other eye. The clinician must ask whether the lights are all present at the same time or whether they change between two and three very quickly.

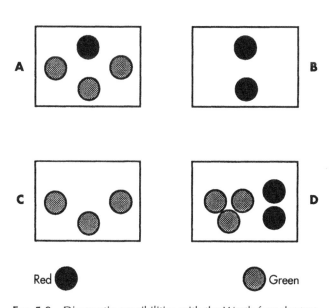

Red ● ● Green

FIG. 5-9 Diagnostic possibilities with the Worth four dot test. **A,** Fusion. The unilateral cover test can be used to differentiate whether it is normal (no manifest deviation) or anomalous (manifest strabismus). **B,** Left eye suppression, **C,** Right eye suppression, **D,** Diplopia (normal correspondence or unharmonious anomalous correspondence).

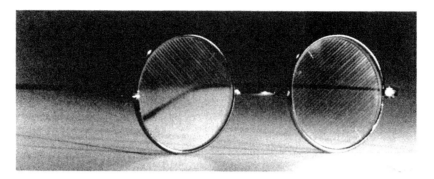

FIG. 5-10   Bagolini striated lenses.

The hand-held flashlight allows for estimating the size of the suppression zone by varying the test distance. The farther away the target is presented, the smaller the angle it will subtend on the retina. At 33 cm, the angular size subtended by the outside edges of the target will project approximately a 6-degree area of the retina and test peripheral fusion, whereas at 6 m, the target will project approximately 1.5 degrees and test macular or bifoveal fusion. If the suppression zone is very small, the image of the target may fall completely within it at distance fixation but outside it at near fixation. Estimation of the size of the suppression zone can be made by determining how far the flashlight must be removed from the patient and therefore how small the retinal image becomes before suppression occurs. For example, if the patient reports only two or three dots at 6 m, then the size of the suppression zone is larger than 1.5 degrees, but if the patient reports seeing all four dots at 33 cm, then the suppression zone is smaller than 6 degrees. It is best to begin testing at near and recede from the patient. In our experience, most suppression zones in esotropia are detected when the flashlight is held 2 to 5 feet from the patient. Repeating the Worth four dot test while the patient with constant strabismus is wearing prisms equivalent to the angle of deviation can help determine the potential for normal binocular vision.

A limitation of the Worth four dot test is the high degree of binocular dissociation produced by the red-green glasses. A heterophoria may change to a strabismus under the red-green glasses, and the patient will be diplopic or suppress. The test also produces retinal rivalry, which may cause false positive results. Using a polarized Worth four dot test has been recommended because it tests under more natural conditions of viewing.[22,23] More significant is that as many as 20% of patients with strabismus exhibit either changing fusion status (i.e., from suppression to fusion) or changing laterality of suppression when placing the red lens before the left eye and the green lens before the right eye.[24] This may be caused by the difference in lumi-

nance between the red and green images. Testing twice, with the red-green glasses reversed between trials will prevent misinterpretation of binocular status and may provide diagnostically useful information.

Bagolini Striated Lenses

These consist of a pair of plano lenses that are etched with barely perceptible striations. The striations act as a Maddox rod and produce a luminous streak 90 degrees away from the striations when the patient views a point source of light. These clear plano lenses are relatively nondissociating, and binocular functions are not disrupted as the patient looks through them. The patient's vision is clear. The striations are placed at 45 degrees and 135 degrees in front of the eyes (Fig. 5-10). Because the Bagolini striated lens test requires a degree of maturity, we seldom use it in patients under age 7. A point light source is viewed by the patient at 6 m and 33 cm.

The test is used for suppression by asking if lines radiating in both directions from the light are seen. The patient with normal binocular vision will see the lines intersect at the point light source, forming a complete X (Fig. 5-11). Because the patient's and clinician's viewpoints are mirror images, it is best to have the patient draw what he or she sees. If the patient has suppression in one eye, a gap will be present in the streak seen by the deviating eye. The gap constitutes the portion of the line falling on the suppression zone. The more extensive the gap, the larger the suppression zone. If the gap is small, it can easily be overlooked. When the fixating eye is covered, the gap in the streak disappears, and the entire streak then passes through the center of the fixation light. Total suppression of one eye results in either one or the other streak being seen.

If the strabismic patient sees two lights, this indicates diplopia without suppression. In esotropia the image on the retina is nasally displaced, and the patient reports the lights as being displaced uncrossed in space. In exotropia the image on the retina is temporally dis-

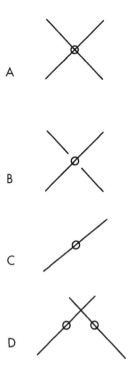

FIG. 5-11 Diagnostic possibilities with Bagolini striated lens test. **A,** Bifoveal or anomalous binocular vision. **B,** Central suppression in one eye. **C,** Complete suppression in one eye. **D,** Diplopia (normal correspondence or unharmonious anomalous correspondence).

placed, and the patient sees the two lights as being crossed in space.

Binocular Perimetry

The suppression zone can be mapped more precisely in patients by binocular perimetry or binocular scotometry. Fixation is controlled by the preferred eye, and only the deviating eye is able to see the target. The apparatus, a Hess-Lancaster screen, is used while the patient views with red-green glasses. The red target projector is placed in the center of the screen and is the color that matches the filter in front of the fixating eye. The green target projector is moved over the entire area of the screen. The suppression zone is demonstrated when the roving green projected test target disappears as it approaches the fixation target. The zone can be plotted by moving the light from the periphery inwards along each isopter, recording when it disappears and when it reappears.

The Brock posture board is based on a similar principle by which the patient also wears red-green glasses (red over the deviating eye). The patient views a fixation mark on top of a red translucent plastic screen. A bright penlight that is only visible to the deviating eye is projected from beneath the red screen to map out suppressed regions of the visual field.

Binocular perimetry is a time-consuming process that requires accurate observation on the part of the patient and constant checking to see that the angle of strabismus has not changed during the test. The method described can rarely be used with young children, which limits its usefulness.

Prisms

The use of prisms is based on the presumption that patients with strabismus will recognize diplopia when the image falls outside the limits of the suppression zone. The conditions of this test approximate those of everyday vision. The patient fixates a light at 6 m. Prisms (prism bars or Risley rotary prisms) are placed in front of the deviating eye base-up, base-in, base-down, and base-in, increasing in strength in each direction, until the patient becomes aware of diplopia. The presence of diplopia defines the boundary of the suppression zone from the zero measure point. The temporal border of the suppression zone is determined with base-out prisms, the nasal border with base-in prisms, and the vertical borders with base-up and base-down prisms. During this test it is important to establish that the eye behind the prism does not move, or the test results may be misinterpreted. The dimensions of the suppression zone vary according to the conditions of the test. Any dissociation may disrupt the suppression mechanism. If a red lens is also placed in front of the deviating eye, the suppression zone can become smaller and may disappear entirely.

A variation of the above is the 4-PD base-out prism test. We use it to detect suppression in cases of unexplained amblyopia and/or reduced stereopsis when the results of the cover test are equivocal, such as in microtropia. With suspected small-angle exotropia, base-in prisms can be used instead of base-out prisms. The 4-PD base-out prism test is the only clinically objective test for central suppression. The patient's cooperation is limited to maintaining fixation on a target.

> **✿ CLINICAL PEARL**
>
> The 4-PD base-out prism test is used to detect suppression in cases of unexplained amblyopia and/or reduced stereopsis when the results of the cover test are equivocal, such as in microtropia.

While the patient views a fixation light at 6 m, a 4-PD base-out prism is quickly placed before each eye separately. The clinician observes the eye without the prism. In patients without suppression the introduction of the small prism before one eye results in a binocular refixation movement followed by a monocular fusional movement in the opposite eye (Fig. 5-12, *A*). The eye behind the prism will make a barely perceptible inward movement to replace the image on the fovea. The opposite eye abducts and then adducts. This biphasic move-

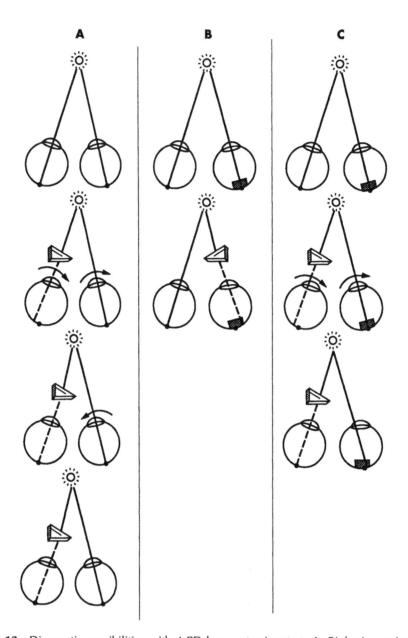

Fig. 5-12 Diagnostic possibilities with 4-PD base-out prism test. **A,** Biphasic version and vergence movements with normal binocular vision. **B,** Absence of movements when prism is placed before suppressed eye. **C,** When prism is placed before nonsuppressed eye, version movement occurs without vergence movement. (From Nelson LB, Catalano: *Atlas of ocular motility,* Philadelphia, 1989, WB Saunders.)

ment occurs in accordance with Hering's law. The test is repeated, changing the prism to base-out in front of the opposite eye. The essential finding is a difference in the response between the eyes if suppression is present.

In patients with suppression the complete biphasic response does not occur. A prism placed over the suppressing eye will not cause movement of either eye. The prism displaces the object of regard within the small suppression zone, and the patient does not ob-

serve the effect of the prism (Fig. 5-12, *B*). Because no diplopia is induced, there is no stimulus to relocate the object, and neither eye shifts. If the prism is placed in front of the fixating eye, this eye turns in and the opposite eye simultaneously turns out. The inward fusional movement of the opposite eye does not occur, because the shift of the object in the suppression zone is not appreciated by the patient (Fig. 5-12, *C*). If neither eye moves, no clear conclusion can be made.

Atypical and variable responses are frequent with this test both for patients with and without suppression.[25-27] In patients with normal binocular vision the fusional movement of the eye without the prism may not occur because of poor vergence facility. It sometimes helps to ask the patient to look at the target if he or she sees it jump (not everyone automatically looks at the jump of the target). False negative responses in patients with strabismus may occur in the form of fusional movements, as a result of either peripheral fusion (the image is displaced out of the suppression zone) or anomalous correspondence. Supposedly, with less than 3 PD of esotropia, this fusional movement can occur.[28] We have observed that the suppressed eye will move and not recover when the prism is placed in front of the nonsuppressed eye, even if the direction of the prism base is opposite to that of the deviation (i.e., base-in prism for esotropia), suggesting a larger suppression zone. In addition, without other diagnostic testing the 4-PD base-out prism test does not allow differentiation of suppression, strabismus, amblyopia, a lesion of the macula, or monocular blindness. Caution should be used when making a diagnosis of suppression based solely on this test.

Synoptophore

The synoptophore (major amblyoscope, troposcope) functions as a haploscopic test in which separate targets are presented to each eye. The patient sees only one of the targets with each eye through a tube that can be adjusted horizontally, vertically, and torsionally. The amounts of deviation can be read from the instrument scales on the tubes.

The synoptophore is optically designed to simulate optical infinity (Fig. 5-13). The targets are located at the focal distance of a +6.50-D or +7.00-D convex lens. Concave lenses (2.50 or 3.00 D) can be added to test at near. The tubes are angled, and mirrors bend the image of the targets so that they project into each eye. The clinician controls the illumination of the targets, which can be presented either simultaneously or alternately.

Different types of targets, either superimposition, fusion, or stereoscopic, can be used to measure suppression (Fig. 5-14). Superimposition targets are called *first degree,* fusion targets are called *second degree,* and stereoscopic targets are called *third degree.* These *degrees of fusion,* as defined in Chapter 1, are not a continuum but actually test different things. First degree measures the angle of deviation and retinal correspondence; second degree measures sensory and motor fusion, and third degree measures stereopsis. Because the examining conditions should approximate everyday visual conditions as closely as possible, fusion, or second-degree, targets are preferred to measure sup-

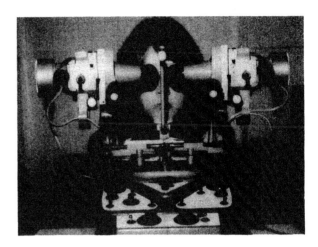

Fig. 5-13 Synoptophore.

pression. These targets are identical except for one detail. For example, the target may be a rabbit that is identical in every detail on the right and left side, except that the flower is lacking from the right side and the tail from the left side. The report that the rabbit has both a flower and a tail indicates fusion with no suppression, whereas the absence of one indicates suppression. To measure the extent of the suppression zone, one tube is rotated in the horizontal direction at which the unique part of the target carried by the moving tube disappears and reappears. The size of the targets can be varied to test for peripheral, parafoveal, and foveal suppression. The absence of stereopsis appreciation when using stereoscopic targets also indicates suppression.

A criticism of the synoptophore for the examination of suppression is that it greatly changes the conditions of natural vision. It can detect suppression at a different level than experienced in everyday life. Suppression elicited by the synoptophore is deeply ingrained. An advantage of the synoptophore is that the tubes can be set at the patient's angle of deviation, allowing control of the retinal areas being stimulated. In constant strabismus, detection with the synoptophore of the presence of second-degree fusion at the objective angle with some vergence range indicates that a functional result with normal fusion should be obtainable with therapy.

> **CLINICAL PEARL**
>
> In constant strabismus, detection with the synoptophore of the presence of second-degree fusion at the objective angle with some vergence range indicates that a functional result with normal fusion should be obtainable with therapy.

A   **B**   **C**

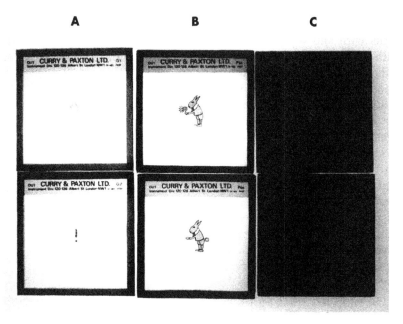

FIG. 5-14 Targets for synoptophore. **A,** First degree: superimposition. **B,** Second degree: fusion of common borders. **C,** Third degree: stereopsis.

Tests for Stereopsis

Stereotests are used to indirectly measure suppression. Bifoveal fusion without suppression is essential for high-grade stereoacuity. Stereoacuity of 60 seconds of arc or better will not be achieved without accurate bifoveal alignment. However, lower degrees of stereopsis may be present simultaneously with small-angle strabismus and suppression.[29,30] Generally, the larger and deeper the suppression,[29] the poorer the stereopsis. Although stereotesting is minimally dissociating, it is sometimes the only test in which patients, especially those with exotropia, will pull their eyes straight and report fusion.

✾ CLINICAL PEARL

Stereoacuity of 60 seconds of arc or better will not be achieved without accurate bifoveal alignment.

Clinical evaluation of stereopsis is mostly done at near viewing distances and involves measuring both contour (local) and random-dot (global) stereopsis. Patient performance will often differ on these two types of stereotests.[31] In contour or non–random-dot stereotests, localized features of objects are extracted from a visual scene and assigned relative depth values. These tests use a simple disparity stimulus, such as a stereogram, with two parallel vertical line segments seen by each eye, with slightly different lateral separations. Contour stereotests involve binocular fusion of a single dot or line segment. Stereotests that measure contour stereopsis, because of possible monocular clues, may in certain cases overestimate the level of stereopsis.[32-34]

Random-dot stereotests consist of targets containing a computer-determined random arrangement of dots with no information about form or depth. The targets appear identical except that a certain part of one target is displaced horizontally with respect to the others.[35] Random-dot stereopsis involves binocular fusion of a set of dots or lines. These stereotests supposedly eliminate the artifact of monocular nonstereoscopic clues. They are more sensitive than contour stereotests. Although some patients with binocular vision disorders may demonstrate stereopsis when using contour stereotests, they have much more difficulty responding to random-dot stereotests.

The commonly used clinical stereotests include the Titmus, Randot, TNO, Frisby, Random-dot E, and the Lang (Table 5-1). Unlike laboratory testing, none control parameters such as location of fixation, duration of presentation, luminance, and adaptation effects. With constant strabismus, measuring stereopsis while the patient wears prisms equivalent to the angle of deviation can help determine the potential for normal binocular vision.

The Titmus stereotest (Fig. 5-15) historically has been the most widely used. It measures contour stereopsis. The test is performed at 40 cm and requires polarized glasses. The disparity ranges from 3000 to 40 seconds of arc. Shortening or extending the test distance somewhat will have very little effect on the relative demand of the test. The targets comprise a housefly, animals, and sets of circles, one target that is disparate from each set. The Titmus test gives some monocular (lateral displacement) clues, especially when viewing the first three sets of circles; it is easy to see

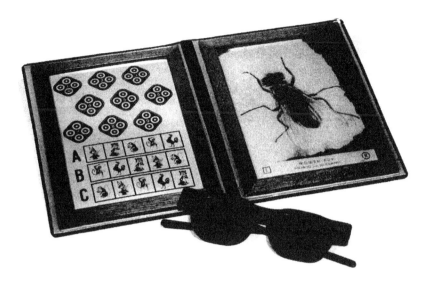

FIG. 5-15   Titmus stereotest.

TABLE 5-1   FEATURES OF CLINICAL STEREOTESTS

Test	Stereopsis Type	Range	Filters	Distance	Comments
Titmus	Contour; crossed and un-crossed disparity	3000-40 sec	Polaroid	40 cm	Monocular clues are common; may overestimate stereoacuity
Randot	Contour and random-dot; crossed and uncrossed disparity	500-20 sec	Polaroid	40 cm	Some monocular clues
Frisby	Random-dot; crossed and uncrossed disparity	600-15 sec	None	Varies	Tedious; motion parallax may give monocular clues
TNO	Random-dot; crossed and uncrossed disparity	480-15 sec	Red-green	40 cm	Free of monocular clues
RDE	Random-dot; crossed and uncrossed disparity	504-50 sec	Polaroid	Varies	May underestimate stereoacuity; good as a screening test
Lang	Random-dot; crossed disparity	1200-500 sec	None	40 cm	May underestimate stereoacuity; good as a screening test
B-VAT II	Contour and random-dot; crossed disparity	240-15 sec	Liquid crystal	6 m	Distance stereopsis thresholds are generally higher than near thresholds

monocularly that one circle is displaced. Some of the circles may be selected because they look different and not because they are seen stereoscopically. Hence, stereopsis derived from the Titmus test may not always be valid. The patient's response, when questionable, can be confirmed either by covering one eye, or by turning the target through 180 degrees when the disparity becomes uncrossed (the target appears farther from the rest) or through 90 degrees when there is no stereoscopic effect. Interestingly, even under monocular conditions some patients have achieved 40 seconds of arc.[32] Because of this, we rarely use the Titmus test in our clinic.

The Randot stereotest (Fig. 5-16), like the Titmus, is done at 40 cm and with the patient wearing polarized glasses. It consists of three parts, or subtests: (1) six large areas containing geometric forms (500 and 250 seconds of arc), (2) three lines of five different animals in different sequences in decreasing image disparity (400 to 100 seconds), and (3) a series of 10 circles in different sequences, in decreasing image disparity (400 to 20 seconds). The geometric forms test for random-dot stereopsis. The animal subtests and circle subtests are similar to the Titmus and measure contour stereopsis.

The TNO stereotest (Fig. 5-17) measures random-

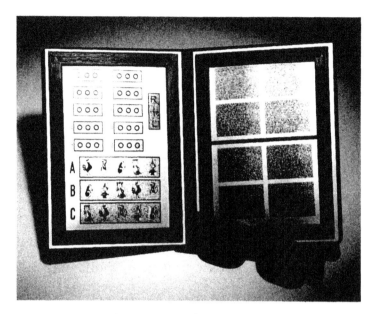

FIG. 5-16 Randot stereotest.

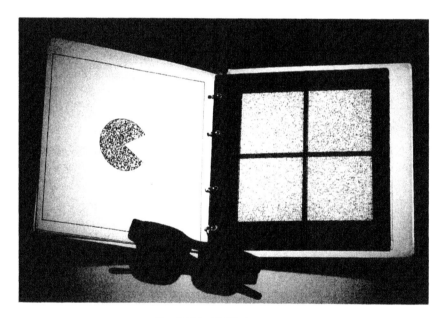

FIG. 5-17 TNO stereotest.

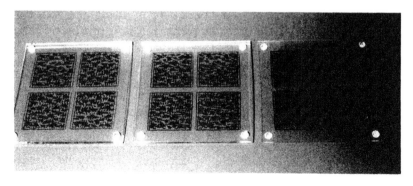

FIG. 5-18 Frisby stereotest.

dot stereopsis exclusively.[36] It employs random-dot stereograms devoid of any monocular clues in a graded manner. The patient wears a pair of red-green glasses and views a series of plates in a booklet at 40 cm. The TNO test consists of screening plates and quantitative plates to measure stereoacuity thresholds. The screening plates consist of a butterfly and geometric shapes. When viewed monocularly the pictures just appear to be random red and green dots; binocularly, the images appear to stand out. The quantitative plates each show a circle from which a 60-degree wedge or sector has been deleted. The patient is instructed to point to the sector. The stereograms vary in the orientation of the sector. The disparities range from 480 to 15 seconds of arc.

The Frisby stereotest consists of three plastic transparent test plates (Fig. 5-18).[37,38] Each plate is a different thickness (6 mm, 3 mm, or 1 mm) and contains four squares of small curved random shapes; one square contains a "hidden" circle that is printed on the back surface of the plate. No single square is distinctive; each looks much like the other three. The stereopsis is created by an actual physical separation of the circle from the background, which corresponds to the thickness of the test place. Either crossed (circle seen in front of the background) or uncrossed (circle seen behind the background) disparities can be tested. The test plates can be presented in any orientation. By rotating the plates the validity of the patient's responses can be confirmed. The test does not require either Polaroid or red-green glasses. The disparities range from 600 to 15 seconds of arc.

The level of stereopsis depends on the thickness of the test plate and the distance of the plate from the observer. The thicker the test plate and/or the shorter the viewing distance, the lower the stereoacuity. A tape is used to measure the distance from the eyes. We test at 40 cm. The test begins by asking the patient to indicate the circle on the thickest plate, progressing to the thinner plates if the response is correct. A patient with normal binocular vision sees one square appearing to have a circular indentation. The patient with suppression will not perceive the circle; all four squares will look the same.

Some patients with monocular vision whom we have examined have performed well on this test. The plates must be held parallel to the plane of the patient's face, otherwise motion parallax can reveal the circle. False positives can also occur if the patient's head is moved slightly or there is a shadow that moves across the plate.

The Random-dot E stereotest (RDE) consists of three 8- by 10-cm cards that are shown to a patient wearing Polaroid glasses (Fig. 5-19).[39] One card is a demonstrator and has a model showing an embossed *E* in the center, a second card is a blank, and a third card has an *E* that when seen stereoscopically with Polaroid

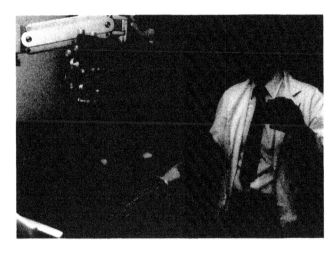

FIG. 5-19   Random-dot E stereotest.

glasses appears raised (crossed disparity) or recessed (uncrossed disparity), depending on the position of the card. For training purposes the patient is first shown the card with the model *E*. The other two cards are next shown, usually at 50 cm. The RDE uses a forced-choice paradigm. For a correct response, the patient must tell or point to the card with the *E* on it. Four trials are given. At 50 cm, the disparity is 604 seconds of arc. By moving the test card farther away, the disparity is reduced. For example, when testing at 1 m, the disparity is 252 seconds of arc, whereas at 2 m, the disparity is 126 seconds of arc. These values probably underestimate the patient's stereoacuity because moving the target farther away reduces the visual angle of the test target, making it harder to see because of nonstereoscopic reasons, as well as reduced disparity. To demonstrate 50 seconds of arc the patient must be able to discriminate the *E* at a distance of 16 feet. Accordingly, we prefer not to quantify stereothresholds with this test and administer it on a pass/fail basis. A pass usually requires the patient to identify the *E* at least four times in succession. Because it is quite simple and does not require a verbal response, the RDE has been advocated in vision screening for nursery-school and grade-school children.[38-42] The child either sees the figure or does not and is not required to recognize the stimulus as the letter *E*.

The Lang stereotest is a recently developed random-dot stereotest consisting of a single 9.5- by 14.5-cm card (Fig. 5-20). Similar to the Frisby test, it does not require either Polaroid or red-green glasses. The three easily recognizable figures (car, star, and cat) are created by a lateral displacement of a group of dots seen by each eye. The random-dot technique is combined with a panography technique in which cylindric screens provide a separate image to each eye. At a test distance of 40 cm, three disparities are present (car,

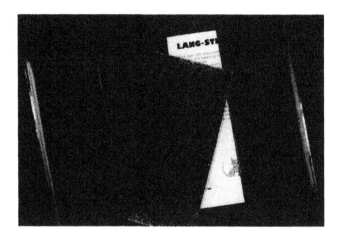

FIG. 5-20 Lang stereotest.

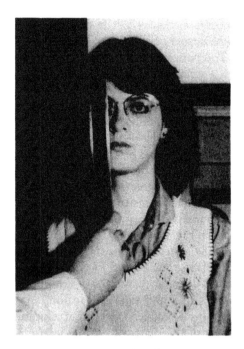

FIG. 5-21 Bagolini filter bar.

550 seconds; star, 600 seconds; and cat, 1200 seconds). The patient names or points to the target. The targets are seen only in crossed disparity. The card on which the targets are printed must be held parallel to the plane of the patient's face; otherwise, monocular clues are given. Larger test distances can interfere with the isolation of the figures and give false negatives, similar to the RDE stereotest. Because of the relatively gross disparities, the Lang stereotest is more suitable for screening purposes than for measurement of stereoacuity threshold.[43,44]

The preceding tests all measure stereopsis at near viewing distances. Clinicians rarely measure stereopsis at distance. The measuring of stereopsis at distance may be useful for patients with good fusion ability at near and binocular vision disturbances at distance, such as in divergence excess type of intermittent exotropia.[45] In the past, when testing distance stereopsis the Polaroid vectographic slide was most often used.[46] The Mentor Binocular Vision Testing System (B-VAT II) can also be used to measure stereopsis at distance. In this computerized system, liquid crystal binocular glasses are connected to a high-frequency microprocessor. The glasses are constructed with a separate aperture for each eye, consisting of a liquid crystal shutter that can transmit or block out light. The shutter signal sent by the microprocessor is synchronized with the presentation of two disparate images that can be presented independently to either eye. The images alternate at a rate of 60 cycles/sec, which is faster than binocular alternating critical flicker fusion and allows the patient to perceive the images as continuous. The amount of disparity of the stereoscopic targets permits measurements at 240, 180, 120, 60, 30 and 15 seconds of arc. Both contour and random-dot stereopsis can be measured. With this system the distance stereothresholds tend to be lower for patients with heterophoria than for patients with intermittent stra-

bismus.[47] Improvement in stereopsis with the B-VAT II has been reported following treatment of intermittent exotropia.[48]

Bagolini Filter Bar

The Bagolini filter bar measures the depth, or intensity, of suppression. The depth of suppression refers to the ease with which the suppression can be "broken through," or overcome, and the patient made aware of diplopia. Suppression is not equally deep in all patients nor is its depth related to the size of the suppression zone or the magnitude of the strabismus. In some patients with strabismus, suppression may be readily overcome and normal binocular vision achieved by eliminating the strabismus with either prisms, added lenses, orthoptics/vision therapy, or extraocular muscle surgery. In other patients in whom suppression is deep, such therapy is less likely to be beneficial.

The Bagolini filter bar (Fig. 5-21) consists of a long narrow bar of 17 gradations of red gelatine filter of increasing darkness used to dissociate the two eyes. The patient views a fixation light at 6 m. The filter bar is placed before the fixating eye, beginning with filter 1, the least dense. The clinician attempts to overcome the suppression by gradually increasing the degree of binocular dissociation. The darkness of the filter is increased one step at a time. The patient indicates as soon as he or she sees diplopia. The darkness of the red filter necessary to cause diplopia of the fixation light is a measure of the density of suppression. In some patients, light red filters are more effective in eliciting diplopia, whereas in others the retinal illumination must be reduced by darker filters before the patient experiences diplopia. The darker the filter necessary to make the patient aware of the diplopia, the deeper is the suppression.

VARIABLES AFFECTING SUPPRESSION

Suppression is usually not "all or none." Some patients with strabismus have it under all seeing conditions; whereas others have it only under certain seeing conditions. Certain conditions make it more likely that the patient will suppress, and other conditions make it less likely. Altering the patient's fixation pattern during the examination may change, diminish, or eliminate entirely any suppression. The eye that takes fixation during testing should always be the habitually fixating eye. With the synoptophore, for example, placing the tube before the deviating eye at the orthoposition rather than placing the tube before the fixating eye at the orthoposition frequently disrupts suppression.

In that regard a switch in the fixation preference can cause diplopia in adult patients with a history of childhood strabismus.[49-53] This is more likely in unilateral strabismus with amblyopia than in alternating strabismus without amblyopia, in which suppression occurs regardless of the fixating eye. Generally, when vision of 20/40 or worse exists in the amblyopic eye, the ability to transfer the suppression to the preferred eye when the amblyopic eye fixates is not present. This switch in fixation can be secondary to asymmetric cataract development, as indicated by the following case.

 CLINICAL PEARL

A switch in the fixation preference can cause diplopia in adult patients with a history of childhood strabismus.

CASE 2

An 89-year-old woman presented with the complaint of intermittent diplopia of 2-weeks duration.[52] There was no history of trauma or recent illness. She had a long history of exotropia and amblyopia in the left eye, and had undergone strabismus surgery many years earlier.

Corrected visual acuities with OD +1.75 sphere and OS −0.50 −3.00 × 180 were 20/80 and 20/400 for the right and left eyes, respectively. Cataractous lens changes, greater for the right eye, were noted with biomicroscopy. Ophthalmoscopy revealed mild macular degeneration in both eyes. With the Krimsky test, a constant left 40-PD exotropia was measured. Version testing revealed medial rectus restriction in the left eye. Fusional ability could not be demonstrated.

Despite the difference in visual acuity between the two eyes, the patient would occasionally fixate with the left eye. When this occurred, she had diplopia. When she fixated with the right eye, diplopia was not present.

Diplopia as a result of a fixation switch can also occur in patients with strabismus and anisohyperopia in which a myopic refractive shift develops over time only in the less hyperopic eye.[54] When the patient takes up fixation with the hyperopic eye, especially for distance vision, it may be impossible to suppress the image in the newly myopic eye that has been used for many years as the fixating eye. This usually happens in adolescence but also may begin in early adult life. Diplopia caused by a fixation switch may also occur in the adult with childhood-onset strabismus who is given either an incorrect refractive correction or a monovision contact lens fit.[55]

Training and repeated testing may alter suppression. Even though repeated examinations are desirable, the results of the first examination are usually more indicative of the patient's habitual suppression. An untrained patient gives more valuable information as to the character of suppression than a patient who is aware of various possibilities in the procedure. Repeated testing tends to reduce the suppression zone as a result of training effect. Similarly, the attention of the patient can alter suppression. Attention is the opposite of suppression. If greater attention is attracted to the target of one eye by changing the target's color, clarity, or movement, the results of the examination are greatly modified.

SUPPRESSION AND IGNORING

The absence of diplopia in a patient with strabismus does not always imply that suppression has developed and that the strabismus commenced in early childhood. Some patients who develop strabismus later in life learn to disregard the fainter diplopic image, especially if it is out in the periphery. Further questioning by the clinician usually reveals that the patient actually does see double. This is described as *visual ignoring*. Whereas suppression is a subconscious cortical reflex that eliminates visual processing and recognition of visual information from some or all of the visual field, visual ignoring is thought to represent a psychologic phenomenon based on a conscious disregard of a perceived image.[20,35,57] It probably falls somewhere between conscious and unconscious thought. Visual ignoring is similar to the lack of awareness of physiologic diplopia in patients with normal binocular vision. Ignoring, rather than suppression, of diplopia seems to be the mechanism used by some patients with Duane's and Brown's syndromes.

 CLINICAL PEARL

The absence of diplopia in a patient with strabismus does not always imply that suppression has developed and that the strabismus commenced in early childhood.

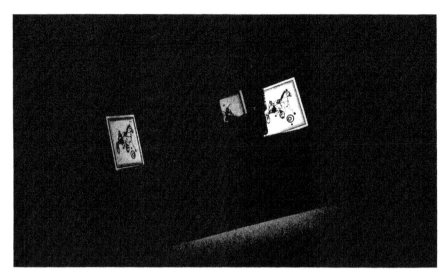

FIG. 5-22 Variable mirror stereoscope/cheiroscope.

Differentiating between suppression and ignoring is important because it helps the clinician to differentiate a long-standing strabismus from a more recently acquired strabismus. The Bagolini filter bar or prisms can be used for this differentiation. With the Bagolini filter bar, a light red filter (i.e., 1 to 3) before the fixating eye while the patient views a muscle light will make the patient who is ignoring aware of diplopia. Much denser filters are generally necessary with suppression. With prisms that partly compensate for the amount of deviation, the patient who ignores will notice diplopia, whereas the patient who suppresses will likely not, because the second image is still within the suppression zone.

TREATMENT

Strabismic suppression is a neurosensory adaptation that spares the patient from diplopia. It serves a useful function for patients in whom restoration of normal binocular vision is unattainable. With other patients, suppression prevents an obstacle that must be overcome to obtain a functional cure. The elimination of suppression does not guarantee the achievement of fusion with prisms, added lenses, orthoptics/vision therapy, or muscle surgery. It must be remembered that once suppression is eliminated in visual adults, it is no longer available. This may be overlooked by advocates of treatment. We have examined adults with a history of childhood strabismus who presented with intractable diplopia.[58] A common factor for many was muscle surgery, occlusion, and/or orthoptics/vision therapy when they were older.

We use suppression therapy mostly in patients with intermittent strabismus, anisometropic amblyopia, and constant strabismus with normal fusion potential. The therapeutic approaches include using the synoptophore

or similar haploscopic instruments, prisms, anaglyphic and Polaroid techniques, cheiroscopic tracings, and teaching the recognition of physiologic diplopia.

 CLINICAL PEARL

Suppression therapy is used mostly in patients with intermittent strabismus, anisometropic amblyopia, and constant strabismus with normal fusion potential.

The synoptophore involves stimulation of the suppressed region of the retina of the deviated eye by moving targets of various types and sizes back and forth across the suppression zone while the patient attempts to see diplopically. Rapid alternate flashing and varying of target brightness can be used to treat suppression. Target illumination can be varied in the synoptophore so that the fixating eye's target is less brightly illuminated and/or the suppressing eye's target is more brightly illuminated. More conducive for home training is the variable mirror stereoscope/cheiroscope (Fig. 5-22). This is a modest version of the synoptophore that is W-shaped with a separate mirror on each side. It is accompanied by a variety of targets, some requiring superimposition, some requiring fusion, and some requiring stereopsis. The separation of the targets is controlled by positioning of the stereoscope's mirror panels and allows for the targets to be positioned at the angle of deviation in constant strabismus. The variable prismatic stereoscope is used more frequently for vergence therapy than for suppression therapy.

As indicated earlier, prisms can be used to move the image out of the suppression zone. A 10-PD vertical prism is placed before the deviating eye while the patient views a fixation target at 6 m. Vertical prisms rather than horizontal prisms are used, because the vertical extent of the suppression zone is smaller. Most

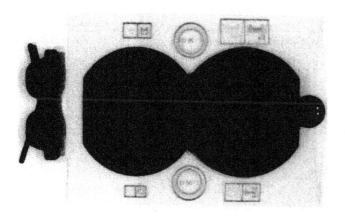

FIG. 5-23 TV trainers (these can be red/green or Polaroid).

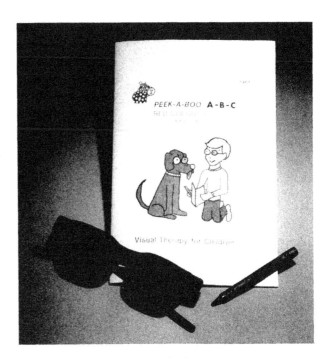

FIG. 5-24 Anaglyphic tracings.

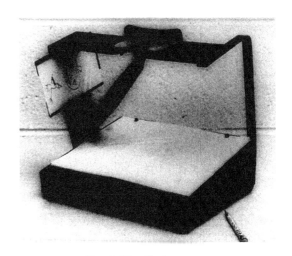

FIG. 5-25 Cheiroscope.

all patients with esotropia can appreciate diplopia this way. The prism strength can be reduced slowly while the patient tries to maintain diplopia of the fixation target. Colored filters can be used to make it more difficult for the patient to suppress.

Anaglyphic techniques require that the patient wear red-green glasses. The most popular is the TV trainer (Fig. 5-23). It does not require a great deal of instruction to use and is particularly useful for young children with divergence excess type of intermittent exotropia. The TV trainer comprises a single plastic sheet, part of which is all red, another portion, all green. The plastic sheet is attached to a television screen with a suction cup. The eye behind the red filter sees only the red portion, and the eye behind the green filter sees only the green portion. If the patient does not suppress, none of the television screen will be blacked-out. With suppression, half of the screen will be blacked-out, depending on which eye is suppressed. Polaroid TV trainers are also available.

With anaglyphic tracings, the patient, while wearing the red-green glasses, traces or draws with a red crayon or pencil (Fig. 5-24). Because the drawing is done on a white background, only the eye with the green filter will see the red markings. When the green filter is placed before the suppressed eye and the patient is asked to trace over a black line drawing with the red crayon, both eyes will perceive the black line drawing but only the suppressed eye will see the lines drawn with the red crayon. Tasks such as connect-the-dots mazes and filling in the letter *o* in the newspaper can be used.

Error with anaglyphic techniques can arise when the color of the filters does not match that of the targets. When this happens the target is not completely extinguished by the filter and is seen by both eyes. Also, if the patient rapidly alternates fixation, he or she may not report any portion of the television screen or drawing missing.

Cheiroscopic tracings use a stereoscope, either a Wheatstone or Brewster type, to treat suppression (Fig. 5-25). A picture viewed in a mirror by one eye is projected onto a drawing surface visible only to its fellow eye. The picture is placed in front of the fixating eye. The other eye views a blank sheet of paper. The patient is asked to trace with a colored pencil over the stimulus perceived with the suppressed eye. As the patient does this, he or she will be stimulating one eye under conditions of binocular vision. Patients with normal binocular vision will project the stimulus onto the drawing surface and be unaware of which eye is perceiving the picture and which eye is projecting it. With

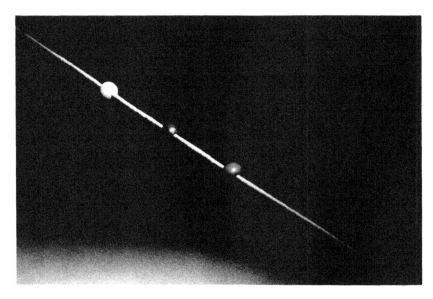

FIG. 5-26 Brock string.

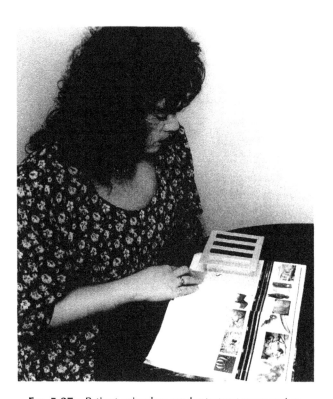

FIG. 5-27 Patient using bar reader to treat suppression.

suppression the pencil and/or drawing will disappear. Large targets with simple line drawings are used first, followed by smaller and more complex targets.

The recognition of physiologic diplopia is very useful in treating suppression. The presence of normal single binocular vision without suppression is confirmed when physiologic diplopia is recognized by the patient.

The Brock string, or beads-on-string, (Fig. 5-26) is the technique most frequently used to train physiologic diplopia. It provides the patient with a precise method for monitoring where the patient's eyes are directed. The procedure calls for a string to be held taut, with one end held by the patient at the bridge of the nose and the other end attached to a stationary object, such as a doorknob. Mounted on the string are three moveable beads. The patient with normal single binocular vision fixating at the farthest bead will see two strings that converge to a point in the form of a horizontal V at the fixation target. The strings and the nonfixated beads are seen in crossed physiologic diplopia. The presence of diplopia of the strings and beads act as a suppression clue and monitors the exactness of bifixation. If the string on the right side is missing, the patient is suppressing the left eye, whereas if the string on the left side is missing, the patient is suppressing the right eye. When the patient fixates the middle bead, the two strings now form a horizontal X. The diplopia is crossed for the bead and string in front of the fixation target and uncrossed for the bead and string beyond the fixation target. Red-green glasses can be used to assist the patient with recognizing physiologic diplopia.

Bar reading also uses physiologic diplopia recognition to treat suppression. Although bars are available commercially (Fig. 5-27), a wooden tongue depressor or any vertically oriented object and a printed page can be used. The print is usually a size larger than the best visual acuity of the patient. The bar reader is held vertically by the patient at a distance from the page so that its width causes the fields of both eyes to be obstructed but not overlapped when it is held between the eyes and the print. With normal single binocular vision, the patient will see the print behind the bar on the left side of the page with the left eye and the print on the right with the right eye. The patient should be able to read without the bar reader obscuring the print. At the same time, the patient should perceive the bar reader in crossed diplopia. Suppression exists when the bar reader covers any of the print. If suppression is unilateral, the bar reader will remain on one side of the page, whereas if there is alternating suppression, the bar reader will jump from one side to the other. With patients with intermittent strabismus, the print may become blurred if the patient elects to alter accommodation to control the deviation. Anaglyphic and Polaroid bar readers are also available (Fig. 5-28).

RETINAL CORRESPONDENCE IN STRABISMUS

Patients with strabismus either maintain normal retinal correspondence or develop anomalous correspondence. Normal correspondence exists when the foveae of the two eyes, despite the strabismus, continue to form a pair of corresponding points.[59] The primary line of sight of the two eyes is still subjectively perceived in the same visual direction. With normal correspondence, a patient with esotropia viewing a fixation light at 6 m with a red-green filter will see a red and green light projected homonymously and separated by an amount equal to the angle of deviation, assuming any suppression is disrupted with the filters.

 CLINICAL PEARL

Normal correspondence exists when the foveae of the two eyes, despite the strabismus, continue to form a pair of corresponding points.

When strabismus develops in early childhood the normal relationship between the two foveae can become disrupted. Anomalous or abnormal retinal correspondence is the condition in which normally noncorresponding areas acquire the same visual direction and their stimulation gives rise to different subjective visual directions.[60] Equal visual direction is established for certain retinal regions that are disparate in normal vision. The foveae of the two eyes no longer form a pair of corresponding points. The fovea of one eye has a common visual direction with an extra foveal point or area in the other eye. Anomalous correspondence adapts the sensory visual system to the motor condition created by the strabismus. A patient with esotropia with anomalous correspondence viewing a fixation light at 6 m with red and green filters, sees either red and green homonymously projected lights separated by less or more than the amount of the angle of deviation, red and green heteronomously projected lights, or a single "fused" red-green light, assuming any suppression is disrupted with the filters.

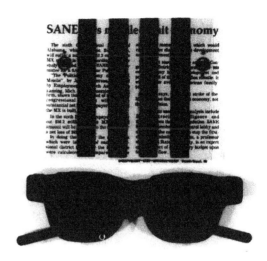

FIG. 5-28 Bar reader (these can be red, green, or Poloroid).

 CLINICAL PEARL

Anomalous or abnormal retinal correspondence is the condition in which normally noncorresponding areas acquire the same visual direction and their stimulation gives rise to different subjective visual directions.

Similar to suppression, anomalous correspondence may or may not be accompanied by amblyopia, develops only in very young patients, and is entirely a binocular phenomenon.[61] When the eyes are used monocularly, there is no change in visual direction of any retinal area. Also in a manner similar to suppression, anomalous correspondence is not necessarily "all or none"; it has levels of severity.

Three angles are involved in determining the correspondence status of a patient with strabismus. The objective angle *(H)* is the angle between the two primary lines of sight when one eye is fixating. Represented by *zF*, in which *z* is the zero measure point and *F* is the fovea of the strabismic eye, the objective angle is the amount of prisms in place when there is no longer any shift of the eyes with the alternate cover test. The subjective angle *(S)* is the angle between the primary line of sight in the fixating eye and the line of sight in the nonfixating eye, which corresponds to the primary line of sight in the fixating eye. Represented by *za*, in which *z* is the zero measure point and *a* is the anomalous point or area that corresponds to the fovea of the fixating eye, the subjective angle is the angular separation in subjective visual space between the diplopic images of a single target. The angle of anomaly *(A)* is the difference between the objective and subjective angles. It is the angle separating the anomalous point *a* and the anatomic fovea of the strabismic eye and is represented by *aF*.

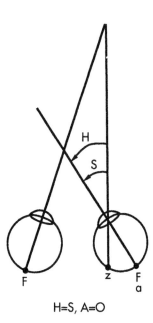

H=S, A=O

FIG. 5-29 Normal correspondence. Subjective angle *(za)* is in same direction and equal to objective angle *(zF)*.

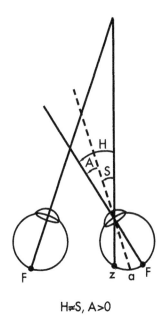

H≠S, A>0

FIG. 5-30 Unharmonious anomalous correspondence. Subjective angle *(za)* is in same direction but significantly smaller than objective angle *(zF)*.

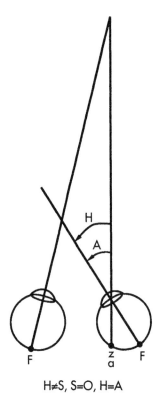

H≠S, S=O, H=A

FIG. 5-31 Harmonious anomalous correspondence. Subjective angle *(za)* is zero.

In normal correspondence (Fig. 5-29), the objective angle and subjective angle are equal and there is no angle of anomaly. Anomalous correspondence exists when the objective angle does not coincide with the subjective angle and there is an angle of anomaly. Anomalous correspondence is either unharmonious or harmonious. In unharmonious anomalous correspondence the subjective angle is in the same direction and smaller than the objective angle (Fig. 5-30). The angle of anomaly is also smaller than the objective angle. This is an incomplete adaptation, because the anomalous point (point *a*) in the deviating eye falls between the fovea and the area stimulated by the object of regard (point *z*). A patient with esotropia with unharmonious anomalous correspondence viewing a fixation light at 6 m with red-green filters sees red and green homonymously projected lights separated by less than the amount of deviation. In harmonious anomalous correspondence, the fovea of the fixating eye acquires a common visual direction with the area in the retina of the deviated eye on which the fixation point is imaged, the zero measure point (Fig. 5-31). The shift in visual directions has fully offset the amount of deviation. The subjective angle is zero, and the angle of anomaly coincides with the objective angle. A patient with esotropia with harmonious anomalous correspondence viewing a fixation light at 6 m with red-green filters sees a single fused red-green light. Subjective fusion occurs when the retinas are stimulated as they normally are in a patient with strabismus. Harmonious anomalous correspondence can provide a form of binocular vision in the presence of strabismus. From a practical point, this sensory adaptation may be of benefit, particularly in patients with small angles of strabismus.

CLINICAL PEARL

Harmonious anomalous correspondence can provide a form of binocular vision in the presence of strabismus.

Whether unharmonious anomalous correspondence truly exists has been questioned. It seems illogic that anomalous correspondence would only be a partial adaptation. Whereas the sensory adaptation in harmonious anomalous correspondence is most successful and useful in everyday life, unharmonious anomalous correspondence does not occur because of incomplete compensation for the deviation of the eye. Unharmonious anomalous correspondence possibly represents an artifact produced by the conditions under which the patient is examined. For example, unharmonious anomalous correspondence is more frequently diagnosed with the synoptophore examination than with the other tests. This can be attributed to the proximal convergence that is induced with the synoptophore and other stereoscopes.[62] The sensation of nearness brought on by the targets being close to the eyes may cause the eyes to converge, artificially changing the angles of deviation. A patient with 20-PD esotropia may show a subjective angle of zero with other tests yet with the synoptophore show an equal increase in both objective and subjective angles (e.g., H = 30 PD, S = 10 PD), giving an "unharmonious" anomalous correspondence.

Unharmonious anomalous correspondence may also represent an in-between stage in the evolution of harmonious anomalous correspondence. The development of harmonious anomalous correspondence may occur over time, with the angle of anomaly gradually increasing until full compensation for the deviation is achieved. The fovea of the fixating eye establishes correspondence with various areas and eventually with the zero measure point in the strabismic eye. The process continues with the anomalously corresponding point moving across the retina until it becomes harmonious. This is envisaged as a slow process that may never actually be completed. However, if unharmonious anomalous correspondence is an intermediate stage, it would be diagnosed more in younger than older patients with strabismus, which does not appear to be the case. Furthermore, we have not observed increases in the angle of anomaly over time with our patients.

This is not to say that the unharmonious type of anomalous correspondence is not a true clinical entity. It can develop from strabismus with well-established anomalous correspondence. In these cases a sudden change in the angle of the strabismus occurs. For example, an adult with esotropia since childhood and harmonious anomalous correspondence develops a lat-

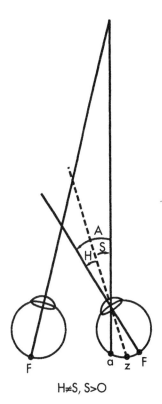

FIG. 5-32 Surgically induced unharmonious anomalous correspondence. Postoperatively, patient with residual esotropia perceives crossed diplopia as if exotropic.

eral rectus paresis. The objective angle increases, and the subjective angle increases by an equivalent amount. The patient will be diplopic (uncrossed and by an amount significantly less than the objective angle), assuming a suppression zone was adapted to the original angle of strabismus.

Another possibility is the situation in which the angle of strabismus is suddenly decreased by extraocular muscle surgery, prisms, or a large shift in the refractive error. In this case the newly formed subjective angle is in the opposite direction to the new objective angle.[63,64] Crossed diplopia in patients with esotropia and uncrossed diplopia in patients with exotropia occurs and is caused by persistence of anomalous correspondence. This is also referred to as *paradoxic anomalous correspondence, type I*. Assume, for example, the patient has esotropia with harmonious anomalous correspondence before extraocular muscle surgery and after surgery has a smaller esotropia (Fig. 5-32). Because the zero measure point is now temporal to point *a*, the patient projects with crossed diplopia, despite still being esotropic. In children, diplopia of this nature likely disappears in a few days. Other patients may not report diplopia spontaneously because the image of the point of fixation (the zero measure point) is still within a suppression zone.[65] With testing conditions that are dissociative enough to disrupt suppression, the paradoxic diplopia can usually be measured.

The subjective angle can exceed the objective angle in unharmonious anomalous correspondence. This occurs in individuals with strabismus with prior harmonious anomalous retinal correspondence who develop consecutive deviations, that is, usually following surgery those with esotropia instead have exotropia and those with exotropia instead have esotropia. This is referred to as *paradoxic anomalous correspondence, type II.*

Covariation

Patients with strabismus with anomalous correspondence may exhibit a certain amount of plasticity.[66] Instead of developing unharmonious anomalous correspondence following a change in the strabismic angle, as described above, some patients maintain harmonious anomalous correspondence. Covariation occurs when the objective angle and the angle of anomaly change in concert while the subjective angle remains zero.[67] With covariation, cortical adjustment is adapted to match the directional values of the retinal elements to the new ocular alignment. A new system of harmonious anomalous correspondence develops after the change in the objective angle. The angle of anomaly becomes zero (normal correspondence) when the eyes become perfectly aligned. Whether covariation takes place mostly as a result of sensory fusion or motor fusion is unclear.[66,68,69] If it occurs from sensory fusion and the angle of anomaly changes to conform with the new angle of deviation, covariation is more likely to occur in patients who are visually immature. The reestablishment of harmonious anomalous correspondence would be expected in young children, whereas unharmonious anomalous correspondence with paradoxic projection would be more likely in older patients who have had a change in the objective angle.

Horror Fusionis

Horror fusionis, or horror fusionalis, is a rare condition in which there is an active aversion to fusion. In determining the subjective angle with the synoptophore, the images approaching superimposition or fusion slide or jump past each other without apparent fusion or suppression.[70] The two foveae actually repel each other. Patients with horror fusionis apparently alter their angle of strabismus by performing ocular movements to avoid fusion as the images approach. Horror fusionis is usually associated with intractable diplopia. Rutstein and Bessant[58] describe five adults with horror fusionis. All had strabismus since early childhood and had been treated earlier with extraocular muscle surgery, occlusion, and/or orthoptics/vision therapy. The diplopia for all patients had existed for many years and was not amenable to any form of treatment.

A condition similar to horror fusionis has been reported in adults with previously normal binocular vision. Known as *central fusion disruption,* it develops after mechanical, vascular, or inflammatory central nervous system insult or when a cataract is left in situ for many years.[71-73] Unlike horror fusionis, central fusion disruption consists of a defect of motor fusion and not sensory fusion. The patient alternates between crossed and uncrossed diplopia at the angle of deviation and usually notices a vertical "bobbing" of the second image. Motor fusion can be achieved for only a moment with the synoptophore or prisms but cannot be maintained, even though sensory fusion exists. We have seen central fusion disruption develop in adults following head trauma (see Chapter 7, Case 5) and in adults with uncorrected aphakia. Central fusion disruption and horror fusionis must be differentiated from the diplopia caused by bilateral superior oblique paresis. With the latter, compensating for the large excyclodeviation in the synoptophore frequently permits stable fusion.[71,74]

CLINICAL DIAGNOSIS OF ANOMALOUS CORRESPONDENCE

There are several tests for retinal correspondence. In accordance with the definition of anomalous correspondence the tests involve either determining the subjective angle and comparing it to the objective angle or measuring the angle of anomaly directly. The former tests determine simultaneously the visual directions of the fovea of the fixating eye and a peripheral element of the deviating eye. The latter tests determine the visual directions of the two foveae simultaneously. Testing retinal correspondence requires the proper refractive correction, adequate patient understanding and cooperation, and knowledge of the patient's fixation status and eye position. It must be remembered that any subjective fusion test in which fusion is reported in the presence of constant strabismus indicates anomalous correspondence.

Comparing the Subjective Angle to the Objective Angle

Tests measuring the subjective angle include the red lens, synoptophore, Worth four dot, and Bagolini striated lenses.

Red Lens Test

This test is also described with incomitant deviations in Chapter 10 under Diplopia Fields. It is a simple and quick method of determining the state of correspondence. A red lens and a 10-PD prism (base-up or base-down) is placed before the fixating eye while the patient views a fixation light at 6 m. The vertical prism displaces the image on a retinal area that is not suppressed, resulting in easily recognized diplopia. The horizontal separation of the vertically displaced images is used to assess the presence of normal or anomalous correspondence.

The patient is asked to describe the position of the two lights. If there is no horizontal separation, the subjective angle is zero and harmonious anomalous correspondence exists. If the patient has uncrossed diplopia, base-out prisms are added until the red and white lights are vertically aligned. Base-in prisms are added for crossed diplopia. If the amount and direction of prism necessary to align the lights is commensurate with the objective angle as measured with the alternate cover test with prisms at the same fixation distance and with the same eye fixation, normal correspondence exists, whereas if they differ by more than 4 PD, unharmonious anomalous correspondence exists.

Synoptophore Test

To determine the status of retinal correspondence, the objective angle is first measured. Superimposition or first-degree targets, such as the soldier and house, are used. The use of larger targets is generally easier for the patient. The target with the lion should be in front of the nonpreferred eye, and the target with the cage should be placed before the preferred eye. The tube before the preferred eye is locked at the orthoposition. The patient is asked to fixate on the center of each target. The examiner moves the tube before the deviating eye while alternately turning the illumination before each eye on and off. Horizontal deviations are compensated for by moving the synoptophore tubes, and vertical deviations are compensated for by elevating or depressing the targets. The absence of any fixation movement discloses the objective angle, as indicated on the scale of the instrument. Assuming central fixation, the target for the right eye is directed at the right fovea and the target for the left eye is directed at the left fovea, so that when either eye is shown, its target does not have to move to fixate it. Because the two targets are presented alternately, this is the same angle found with the alternate cover test with prisms. With eccentric fixation, the objective angle is offset by that amount.[75] When one eye is deeply amblyopic without the capacity for central fixation, the objective angle can be determined by shifting the synoptophore tube in front of the amblyopic eye until the corneal reflex is centered in the pupil.

The subjective angle is determined by having the clinician or the patient move the tube before the deviating eye until the targets appear superimposed. The patient fixates on the target before the preferred eye. Objective and subjective angles that are equal indicate normal correspondence, whereas those that are dissimilar by more than 4 PD indicate anomalous correspondence.[65] A subjective setting of zero by a strabismic patient indicates harmonious anomalous correspondence, whereas a subjective setting somewhere between zero and the objective angle indicates unharmonious anomalous correspondence. Frequently, the subjective angle will not be definite, particularly for patients with long-standing strabismus. These patients experience some difficulty in superimposing the targets at the subjective angle. As the soldier on the target approaches the house and is seen on one side of the house, he suddenly disappears because of suppression and crosses over to reappear as he leaves the other end of the house. True superimposition of the two targets is not possible. This procedure can be modified to avoid suppression by briefly flashing the target before the suppressed eye at different positions. Bracketing the measurements from left to right and vice versa helps to refine the measurement. If this suppression and crossover occurs within ±4PD of the objective angle, retinal correspondence is considered to be normal. If not, it is anomalous.

Once the subjective angle has been determined and the targets are superimposed, the retinal correspondence can be confirmed by briefly extinguishing the target before the preferred eye and watching for any movement of the other eye (unilateral cover test). No movement indicates normal correspondence, and movement indicates anomalous correspondence. The status of the retinal correspondence can also be confirmed when the tubes of the synoptophore are set at the objective angle and imaged on both foveae. In the presence of normal correspondence, superimposition of the targets will occur. In anomalous correspondence there is diplopia. Patients with esotropia who have anomalous correspondence will perceive the targets as being diplopic and crossed and those with exotropia and anomalous correspondence will see them as being diplopic and uncrossed.

Worth Four Dot Test

In evaluating retinal correspondence with the Worth four dot test, the clinician must ensure that the four dots, or lights, are large enough to test the patient peripheral to any suppression zone that may exist. Because suppression interferes more with testing at distance, this is best accomplished by testing at near. The response of four dots in the presence of constant strabismus indicates a subjective angle of zero and harmonious anomalous correspondence (Fig. 5-9, *A*). This is most likely to occur in small-to-intermediate angles of esotropia.

The position of the eyes during testing must always be known. The Worth four dot test may be difficult to interpret because with the red-green glasses the clinician cannot be absolutely certain a strabismus exists at the moment a patient reports fusion. For example, a child with refractive accommodative esotropia might not be accommodating accurately on the lights. The child may therefore have straight eyes during testing and have normal correspondence. Conversely, if the child does accommodate and becomes esotropic during testing while still reporting fusion, anomalous correspondence exists. The clinician can look over the top of the glasses at the time of testing and perform the unilateral cover test.

If the patient reports five dots simultaneously (Fig. 5-9, *D*), a subjective angle exists and prisms can be used to differentiate normal from anomalous correspondence. Normal correspondence is diagnosed if the lights are superimposed into four, with prisms equal to the objective angle, and the unilateral cover test reveals no movement. The diagnosis of unharmonious anomalous correspondence is made if a significantly different prism (more than 4 PD) allows superimposition into four lights and with that prism the unilateral cover test shows movement. As indicated earlier, patients with rapid alternating suppression occasionally report seeing five lights simultaneously. This can be checked by observation of the behavior of the eyes behind the red-green glasses.

Bagolini Striated Lenses

Because this procedure is performed under nearly normal seeing conditions and is a minimally dissociative test, the Bagolini test is very sensitive in detecting anomalous correspondence. If the patient with strabismus sees two lines crossing at the light (Fig. 5-11, *A*), forming a symmetric X, the subjective angle is zero and harmonious anomalous correspondence is present. This frequently is accompanied by a central gap in one line, indicating a coexisting suppression (Fig. 5-11, *B*). As with the Worth four dot test, the position of the eyes must be known during testing. If there is a question of a very small angle of deviation or of the eyes being parallel, the unilateral cover test will make the diagnosis.

Lines with two distinct lights indicate a non-zero subjective angle with normal correspondence or with unharmonious anomalous correspondence (Fig. 5-11, *D*). Prisms are added base-out for uncrossed lights or base-in for crossed lights, until a single light is seen centered at the intersection of the X. The unilateral cover test is then performed. Absence of a strabismus of the deviating eye when the preferred eye is covered indicates normal correspondence. Persistence of strabismus indicates unharmonious anomalous correspondence.

Measuring the Angle of Anomaly Directly

These tests allow the measurement of retinal correspondence using entoptic imagery, either with afterimages alone or the Haidinger brushes and afterimages.

Hering-Bielschowsky Afterimage Test

For the patient with normal correspondence, afterimages produced successively on the foveae of the two eyes appear in their common visual direction regardless of whether the eyes are open or closed and regardless of the relative position of the eyes. This is the basis of the Hering-Bielschowsky afterimage test. Each eye is stimulated separately to specifically determine and label the visual direction of each fovea. It is performed by successively stimulating one eye with a hand-held linear electronic flash device while the other eye is occluded. The center of the line is blacked out and serves as a fixation target. Fixation is required only long enough for the electronic flash to be emitted. The afterimage test is a fovea-to-fovea test. The objective is to apply a vertical afterimage across the fovea of one eye and a horizontal afterimage across the fovea of the other eye. The clinician should stand a known distance from the patient. The vertical afterimage is first generated preferably in the right eye, with the left eye occluded, and then the horizontal afterimage is generated in the left eye, with the right eye occluded (Fig. 5-33).

After stimulation of both eyes, the two linear afterimages are seen simultaneously. In a dark room or with the eyes closed, they are seen as bright lines against a dark background (positive afterimages). In a lighted room with the eyes open, they are seen as dark lines against a bright background (negative afterimages). If the patient has trouble seeing them simultaneously, the patient should blink rapidly. Turning the room lights on and off quickly achieves the same effect. The patient should sketch the relative orientation of the two afterimages. If both foveae maintain the same visual direction, the central gaps, which correspond to the fovea of each eye, will be superimposed and the patient will see a perfect cross, indicating normal correspondence (Fig. 5-34, *A*). If the vertical afterimage appears to the left or to the right of the gap in the horizontal afterimage, the two foveae have different visual directions and anomalous correspondence is present. In esotropia with anomalous correspondence the patient will draw the afterimages as crossed (Fig. 5-34, *B*), whereas in exotropia with anomalous correspondence the patient will draw the afterimages as uncrossed (Fig. 5-34, *C*). The distance between the gaps can be measured and represents the angle of anomaly.

It is important when doing the test that the patient precisely fixate the center of the line, because fixation errors can simulate anomalous correspondence. Caution should be used in patients with eccentric fixation, because this will invalidate the angle of anomaly. Visuoscopy should be done before determining correspondence in all patients with amblyopia. In rare cases in which the angle of anomaly equals the angle of eccentric fixation the patient will see a perfect cross, as occurs in normal correspondence.

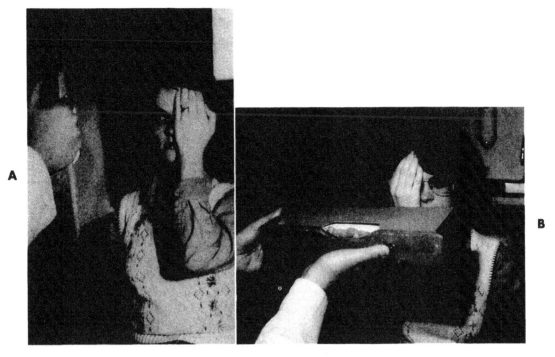

FIG. 5-33 **A** and **B,** Hering-Bielschowsky afterimage test.

Haidinger Brush Afterimage Transfer Test

This test is another procedure that measures the angle of anomaly directly using entopic imagery. Because it also monitors fixation, this test can be used to determine the retinal correspondence in patients with strabismic amblyopia with small angles of deviation and with eccentric fixation.

While the amblyopic eye is occluded, an afterimage is placed vertically on the fovea of the other eye. The occluder is then switched to the nonamblyopic eye. The patient is asked to fixate on a target (usually a dot) while viewing the Macular Integrity Tester with a cobalt blue filter. The amblyopic eye should see the fixation target, the Haidinger brushes, and the transferred afterimage. Some patients may not be able to perceive the transferred afterimage, however.

The diagnostic possibilities are illustrated in Fig. 5-35. With normal correspondence the transferred afterimage and the Haidinger brushes coincide; with anomalous correspondence, they are separated. The amount of separation between the transferred afterimage and the Haidinger brushes can be measured and represents the angle of anomaly. Displacement of the fixation point and the Haidinger brushes, as mentioned previously, is diagnostic of eccentric fixation.

TEST EVALUATION AND DEPTH OF ANOMALY

Estimates of the incidence of anomalous correspondence range from 10% to 90% of the population with strabismus.[76] This is the result in part of the observation that the status of retinal correspondence

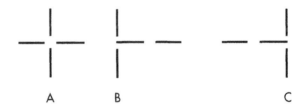

A	B	C

FIG. 5-34 Diagnostic possibilities with Hering-Bielschowsky afterimage test. Vertical afterimage was presented to right eye, horizontal afterimage to left eye. **A,** Normal correspondence (can also be anomalous correspondence when angle of eccentric fixation equals angle of anomaly). **B,** Anomalous correspondence (right esotropia). **C,** Anomalous correspondence (right exotropia).

varies considerably with the method of measurement.[77-84] Anomalous correspondence is rarely completely present or completely absent in a given patient. Many patients will display anomalous correspondence in certain test situations and normal correspondence in other test situations. Differences in retinal correspondence status for a patient when using different tests is possibly the result of fixation errors, changes in the position of the eyes between tests, and measurement errors.[82] More likely, it is the degree of dissociation that exists with different tests. Depending on their degree of dissociation or interference with binocular vision input, sensory tests may either detect or fail to detect anomalous correspondence in a given patient. Factors

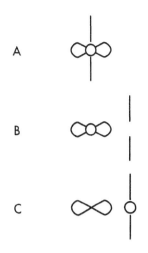

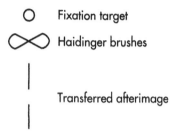

Fixation target

Haidinger brushes

Transferred afterimage

FIG. 5-35 Diagnostic possibilities with Haidinger brush afterimage test. **A,** Normal correspondence and central fixation. **B,** Anomalous correspondence and central fixation. **C,** Anomalous correspondence and eccentric fixation.

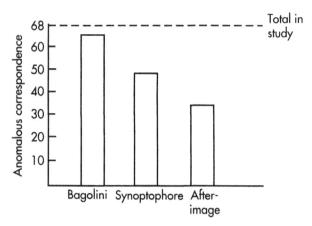

FIG. 5-36 Number of patients with anomalous correspondence using Bagolini striated lenses, synoptophore, and Hering-Bielschowsky afterimage test. (Modified from Rutstein RP, Daum KM, Eskridge JB: Clinical characteristics of anomalous correspondence, *Optom Visi Sci* 66:42, 1989.)

that influence the amount of dissociation include differences between the images stimulating the two retinas, the use of static or dynamic test backgrounds, the position of the images on the retina, the size and nature of fusional clues, and the level of illumination and stimulus intensity under which the test is performed.

✿ **CLINICAL PEARL**

The status of retinal correspondence varies considerably with the method of measurement.

The less dissociative the sensory test (test situation is close to normal seeing conditions), the more likely is the patient to give an anomalous correspondence response, whereas the more dissociative the test, the more likely the response will be normal. The Bagolini striated lens test is the least dissociative, and the tests using afterimages are the most dissociative. Over 90% of patients with strabismus show anomalous correspondence with the Bagolini lenses, and approximately 50% show it with the Hering-Bielschowsky afterimage test (Fig. 5-36).[85]

Patients with strabismus should be assessed with more than one test to determine the depth of anom-

alous correspondence. A patient demonstrating anomalous correspondence only with the Bagolini striated lens test has superficial anomalous correspondence, whereas a patient also demonstrating anomalous correspondence with the Hering-Bielschowsky afterimage test has deep anomalous correspondence. The prognosis for converting to normal correspondence and achieving a functional cure with therapy is presumably better in the former case than it is in the latter case. As with suppression, the more long-standing and more constant the strabismus, the deeper will be the anomalous correspondence. Adults with deep anomalous correspondence, however, are at no greater risk for developing diplopia when treated surgically than are patients with superficial anomalous correspondence.[86]

CONDITIONS FAVORING ANOMALOUS CORRESPONDENCE

Additional factors, aside from the nature of the testing procedure, that affect the status of retinal correspondence include the age of onset and the magnitude and stability of the strabismus.

Age of Onset of the Strabismus

Similar to amblyopia and suppression, anomalous correspondence develops only in strabismus that begins in early childhood. Visually mature patients who acquire strabismus are incapable of developing anomalous correspondence. The earlier the age of onset of strabismus, the greater the chance for development of anomalous correspondence. Katsumi, Tanaka, and Uemura[61] evaluated retinal correspondence status using the synoptophore for 391 patients. When the strabismus began in the first year of life the incidence of anomalous correspondence was 62%; when it began in the second year, it was 48%; when it began in the third year it was 35%; and when it began in the fourth year, the incidence of anomalous correspondence was 33%. Normal correspondence was always found when the strabismus began after age 4.

Magnitude of the Strabismus

Anomalous correspondence is more likely to develop in small-angle and intermediate-angle strabismus rather than large-angle strabismus.[79,87] In animal experiments, it has been reported only with angles of strabismus less than 10 degrees (17.5 D).[88] Clinically, anomalous correspondence is a frequent finding in microtropia. The closer the zero measure point is to the fovea of the strabismic eye, the greater chance for it to develop the same subjective visual direction as the fovea of the fixating eye. When the angle of strabismus is less than 10 D, anomalous correspondence is present in over 90% of the cases, whereas when the deviation is 30 PD to 40 PD, anomalous correspondence is essentially nonexistent.[79] This inverse relationship between the magnitude of the strabismus and the incidence of anomalous correspondence is more likely to be found with the Bagolini striated lenses than with the synoptophore or the use of afterimages.[85]

Stability of the Strabismus

A constant and stable strabismus facilitates the development of anomalous correspondence, because the same retinal visual stimulation will be maintained. Esotropia more than exotropia is associated with deep anomalous correspondence. As many as 85% of children in our clinic who have esotropia that is not totally accommodative have some degree of anomalous correspondence.

Anomalous correspondence is more likely in comitant than incomitant strabismus. The instability and changes in size of the deviation according to the direction of gaze and the compensatory head posture with incomitant strabismus make anomalous correspondence more unlikely. Anomalous correspondence is mainly associated with horizontal strabismus and not vertical strabismus. We do occasionally see patients with vertical deviations and anomalous correspondence. In these cases the anomalous correspondence is usually superficial. Anomalous correspondence has been reported in patients with congenital absence of the superior oblique muscle.[89]

On the other hand, anomalous correspondence is quite flexible, enabling patients who have intermittent and incomitant forms of strabismus to maintain visual comfort, despite varying angles of deviation. Anomalous correspondence can coexist with normal correspondence in the same patient. For example, a patient with intermittent exotropia may have normal correspondence and bifoveal fusion when aligned and

anomalous correspondence when exotropic.[5,67,90] Anomalous correspondence coexisting with normal correspondence can also occur with A or V patterns. A patient with a V-pattern esotropia may exhibit normal correspondence and bifoveal fusion in upgaze, in which the eyes are straight, and anomalous correspondence in downgaze, in which the eyes are esotropic.

BINOCULAR VISION IN ANOMALOUS CORRESPONDENCE
Fusional Movements

It has been known for some time that when given prisms a patient with anomalous correspondence is likely to move his or her eyes in a manner that resembles fusional vergence in normal patients.[91-93] This frequently encountered convergence elicited by base-out prisms in patients with esotropia has been interpreted as an attempt on the part of the patient with anomalous correspondence to maintain the rudimentary fusion despite the prisms. These fusional movements produce changes in the angle of anomaly that return retinal correspondence to its state before wearing of the prisms. Referred to as *anomalous fusional movements,* they are much slower (i.e., minutes, hours, and even days) and not as precise (smaller than the amount of the prism) than normal fusional movements and are usually invisible to the naked eye.[94] These anomalous fusional movements are the basis of prism therapy for treating anomalous correspondence.

Instead of being actual fusional movements, however, these movements may represent manifestations of covariations of the angle of anomaly, the repeated changes that can occur in the angle of strabismus without upsetting the fully compensated state of harmonious anomalous correspondence. Patients with anomalous correspondence have a larger area of horizontal single binocular vision (pseudo Panum's area) than patients with normal binocular vision.[95] This allows for a point-to-area rather than a fixed point-to-point sensory relationship between the two retinas. An infinite number of retinal elements between the fovea of the fixating eye and an area on the retina of the deviating eye are capable of forming a common visual direction. With each change in the strabismic angle the harmonious anomalous correspondence persists. This can explain the maintenance of harmonious anomalous correspondence following extraocular muscle surgery in some cases, as well as its maintenance in up and down gaze in patients with A or V patterns.[96,97] It can also explain how some patients with anomalous correspondence can maintain gross fusion while the tubes of the synoptophore are moved, although their eyes do not move.

Stereopsis

Stereopsis is thought to be one of the advantages of patients with strabismus who have anomalous correspondence vs. patients with strabismus who have only suppression.[29,98-100] Stereopsis is more likely to be present when using contour stereotests.[101] Some investigators, using the Titmus stereotest, have reported high-grade stereoacuity (60 seconds of arc or better) in small-angle strabismus with anomalous correspondence.[102,103] Such levels of stereoacuity clearly cannot differentiate these patients from those with normal binocular vision. These patients were either incorrectly diagnosed or were using clues other than binocular retinal disparity. Patients with anomalous correspondence generally have a disparity discrimination function 3 times worse than normal patients.[104] Most investigators have reported no better than 200 seconds of arc with the Titmus stereotest with similar patients.[29]

The presence of random-dot or global stereopsis with anomalous correspondence is more doubtful. Hansell[30] measured stereopsis using the Titmus, TNO, and Lang stereotests in 91 patients with anomalous correspondence. For the patients with a history of treated infantile esotropia (onset at or before 6 months of age), as many as 25% had contour stereopsis, whereas none had random-dot stereopsis. For the patients with treated acquired strabismus (onset after 6 months of age), 69% with deviations of 6 to 19 PD and 100% with deviations less than 6 PD had contour stereopsis. Of the patients with the smaller acquired deviations, 31% also had random-dot stereopsis. Random-dot stereopsis appears to be a possibility with anomalous correspondence only when the strabismus begins after 6 months of age and when the strabismus is very small.

Despite having only rudimentary stereopsis at best, many patients with anomalous correspondence possess an ability to judge distances that is similar to patients with normal binocular vision.[105] Anomalous correspondence supposedly provides these patients with useful clues in their daily life.

PATHOPHYSIOLOGY

The site of anomalous correspondence is cortical.[88] Shlaer raised kittens wearing 4-PD vertical prisms and found a compensating shift of slightly less than 4 D in the mean disparity in cortical cells.[106] Binocular cortical interaction has been confirmed in humans with the visual evoked potential (VEP).[107-110] In patients with strabismus who have small-angle deviations and anomalous correspondence, VEP summation occurs when both eyes are flashed together. The binocular VEP is much larger than the monocular VEP. For patients with large-angle strabismus without anomalous correspondence, summation does not occur and the binocular VEP is the same as the monocular VEP.

Anomalous correspondence probably has its seat where the retinal topology is not exact, that is, where

the binocular receptive fields are very large. Recent studies in cats indicate that cortical cells with anomalous correspondence are not found in the primary visual cortex (area 17) but are found in the lateral suprasylvian gyrus, which contains several areas of secondary visual cortex.[88] They are also found in area 18. Cells in the primary visual cortex tend to have small receptive fields, whereas cells in the lateral suprasylvian gyrus have larger receptive fields.

THEORETIC BASIS

Several theories have been used to explain anomalous correspondence. None of these theories by themselves can account for all the characteristics of anomalous correspondence found in a given patient with strabismus or the differences between strabismics.

Anomalous correspondence has been considered as being either innate or an acquired sensory or motor adaptation. If innate, it is the cause rather than the result of strabismus.[111] This is consistent with the views of Worth, as discussed in Chapter 7, who indicates that some patients have congenitally poor fusion ability.[112] Failure of normal correspondence to assert itself after treatment[113]; a poor correlation between some clinical features of strabismus and the type of retinal correspondence[85]; and the fact that the earlier the onset of strabismus, the greater the incidence of anomalous correspondence[61] give some credence to this theory.

The absence of diplopia in anomalous correspondence has led the majority of clinicians, including ourselves, to consider anomalous correspondence as being an acquired sensory adaptation.[66,114] Its acquisition represents an adaptation of the sensory apparatus of the eyes to the abnormal position of the eyes. Anomalous correspondence evolves only from normal correspondence. The development of anomalous correspondence is a slow process, and at first the relationship is not very deeply rooted. This view is consistent with those of Chavasse,[115] as discussed in Chapter 7, who reported that poor fusion results from disuse of the eyes together. If this is entirely the case, patients with congenital strabismus would rarely develop anomalous correspondence.[116] We and other investigators, however, have examined numerous patients with congenital (infantile) esotropia who have anomalous correspondence.[81,117] The sensory adaptation theory is more convincing for a proportion of small-angle strabismus of constant angle and long duration.

An alternative view is that anomalous correspondence involves a motor adaptation rather than a sensory adaptation to strabismus.[118,119] The innervational pattern associated with the strabismus gives the potential for a change in retinal correspondence. According to Morgan,[119] presence or absence of anomalous correspondence depends on whether the basic underlying innervational pattern to the extraocular muscles is "registered" as altering egocentric direction or whether the pattern is "nonregistered" as altering egocentric direction. A nonregistered eye movement pattern is one in which the neural impulses from the site of origin of an eye movement in the brain communicate only with the extraocular muscles and produce only an eye movement. Accommodative vergence is supposedly nonregistered. In a registered eye movement, these impulses communicate with the perceptual apparatus of the brain responsible for visual direction, as well as with the extraocular muscles and produce both a change in retinal correspondence and an eye movement. A deviation that is the result entirely of a nonregistered eye movement gives normal correspondence, whereas a deviation that is the result entirely of a registered eye movement gives harmonious anomalous correspondence. In a deviation that is the result partly of a registered eye movement and partly of a nonregistered eye movement, an unharmonious anomalous correspondence would result.

According to this theory, accommodative esotropia would not be accompanied by anomalous correspondence (it rarely is) and strabismus caused by an anomaly in the version mechanism would always be accompanied by anomalous correspondence (not necessarily the case). The motor theory does nicely explain covariation in which harmonious anomalous correspondence persists despite the angle of strabismus changing from distance to near, looking up and down, or wearing or not wearing glasses, as well as the changing retinal correspondence (normal when aligned and anomalous when strabismic) that we frequently see in intermittent exotropia.

TREATMENT

Anomalous correspondence is a significant concern in the complete remediation of strabismus. Whether it can be effectively treated is a continuous debate. Many clinicians feel that anomalous correspondence should not be treated at all because it provides a rudimentary form of binocular vision for some patients.[57,62,99] This view seems reasonable, based on the reported efficacy of therapy. In general, deeply established anomalous correspondence rarely responds to treatment. Although the angle of anomaly can be reduced, it can rarely be eliminated. Flom,[121] in reviewing the literature, documented cures in only 11 of 262 patients with esotropia with anomalous correspondence, a cure rate of less than 5%. However, higher rates of success (as much as 50%) have been reported by other clinicians.[122-129]

❖ CLINICAL PEARL

Deeply established anomalous correspondence rarely responds to treatment.

Mallet[62] differentiates anomalous correspondence according to when it should or when it should not be treated. He divides anomalous correspondence into three categories based on its depth. Type A, which constitutes about 80% of all cases of patients with strabismus, is associated with intermediate and larger degrees of strabismus and those of variable angle. With these patients, the anomalous correspondence is superficial and present only with the Bagolini striated lens test. Because these patients project normally with orthoptic/vision therapy instruments such as the synoptophore, Mallett recommends no specific treatment for the anomalous correspondence. The strabismus can be treated with prisms, orthoptics/vision therapy, and/or surgery. Type B anomalous correspondence is more deeply established. Anomalous correspondence is present with the synoptophore, as well as with the Bagolini striated lenses. The angle of strabismus is smaller and much more stable than in type A. According to Mallet, type B requires treatment of the anomalous correspondence if elimination of the strabismus is to be entirely successful. Treatment includes prisms and/or orthoptics/vision therapy. Type C anomalous correspondence occurs in small-angle strabismus (microtropia) that is stable and has a very early onset. These patients have anomalous correspondence also with the Hering-Bielschowsky afterimage test. According to Mallet, patients with type C anomalous correspondence have a very useful, although rudimentary, binocular vision, and the anomalous correspondence does not require treatment.

The methods for restoring normal correspondence include occlusion, surgery, prisms, and orthoptics/vision therapy.

Occlusion

Occlusion is used prophylactically in the young patient with strabismus. The technique consists of constant and total occlusion therapy on an alternate-day basis, as is done in amblyopia. It is generally applied as soon as the child starts to manifest the strabismus and is not terminated until other treatment is provided to perfectly align the eyes. Because anomalous correspondence exists only during binocular viewing, occlusion therapy provided early enough may prevent its development. We have no evidence that such therapy is effective in disrupting an already existing anomalous correspondence, however.

Surgery

Normalization of anomalous correspondence has been reported to occur following extraocular muscle surgery in approximately one-fifth of all patients.[61,65,130-132] Normal correspondence has also been achieved in some patients treated with botulinum toxin rather than conventional surgery.[133] Reducing the strabismic angle and leaving a residual angle falls short of eliminating the anomalous correspondence. Hugonnier[130] reports on 70 patients with esotropia with anomalous correspondence. After surgery, 46 patients became exotropic and 24 patients remained esotropic. Of the patients with exotropia, 32 (70%) developed normal correspondence. For all those with esotropia, anomalous correspondence persisted. Katsumi, Tanaka, and Uemura[61] surgically treated 66 patients with esotropia with anomalous correspondence. Normalization of retinal correspondence occurred in 14 (21%) patients. Twelve of these patients (86%) had a final ocular alignment of either orthotropia or exotropia. When esotropia remained, most patients had a tendency to develop harmonious anomalous correspondence and normal correspondence did not occur.

Normalization of anomalous correspondence may occur when a consecutive strabismus develops over time without surgery. Rutstein and others[65] studied the changes in retinal correspondence for patients with constant strabismus whose ocular alignment was altered either surgically or spontaneously over a period of years. Patients with normal correspondence maintained it after the change in ocular alignment. Of the 21 patients with anomalous correspondence, 14 maintained anomalous correspondence and 7 developed normal correspondence. For all the patients achieving normal correspondence, the direction of the strabismus also changed (i.e., esotropia to exotropia).

Based on these reports and our clinical experience, an important factor in normalizing retinal correspondence with extraocular muscle surgery is the final eye position. The eye position must be either exactly parallel or slightly overcorrected to develop normal correspondence. Even so, this does not always guarantee achieving normal correspondence. In addition, although retinal correspondence may become normalized, rarely do these patients also achieve normal binocular vision (see the following Case, as well as Chapter 8, Case 2).

CASE 3

A 25-year-old man was referred for strabismus. Ocular history revealed strabismus surgery at 8 months and 6 years for an infantile esotropia. Occlusion and orthoptics/vision therapy were performed from ages 4 to 6. He presently denied diplopia, but was concerned about the way his eyes appeared.

Our examination showed visual acuities of 20/30 OD and 20/20 OS. The patient was emmetropic. A 30-PD constant right exotropia with a dissociated vertical deviation was present at distance and near. The patient suppressed the right eye with both the Worth four dot and Bagolini striated lens tests. With the synoptophore, an objective angle of 30 D base-in and a subjective angle of 30 PD base-out were measured, indicating paradoxic anomalous correspondence. Surgical therapy was undertaken.

Following surgery, the patient manifested a 6-PD esotropia at distance and near with the dissociated vertical deviation. He denied diplopia. With the synoptophore, both objective and subjective angles were 8 D base-out, indicating normal correspondence. Suppression prevented any demonstrable second-degree fusion.

Prisms

The responses observed in strabismus during prism wear have led to development of various therapeutic techniques. Prism therapy for anomalous correspondence, interestingly, has been advocated mostly by European clinicians.[125,134-139] It involves the use of compensating, overcorrecting, reverse, or vertical prisms. Fresnel press-on prisms are placed, usually before the dominant eye, in which the slight reduction in acuity maintains the acuity gained with amblyopic therapy. The goal is to break down the harmonious anomalous correspondence developed in response to the strabismus. Compensating prisms provide stimulation of both foveae and it is hoped that normal correspondence can be reestablished. However, as mentioned before, prisms in many cases result in the angle of deviation increasing, sometimes by as much as the original angle of strabismus. The strabismus reappears after it has been prismatically corrected, presumably as a result of the motor fusional response evoked by the anomalous correspondence. Because of this, overcorrecting, or reverse, prisms are preferred. Prisms of power greater than the strabismic angle image the target of interest on the opposite hemiretina of the deviating eye. With esotropia, base-out prisms are gradually increased in strength until the patient is unable to compensate or make anomalous fusional movements for them.[140] The eyes return to the original angle of esotropia, but the retinal images now are being received on retinal areas that are neither normally corresponding nor associated with the previous harmonious anomalous correspondence. A prismatically induced unharmonious anomalous correspondence is created. Normal correspondence may eventually be obtained. The prism power required to achieve this may be 20 to 40 PD in excess of the angle of deviation. This, together with the eyes appearing to be even farther displaced inward, ensures a poor cosmetic appearance. To avoid this, reverse prisms can create a similar effect. Using base-in prisms for esotropia that are too strong for the patient to overcome with a divergent fusional movement (i.e., 16 D), noncorresponding retinal areas are stimulated with the breakdown of harmonious anomalous correspondence. The appearance is slightly improved because of the patient's eyes being displaced temporally and therefore appearing less esotropic. Vertical prisms worn base-up and base-down on alternate days have also been used. Regardless of the direction of the prism, the

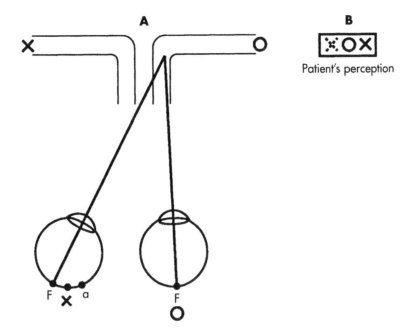

Patient's perception

FIG. 5-37 Monocular diplopia (binocular triplopia) resulting from orthoptics/vision therapy. **A,** Target *X* stimulates area on nasal hemiretina and is projected both homonymously (normal correspondence) with respect to fovea (*F*) of deviating eye and heteronymously (anomalous correspondence) with respect to point *a* in deviating eye. **B,** Image projected normally is less distinct than image projected anomalously.

prism power is gradually reduced over time as the retinal correspondence normalizes.

Although the theoretic basis for prism therapy is sound, we are not convinced of its efficacy. Converting to normal correspondence does not seem to occur for most of our patients. This may be the result of poor compliance. Prism therapy is time-consuming, and many times the patient is diplopic during therapy. We have used prism therapy in patients with anomalous correspondence who experience a sudden change in the habitual angle of strabismus without a corresponding change in the angle of anomaly. For example, as described earlier, an adult with childhood-onset esotropia and harmonious anomalous correspondence who develops a lateral rectus paresis will have diplopia. Sensory testing will reveal unharmonious anomalous correspondence. Prisms equal to the new subjective angle usually eliminates the diplopia.

Orthoptics/Vision Therapy

The efficacy of orthoptics/vision therapy for treating anomalous correspondence can be as high as 50%, according to Wick and Cook.[127] Traditional methods involve procedures using the synoptophore or other Wheatstone type of stereoscopes, such as the variable-mirror stereoscope. Superimposition targets are presented at the objective angle, and antisuppression therapy in the form of alternate flashing is given. Normal correspondence can also be stimulated by setting the

tubes of the synoptophore at the objective angle and moving the tube in front of the deviated eye laterally across the foveal region a few prism diopters to stimulate the normal use of the fovea. At first the patient projects the targets anomalously, but hopefully is soon localized correctly. Occlusion therapy is usually carried out when the patient is not performing the procedure. Vergence therapy based on covariation, rather than antisuppression therapy, has been used to treat anomalous correspondence in patients with small-angle esotropia.[140,142] This method is described in Chapter 8.

Transient monocular diplopia and binocular triplopia may develop while the patient is undergoing orthoptics/vision therapy for anomalous correspondence. Anomalous and normal retinal correspondence may compete with each other to localize the image in the strabismic eye. One retinal point receiving the fixing object will localize it in two directions. As illustrated in the case of a patient with esotropia with anomalous correspondence (Fig. 5-37), after undergoing therapy, the target *(x)* will project both anomalously with respect to the point *a,* as well as normally with respect to the fovea in the esotropic eye. The patient will see two images when the nonstrabismic eye is covered and three images in binocular viewing. Characteristically, the normally projected image is the dimmer of the two. With time and the establishment of normal correspondence, the anomalously projected image fades and the normally projected image becomes brighter.

REFERENCES

1. Smith EL and others: The relationship between binocular rivalry and strabismic suppression, *Invest Ophthalmol Vis Sci* 2B:80, 1985.
2. Smith EL and others: Intraocular suppression produced by rivalry stimuli: a comparison of normal and abnormal binocular vision, *Optom Vis Sci* 71:473, 1994.
3. Jampolsky A: Characteristics of suppression in strabismus, *Arch Ophthalmol* 54:683, 1955.
4. Parks MM: *Ocular motility and strabismus,* New York, 1975, Harper & Row.
5. Cooper J, Record CD: Suppression and retinal correspondence in intermittent exotropia, *Br J Ophthalmol* 70:673, 1986.
6. Pratt-Johnson J, Wee HS: Suppression associated with exotropia, *Can J Ophthalmol* 4:136, 1969.
7. Melek N and others: Intermittent exotropia: a study of suppression in the binocular visual field in 21 cases, *Binoc Vis Eye Muscle Surg* 7:25, 1992.
8. Pratt-Johnson JA, MacDonald AL: Binocular visual field in strabismus, *Can J Ophthalmol* 11:37, 1976.
9. Pratt-Johnson JA, Tillson G: Suppression in strabismus: an update, *Br J Ophthalmol* 68:174, 1984.
10. Pratt-Johnson JA, Tillson G, Pop A: Suppression in strabismus and the hemiretinal trigger mechanism, *Arch Ophthalmol* 101:218, 1983.
11. Mehdorn E: Suppression scotomas in primary microstrabismus: a perimetric artifact, *Doc Ophthalmologica* 71:1, 1989.
12. Pratt-Johnson JA: Fusion and suppression: development and loss, *J Pediatr Ophthalmol Strab* 29:4, 1992.
13. Hallden U: Suppression scotomata in concomitant strabismus with harmonious anomalous correspondence, *Acta Ophthalmol* 60:828, 1982.
14. Campos EC: Binocularity in comitant strabismus: binocular visual field studies, *Doc Ophthalmol* 53:243, 1982.
15. Schor CM, Terrell M, Peterson D: Contour interaction and temporal masking in strabismus and amblyopia, *Am J Optom Physiol Opt* 53:217, 1976.
16. Romano JA, Romano PE: Rapid sensory adaptations in three 5-year old children, *Am Orthopt J* 71, 1978.
17. Franceschetti AT, Burian HM: Visually evoked responses in alternating strabismus, *Am J Ophthalmol* p 1292, 1971.
18. Hess RF: The site and nature of suppression in strabismic amblyopia, *Vision Res* 31:111, 1991.
19. Wright KW and others: Suppression and the pattern visual evoked potential, *J Pediatr Ophthalmol Strab* 23:252, 1986.
20. Wright KW, Fox BES, Eriksen KJ: PVEP evidence of true suppression in adult onset strabismus, *J Pediatr Ophthalmol Strab* 27:196, 1990.
21. van Balen ATM: The influence of suppression on the flicker ERG, *Doc Ophthalmol* 28:440, 1964.
22. Arthur BW, Keech RV: The polarized three dot test, *J Pediatr Ophthalmol Strab* 24:305, 1987.
23. Arthur BW, Marshall A, McGillivray D: Worth vs. Polarized Four-dot test, *J Pediatr Ophthalmol Strab* 30:53, 1993.
24. Simons K, Elhatton K: Artifacts in fusion and stereopsis testing based on red/green dichoptic image separation, *J Pediatr Ophthalmol Strab* 31:290, 1994.
25. Romano PE, von Noorden GK: Atypical responses to the four-diopter prism test, *Am J Ophthalmol* 67:935, 1969.
26. Bagolini B, Campos EC, Chiesi C: The Irvine 4 diopter prism test for the diagnosis of suppression: a reappraisal, *Binoc Vis Eye Muscle Surg* 1:77, 1985.
27. Frantz KA, Cotter SA, Wick B: Re-evaluation of the four prism base-out test, *Optom Vis Sci* 69:777, 1992.
28. Dale RT, Guyton DL: The influence of peripheral fusion on the 4-prism diopter base-out test, *Invest Ophthalmol Vis Sci* 20(suppl):199, 1979.
29. Rutstein RP, Eskridge JB: Stereopsis in small-angle strabismus, *Am J Optom Physiol Opt* 61:491, 1984.
30. Hansell R: Stereopsis and ARC, *Am Orthopt J* 41:122, 1991.
31. Cooper J: Clinical stereopsis testing: contour and random dot stereograms, *J Am Optom Assoc* 50:41, 1979.
32. Cooper J, Warshowsky J: Lateral displacement as a response cue in the Titmus stereotest, *Am J Optom Physiol Opt* 54:537, 1977.
33. Archer SM: Stereotest artifacts and the strabismus patient, *Graefes Arch Clin Exp Opthalmol* 226:313, 1988.
34. Schweers MA, Baker JD: Comparison of Titmus and two Randot tests in monofixation, *Am Orthopt J* 42:135, 1992.
35. Dale RT: *Fundamentals of ocular motility and strabismus,* New York, 1982, Grune and Stratton.
36. Okuda FC, Apt L, Wanter BS: Evaluation of the TNO randomdot stereogram test, *Am Orthopt J* 27:124, 1977.
37. Frisby JP: Random-dot stereograms, *Br Orthopt J* 31:1, 1974.
38. Manny RE, Martinez AT, Fern KD: Testing stereopsis in the preschool child: is it clinically useful, *J Pediatr Ophthalmol Strab* 28:223, 1991.
39. Rosner J: Effectiveness of the random-dot E stereotest as a preschool vision screening instrument, *J Am Optom Assoc* 48:1121, 1978.
40. Hope C, Maslin K: Random-dot stereogram E in vision screening of children, *Aust N Z J Ophthalmol* 18:313, 1990.
41. Hammond RS, Schmidt P: A Random Dot E stereotest for the vision screening of children, *Arch Ophthalmol* 104:54, 1986.
42. Ruttum MS, Nelson DB: Stereopsis testing to reduce over-referral in preschool vision screening, *J Pediatr Ophthalmol Strab* 28:131, 1991.
43. Smith GM: Evaluations of the Frisby screening plate and Lang II stereotest in primary vision screening in pre-school children, *Br Orthopt J* 52:1, 1995.
44. Franceschetti A and others: The Lang stereotest for screening of pre-school children, *Klin Monatsbl Augenheilkd* 204:363, 1994.
45. Stathacopoulos RA and others: Distance stereoacuity: assessing control in intermittent exotropia, *Ophthalmology* 100:495, 1993.
46. Parks MM: The monofixation syndrome, *Trans Am Ophthalmol Soc* 67:603, 1969.
47. Rutstein RP, Fuhr PD, Schaafsma D: Distance stereopsis in orthophores, heterophores, and intermittent strabismics, *Optom Vis Sci* 71:415, 1994.
48. O'Neal TD, Rosenbaum AL, Stathacopoulos RA: Distance stereo acuity improvement in intermittent exotropic patients following strabismus surgery, *J Pediatr Ophthalmol Strab* 32:353, 1995.
49. Boyd TAS and others: Fixation switch diplopia, *Can J Ophthalmol* 9:310, 1974.
50. Karas Y, Budd GE, Boyd TAS: Late onset diplopia in childhood onset strabismus, *J Pediatr Ophthalmol Strab* 11:135, 1974.
51. Pratt-Johnson JA: Sensory phenomena associated with suppression, *Br Orthopt J* 26:15, 1969.
52. Rutstein RP: Fixation switch: an unusual cause of adolescent and adult onset diplopia, *J Am Optom Assoc* 56:862, 1985.
53. Smith KG and others: Fixation switch diplopia: an evaluation of suppression, *Am Orthopt J* 41:90, 1991.
54. Richards R: The syndrome of antimetropia and switched fixation in strabismus, *Am Orthopt J* 41:96, 1991.
55. Kushner BJ: Fixation switch diplopia, *Arch Ophthalmol* 113:896, 1995.
56. Deleted in galleys.
57. von Noorden GK: *Binocular vision and ocular motility: theory and management of strabismus,* St Louis, 1996, Mosby.
58. Rutstein RP, Bessant B: Horror fusionis: a report of 5 cases, *J Am Optom Assoc* 67:733, 1996.

59. Flom MC: Corresponding and disparate retinal points in normal and anomalous correspondence, *Am J Optom Physiol Opt* p 656, 1980

60. Daum KM: Anomalous correspondence. In Eskridge JB, Amos JF, Barteltt JD, editors: *Clinical procedures in optometry,* Philadelphia 1991, JB Lippincott.

61. Katsumi O, Tanaka Y, Uemura YL: Anomalous retinal correspondence in esotropia, *Jpn J Opthalmol* 26:166, 1982.

62. Mallett RFJ: Anomalous retinal correspondence: the new outlook, *Ophthalmic Opt* p 606, 1970.

63. Robertson KM: Diplopia after extraocular muscle surgery for exotropia: two case reports, *Can J Optom* 57:22, 1995.

64. Azar RF: Post-operative paradoxical diplopia, *Am Orthopt J* 15:64, 1965.

65. Rutstein RP and others: Changes in retinal correspondence after changes in ocular alignment, *Optom Vis Sci* 68:325, 1991.

66. Hallden U: Fusional phenomena in anomalous correspondence, *Acta Ophthalmol Suppl* 37:1, 1952.

67. Daum KM: Covariation in anomalous correspondence with accommodative vergence, *Am J Optom Physiol Opt* 59:146, 1982.

68. Kerr KE: Instability of anomalous retinal correspondence, *J Am Optom Assoc* 39:1107, 1968.

69. Kerr KE: Accommodative and fusional vergence in anomalous correspondence, *Am J Optom Physiol Opt* 57:676, 1980.

70. Kramer L: Horror fusionis, *Am Orthopt J* 10:63, 1960.

71. London R, Scott SH: Sensory fusion disruption syndrome, *J Am Optom Assoc* 58:544, 1987.

72. Pratt-Johnson JA, Tillson G: Acquired central disruption of fusional amplitude, *Ophthalmology* 86:2140, 1979.

73. Sharkey JA, Sellar PW: Acquired central fusion disruption following cataract extraction, *J Pediatr Ophthalmol Strab* 31:391, 1994.

74. Kushner BJ: Unexpected cyclotropia simulating disruption of fusion, *Arch Ophthalmol* 110:1415, 1992.

75. Eskridge JB: The complete cover test, *J Am Optom Assoc* 44:602, 1974.

76. Mallett RFJ: Binocular vision in strabismus, *Ophthalmic Opt* 9:812, 1969.

77. Lambert SJ, Murray JMC, Ryan JB: Effect of target size of anomalous sensory responses in the Bagolini striated lens test, *Am J Optom Physiol Opt* 64:173, 1987.

78. Daum KM: Analysis of seven methods of determining anomalous correspondence, *Am J Optom Physiol Opt* 59:870, 1982.

79. Bagolini B: Sensory anomalies in strabismus (suppression, anomalous correspondence, amblyopia), *Doc Ophthalmol* 41:1, 1976.

80. Jennings JAM: Anomalous retinal correspondence: a review, *Ophthalmic Physiol Opt* 5:537, 1985.

81. Burian HM, Luke NE: Sensory retinal relationships in 100 consecutive cases of heterotropia, *Arch Ophthalmol* 84:16, 1970.

82. Flom MC, Kerr KE: Determination of retinal correspondence: multiple testing results and the depth of anomaly concept, *Arch Ophthalmol* 77:200, 1967.

83. Yamashita M, Tokoro T: Retinal correspondence under dynamic background, *Optom Vis Science* 10:737, 1995.

84. Deguchi M and others: Study of retinal correspondence in esotropia with phase difference haploscope, *Acta Soc Ophthalmol Jpn* 97:981, 1993.

85. Rutstein RP, Daum KM, Eskridge JB: Clinical characteristics of anomalous correspondence, *Optom Vis Sci* 66:420, 1989.

86. Flanders M, Beneish R: The risk of postoperative diplopia in adult surgical correction of childhood strabismus, *Binoc Vis Eye Muscle Surg* 10:243, 1995.

87. Pasino L, Maraini G: Importance of natural test conditions in assessing the sensory state of the squinting subject with some clinical considerations on anomalous retinal correspondence, *Br J Ophthalmol* 48:30, 1964.

88. Grant S, Berman NE: Mechanism of anomalous retinal correspondence: maintenance of binocularity with alteration of receptive field position in the lateral suprasylvian visual area of strabismic cats, *Vis Neurosci* 7:253, 1991.

89. Matsuo T and others: Vertical abnormal retinal correspondence in three patients with congenital absence of the superior oblique muscle, *Am J Ophthalmol* 106:341, 1988.

90. Cooper J, Feldman J: Panoramic viewing, visual acuity of the deviating eye and anomalous retinal correspondence in the intermittent exotrope of the divergence excess type, *Am J Optom Physiol Opt* 56:422, 1979.

91. Burian HM: Fusional movements in permanent strabismus, *Arch Ophthalmol* 26:626, 1941.

92. Carniglia PE, Cooper J: Vergence adaptation in esotropia, *Optom Vis Sci* 69:308, 1992.

93. Bagolini B: Sensory anomalies in strabismus, *Br J Ophthalmol* 58:313, 1974.

94. Campos EC and others: Recording of disparity vergence in comitant esotropia, *Doc Ophthalmol* 71:63, 1989.

95. Bagolini B, Capobianco NM: Subjective space in comitant squint, *Am J Ophthalmol* 50:430, 1965.

96. Heleveston EM, von Noorden GK, Williams F: Retinal correspondence in the **A** or **V** pattern, *Am Orthopt J* 20:22, 1970.

97. Ciancia AO: Sensorial relationship in **A** and **V** syndromes, *Trans Ophthalmol Soc U K* 82:243, 1962.

98. Dengler B, Kommerell G: Stereoscopic cooperation between the fovea of one eye and the periphery of the other eye at large disparities. Implications for anomalous retinal correspondence in strabismus, *Graefes Arch Clin Exp Ophthalmol* 231:193, 1993.

99. Lang J: Anomalous retinal correspondence update, *Graefes Arch Clin Exp Ophthalmol* 226:137, 1988.

100. Marsh WR, Rawlings SC, Mumma JV: Evaluation of clinical stereoacuity tests, *Ophthalmology* 87:1265, 1980.

101. Cooper J, Feldman J: Random dot stereogram performances by strabismic, amblyopic and ocular pathology patients in an operant-discrimination task, *Am J Optom Physiol Opt* 55:593, 1978.

102. Hill M, Perry J, Wood ICJ: Stereoacuity in microtropia. In Moore S, Mein J, Stockbridge L, editors: New York, 1976, Stratton Intercontinental.

103. Henson DB, Williams DE: Depth perception in strabismus, *Br J Ophthalmol* 64:343, 1980.

104. Nelson JI: A neurophysiological model for anomalous correspondence based on mechanisms of sensory fusion, *Doc Ophthalmol* 51:3, 1981 (review).

105. Campos EC, Aldrovandi E, Bolzani R: Distance judgment in comitant strabismus with anomalous retinal correspondence, *Doc Ophthalmol* 67:223, 1987.

106. Shlaer R: Shift in binocular disparity causes compensatory change in the cortical structure of kittens, *Science* 173:285, 1971.

107. Chiesi C, Sargentini AD, Bolzani R: Binocular visual perception in strabismics studied by means of visual evoked responses, *Doc Ophthalmol* 58:51, 1984.

108. Campos EC: Anomalous retinal correspondence: monocular and binocular visual evoked responses, *Arch Ophthalmol* 98:293, 1980.

109. Campos EC, Chiesi C: Binocularity in comitant strabismus. II. Objective evaluation with visual evoked responses, *Doc Ophthalmol* 55:277, 1983.

110. Bagolini B and others: Binocular interactions and steady-state VEPs: a study in normal and defective binocular vision. II. *Graefes Arch Clin Exp Ophthalmol* 232:737, 1994.

111. Adler FH, Jackson FE: Correlations between sensory and motor disturbances in convergent squint, *Arch Ophthalmol* 72:283, 1974.

112. Worth C: *Squint: its causes, pathology and treatment,* ed 6, London, 1929, Bailliere, Tindall, and Cox.

113. Bedrossian EH: Anomalous retinal correspondence in alternating strabismus, *Arch Ophthalmol* 52:663, 1954.

114. Burian HM: Sensorial retinal relationships in concomitant strabismus, *Arch Ophthalmol* 37:336, 1947.

115. Chavasse FB: *Worth's squint on the binocular reflexes and the treatment of strabismus,* ed 7, Philadelphia, 1939, P Blakiston & Son.

116. Parks MM: Sensory adaptations in strabismus. In: *Symposium on strabismus,* St Louis, 1971, Mosby.

117. von Nooden GK: A reassessment of infantile esotropia, *Am J Ophthalmol* 105:1, 1988.

118. Boeder P: "Response shift" vs. anomalous retinal correspondence, *Am Orthopt J* 28:44, 1978.

119. Morgan MW: Anomalous correspondence interpreted as a motor phenomenon, *Am J Optom Arch Am Acad Optom* 38:131, 1961.

120. Deleted in galleys.

121. Flom MC: Treatment of binocular anomalies in children. In Hirsch MJ, Wick RE, editors: *Vision of children: an optometric symposium,* Philadelphia, 1963, Chilton.

122. Schellenbeck R, Schmit I: Zum Problemdes Korrespondenzwandels durch Schieloperation, *Klin Monatsbl Augenheilkd* 172:246, 1979.

123. de Decker W: Results of surgery versus prism tolerated over correction therapy of anomalous correspondence. In Fells P, editor: *International Strabismological Association at Marseilles, France,* Marseilles, 1974, Masson.

124. Etting GL: Strabismus therapy in private practice: cure rates after three months of therapy, *J Am Optom Assoc* 49:1367, 1978.

125. Pigassou-Albouy R, Garipuy J: The use of overcorrecting prisms in the treatment of strabismic patients without amblyopia or with cured amblyopia, *Graefes Arch Klin Exp Ophthalmol* 186:203, 1973.

126. Grisham JD: Treatment of binocular dysfunction. In Schor C, Ciufffreda KJ, editors: *Vergence eye movements: basic and clinical aspects,* Boston, 1983, Butterworth-Heniemann.

127. Wick B, Cook D: Management of anomalous correspondence: efficacy of therapy, *Am J Optom Physiol Opt* 64:405, 1987.

128. Cook DL: Considering the ocular motor system in the treatment of anomalous retinal correspondence, *J Am Optom Assoc* 55:103, 1984.

129. Ludlam WM: Orthoptic treatment of strabismus, *Am J Optom Arch Am Acad Optom* 38:363, 1961.

130. Hugonnier R: The influence of operative overcorrection of an esotropia on abnormal retinal correspondence. In Arruga A, editor: *International Strabismus Symposium,* New York, 1968, S Karger.

131. Uemura Y: Indications and limitations of orthoptics, *Jpn Rev Clin Ophthalmol* 67:1113, 1973.

132. Flom MC, Kirschen DG, Williams AT: Changes in retinal correspondence following surgery for intermittent exotropia, *Am J Optom Physiol Opt* 59:146, 1982.

133. Fukai S and others: Studies on botulinum therapy for esotropia improvement of retinal correspondence, *Acta Soc Ophthalmol Jpn* 97:757, 1993.

134. Mallett RFJ: The use of prism in the treatment of concomitant strabismus, *Ophthalmic Opt* 19:793, 1979.

135. Berard PV: Constant wearing of prisms in treatment of concomitant strabismus, *Int Ophthalmol Clin* 4:272, 1971.

136. Toder F: Prismen in der Behandlung des Strabismus, *Klin Monatsbl Augenheilkd* 166:737, 1972.

137. Beard PV: The use of prisms in the pre and post-operative treatment of deviation in constant squint. In Fells P, editor: *The First Congress of the International Strabismological Association, Acapulco, 1970,* St Louis, 1971, Mosby.

138. Stangler-Zuschrott E: Acht Jahre Prismenbehandlung des Strabismus Covergens alternans, *Klin Monatsbl Augenheilkd* 177:835, 1980.

139. Amigo G: Diagnosis and treatment of anomalous correspondence, *Aust J Optom* 65:100, 1982.

140. Caloroso EE, Rouse MW: *Clinical management of strabismus,* Boston, 1993, Butterworth-Heineman.

141. Wick B: Visual therapy for esotropia with anomalous correspondence, Paper presented at the American Academy of Optometry, Dec, 1984.

142. Wick B: Visual therapy for small-angle esotropia, *Am J Optom Physiol Opt* 51:490, 1974.

Heterophoria and Vergence Anomalies

Similar to accommodative dysfunction, anomalies of the vergence system cause a variety of symptoms, such as blur, headaches, eyestrain, and diplopia.[1] Vergence dysfunction has also been shown to decrease visual performance.[2] Vergence dysfunction can be broadly divided into the categories of problems related to exodeviations, esodeviations, or hyperdeviations. The exodeviations are more commonly found and typically are more amenable to treatment. Esodeviations are less frequent and often are related to uncorrected

hyperopia. The full extent of a binocular problem is usually less obvious with an esodeviation, because an extended lag of accommodation masks the true magnitude of the esodeviation. Small esodeviations therefore are more significant than small exodeviations. Hyperdeviations usually are incomitant if they are more than a few prism diopters in magnitude and generally are treated with prisms.

TESTING VERGENCE FUNCTION
HETEROPHORIA
Cover Test

The cover test is the most important clinical test of binocular visual function (Fig. 6-1) and is used to classify anomalies as being esophoria or exophoria, esotropia or exotropia, and hyperphoria or hypertropia. It is also used to classify the Duane's categories, such as convergence insufficiency or excess or divergence insufficiency or excess.[3-7] The unilateral (or cover-uncover) test is used to detect the presence or absence of a strabismus. If the patient is strabismic, the test is used to determine the frequency of the deviation (intermittent or constant) and, if constant, the laterality of the deviation (unilateral or alternating). After the unilateral test the alternate cover test is used to ascertain the magnitude and direction of the deviation.

von Graefe Technique

The von Graefe technique uses variable prisms (which are usually attached to the phoropter) to determine the magnitude of a phoria at either distance or at near or both, as desired. The von Graefe technique is accomplished using one rotary prism to cause diplopia (diplopia prism) and using another rotary prism to measure the deviation (measuring prism) when the diplopic images are aligned. Although lateral or vertical deviations can be measured, the von Graefe technique is less useful than the cover test because it provides less information, takes more time to complete, is performed with an instrument that may effect visual perception, and requires more equipment. However, the von Graefe test often detects spurious vertical devi-

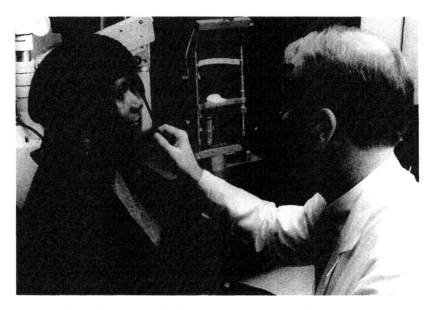

FIG. 6-1 The cover test is the most important test of binocular vision.

ations related to head tilts (causing optically induced vertical deviations) or small offsets of the prisms.

Maddox Rod

Although the Maddox rod also can be used to assess an angle of deviation at distance or near lateral, vertical, or cyclodeviations, we use it mostly for measuring small vertical deviations at the near point in straight ahead and down gazes. It is a quick, easy, and accurate procedure. The double Maddox rod test is used for the measuring of cyclodeviations (see Chapter 10).

Synoptophore

The synoptophore, a type of haploscope, provides a very convenient method of assessing angles of deviation, retinal correspondence, stereopsis, and vergences on patients with complex binocular visual problems (see Chapter 5).

VERGENCES

Vergences are disconjugate movements of the eyes and include horizontal, vertical, and cyclofusional movements.[8-16] Vergence measurements usually include blur, break, and recovery findings. The blur finding is specified when the stimulus first becomes blurry while fusion is maintained and is related to changes in accommodative level to maintain fusion. The break finding is the point at which fusion is first lost, and the recovery finding describes the prism in place when refusion occurs. Standards for vergences have been established by many investigators.[8-10,17-22] Vergence movements can occur with similar or dissimilar stimuli and are larger, with slower, larger, more complex stim-

uli.[12,17,24-28] Various nonoptical factors can affect vergences.[29-31] Vergence amplitude remains stable after adapting to a particular prism.[32]

Prism Bar

We prefer vergences assessed by prism bars over other types.[33] Prism bars allow observation of the eyes during the measurement process.

Risley Prisms

Vergence ranges using Risley prisms with a phoropter tend to measure a few prism diopters larger than those determined with prism bars, whereas those determined using a hand-held Risley prism are similar to those obtained by prism bars.[18]

Synoptophore

Vergence amplitude can be measured at any distance and direction of gaze using second-degree fusion targets (common borders) on the synoptophore. The selected second-degree fusion target should be used consistently for a given patient, because vergence ranges vary with target size. An advantage of the synoptophore is the large range over which vergences can be tested (up to about 120 PD).

Other Devices

Vergences also can be measured using devices such as loose prisms, tranaglyph, vectograms, the variable-mirror stereoscope/cheiroscope, the Computer Orthopter, and so on.[22]*

---

*Variable-mirror stereopscope/cheiroscope, Bernell Corp., South Bend, Ind.; Computor Orthopter, Teletherapy, Inc., Indianapolis, Ind.

VERGENCE FACILITY

Some patients may show slow vergence facility and have restricted vergence ranges. The criterion value for dysfunction varies depending on the population.[34-35] Similar to testing accommodative facility, vergence facility is performed using flipper prisms while viewing a target, typically at the near point. The patient is instructed to fuse and clear the targets as quickly as possible, and the number of cycles that can be completed within a specified period is determined. Unfortunately, there has not been agreement as to the appropriate prism values to use for testing vergence facility. Mean population values vary from about 5 to 8 cpm with 8 PD BI and 8 D BO.[35] With 16 PD BO and 4 PD BI, mean normal values are 8 cpm for ages 5 to 8 and 11 to 13 cpm for ages 9 to 14.[36]

NEGATIVE AND POSITIVE RELATIVE ACCOMMODATION

The positive and negative relative accommodation tests (PRA and NRA, respectively) are indirect measures of vergence function. To perform the NRA test a patient typically views small print (20/30) placed at 40 cm through the phoropter. In +0.25-D steps, plus lenses are progressively added binocularly, until the first sustained blur occurs. The amount of plus lenses added to blur is the NRA value. Minus lenses are added to the same set-up, until first sustained blur occurs to determine the PRA, and the amount of minus lenses added is the PRA value.

During the relative accommodation tests, the convergence demand remains fixed, but the phoria varies according to the AC/A ratio and accommodation varies according to the lens in place during these tests. The NRA and PRA are relative tests of both accommodation and vergence because both are active during measurement. As plus lenses are added during the NRA, accommodation is then relaxed. As accommodation relaxes, the phoria becomes progressively more exophoric because less accommodative vergence is in play. To remain fused during the NRA therefore positive fusional vergences must be increased to deal with the increased exophoria. A high NRA value tends to indicate either a good positive vergence system, an initially esophoric patient, or a patient who was over-minused (if the NRA is over +2.50 D). The usual value for the NRA is about +2.00 D. The PRA measurement indirectly determines negative vergence ability. High PRA values indicate an initially exophoric patient, a good negative fusional vergence system, or a patient who was over-plussed refractively. The PRA is often about -2.50 D. The NRA and PRA can be used to determine an add for a patient with presbyopia.

BINOCULAR CROSS CYLINDER

Although the binocular cross cylinder (BCC) test assesses the accommodation response, it is influenced by factors such as the patient's phoria, vergence capability, and refractive and accommodative status (see Chapter 3). A common finding for the binocular cross cylinder is +0.50 or +0.75 D. A high cross cylinder finding (+1.00 D or more) often indicates an individual who is esophoric, has poor negative vergences, is over-minussed refractively, or has presbyopia. Low or negative cross cylinder findings indicate a patient who is exophoric, has poor positive vergences, or is over-plussed.

DYNAMIC RETINOSCOPY

The technique for dynamic retinoscopy using the MEM and Nott methods also has been discussed previously (see Chapter 3). The accommodative lag may be large (i.e., +1.00 D or more) in a patient with uncorrected hyperopia who has accommodative insufficiency, is significantly esophoric, has a poor negative vergence system, is over-minused, or has presbyopia. A low or negative lag can indicate a patient that is significantly exophoric, has a poor positive vergence system, or is over-plussed.

 CLINICAL PEARL

The accommodative lag may be large (i.e., +1.00 D or more) in a patient with uncorrected hyperopia who has accommodative insufficiency, is significantly esophoric, has a poor negative vergence system, is over-minused, or has presbyopia. A low or negative lag can indicate a patient that is significantly exophoric, has a poor positive vergence system, or is over-plussed.

FORCED-VERGENCE FIXATION DISPARITY CURVES

Fixation disparity (in minuntes of arc) is the small error in fixation that occurs under binocular conditions.[37] Fixation disparity errors are significantly different from errors of fixation that occur with strabismus, because the largest fixation disparity (10 to 25 minutes of arc) is a fraction of a prism diopter. A variety of literature indicates that the fixation disparity curve and its components are useful clinically.[38-47] The slope of the curve, the X and Y intercept values, as well as the type of the curve, can play a role with regard to the diagnosis and treatment of binocular dysfunction[38-44, 48-52] (Fig. 6-2). A type I curve is relatively flat as it crosses the Y axis and symmetrically changes in both the base-in and base-out prism directions. Type II curves drop rather steeply in the base-in area and flatten in the base-out direction. Type III curves drop off on the base-out side of the graph from a relatively flat base-in side. A type IV curve is flat on both the base-in and base-out sides of the curve.

The parameters from fixation disparity curves that have been shown to be of diagnostic value are the

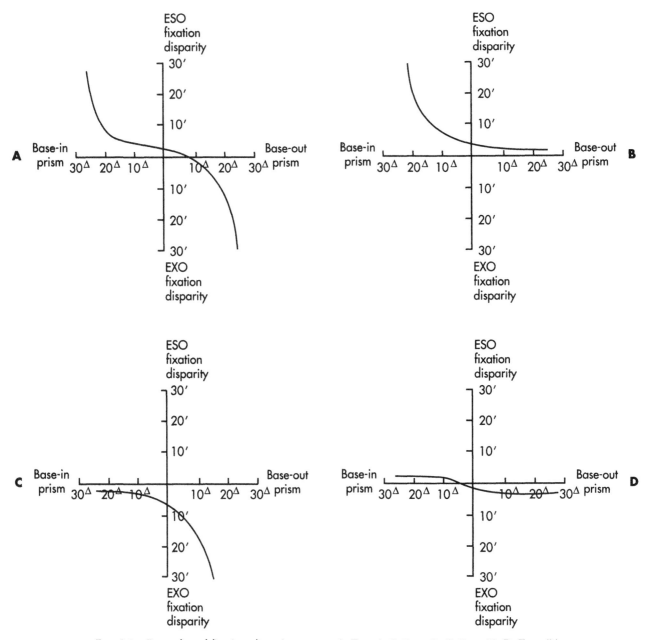

FIG. 6-2 Examples of fixation disparity curves. **A,** Type I. **B,** Type II. **C,** Type III. **D,** Type IV. (Modified from Sheedy JE: Actual measurement of fixation disparity and its use in diagnosis and treatment, *J Am Optom Assoc* 51:1079, 1980.)

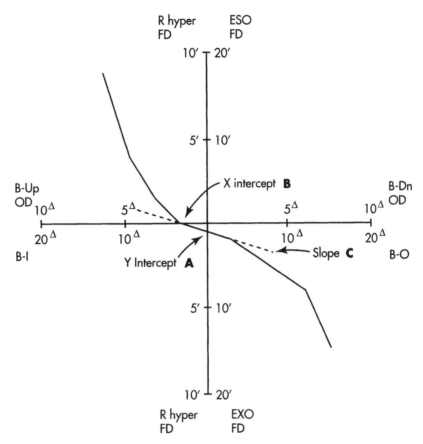

FIG. 6-3 Parameters of fixation disparity curve (besides type of curve) that are useful in diagnosis. **A,** Fixation disparity value, *Y* intercept, in minutes of arc. **B,** Associated phoria, *X* intercept, in PD (Δ) BO or BI. **C,** Slope of the curve at the *Y* axis. (Modified from Sheedy JE: Actual measurement of fixation disparity and its use in diagnosis and treatment, *J Am Optom Assoc* 51:1079, 1980.)

curve type (Fig. 6-2), the fixation disparity (*Y* intercept), the associated phoria (*X* intercept), and the slope of the curve at the *Y* axis (Fig. 6-3).[41-42,52] The fixation disparity curve type varies somewhat, as a function of the testing apparatus (Table 6-1).[37, 53-55]

Fixation disparity curves can be influenced by adaptation to prisms,[56-58] contours in the field of view,[43] the size of the target used as a fusion lock,[38,55,59-60] stress on the fast fusional vergence system,[58] and other factors.[46,61-63] Increased vergence capabilities, greater fusional efficiency, greater amounts of blur, and dissimilarity of the images presented to the eyes during measurement all cause a change in the fixation disparity.[64-65] Orthoptics/vision therapy can also affect the curve.[66]

DISPAROMETER

The Sheedy Disparometer can be used to assess fixation disparity (Fig. 6-4).[41-42, 67] Using Polaroid filters, a subject views a pair of vernier lines (also polarized). To measure the horizontal fixation disparity the clinician rotates a knob to present the pair of vertical vernier lines while the subject judges whether the top line is to the left or to the right of the bottom line. The

TABLE 6-1 DISTRIBUTION OF FIXATION DISPARITY CURVE TYPES

Fixation Curve Type	Distance		Near	
	Ogle* %	Saladin and Sheedy† %	Ogle* %	Saladin and Sheedy† %
I	57.5	68.3	57.2	58.2
II	30.0	26.7	22.1	27.6
III	9	0	13.4	8.2
IV	3.4	5	4.9	7.2

Modified from Ogle KN, Martens TG, Dyer JA: *Oculomotor imbalance in binocular vision and fixation disparity,* Philadelphia, 1969, Lee and Febiger; Sheedy JE, Saladin JJ: Association of symptoms with measures of oculomotor deficiencies, *Am J Optom Physiol Opt* 55:670, 1978.
*Data from Buzzelli AR: Vergence facility: developmental trends in a school age population, *Am J Optom Physiol Opt* 63:351, 1986.
†Data from Sheedy JE, Saladin JJ: Phoria, vergence, and fixation disparity in oculomotor problems, *Am J Optom Physiol Opt* 54:474, 1977.

judgment of the position of the lines should be completed within 15 seconds to minimize voluntary influences and to minimize adaptation to the prisms. The amount of fixation disparity is bracketed. The fixation disparity curve is determined by placing equal increments (3 PD total) of a prism before the eyes, repeating the measurement at each point and plotting the fixation disparity value at each point vs. the additional prism demand.

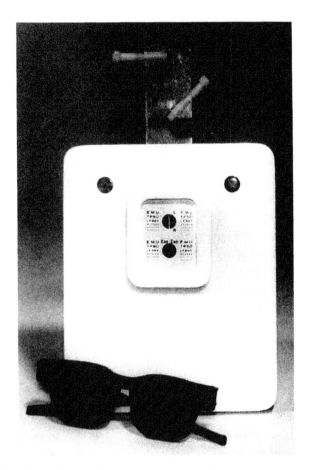

FIG. 6-4 Sheedy Disparometer is a useful way to measure fixation disparity.

WESSON CARD

The Wesson card is also used to measure fixation disparity (Fig. 6-5).[68] The Wesson card is a 4- by 6-inch laminated card with a series of 2-mm colored line stimuli at its center, which are seen by one eye. Through Polarized filters, the other eye sees a 3-mm arrow immediately below the colored line series. This is surrounded by a 1-cm black square that serves as a fusion lock. The patient holds the card at a distance of either 25 or 40 cm and is instructed to report the color seen and to which side the arrow points. Using this information the clinician reads the fixation disparity value off of a table on the upper right portion of the card. To construct a fixation disparity curve, this process is repeated with a series of prisms held before the eyes. Typically, this is done in 3-PD increments, alternating base-in and base-out until either suppression or diplopia occurs. The fixation disparities so determined are plotted, and the various aspects of the curve are determined.

ASSOCIATED PHORIA

The associated phoria is the amount of prism that is necessary to reduce the fixation disparity to zero. At

distance, the Mallett unit and the American Optical vectographic slide allow the measurement of the associated phoria, that is, the amount of fixation disparity necessary to make the fixation disparity zero.[48] The Borish card, Bernell test lantern, Disparometer, and Wesson card can be used to measure this value at the near point.[48] The associated phoria is a good technique for determining the amount of prism to prescribe for a binocular deviation, and particularly for vertical deviations.

 CLINICAL PEARL

The associated phoria is a good technique for determining the amount of prism to prescribe for a binocular deviation, particularly vertical deviations.

COMPARISON OF RESULTS FROM DIFFERENT TECHNIQUES

The results from one technique for fixation disparity do not reliably correlate with results from other techniques, with some exceptions. The Mallett unit and AO vectographic slide at distance and the Borish card and the Bernell test lantern are well correlated (r =

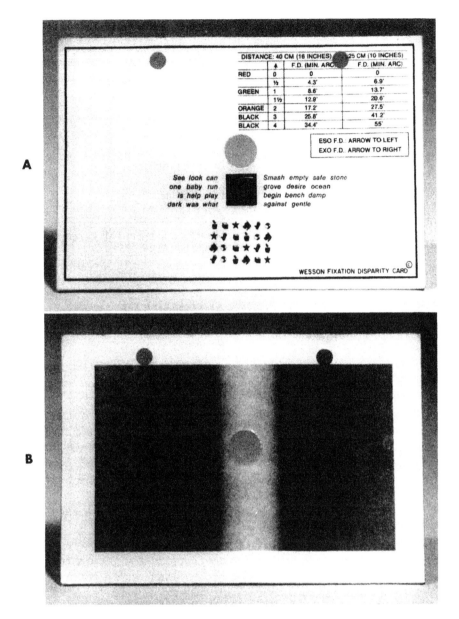

FIG. 6-5 Wesson fixation disparity card provides easy method of measuring fixation disparity. **A,** Front of card showing fixation disparity measurement. **B,** Difference of Gaussians (DOG) target on reverse of card.

0.79, 0.88, respectively).[48] The Sheedy disparometer correlates less well with each of the above (r = 0.38). The Wesson card and the disparometer provide different results; norms established with one device probably cannot be used with the other.[48,69,70] The Disparometer and the Mallett unit also provide different results.[71]

AC/A RATIOS

The two types of AC/A ratios are the distance-near ratio and the gradient ratio. They describe the relationships between changes in vergence (PD) that occur in conjunction with changes in accommodation (D). The distance-near AC/A typically is nearly twice as large as the gradient AC/A, probably because of proximal effects. Proximal vergence affects only the near phoria during the distance-near AC/A test, whereas it is present to an equal extent during the two measurements of the two phorias in the gradient AC/A determination. The gradient AC/A should be used whenever lens additions are involved because it is most specific for that application. Typical AC/A ratios are about 3 to 5 PD/D. The AC/A ratio is useful in a variety of situations, such as determining the magnitude of an add for a patient with an esophoria at the near point.

The distance-near AC/A is typically calculated using the formula[72]:

$$AC/A = IPD + (NFD)(H_n - H_d)$$

where AC/A is expressed in PD/D; IPD (interpupillary distance) is in cm; NFD (near fixation distance) is in meters; H_n (near phoria) in PD, eso is plus and exo is minus; and H_d (distance phoria) in PD, eso is plus and exo is minus.

Consider an example of an individual with 6-cm IPD viewing a target at 40 cm. With a distance phoria of 2 PD exophoria and a near esophoria of 4 PD:

$$AC/A = 6 + 0.40(4 - -2) = 6 + 2.4 = 8.4 \text{ PD/D}.$$

Bearing in mind the definition of the AC/A, that is, it is the change in vergence over the change in accommodation, the AC/A can be easily calculated using the gradient method. For example, the phoria while viewing a target at 40 cm is 6-PD exophoria. If, while viewing the same target, -2.00-D lenses are added before both eyes and the phoria is changed to ortho, the AC/A ratio is 3 PD/D (change in vergence, 6, in PD; change in accommodation, 2, in D).

CA/C RATIOS

The CA/C ratio is the convergence accommodation (D) that occurs in response to changes in vergence (PD). The CA/C ratio typically is not measured clinically, although systems have been devised.[73] A DOG (difference of Gaussians) target is presented to the eyes (see Fig. 6-5), opening the accommodative loop so that changes in accommodation in response to changes in vergence can be assessed. Accommodation is assessed via dynamic retinoscopy without prism and then after a given amount of prism has been added (6 PD). Schemes have been developed to plot both the AC/A and CA/C on the same graph.[73,74]

STEREOPSIS

Stereopsis is the binocular recognition of disparity. Some patients with large phorias, intermittent strabismus, poor vergence ability, severe symptoms, and poor performance can summon resources to obtain a good level of stereopsis while the test is being performed (see Chapter 5). Operant conditioning techniques may allow a greater percentage of children to be tested for stereopsis.[75,76]

❖ CLINICAL PEARL

Some patients with large phorias, intermittent strabismus, poor vergence ability, severe symptoms, and poor performance can summon resources to obtain a good level of stereopsis while the test is being performed.

TABLE 6-2 **SYMPTOMS REPORTED BY PATIENTS WITH CONVERGENCE INSUFFICIENCY (n = 110)**

Symptom	Frequency	Percentage (%)
Headaches	59	54
Diplopia	52	47
Blur	52	47
Asthenopia	40	36
Fatigue	21	19
Reading problems	11	10
None	4	4
Photophobia	3	3
Other	2	2

Modified from Daum KM: Convergence insufficiency, *Am J Optom Physiol Opt* 61:16, 1984.

ANOMALIES OF HETEROPHORIA/FUSIONAL VERGENCES

EXOPHORIAS

Duane was among the first to classify exophoria into three basic types: convergence insufficiency; basic, or equal, exodeviations; and divergence excess.[77-79] Other factors, besides the angle of deviation at distance compared with that found at near, are also important, but 10 PD is often chosen as the cutoff point, although that is probably too large. A similar criterion exists for intermittent exotropia (see Chapter 9).[80-82]

Convergence Insufficiency
Definition

Convergence insufficiency (CI) usually involves a high exophoria or intermittent exotropia in near vision in association with a relatively orthophoric condition in distance viewing, the AC/A ratio being rather low (Fig. 6-6).[79] von Graefe first defined CI around the turn of the century.[77,78] The essence of the anomaly is an inability to maintain convergence to meet the visual near point demand, which causes symptoms.[80-83]

Symptoms

CI causes a variety of symptoms (Table 6-2), such as ocular fatigue, asthenopia, and headaches, especially frontal[77,78,84-86]; blur and diplopia,[77,78,86-91] which are especially apparent with near work[80,84,92-94]; and cause a loss of concentration[95] or sleepiness.[90] The symptoms do not generally appear before age 10[90]; often occur near the end of the day[84,93]; and do not occur as frequently when the load is light and/or the patient is well rested.[96]

Infrequently, patients' complaints include tearing,[97,98] nausea or dizziness,[80-82,84,93] or reports of poor depth perception.[90] Various psychogenic difficulties may be present[80,91,92] and, if severe, may be associated with neurotic tendencies.[90,99-102]

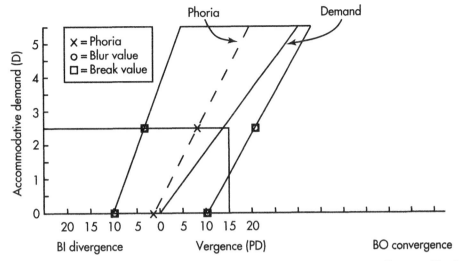

FIG. 6-6 Graphic analysis of zone of binocular vision for convergence insufficiency. Phoria at near is significantly exo, whereas compensating positive vergences are low.

TABLE 6-3 **A CLINICAL SURVEY OF CONVERGENCE INSUFFICIENCY**

Parameter	Distance	Number	Mean	Standard deviation
Angle of deviation (PD)	6 M	59	3.8	5.3
	40 cm	71	12	6.8
AC/A (PD/D)	NA	58	2.7	1.3
Negative vergences	6 M	17	6/7/5	4/4/3
	40cm	26	12/17/12	7/7/5
Positive vergences	6 M	28	10/15/9	6/7/7
	40 cm	65	12/18/12	6/8/8
NPC (cm)	NA	20	7.4	48
Amplitude of accommodation (D)	NA	44	8.9	2.7
Stereopsis threshold (sec)	40 cm	21	39.1	27

On occasion, ascertaining a patient's symptoms can be very challenging because there are other sources of these same problems[1,40,103-105] (glare, presbyopia, refractive error, stress and fatigue[103]), and visual comfort is variable and both task- and time-dependent.[104] Of 57 patients presenting with diplopia as a chief complaint, five had CI, whereas the remainder were afflicted with a variety of neurologic anomalies.[106]

Some patients with severe CI may not report symptoms because of their avoidance of near work[90,107]; however, most patients are symptomatic (85%, 75%) and sometimes reports are out of proportion to the signs.[87,92,108] Children may not report symptoms for a variety of reasons.[90] Individuals with CI may suffer from poor performance.

Signs
The most common features of CI are an exodeviation at near in concert with a receded NPC value and

reduced positive vergences (Table 6-3).[89] Often, accommodative function is somewhat reduced

 CLINICAL PEARL
The most common features of CI are an exodeviation at near in concert with a receded NPC value and reduced positive vergences.

Phoria, AC/A, Vergences, and Sheard's Criterion. The condition usually involves a phoria at both distance and near (78%); however, sometimes an intermittent exotropia at the near point occurs (20% of cases).[89] The median-distance exodeviation of 16 studies of CI was 2 PD.[103] The median near heterophoria of 20 studies was about 10 PD.[103] The AC/A ratio therefore is typically low; most studies have mean AC/A ratios for CI below standards for the population.[103]

An exodeviation is neither necessary nor sufficient for CI.[83,90,100,109-111] In one study only 78% had exodeviation and 3% had esodeviation; in another, 63% had an exodeviation.[84,85] Near deviations in cases of CI related to trauma may be large (6 to 20 PD in a series of 23 patients).[112] Vertical deviations are not usually important in CI.[89,95]

 CLINICAL PEARL

An exodeviation is neither necessary nor sufficient for CI.

Vergence levels at the near point are at or below the expected population levels for CI.[97,101,103,107,113-115] Despite difficulties in determining the proper criterion level to constitute low vergences (8 to 10 PD, 12 PD, 10 to 20 PD, or 15 PD), there is a consensus that reduced positive vergences frequently indicate symptoms.[80,84,87,90,93,94] Sometimes reduced vergence levels alone signal a convergence problem, and the heterophoria and NPC measures may be normal.[94]

Patients with CI often fail to meet Sheard's criterion (see below).[103,116] Although individuals may meet Sheard's criterion and still have convergence insufficiency, the inability of the vergence system to handle the phoria is critical to the generation of CI.[54,110]

Near Point of Convergence. The near point of convergence in CI is frequently remote, ranging from 6.9 to 41.3 cm, which is a consistent finding.[84,90,107,117,118] Repeated measurement of the NPC sometimes demonstrates an otherwise not noticeable reduction in the NPC value.[109,119,120] The NPC value does not necessarily strongly correlate with the magnitude of the near phoria and is not always reduced.[110,118,121-123] Patients with CI often are unable to voluntarily cross their eyes.[99,100] The NPC is directly affected in anoxic states.[113]

Accommodation. In CI, accommodative amplitude (and sometimes accommodative facility) usually is lower than would be expected for a patient's age.[90,114,117,124-128] A subgroup of CI with severely reduced accommodative amplitude may exist and has a poor prognosis.[114,117,127,128] Accommodation weakness may be a causative factor for CI.[75-76,114,125,129]

Fixation Disparity. Fixation disparity signs related to CI include a base-in- and variable-associated phoria, as well as a fixation disparity that is 6 minutes of arc exo or greater, with a slope as it crosses the Y axis greater than 45°.[54] The fixation curve is variable on the base-out side and, if voluntary convergence is being used, the fixation disparity is eso, whereas the phoria is exo.

Amblyopia, Suppression, Anomalous Correspondence, and Stereopsis. Amblyopia is not a feature of convergence insufficiency.* No consensus regarding suppression in CI has been reached. Some have sug-

gested that suppression is common[90,104] and important,[130] whereas others have suggested that suppression is minor[84,104] or absent.[108,131] Suppression may develop over time to eliminate diplopia in cases deteriorating to intermittent exotropia. Suppression occurs 3 times more frequently in patients with CI than in a control group.[132] There have been no reports of anomalous correspondence in CI.[103] Stereopsis is typically normal in CI.[85,90]

Refractive Status. No author has suggested any correlation between the type or magnitude of refractive error and CI.*

Prevalence

Crude prevalence rates of a particular anomaly may be misleading.[140] They are very difficult to compare in cases of convergence insufficiency, because most authors have tended to use their own definitions (or study design) of CI, so that consistency is lacking. Crude estimates of the prevalence of convergence insufficiency in the population range from 1.3% to 37%, depending on the population and the assessment technique, at 1.3% of 1296 school children[141]; 1.75% of 10,022 patients[80]; 2.6%,[100] 2.8%,[90,104,124,140] 1% of normal children and 15% of adults[82]; 11% of patients age 40 and younger[88]; 25% of 500 patients (75% exhibiting symptoms)[92]; and 37% of 200 patients, 20% of 455 patients,[132] and 35% of 710 patients.[142] Most studies have found a prevalence of around 3% to 5%,[143] with 3.8% of 11,600 patients,[95] 3.1% of 3075 patients, and 4.9% of 1386 patients,[91] or 4%.[124] CI is possibly the most common binocular visual anomaly[89]; 62% (110) of a sample of 177 individuals classified as having binocular visual difficulties as a result of exodeviations had CI.[104]

Sex. The syndrome is more often seen in females, usually in a ratio of 3:2;[†] however, this does not occur in all studies.[118,124] A retrospective study of 110 patients with convergence insufficiency includes 72 females (65%) and 38 males (35%).[89] Some have speculated that the differences may be related to anemia secondary to gynecologic problems.[145] Epidemiologic studies have yet to show the prevalence in the general population, and factors such as access to care and the likelihood of seeking care are important in an assessment of its true prevalence.

Age. CI can occur at any age; however, certain age groups are more or less likely to manifest the condition.[85] Most patients with CI are ages 10 to 29 or slightly older.[80,84,87-90,92] The prevalence is generally considered to be low in children under age 10.[80,84,92,95,115] However, the condition may be more

*References 1, 49, 86, 88, 110, 120, 124, 131, 133-136

*References 84-88, 90, 92, 96, 99, 100, 103, 107, 114, 120, 130, 133-135, 137-139.
†References 80, 84, 85, 88, 90, 107, 110, 113-115.

prevalent among children who read poorly.[140,146,147] Patients with presbyopia who have CI often manifest a substantial exophoria at near.[38,90] Exophoria at near in presbyopia is less likely to cause symptoms, and it has been speculated that individuals with presbyopia may have far greater use of accommodative vergence to compensate.[38] Clinics such as a Veteran's Administration Hospital may see disproportionate numbers of elderly patients with CI.[148]

Associated Conditions

CI usually occurs without association with any condition except accommodative dysfunction, although it has been associated with a great number of other things in the literature. Even so, conditions associated with CI include diphtheria[134,135]; mononucleosis[134,135]; neuroses or psychogenic factors[85,95,97-101,130,145]; accommodative insufficiency[124-127,149]; paralysis of the medial recti[80]; decompression sickness[150]; hypopituitarism[128]; hyperthyroidism[128]; reading or school difficulties[146,147,151,152] or not[118]; dyslexia[152,153]; aphakia[154]; anemia[145]; cerebral vascular accident[155]; lesions of the occipital or superior colliculus area[127,156]; parietal lobe tumors[157]; encephalitis[127,128,156]; multiple sclerosis[127,156]; medication side effect[116,128,132,158]; head trauma[112,137,138,159]; fatigue[89]; chronic fatigue and immune dysfunction syndrome (suspected)[160]; malingering[84]; overcorrected hyperopia, under-corrected myopia, and presbyopia[80]; anoxia[113,150,161,162]; febrile illness[84]; hepatitis, mononucleosis, and diphtheria[128]; heart disease, sinusitis, and asthma[97]; Parkinson's disease[163]; aging[164]; and idiopathic.[89] Poor working conditions and associated fatigue may cause the syndrome to become manifest.

Etiology

Many etiologies have been suggested for CI but its cause is unknown, and in most patients it is not possible to establish a definite etiology.[82,88-90,103,130] The etiology of CI is usually assumed to be of central origin, causing a deficiency in the AC/A ratio, that is, a breakdown of the interaction between accommodation and convergence or deficient convergence.[80,83,90,125,130] Fatigue is a very common factor in the development of CI.[96]

CI may result from excessive adaptation of accommodation and low adaptation of convergence.[165] Proximal accommodation may be a strong factor in that it may not effectively stimulate accommodative vergence. CI may occur as a result of fatigue in the slow vergence adaptation mechanism.[54] Disparity detectors become insensitive to blur, so that voluntary convergence is used to reduce demands on the system.

As is also true in accommodative insufficiency, uncorrected refractive error (such as against-the-rule astigmatism or anisometropia) also may lead to a decreased output from the disparity detectors in the vergence controller loop.[51] Over time this lack of sensitiv

ity may lead to a larger fixation disparity in an effort to stimulate convergence. This in turn may lead to suppression and a decrease in the blur detector output of the accommodative loop, so that voluntary accommodative vergence must be summoned to avoid blur and diplopia.[54]

Fatigue and anxiety also may fatigue the slow vergence adaptive component.[54] If this occurs, the disparity feedback loop may respond by increasing the exo fixation disparity, which also fatigues the system, again leading to suppression, a break down in the blur detector output, and, finally, the use of voluntary convergence to maintain binocular vision. The use of voluntary convergence leads to suppressed sensitivity of the blur detectors, because the information they supply is no longer being used.[54] The use of voluntary convergence over an extended period compromises the reflex-driven oculomotor system.[54]

A very wide interpupillary distance causes an excessive demand for convergence and may cause CI.[81] Improper development of the vergence mechanism also could cause CI.[80,81,99,101]

Organic Etiologies. Although they are much rarer, exceptions exist in which CI appears related to some type of direct organic etiology.* These are CI related to trauma,[112,137,138] parietal lobe tumors,[157] anemia or decompression sickness,[150] aphakia,[154] or anoxia caused by altitude[113] or vascular insufficiency.[155] Some have speculated that an altered metabolic state of the extraocular musculature secondary to anemia, toxemia, or endocrine disorders may cause CI.[81,161,162] Other causes considered for CI include head trauma, encephalitis, intoxication, malnutrition, debility, hepatitis, or mononucleosis.[128,137] Precise mechanisms for these suspected etiologic factors have not been discovered.

The nature of the loss in trauma and decompression sickness is assumed to be central in origin.[101,150] Accommodative dysfunction is an etiologic factor in a great many cases of CI.[90,114,127,129,166]

Diagnosis

If a patient presents with symptoms, a receded NPC, an exophoria at the near point, and reduced positive vergences, the diagnosis of convergence insufficiency is straightforward.[110] The diagnosis is more difficult if the patient lacks symptoms or if the above appear to be in the normal range.[110,120]

There may be two types of CI, depending on the accommodative ability.[77,78,114,127,128] Those with severely reduced accommodative ability are more symptomatic and the prognosis is poorer.[114,125,127] We believe that there is a continuum of accommodative ability in these cases, ranging from patients with CI

---

*References 81, 112, 118, 137, 138, 145, 150, 154, 155.

and severely comprised accommodation to patients with CI and normal accommodation. One study found that 40% of patients with CI had accommodative dysfunction.[124]

In many cases the diagnosis of CI is complicated by confounding sources of eye strain, such as stress, fatigue, refractive error, and so on. Additionally, the diagnosis may be hindered by problems in comparing findings with population norms, undiscovered subpopulations, and poor reliability of certain clinical findings.[167] Many papers have intentionally studied unusual or specific subpopulations.*

In certain cases in which there is a question, often the phoria is low and the vergences appear borderline and there is substantial variation in the vergence capability. Vergences are often sufficient at one time and not at others, such as when the patient is tired.

Sudden changes in the clinical picture may indicate a serious systemic disease.[157] Neurologic examination should be completed on each patient, and papilledema, afferent pupillary defect signs, and vomiting, particularly with sudden onset, should be regarded with extreme caution.

Treatment

The first step in treating any visual anomaly is to correct any significant refractive error.[54,170] This is especially relevant in CI, because blur may decrease the sensitivity of the accommodative loop blur detector, which eventually fatigues the vergence system via the interaction between the accommodative and vergence loop.[54] A second step is to deal with the etiology of the condition, if it is discoverable. Although frequently no cause is obvious, many patients who suffer from overall fatigue and overwork should be counseled regarding sequelae of these factors and the significance of minimizing them. To the extent that fatigue is a factor in CI, it must be removed as much as possible.[96]

CI is successfully treated using orthoptics/vision therapy, which is the treatment of choice for this condition by optometrists, orthoptists, and ophthalmologists, even for patients with presbyopia.†

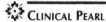 CLINICAL PEARL

> CI is successfully treated using orthoptics/vision therapy, which is the treatment of choice for this condition by optometrists, orthoptists, and ophthalmologists, even for patients with presbyopia.

Orthoptics/vision therapy treatment techniques are aimed at improving vergences and accommodative ability.[90,99] Orthoptic/vision therapy treatment techniques and instruments include Brock string training, vectograms, tranaglyphs, stereoscopes, computerized orthoptic programs, prism or lens flippers, chiastopic fusion techniques (lifesaver cards, eccentric circles), push up training, and Aperture Rule trainer.*[1,84,89,136] In-office treatment on the synoptophore and computerized systems are also helpful.[131]

The Brock string (see Chapter 5) can be used initially for these patients.[170] This helps the patient use voluntary convergence to grossly align the eyes while recognizing physiologic diplopia. The Brock string also helps with any suppression that may be encountered that may impede therapy.[54,175]

Training with flip lenses helps train the accommodative system and hone the accommodative controller response to blur.[54] In patients over age 40, accommodative training is omitted. Base-out vergence training, first for amplitude (range) (e.g., Vectograms) and then for facility (quality) (e.g., the Aperture Rule*) should then be instituted.[54] Training should continue so that the patient can master each of the twelve cards of the Aperture Rule within 2 seconds for each fusion step.[54]

Near-point lenses may be useful if significant accommodative dysfunction is present.[117] Accommodative dysfunction in the form of reduced amplitude of accommodation and an extended lag of accommodation suggest the use of plus lenses at the near point. Although they would tend to increase the exophoria at the near point via the AC/A interlink to vergence, these patients have low AC/As, which minimizes these effects.

Surgery is rarely recommended for dealing with CI.[77,78,108,134,135] The surgical technique is a symmetric bimedial rectus resection and should be reserved for extreme and severe cases of convergence insufficiency.[80,83,108,126,135] The technique is described in detail in Chapter 11.

Success with Treatment. The mean length of treatment of CI ranges from about 4 weeks to 16 weeks.[86,174] Older ages of patients may be associated with shorter lengths of treatment and relatively few visits (e.g., a regimen of 12 visits).[90]

Several factors change with the application of orthoptics/vision therapy.[89] The positive vergences at both distance and near should increase significantly (about 10 to 15 PD on average; Fig. 6-7; p = 0.01 to 0.0001).[89] The near angle of deviation may decrease slightly (from an average of 12 PD exo to 10.7 PD exo, p = 0.0007) while the AC/A increases (mean 2.7:1 to 3.2:1, p = 0.016); the NPC should improve (mean 7.4

---

*References 1, 77, 78, 80, 82-84, 93, 97, 108, 117, 128, 131, 142, 169-174.
†References 80, 86, 94, 106, 112, 114, 125, 127, 129, 131, 132, 134, 137, 138, 145, 148, 150, 154, 161, 168, 169.

*Bernell Corp., South Bend, Ind.

to 4.3 cm, p = 0.003), as should the amplitude of accommodation (mean 8.9 to 11.4 D, p = 0.0001).

Changes in the angle of deviation and AC/A ratios with orthoptics/vision therapy or optical treatment have been noted.[176-179] These changes in the angle of deviation and the AC/A ratio have not been found to be related to changes in the lag of accommodation, practice effects, or proximal convergence.[177] The mechanism is unclear and its permanence is unknown.[89]

A review of 1931 patients with CI suggested that 91% had significant improvement with orthoptics/vision therapy (Table 6-4).[83] An overall weighted average cure rate has been suggested as 72%.[83] Other documentation regarding orthoptics/vision therapy for CI also has been presented.[136,180] One hundred patients with CI who did not meet Sheard's criterion[116] received a combination of in-office and at-home therapy for their conditions; after treatment, 84 met the criterion.[136]

Some studies of CI have been impeccably designed in their evaluation of treatment effects. A matched-subjects control group cross-over design was used to evaluate the automated vergence treatment of seven patients with CI.[1] A statistically significant reduction in symptoms and an increase in vergence range was demonstrated during the period when training occurred but not during the control period. Bowman and others (as cited in Grisham[83]) also have completed a study with an objective assessment of vergence training of patients with CI. Both of these studies used control groups.

CI can be successfully treated in the elderly.[148,169] An examination of 191 patients with presbyopia with CI and symptoms suggested that 92% of the patients were successfully treated using a mixture of home and in-office training.[169] The treatment period averaged about 10 weeks, although longer treatment was necessary for older patient groups. Follow-up at 3 months suggested that additional training was necessary for 48% of the previously successfully treated patients. Another study achieved similar results (96% success) with 28 CI patients over the age of 60.[148]

Complete remediation of signs and symptoms is important in maintaining relief from CI, because patients who were only partially successful were most likely to regress.[181] Training results persist for at least 1 to 2 years if the patient has met strict criteria for a functional cure.[83]

Certain patients do not respond well to the treatment of CI with standard orthoptics/vision therapy, lenses and/or prisms, or other forms of therapy, such as surgery or special orthoptics/vision therapy techniques.* Failure of orthoptics/vision therapy may suggest a systemic etiology or component to the condition.[85,111] Patients with a traumatic etiology to CI

---
*References 86, 108, 117, 127, 134, 135, 174.

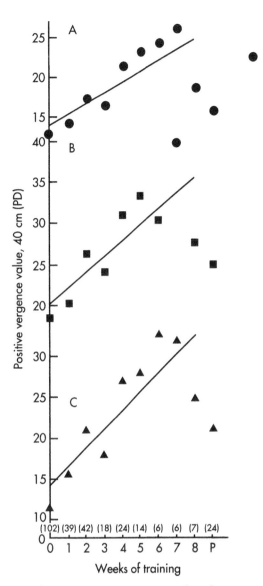

FIG. 6-7 Change in positive vergence values for convergence insufficiency patients at near over weeks of training. Numbers in parentheses above abscissa represent number of points used in computing mean. Points associated with *P* are values recorded at progress check an average of 8.6 months after training. No training was given in interim. **A,** Blur values (●). **B,** Break values (■). **C,** Recovery values (▲). (Modified from Daum KM: Convergence insufficiency, *Am J Optom Physiol Opt* 61:16, 1984.)

have a poorer prognosis than would otherwise be the case.[112]

Surgery, although reserved for cases of intractable symptoms and large deviations, has occasionally been helpful; however, contradictory results have been reported.[17,108,134,135,182] After surgery, patients frequently present with a short-lived consecutive esotropia and diplopia that can last several months.[108,134,135] Unfortunately, recurrence of the exodeviation and symptoms

TABLE 6-4 VISION THERAPY RESULTS WITH CONVERGENCE INSUFFICIENCY

Author(s), Year	Number	Cured (%)	Improved (%)	Failed (%)
Lyle and Jackson	300	83	10	7
Mann	142	68	30	3
Cushman and Burri	66	66	30	4
Hirsch	48	77	12	10
Duthie	123	88	6	6
Mayou	480	72	5	5 (16)*
Mayou	100	93	5	2
Mayou	87	92	6	2
Mellick	88	77	10	12
Passmore and MacLean	100	82	18	0
Norn	65	9	60	30
Hoffman and others	17	88	—	12
Pantano	207	53	3	4
Daum	80	41	56	3
Cohen and Sodden	28	96	4	—
Weighted average cure rate, 72%				
Weighted average improved rate, 19%				
Weighted average fail rate, 9%				
Total number of patients, 1931				

Modified from Grisham JD: Visual therapy results for convergence insufficiency: a literature review, *Am J Optom Physiol Opt* 65:448, 1988.
See references 80, 90, 91, 93, 95, 96, 99, 103, 104, 147, 151, 176, 185.
*( ) Dropped out.

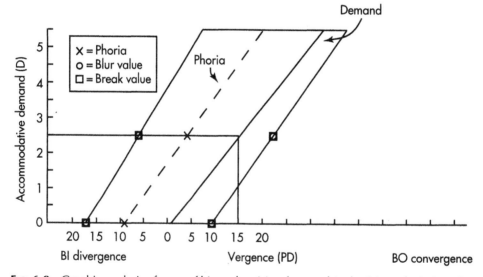

FIG. 6-8 Graphic analysis of zone of binocular vision for equal (or basic) exodeviations. Exophoria at distance and near is approximately the same.

occurred in five of six patients in one study.[135] Other studies report alleviation of symptoms.[135]

Summary

Convergence insufficiency is a syndrome commonly seen in patients who complain of headaches, blur, diplopia, and asthenopia. Some or all of the following occur: (1) the angle of deviation usually is exophoria and is much larger at near than at distance; (2) the AC/A ratio is low; (3) the positive vergences at near are inadequate to compensate for the angle of deviation; (4) the NPC value is receded; (5) the accommodative amplitude may be reduced; (6) the stereopsis threshold is good; and (7) suppression, if present, is likely to be intermittent in nature.

Equal (Basic) Exophoria
Definition

Equal (basic) exophoria is a condition in which the exophoria is approximately the same at distance and at near (Fig. 6-8).[77,78,80]

Symptoms

Typical symptoms reported by patients with equal exophoria are blur, asthenopia, headache, and diplopia (Table 6-5).[183] These symptoms can occur with either distance or near tasks or both. They are not always strongly associated with the use of the eyes. Because the deviations are occasionally large, diplopia is reported often.

Signs

Heterophoria and Vergences. The angles of deviation of individuals with basic exophorias tend to be large (10 to 15 PD or greater) and may show intermittent strabismus.[183] Vertical deviations occur rather frequently in patients with exodeviations (up to 60% of the time).[95] Vergences often are about at population norms; however, considering the deviation, they are substantially below that necessary to compensate for the deviation.

Accommodation. Although sometimes associated with defective accommodation, accommodative function is generally good in basic exophoria.[127]

Prevalence

The prevalence of basic exophoria has not been established. One study of individuals with binocular visual dysfunction caused by exodeviations suggests that 28% (49 of 177) had equal exophoria.[104]

Sex and Age. There is a slightly stronger predilection for women than men in basic exodeviations (females 55%, males 45%, n = 49).[183] There is little literature suggesting a particular age prevalence for basic exodeviations.[183]

TABLE 6-5 SYMPTOMS REPORTED BY PATIENTS WITH EQUAL EXODEVIATIONS (n = 49)

Symptom	Frequency	Percentage (%)
Diplopia	19	39
Asthenopia	14	29
Headaches	13	26
Blur	7	14
Reading problems	7	14
Fatigue	6	12
None	5	10
Feels eyes deviate	3	6
Photophobia	2	4

Modified from Daum KM: Equal exodeviations: characteristics and results of treatment with orthoptics/vision therapy, *Aust J Optom* 67:53, 1984.

Etiology

Strictly speaking, the etiology of basic exophoria is unknown. A passive tendency for the eyes to diverge for anatomic reasons (inclination of the orbits, etc.) may cause this divergence.[82] The suggestion of an anatomic etiology seems largely to be related to the lack of an accommodative component to the problem. Basic exophorias also may have many of the same etiologic factors as divergence excess. The proximal adaptation thought to cause the decreased near deviation either has not occurred or is much less in magnitude. Refractive status is not strongly associated with this condition.[82]

Diagnosis

Clinicians often can overlook symptoms reported by patients with basic exophorias if the deviation is not large (i.e., if the deviation is 10 PD or less). Because the vergence levels are often at or near normal levels, a comparison of the deviation with the vergence is helpful (Sheard's criterion).[116] Probing for possible symptoms related to binocular vision is the key to diagnosis of this particular anomaly. When the deviation is large, this is not usually a problem, but in borderline cases, sorting out symptoms associated with the exodeviation from those caused by stress, fatigue, and so on, may be challenging.

Treatment and Results of Treatment

A large-scale controlled clinical trial has not been completed to suggest the best method of treatment.[184] The treatment of basic exophoria includes the use of prisms,[185] lenses or orthoptics/vision therapy,[186] and, on rare occasions, surgery.[17,182,187] We recommend as first measures the use of orthoptics/vision therapy directed at increasing positive vergences or prisms equal to the associated phoria. There have not been many

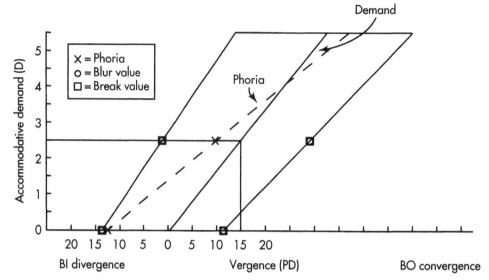

Fig. 6-9 Graphic analysis of zone of binocular vision for divergence excess. Exophoria at distance is much larger than that found at near.

studies that assess the results of treating basic exophorias.[183,188] Overminus lenses also have been used effectively.[189]

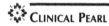

> **CLINICAL PEARL**
>
> We recommend as first measures the use of orthoptics/vision therapy directed at increasing positive vergences or prisms equal to the associated phoria.

Divergence Excess Exophoria
Definition
The syndrome of divergence excess exophoria (DE) has been defined using several criteria.[190,191] Most criteria include an exophoria at distance associated with significantly less exophoria or orthophoria at the near point (Fig. 6-9).[77-79,192] The stimulus AC/A is somewhat high to very high. DE has many features that distinguish it from other types of binocular anomalies, including questions about the magnitude of the AC/A ratio, the presence of an intermittent form of anomalous correspondence (if strabismic), the angle of deviation being outside of the zone of single clear binocular vision, as well as other findings. Patients with DE are very likely to have an intermittent exotropia, mainly at distance. A complete review of the features of these patients is presented in Chapter 9.

Symptoms
Individuals with DE are most likely to complain of diplopia (89%) and/or asthenopia or photophobia.[193-196] Often no near difficulties are reported, and the presentation is because another person, such as a grandparent or school teacher, notices an occasional eye turning.

Signs
Angle of Deviation and AC/A Ratio. In DE the exophoria is substantially higher at distance than at near. Curiously, the distance angle of deviation is often so large as to appear outside of the zone of single clear binocular vision.[192,197-199] This occurred in 8 of 11 cases in one series.[193] Only a small percentage of these patients have an associated primary vertical deviation, and about a third have inferior oblique overactions.[95,192,193,200]

There has been substantial discussion about the AC/A ratio in patients with DE patients.[190,201] Although the stimulus AC/A appears elevated, the response AC/A ratio is in the normal range or slightly above it, at 3 to 9:1.[192,202] Proximal convergence and stimulus aftereffects likely explain the difference.[202]

Fixation Disparity. Although there is an exodeviation at near with DE, the fixation disparity is often an eso fixation disparity.[198] This is another factor suggesting that the dissociated and associated states in these patients are dissimilar.

Vergences. The distance divergence ability and the positive vergence ability at both distance and near are likely to be substantial.[193,203,204] The negative vergences at distance are often 15 to 20 PD or more to the break finding, a value more than twice Morgan's norms.[19,20] Positive vergences at distance and at near, although they generally do not meet Sheard's criterion, are still at or above norms for the population.[19,20,192] This suggests that vergences are not a simple measure of the potency of the fusional vergence system to withstand the stresses put upon it.

Stereopsis, Suppression, and Anomalous Retinal Correspondence. Stereopsis is generally excellent for these patients.[192,205,206] Suppression, or anomalous correspondence, can occur when there is an associated intermittent strabismus (see Chapter 9).[190,192,194,207]

Types of Divergence Excess. There are likely two types of DE (see Chapter 9).[191]

Prevalence

Divergence excess is less commonly seen than other forms of exophoria/vergence dysfunction.[82,104,207] The prevalence in the general population has not been determined. Estimates have ranged from about 0.5% to 4% prevalence.[192]

Gender and Age. DE may be more common in women (94%, 61%, 60% to 70%).[1,192,193,195,207] DE is the exodeviation of childhood.[192] Most frequently, a distance deviation becomes obvious in grade school.

Etiology

The etiology of DE exophoria is unknown.[82,190] It has been classically considered by Duane to be a result of an active divergence of the eyes.[190,208] Other factors that have been suggested as the etiology for this condition include factors related to anatomic and mechanical conditions; AC/A ratio; near-point stress; phylogenetic, hemiretinal suppression of genetic origin; genetic anomaly; and a congenital anomaly with a functional origin.[190,192] There is no association between this condition and refractive error.[194]

Movement between the divergence excess and basic exophoria classifications is possible, although there is no literature clearly defining this event.[190] A hereditary factor in DE has been recognized by several authors[80,203,209-213] DE can result from aphakia, with or without a traumatic cause.[154]

Diagnosis

The diagnosis is in accordance with the signs and symptoms, which often vary, depending on the testing completed.[190] Patients with larger deviations and severe binocular disruptions have a poor prognosis.[214]

Treatment

The principal forms of treatment of DE are orthoptics/vision therapy, overminus lenses, prismotherapy, and surgery.[82] A large-scale controlled clinical trial has not been completed to suggest the best method of treatment.[184]

Prisms have been advocated in situations in which normal correspondence has been found, although with limited success.[126,185] Overminus lenses have also been used to deal with the distance deviation.[189,215,216] The long-term success of overminus therapy is surprisingly good.[192]

Orthoptics/vision therapy is also used in the treatment of DE, particularly if the angle of deviation is not large.[126,193,217-219] Frequently, the aim of the therapy is to create an awareness of diplopia when the eyes are deviated, that is, antisuppression training.[186,207,217,218] The development of an increased positive fusional vergence range is another goal of therapy.[82,190,207,218] Training also has included ocular motility training, accommodative facility training, and stereoscopic skills training.[218]

Success with Treatment. The success rate for the treatment of DE exophoria varies as a function of the population studied or the technique used. There is substantial disagreement[80-82,220] regarding the success of orthoptics/vision therapy treatment, with many reporting it to be of significant value.* Those with smaller initial angles of deviation are most likely to be successful, assuming the proper age, cognitive factors, and motivation are present. The presence of a vertical deviation is not a significant factor in the outcome.

ESOPHORIAS

Duane classifies esophorias into three basic types: convergence excess; basic, or equal, esophoria; and divergence insufficiency.[77-79] As with exophorias, the criteria for inclusion into one class or the other has varied, but most commonly the phorias at distance and near are compared, although other criteria besides the comparison of the angles of deviation are often included.[80,82] Patients whose near esophoria is substantially more esophoric have convergence excess, those whose distance esodeviation is more esophoric have divergence insufficiency, and those with about the same esodeviation at distance and near have basic esophoria.

Convergence Excess Esophoria
Definition
Convergence excess (CE) is condition with a significant esophoria at the near point and a relatively orthophoric deviation at distance (Fig. 6-10).[77-78,80,126] The AC/A ratio is rather high. If esotropia becomes manifest at near, the condition is referred to as *nonrefractive accommodative esotropia* (see Chapter 8).

Symptoms
Symptoms in CE esophoria are almost entirely near-related and include diplopia, headaches, and asthenopia.[77,78,224] In younger individuals, possibly because of avoidance of near work or an inability to describe their feelings, there may be few symptoms reported, other than a report of occasional diplopia. In

---

*References 126, 186, 190, 193, 207, 221-223.

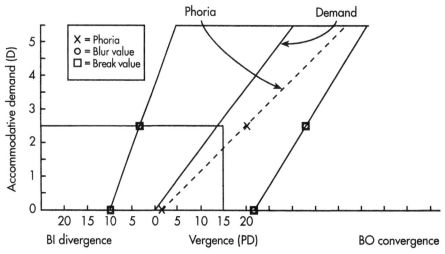

FIG. 6-10   Graphic analysis of zone of binocular vision for convergence excess. Esophoria at near is much larger than that found at distance.

individuals doing a large amount of near work, the symptoms can be rather severe and appear as burning, pulling, lack of concentration, blur, and diplopia after 15 to 20 minutes of near work. These especially show up when near-related tasks are increased, such as starting school, a new job, and so on.

Signs

Individuals with CE are prone to underaccommodate at the near point, so that the near esophoria is lessened. The presenting signs of CE significantly depend on the patient correctly accommodating to a near-point target, otherwise the esophoria may be very small or absent. An inaccurate diagnosis will occur unless the individual accommodates as he or she is urged to keep the print clear. For this reason, small nearpoint fixation targets should be selected for the cover test and the patient instructed to keep them clear.

 CLINICAL PEARL

Individuals with CE are prone to underaccommodate at the near point, so that the near esophoria is lessened.

Angle of Deviation and AC/A. At distance, individuals with CE either have an orthophoria or are slightly esophoric (1 to 3 or 4 PD).[77,78] At the near point, these patients will show a low, moderate, or high esophoria, and therefore the AC/A is high.[77,78] The magnitude of the phoria will vary depending on the material being viewed, which effects the amount of accommodation in play. Vertical deviations can be important in this syndrome (39.8%).[95]

Vergences and Near Point of Convergence. The BI vergences often do not compensate for the phoria (i.e., are of at least twice the phoria).[77,78] The NPC is reduced, although this varies.[77,78]

Accommodation. The most significant test of accommodation for patients with CE is dynamic retinoscopy, because patients with this condition typically show a high lag of accommodation (+1.00 D or greater and may extend to +2.00 D or so on occasion).[224,225] If the lag is greater than +2.50 D for a target placed at 40 cm, the condition must include uncorrected hyperopia. The presence or absence of hyperopia should be determined via a cycloplegic refraction and corrected before considering a diagnosis of CE.

Monocular accommodative amplitudes are usually within the normal ranges for the patient's age. The patient's positive relative accommodation test (PRA) will most likely be reduced.

Sensory Testing. Stereopsis is usually normal; however defects may occur.[226] A long-standing uncorrected CE may diminish or destroy stereopsis if fusion is not maintained at near. On Worth four dot testing the patient may show either uncrossed diplopia or suppression at near, depending on the duration of the problem (typically diplopia initially and suppression later).

Refractive Correction. Hyperopia is strongly associated with esophoria.[77,78,226] Any time an esophoria occurs, hyperopia should be suspected as an etiologic factor, and, before diagnosis, a cycloplegic refraction should be completed. Care should be given to make sure cycloplegia is achieved, especially if the patient's irides are dark.

 CLINICAL PEARL

Anytime an esophoria occurs, hyperopia should be suspected as an etiologic factor, and, before diagnosis, a cycloplegic refraction should be completed.

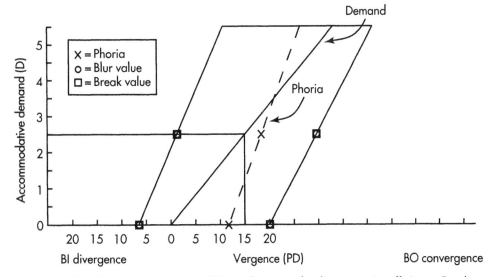

FIG. 6-11 Graphic analysis of zone of binocular vision for divergence insufficiency. Esophoria at distance is much larger than that found at near.

Prevalence

CE esophoria occurs frequently.[77,78] In one study, about 6% of a sample of 119 patients were symptomatic because of a near esophoria.[124] Morgan's normative data[19,20] suggests that 12% of individuals without presbyopia have a significant near esophoria (more than 2 PD).[124]

Sex and Age. No evidence of a correlation of dysfunction with the sex of the patient was found in one study.[121] CE esophoria is much more likely in young people, and many are diagnosed at school age. CE does not go away with age.[227]

Etiology

An obvious factor in the etiology of CE esophoria is a high AC/A ratio. A possible cause for the elevated AC/A and related CE is a system that has an excessive adaptation of convergence and relatively little adaptation of accommodation.[165]

Diagnosis

When there is a significant esophoria at the near point, the diagnosis is uncomplicated.[126] In these cases the clinician can recognize the condition using the cover test. In younger people, objective findings should be taken as sufficient to make the diagnosis, because symptoms often are not reported or near work is avoided. In older people who can reliably report symptomology, the presence or absence of symptoms is useful in discriminating cases with questionable findings. Untreated or poorly treated CE esophoria eventually may decompensate to strabismus, first at near and eventually at distance.[77,78] Prisms at the near point are not typically recommended, because a bifocal is much more predictable and less troublesome.[77,78] A cyclo-

plegic refraction is critical to differentiating CE esophoria from possible contaminating effects of hyperopia.

Treatment

Prescribing for any amount of hyperopia is important.[126] The best solution is to prescribe the distance correction in conjunction with an add for near-point use.[126,225,228-231] Progressive-addition lenses can be effective for near esodeviations, even in children.[228,229,232] Bifocal contact lens corrections have been tried with limited success.[233]

The treatment of CE esophoria anomalies is generally very successful, with over 90% of patients achieving normal binocular function.[234] Orthoptics/vision therapy to increase fusional divergence ranges can also be prescribed but can be difficult.[77,78,126] Surgery is rarely considered.[77,78,235-237] Miotics have also been used in place of spectacles and an add.[237] There are problems with this alternative, including local and systemic side effects, accommodative spasm, and difficulties in getting a consistent dosage (see Chapter 11).[237] The use of miotics is not as effective as a bifocal correction and probably should not be used in treating this condition.[237]

Divergence Insufficiency Esophoria
Definition

Divergence insufficiency (DI) esophoria is a rare condition in which there is a significant esophoria at distance and a much smaller (or absent) esophoria at the near point (Fig. 6-11).[77,78,80,238] The AC/A ratio is therefore relatively normal or low. Cases of DI can be associated with lateral rectus paresis, particularly when esotropia is present (see Chapters 8 and 10).

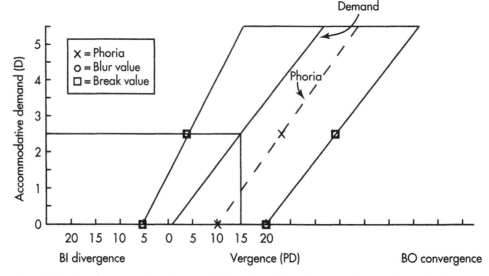

FIG. 6-12 Graphic analysis of zone of binocular vision for equal (or basic) esodeviations. Esophoria at distance and near is approximately the same.

Symptoms

In DI esophoria, the symptoms primarily are distance-related difficulties, such as intermittent diplopia, and include headaches, eyestrain, nausea, dizziness, blurred vision, train and car sickness, difficulty focusing from far to near, and photophobia.[238] Much as with DE problems, the individual may complain of having trouble driving, watching TV, and so on with far viewing. The symptoms are more severe when the patient is tired.[238]

Signs

In DI, there is an esodeviation at distance and a smaller esodeviation at near.[238] The AC/A ratio is low to normal.[238] A true DI is comitant in nature.[238] There are inadequate compensating vergences at distance (and sometimes at near) for DI.[238] Accommodation is normal, as is PRA and NRA testing, because such testing is at the near point.

If the condition is prolonged, suppression can be present at distance. The Worth four dot test usually shows diplopia at distance, if suppression has not developed.

There is no evidence available suggesting that a particular type of refractive error is associated with DI.[238]

Prevalence and Etiology

DI was the least frequently reported of Duane's syndromes.[95] Based on our experience, DI esophoria is very rare. The etiology is unknown.[238] However, a DI type of picture may suggest the presence of a lateral rectus paresis.

Diagnosis and Treatment

A patient presenting with a significantly greater esophoria at distance than near and diplopia should be considered to have a DI esophoria. The correction of hyperopia is important for a patient with an esodeviation.[126,238] Base-out prisms are the treatment alternative of choice for DI esophoria.[126,238] The futility of orthoptics/vision therapy has been noted, although it may have a place in a limited number of cases.[123,238] Prismatic correction has been successfully used by some clinicians.[238] Surgical correction is not recommended.[238]

The procedure of choice in selecting the appropriate prism for distance wear is to prescribe the associated phoria.[238] The best instrument is probably the American Optical distance vectographic slide.[238]

Equal Esophoria
Definition

Equal (basic) esophoria (EE) is the condition in which there is a significant esodeviation of about the same degree at distance and at near, even though the appropriate refractive correction has been provided (Fig. 6-12).[77,78]

Symptoms

The symptoms associated with EE are intimately related to the demands placed on the visual system by the patient. If the demands are distance-related, the symptoms will show up with distance viewing. If the demands are at near, the symptoms will be manifest at near. The symptoms are usually asthenopia, blur, headaches, or diplopia.

Signs
Angle of Deviation and Vertical Deviations.
Patients with an EE have an esophoria at distance and near and therefore an AC/A ratio that approximates the PD. A cycloplegic refraction is important in ruling out esophoria secondary to uncorrected hyperopia. As with CE, the esodeviation also is typically much greater than may be suspected from the cover test, because the accommodative system often produces a large lag that has the effect of reducing the esodeviation and thus symptomology. An increased lag of accommodation obscures the magnitude of the esodeviation, so that a deviation may be much larger if there is accurate and full accommodation. Primary vertical deviations have been frequently reported in esophoric conditions and, if present, should be corrected with prisms.[95]

Vergences. The vergence ranges for patients with EE are normal to low. In many cases the vergences are sufficient to meet either Percival's or Sheard's criterion.[116]

Accommodation. Accommodative amplitude with EE is usually completely normal. The major finding related to accommodation is an extended lag of accommodation of +1.00 D or more to as much as about +2.00 D. The lag of accommodation is larger with bigger and less detailed stimuli.

Suppression and Stereopsis. Patients with EE usually have good stereopsis, intermittent suppression, or diplopia, depending on the size of the deviation and the configuration of the stimulus.

Prevalence
There is relatively little data regarding the prevalence of EE.

Associated Conditions and Etiology
The most common condition associated with esophoria is hyperopia. This should be ruled out in every case with a cycloplegic refraction. Various anatomic, innervational etiologic factors have been suggested with EE, but usually the etiology of a condition is unknown.

Diagnosis
An esodeviation, no matter the magnitude, always should be considered potentially problematic. This is particularly true until two major factors have been examined. These are hyperopia and the lag of accommodation. When an esophoria is discovered, a cycloplegic refraction should be completed to determine if there is uncorrected hyperopia and the effect of its correction. At the same time, a careful examination of the lag of accommodation is critical. Without knowledge of the lag, the near deviation cannot be properly interpreted.

If the lag is greater than about +1.00 D, the near esophoria is actually greater than is shown, because accommodation is not fully active. The magnitude of negative fusional vergences also gives an indication of the significance of the deviation. Percival's criterion (see below) is an appropriate method to use in estimating its significance.

Treatment
The treatment of EE anomalies is generally very successful, with over 90% of patients achieving normal binocular function.[234] Prisms can be used successfully. Maximum plus should always be prescribed with any esodeviation. Orthoptics/vision therapy to increase the negative fusional vergence range is an alternative but is generally difficult. Miotics have been recommended, but because of side effects these should not be used along with the success of lenses and prisms.[239] Surgery should be approached cautiously.[236,239] We do not recommend consideration of surgery until the use of lenses, prisms, and orthoptics/vision therapy have been exhausted.

HYPERPHORIA
Definition
A hyperphoria is a vertical misalignment of the eyes present only in dissociated conditions.

Symptoms
Vertical deviations, even when small in magnitude commonly cause symptoms, including headache, diplopia, loss of place when reading, and fatigue.[240] Vertigo, nausea, and motion sickness also are commonly reported symptoms with vertical phorias.[241,242] Diplopia in a certain direction of gaze often suggests oculomotor system dysfunction (see Chapter 10).[77,78]

Signs
A vertical deviation of even 1 PD can cause significant difficulties, because the vertical vergence system generally produces extraordinarily precise vertical alignment of the eyes[243,244,245] Vertical deviations greater than about 4 PD are usually incomitant and are often related to a dysfunctional cyclovertical muscle. Vertical vergence ranges are much smaller than horizontal vergences.[246] In most small vertical phorias the vertical vergence range is unbalanced and the larger range is in the direction of the vertical phoria (e.g., for a right hyperphoria the right supravergence range will be larger than the right infravergence range).

Stereopsis, accommodation, and other binocular function is typically good. Suppression sometimes occurs under certain conditions; diplopia occurs with larger deviations or, if the deviation is incomitant, in a particular gaze.

Prevalence

There has not been a precise determination of the prevalence of vertical deviations in the general population. Vertical phorias have been suggested to occur in 7% to 25% of the population, or 9%.[241,246,248] Another study reported vertical deviations in 15.5% of controls and 42.1% of individuals with learning-disabilities.[249]

Associated Conditions and Etiology

Several conditions, such as dyslexia[152] and learning disorders[249] have been associated with hyperphoria. Asymmetric orbital placement appears to be a significant factor for small vertical deviations. Other mechanical etiologies, such as an improper insertion of the extraocular muscles, may also cause a vertical deviation.

Although these causes frequently result in strabismus, hyperphorias may arise from anomalies of vertical rectus or oblique muscle function, supranuclear (skew deviation), cranial nerves (oculomotor, trochlear), myoneural junction (ocular myasthenia), or overaction of the inferior or superior oblique muscles, or they may be idiopathic.[123,250] A physiologic hyperdeviation in extreme lateral gaze of 2 PD or more has been described.[250]

Comitant hyperphoria may be associated with combined symmetric pareses and large lateral deviations subsequent to aphakia with or without trauma.[77,78,126,154] Vertical deviations occur in 60% of patients with unilateral pseudophakia.[251] A pseudovertical phoria may occur because of poorly centered spectacle lenses.

Diagnosis

The cover test usually does not permit detection of small deviations, so the vertical Maddox rod test is the best method for determining a vertical deviation. Vertical deviations may cause symptoms even when the vergence range seems adequate.[240,252]

Short-term occlusion of one eye sometimes is used diagnostically to confirm that symptoms are binocular in nature. Vertical deviations cause symptoms only when the patient is binocular and therefore disappear when one eye is covered. At the same time, such occlusion may also cause a latent vertical deviation to become more obvious, because fusional vergence effects sometimes last for a short period after binocularity is interrupted. Occlusion can create minor problems that can mask the beneficial effects of occlusion, such as a reduced field of view, loss of stereopsis, and the uncomfortable effects of wearing a patch.

In some cases it is appropriate to prescribe a trial vertical prism. A convenient option in this respect is a Fresnel press-on prism. If a trial is undertaken, it should be presented to the patient as confirming the hypothesis rather than "trying something to see if it will work."

Treatment

A hyperphoria is usually treated with prisms.[126,240,243,246,247] Orthoptics/vision therapy may be of some value in certain cases.[126,246,253-255]

 CLINICAL PEARL

A hyperphoria is usually treated with prisms.

The amount of prism to prescribe is sometimes difficult to determine.[240] The amount of vertical can vary secondary to a sizable lateral deviation or may vary because of greater dissociation with some measurement devices than others, and the patient may adapt or have adapted to vertical prism.[240] Prescribing vertical prism should include an assessment of the stability and reliability of the vertical deviation and an assessment in straight and down gaze.[240] When possible, the deviation should be measured with the patient fused (an associated phoria), to deal with secondary vertical deviations. Secondary vertical deviations are not present when a patient is evaluated under fused conditions. Rutstein and Eskridge[240] have advocated the prescription of the vertical associated phoria (the amount of prism that reduces the fixation disparity to zero). Our experience suggests that this option is the most successful alternative in choosing a prism.

Directly training vertical vergences is difficult but can be accomplished.[254] One study reports increases in vertical vergence amplitude of up to 2 to 4 PD over a period of 4 weeks of orthoptics/vision therapy.[254] This study eliminated suppression before directly training vertical vergences.

Patients with vertical phorias who desire to wear contact lenses may be interested in vertical vergence training.[247] Cooper[247] reports on four patients who were able to forego prism correction in spectacles in favor of contact lens correction. The minimum prism necessary to eliminate diplopia and provide comfort was prescribed for full-time wear. The orthoptics/vision therapy program began by first maximizing lateral vergence capability with ramp types of devices, such as vectograms, and then using step vergence training to further enhance the vergence system. These patients experienced large increases in horizontal vergence capability and a subsequent ability to forego the wearing of prisms. Cooper speculates that such training for the horizontal vergence system also affected the vertical vergence system by reinforcing fusional reflexes and increasing the adaptive response.[247]

TABLE 6-6 **POPULATION NORMS**

Parameter (Distance)	Study (Mean, Standard Deviation in Parentheses)		
	Morgan*	Saladin-Sheedy†	OEP†
Phoria (PD, 6 M)	1 XP (2)	1 XP (3.5)	0.5 XP
Negative vergences (PD, blur, break and recovery, 6 M)	X/7/4 (−/3/2)	X/8/5 (−/3/3)	X/9/5
Positive vergences (PD, blur, break and recovery, 6 M)	9/19/10 (4/8/4)	15/28/20 (7/10/11)	8/19/10
Phoria (PD, 40 cm)	3 XP (5)	0.5 XP (6)	6 XP
Negative vergences (PD, blur, break and recovery, 40 cm)	13/21/13 (4/4/5)	14/19/13 (6/7/6)	14/22/18
Positive vergences (PD, blur, break and recovery, 40 cm)	17/21/11 (5/6/7)	22/30/23 (8/12/11)	15/21/15

*Data from Morgan MW: The clinical aspects of accommodation and convergency, *Am J Optom Arch Am Acad Optom* 21:301, 1944; Morgan MW: Analysis of clinical data, *Am J Optom Arch Am Acad Optom* 21:477, 1944.
†Data from Grisham JD: In Schor CM, Ciuffreda KJ, editors: *Basic and clinical aspects of vergence eye movements*, Boston, 1983, Butterworth-Heinemann.

DIAGNOSIS OF HETEROPHORIA AND VERGENCE ANOMALIES

THE PROBLEM

Sometimes it is difficult to tell whether a patient's problems are caused by binocular vision dysfunction. Symptoms can be caused by several things, including an anomaly of the heterophoria-vergence relationship, stress or overwork, or ergonomics (poor lighting, bad chair, etc.). Problems with differential diagnosis occur because:

- Symptoms from binocular visual anomalies tend to be nonspecific.[163] Many things cause the eyes to be uncomfortable and result in blur, asthenopia, and headaches. Feelings of eyestrain seem to be related to vergence anomalies, and blurred vision after a period of work seems to be related to accommodative anomalies.[256]
- People are very adaptable and avoid using the eyes if there is a problem. Children, especially, love to do things successfully; if eyestrain or diplopia prevents or inhibits their performance, they will avoid near work.
- There is substantial variation in many of the clinically measured variables, such as vergences. It is difficult to tell if a value is low or the patient is not motivated. There are problems interpreting data where there is a strong voluntary component. Fatigue is another significant factor.
- Models of the oculomotor system do not incorporate all important variables, such as proximal vergence.[30,257] When they do include all factors known to affect binocular vision, a model such as the dual interaction model is very complex to use.

IMPORTANCE OF THE CASE HISTORY

Despite the fact that symptoms generated from various sources tend to be similar and nonspecific, a careful history is often the best way to determine whether the symptoms are visually related or not. This ability is developed through experience. The clinician must determine the extent that the symptoms are associated with the use of the eyes, as opposed to stress or ergonomic factors. The completion of more extensive testing on patients who are symptomatic (rather than on everyone or on no one) to discriminate the cause is the most cost-effective method of delivering eyecare.[258]

APPROACHES TO THE PROBLEM OF DIAGNOSIS

Several different approaches are used in conjunction with the case history in diagnosis of the various binocular vision anomalies. These include normative analysis, graphic analysis, and control theory.[74]

Normative (Expected Values) Analysis

Normative analysis assumes that binocular functions (accommodation and vergence) are related and that as a patient's values deviate from these numbers, especially in a correlated deviation (i.e., low negative vergence and low PRA), then a problem is suspect.[19,20] Several norms for the population have been presented (Tables 6-6 and 6-7).[8,9,19,20,52,259,260]

There are several problems with using normative data.[167] Population averages may not be the optimum value because they tell what the values are rather than what they should be. There may be subpopulations in the sample, related to age, gender, race, and so on; however, the clinician usually does not know how

TABLE 6-7 NORMS FOR OTHER CLINICAL PARAMETERS

Parameter	Value
Dynamic retinoscopy (MEM or Nott)	+0.50 to +0.75 D
Accommodative response	
Binocular cross cylinder	
AC/A (far-near)	5 PD/D
AC/A (gradient)	4 PD/D
Accommodative amplitude	Average (D) = 18.5 - 0.3 (age)
	Low (D) = 15.0 - 0.25 (age)
	High (D) = 25.0 - 0.4 (age)
NRA/PRA (from best correction, *not* the add)	+2.00/ − 2.37 D

Modified from Morgan MW: The clinical aspects of accommodation and convergence, *Am J Optom Arch Am Acad Optom* 21:301, 1944; Morgan MW: Analysis of clinical data, *Am J Optom Arch Am Acad Optom* 21:477, 1944; Grisham JD: In Schor CM, Ciuffreda KJ, editors: *Basic and clinical aspects of vergence eye movements*, Boston, 1983, Butterworth-Heinemann.

many subpopulations exist. There also is poor reliability of some clinical data (e.g., vergences can vary by 10 PD or more) and a finding cannot be discriminated from the normal by less than the normal variation.

One condition in which a diagnostically important subpopulation has been demonstrated is presbyopia. Individuals with presbyopia are likely to manifest a substantial exodeviation at the nearpoint.[38] A population of 10 patients with presbyopia had a mean exodeviation of 8.7 PD, as opposed to a sample without presbyopia of 2.8 PD exo; none of the subjects with presbyopia reported significant symptoms.[38] A different measure of binocularity, the fixation disparity curve, also demonstrated no differences between the two groups. Fixation disparity analyses may provide a truer measure of binocularity for these patients than more traditional analyses.

Despite these problems, normative analysis is a good, first-order way to judge a patient's potential for binocular dysfunction, particularly if the problem is not subtle. Patients who have an esophoria of 2 PD or more, an exophoria of about 6 Δ or more, whose accommodative levels do not reach Hofstetter's minimum standard for their age, whose lag of accommodation is either plano or minus or +1.00 D or more, or whose vergences fall less than 10 PD at the break very frequently will have binocular troubles.

Graphic (Intrasubject) Analysis

Graphic analysis is another common method of investigating relationships between the various factors involved in binocular vision.[261-263] The five fundamental variables of Fry are the distance phoria, the negative fusional convergence value, the positive fusional convergence value, the AC/A ratio and the accommodative amplitude (Fig. 6-13).[53,264] Assuming linear-

ity, these variables completely describe an individual's zone of single binocular vision.

Graphic analysis suffers in common use because the plotting of data is cumbersome. A number of non-linearities can arise, which necessitates plotting more than the fundamental variables to get a sense of things. Graphic analysis also does not, by itself, prescribe what is wrong or what must be done to correct any problems.

Criteria for Normal Binocular Vision
Sheard's Criterion

Sheard's criterion is the most commonly used diagnostic method in binocular vision. Sheard's criterion is that the fusional reserve amount should be twice the fusional demand (phoria), that is, a patient with 6-PD exophoria should have at least 12-PD positive vergence (blur).[33,116] Failure to meet Sheard's criterion correlated well with the presence of symptoms in a group of patients with convergence insufficiency.[136] The criterion can also be used to guide treatment. For example, orthoptics/vision therapy can be used to increase vergence capability to the level necessary to compensate for the phoria, or prism can be prescribed to move the phoria so that the vergence level meets the criterion. The following formula for Sheard's criterion is sometimes used[72]:

Prism = 2/3 (phoria) − 1/3 (compensating vergence)

For example, in a patient with 10-PD exophoria with 15 PD to the positive blur finding:

Prism = 2/3(10) − 1/3(15) = 6.7 − 5 = 1.7 PD

Orthoptics/vision therapy can be used to increase the positive vergence blur finding to 20 PD BO or more, or, alternatively, 1.7 PD BI can be prescribed, so that the resulting phoria is about 8 PD and the blur finding is about 17 PD.

Sheard's criterion seems to work best with exophoria. Several studies suggest that Sheard's criterion is the best single indicator of good binocular function.[39-40,42,264] These same studies have shown that the determination of the best indicator is also partially a function of the way the data are partitioned.

Percival's Criterion

To meet Percival's criterion, the demand should lie within the middle third of the vergence range and hence Percival's rule does not have anything to do with the heterophoria value.[72,33,116] Percival's criterion is generally applied only in cases of esophoria. The following formula is sometimes used[72]:

Prism = NFR + 1/3 ZW

where Prism = prism necessary to meet Percival's criterion if positive (if negative, no prism is necessary,

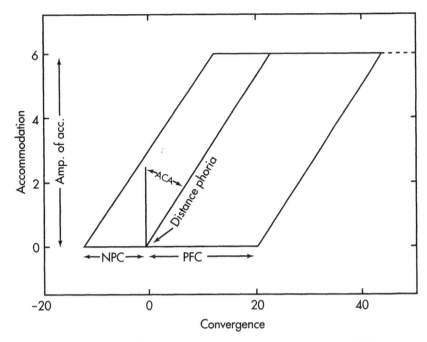

FIG. 6-13 Fundamental variables of graphic analysis: distance phoria, AC/A ratio, positive vergences (PFC), negative vergences (NPC), accommodative amplitude. (Modified from Hofstetter HW: Graphic analysis. In Schor CM, Ciuffreda KJ, editors: *Vergence eye movements: basic and clinical aspects,* Boston, 1983, Butterworth-Heinemann.)

meets criterion); NFR = negative fusional reserve; and ZW = total fusional vergence zone width. For example, if a patient has a negative blur value of 5 PD and a total zone width of 18 PD, then:

$$\text{Prism} = -5 + 1/3(18) = 1$$

that is, 1 PD BO is necessary to meet the criterion.

This criterion does not work well with a large fusional vergence zone. In unusual cases the vergence range may be increased so that the middle third of the zone is shifted and the patient no longer meets the criterion. Percival's criterion suggests that when this occurs the patient should be less comfortable, even though the vergence range has increased. This is a counter-intuitive result, because larger vergence values are always associated with better and more comfortable binocular vision.

Fixation Disparity

Fixation disparity is a steady-state error of disparity-induced vergence.[265] The slope of the fixation disparity curve is a reliable method of discriminating between symptomatic and asymptomatic patients.[52,266] Fixation disparity appears to provide a more accurate measure of binocularity of patients with presbyopia than measurements of phorias and vergences.[38,267] The nature of the vergence system may change with the aging process, whereas fixation disparity curves measured on a given subject tend to remain relatively stable over time, although shifts over a period of months can occur.[38,268,269,270,271] The curve tends to remain stable whether measured in or out of the phoropter.[67]

Fixation disparity variables relate to asthenopia.* Normative data for fixation disparity curves has been provided by several investigators, as well as Sheard's and Percival's criterion.[39,40,52,257,270,272] The order in which variables discriminated in one well-designed study is described in Table 6-8.[40]

The criteria in Table 6-9 can be used to discriminate between normal and abnormal binocular systems.[41] This normative table for fixation disparity is easy to use, although the analysis suffers from problems prone to effect normative analysis. Patients exceeding these measures are more likely to have binocular dysfunction.[69]

Fixation disparity has been considered to be an indicator of stress on the binocular visual system and/or a stimulus to the vergence system under binocular conditions.[265,274] Approximately 25% of the fixation disparity values are in opposite quadrants from what would be expected considering the heterophoria (Fig. 6-14).[53] The differences between heterophoria assessments and fixation disparity suggest that the oculomotor system's binocular status is not easily deduced from findings when the eyes are dissociated.

---

*References 39, 40, 50, 52, 53, 272, 273.

TABLE 6-8 ORDER IN WHICH CLINICAL VALUES WERE DISCRIMINATIVE BETWEEN SYMPTOMATIC AND ASYMPTOMATIC STUDENTS

All Subjects	Exophores	Esophores	Exofixation Disparity	Esofixation Disparity
Sheard blur	Y intercept	Percival break	Sheard blur	FDC slope
FDC type	FDC type	Positive blur	FDC type	Percival recovery
FDC slope	Negative break	Negative break	FDC slope	X intercept
Negative blur	Phoria	Percival recovery	Negative blur	Percival break
Y intercept	Percival blur	FDC slope		
Positive blur		X intercept		
Phoria				
82% correct	92% correct	73% correct	76% correct	96% correct

Modified from Sheedy JE, Saladin JJ: Association of symptoms with measures of oculomotor deficiences, *Am J Optom Physiol Opt* 55:670, 1978.

TABLE 6-9 FIXATION DISPARITY CRITERIA DIFFERENTIATING BETWEEN NORMAL AND ABNORMAL BINOCULAR SYSTEMS

Parameter	Normal	Abnormal
FDC type	I	II, III IV: very abnormal
FDC slope	Lesser −1 min PD or 45°	−1 min/D or 45° or steeper
Y intercept (fixation disparity value, min arc)	Exos: 12 min arc exo FD or less Esos: any eso FD	Exos: more than 12 min arc FD Esos: exo FD
Horizontal associated phoria (X intercept, PD)	0	Any greater than 0, either BI or BO
Vertical FDC: associated phoria (X intercept, PD)	0	Any greater than 0, either BU or BD
Vertical FDC: Y intercept (fixation, disparity value, min arc)	0	Any greater than 0, either min arc, R hyper, or L hyper

Modified from Sheedy JE: Fixation disparity analysis of oculomotor imbalance, *Am J Optom Physiol Opt* 57:632, 1980.

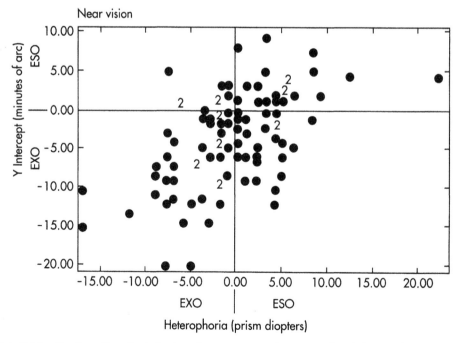

FIG. 6-14 Fixation disparity (minutes of arc, eso or exo) compared with heterophoria values (PD (Δ), eso or exo). (Modified from Saladin JJ, Sheedy JE: Population study of fixation disparity, heterophoria, and vergence, *Am J Optom Physiol Opt* 55:744, 1978.)

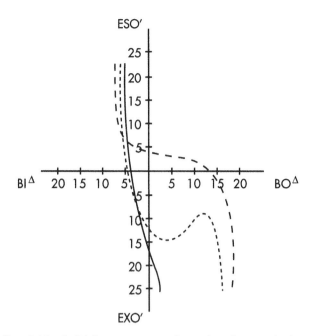

FIG. 6-15 Solid line represents data taken from typical patient with convergence insufficiency. Small-dashed line shows same patient 2 weeks after initiation of training. Large-dashed line shows results of additional 2 weeks of training. (Modified from Saladin JJ: Convergence insufficiency, fixation disparity, and control systems analysis, *Am J Optom Physiol Opt* 63:645, 1986.)

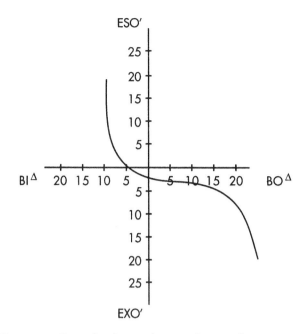

FIG. 6-16 Example of normal 40-cm fixation disparity curve for moderate amount of exophoria. Curve represents smoothed, after-treatment data for case represented in Fig. 6-15. (Modified from Saladin JJ: Convergence insufficiency, fixation disparity, and control systems analysis, *Am J Optom Physiol Opt* 63:645, 1986.)

Vertical Fixation Disparity

The vertical-associated phoria is a reliable method of prescribing for vertical deviations.[252,269,275,276]

Fixation Disparity Analysis and Control Theory

The fixation disparity curve can be broken down into three parts, a central relatively flat portion, an up-sweep portion on the base-in side of the curve, and a down-sweep portion on the base-out side of the curve.[54] These portions represent the slow adaptive vergence component, the operation of an eso disparity vergence controller, and the operation of an exo disparity vergence controller, respectively.[54]

Type II curves may lack a fully functional exo disparity vergence controller, and Type III curves may lack a fully functional eso disparity vergence controller.[54] Changes in vergence capability alters the appearance of the fixation disparity curve (Figs. 6-15 and 6-16).[54]

Control Systems Analysis

Control systems analysis has been used by various investigators in the diagnosis and treatment of binocular defects.[54,277] A major benefit of this analysis is the allowance for time-related accommodative-vergence interactions.[54] The oculomotor vergence system has been modeled as a dual-interactive negative-feedback model

(Fig. 6-17).[278-282] Both accommodation and vergence are negative-feedback systems. The accommodative system is arranged so blur feeds back into the accommodative controller, which alters accommodation to eliminate it.[54] The accommodative system is not sensitive to the sign of the blur, and too much or too little accommodation of the same amount are equivalent stimuli. The vergence system also is a negative-feedback system; however, the aim of the vergence controller is to eliminate disparity.[54] The vergence controller recognizes direction (eso or exo), so that the eyes can be converged or diverged.[54] The forward controller for the vergence system is a leaky integrator, allowing a continual signal to be sent to the ocular muscles so a particular level of vergence can be maintained.[282]

The controllers for both the accommodative and the vergence loops have fast and slow components.[54,283] The fast component has a low-gain and quick-reacting system. Because the gain of the fast component is low, trying to maintain large amounts of innervation is fatiguing. Fixation disparity is the signal from the fast component into the slow component.[54,274] Fixation disparity is the steady-state error for the vergence system, whereas lag of accommodation is the steady-state error for accommodation.[165,284] Together, these provide continual stimuli to assist in maintaining a given accommodative and vergence position.

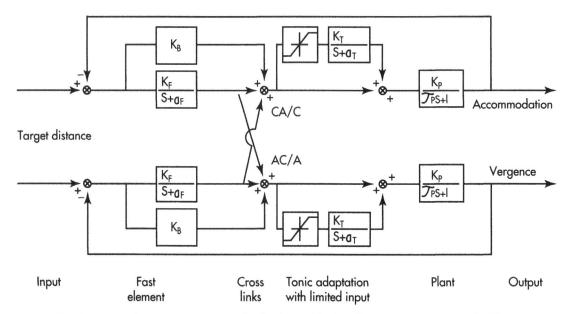

FIG. 6-17 Dual interactive negative-feedback model of oculomotor system. (Modified from Schor CM, Kotulak JC: Dynamic interactions between accommodation and convergence are velocity-sensitive, *Vision Res* 26:927, 1986.)

The slow vergence component has a high gain but a long time constant, that is, it reacts slowly but it has a large capacity to react and does not fatigue easily. The long time constant of the slow component causes the slow component to continue sending similar innervation to the extraocular musculature over an extended period. This may be observed by noting the esophoric shift in the phoria after measuring vergences with base-out prisms.[54] The slow component is responsible for allowing the system to adjust to changes over time.

The accommodative loop and the vergence loop interact with each other.[274,279] The AC/A and CA/C ratios are the measures of the interaction of the accommodative loop with vergence and the vergence loop with accommodation, respectively. The AC/A ratio is the ratio of the innervation in the disparity vergence system to the innervation in the accommodative system.[54] The CA/C ratio is the ratio of the innervation in the vergence controller to that in the accommodative system.[54] Both the AC/A ratios and CA/C ratios are higher when measured under binocular conditions.[165] Various adaptive processes mask these effects under dissociated conditions.[165,279] Imbalances between the AC/A and the CA/C ratios may cause binocular problems.[284] Clinical techniques to assess both the AC/A and the CA/C ratios exist.[285]

There is a complementary relationship between the AC/A and CA/C amplitudes and the tonic adaptation of accommodation and vergence, respectively.[278] Accommodation is more adaptable in patients with low AC/A ratios. Vergence is more adaptable with low CA/C ratios. Moderate AC/A ratios are balanced by moderate CA/C ratios. Whenever one of these ratios is abnormally high, there is an imbalance between accommodative and vergence adaptive abilities. In CE, in which the AC/A is very high, accommodative adaptability is very low and vergence adaptability is correspondingly high. The vergence adaptability adds to the phoria (and the AC/A ratio). The CA/C ratio is highest in patients with low vergence adaptation and high accommodative adaptation. Vergences are related to the fast component of the vergence feedback loop.[265,274] Changes in the vergence capability result in changes in fixation disparity slope.[52]

Summary

There is as yet no single diagnostic system that is used universally or has been found to be perfectly accurate and reliable. Patients will sometimes have symptoms without the "appropriate" anomaly and signs, or they may not have symptoms with all the features of a given anomaly.[110]

MANAGEMENT OF BINOCULAR VISUAL ANOMALIES

The general sequence for treating anomalies of the binocular system is (1) diagnose and manage disease processes appropriately; (2) apply the proper optical correction of ametropia to each eye; (3) deal with any sensory anomalies, such as amblyopia; (4) treat any ac-

TABLE 6-10 STRATEGY FOR MANAGEMENT OF ANOMALIES OF VERGENCE USING THE PYRAMID OF BINOCULAR VISION

Process	Action
Sensory process	Diagnose and manage any disease process
	Correct any significant ametropia
	Treat any amblyopia
	Treat any accommodative anomalies
Integrative process	Treat any suppression
Motor process	Treat any heterophoria/vergence anomalies

BOX 6-1 STRATEGY/ACTION FOR MANAGEMENT OF MOTOR ANOMALIES

ACTION
Determine the benefits of added plus (near only) or minus lenses (near or distance).
Determine the benefits of added prisms.
Consider the application of a program of orthoptics/vision therapy.
Consider the benefits of extraocular muscle surgery.

commodative anomalies; (5) treat any integrative anomalies, such as suppression; and (6) treat any anomalies of heterophoria/vergence (Table 6-10). The pyramid of binocular vision necessitates this sequence because the clinician must treat the most fundamental aspects of the system before treating things dependant on those fundamental aspects.

The management of heterophoria and vergence anomalies also should be dealt with in a particular sequence (Box 6-1). In this respect, we recommend the following sequence: (1) determine the benefits of added plus (near only) or added minus lenses (near or distance), (2) determine the benefits of added ophthalmic prisms for vertical or horizontal deviations, (3) consider the application of a program of orthoptics/vision therapy, and (4) consider the benefits of extraocular muscle surgery. There is more room for adjusting the sequence of management of motor anomalies as a function of both the patient and the doctor's preferences. There is general agreement that surgery should be used only after other alternatives have been exhausted and is generally reserved for strabismus. Typically, patients prefer an optical solution to any problems that they may have, apparently because of convenience. We expend considerable effort educating patients about the benefits of orthoptics/vision therapy.

THE USE OF VERGENCE TRAINING IN SOLVING BINOCULAR VISUAL ANOMALIES
Effects of Vergence Training

Studies of training the oculomotor system have demonstrated that it is possible to produce remarkable effects. For example, the eyes can be trained by matching afterimages to tilted lines to make versional cyclorotatory movements reaching nearly 30 degrees in extent (Fig. 6-18).[286] The cyclorotatory movements occurred at about 0.8 degrees/hr of training. Individuals can also be trained to make monocular vergence movements using a visual feedback technique.[287]

Several studies of the effects of vergence training have included control groups and masking to control bias. A matched-subjects control group cross-over design was used to evaluate the automated vergence treatment of seven patients with convergence insufficiency.[1] A statistically significant reduction in symptoms and an increase in vergence range was demonstrated during the period when training occurred (and not during the control period). Other studies have shown that vergence training is not a function of the Hawthorne (placebo) effect.[1,83] A matched-subjects control group cross-over design has been used to control placebo effects in an evaluation of the effects of fusional vergence training on asthenopia.[1] All seven patients with convergence insufficiency achieved a reduction in asthenopia and an increase in positive fusional vergences over the approximately 10 sessions during the treatment phase of the training. Much smaller increases or no increases were detected after the control phase. This suggests that fusional vergence training is not related to placebo effects.

Using a double-masked, placebo-controlled design, three groups of six subjects were evaluated to determine the most efficacious speed of training when using a computer-controlled vergence training task.[288] Vergence ranges increased significantly for the group using the slowest training rate (0.75 PD/sec). Those training with the faster rate (5 PD/sec) and the control group did not show increases.

Another study examined three groups of reading-disabled students given computer vision training, remedial reading exercises, or a placebo treatment.[83] Only the vision training group showed significant increases in accommodative and vergence facility and near point of convergence over the 10-week training period.

Three young adult subjects with asthenopia underwent objective assessment of vergence ranges using a vergence tracking rate index.[180] Over an 8- to 10-week vergence training period, all three (two with exophoria and one with esophoria) experienced an alleviation of symptoms and increases in both the objective tracking

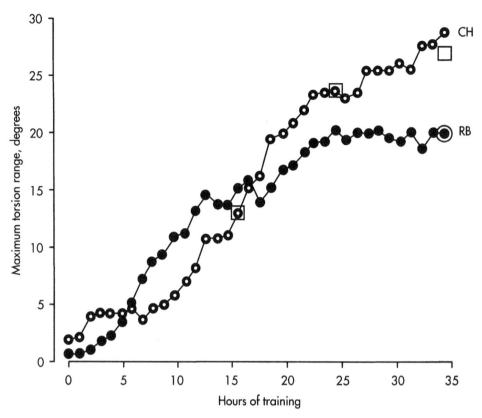

FIG. 6-18 Training of voluntary tonic cycloversion for subjects CH and RB. Hours of training at 1 hr/day vs. total range (degrees) of psychophysically measured torsion is plotted by small symbols. These are maximum tonic ranges that can be held for 5-second duration. Three large squares and large circle are simultaneous measures obtained photographically. (Modified from Balliet R, Nakayama K: Training of voluntary torsion, *Invest Ophthalmol Vis Sci* 17:303, 1978.)

rate index and in clinically-assessed vergence parameters. Another part of the study included six symptomatic subjects and two asymptomatic control subjects completing a vergence training task over a 3-month period. During this period, normal levels of vergences were reached in 2 to 8 weeks and symptoms diminished. Assessments completed at intervals of 3 and 6 months after training showed that the vergence levels remained stable (Fig. 6-19).

Successful increases in vergences should result in flatter fixation disparity curves.[38,169] Small changes in phorias and AC/A ratios may also occur.[89,177,289] Orthoptics/vision therapy improves the ability to adapt to prism, which also strongly correlates with the alleviation of symptoms.[290,291]

Base-out vergence training significantly increases positive fusional vergence ranges; however, base-in (negative) vergences are difficult to train.[153,292-294] One study examined the effects of 50 hours of negative fusional vergence training (two 45-minute sessions per day) over a 7-week period.[295] The negative vergences increased by 5 PD at distance and 9.1 PD at near over

the course of the training. Over the course of training the phorias of both subjects became 3.6 PD more exo than they were at the beginning of the training. Negative relative accommodation values increased for both subjects, and changes in the lag of accommodation and fixation disparity curves also occurred. Negative vergence training is difficult because of the necessary time demands for training.[239]

Over-training vergences seems to produce the best results.[153] Over-training is training after the symptoms are relieved and helps with the maintenance of the training effects over an extended period.

Biofeedback techniques can be used to train positive vergences, particularly with intermittent exotropia.[296-299] Biofeedback may be especially useful if used as an adjunct to conventional therapy.[299] Operant conditioning techniques and an automated convergence system using random-dot stereograms has been used successfully.[75] Random-dot stereograms have the advantage that the fusion cue is not visible unless bifoveal fixation is present.

Not all studies find improvements with orthop-

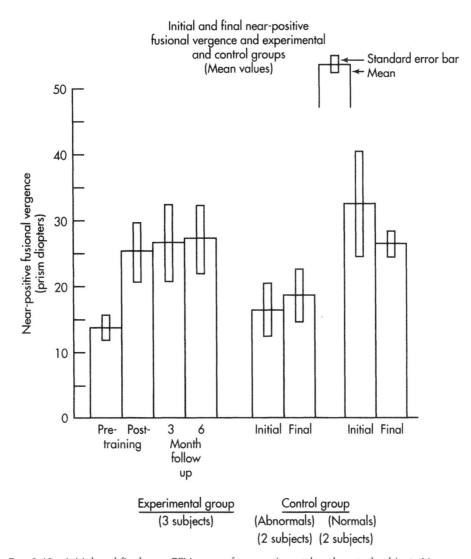

Initial and final near-positive
fusional vergence and experimental
and control groups
(Mean values)

FIG. 6-19 Initial and final near PFV ranges for experimental and control subjects. Vergence-deficient subjects (experimental group) showed significant and persistent changes in fusional convergence after orthoptics/vision therapy, whereas no significant change was seen in untrained control subjects, normal or abnormal. (Modified from Grisham JD and others: Vergence orthoptics: validity and persistence of the training effect, *Optom Vis Sci* 68:441, 1991.)

tics/vision therapy.[300] A masked examination of the effects of training on a test group and a control group of six U.S. Air Force pilots failed to document improvements in vergences, accommodative amplitude, or stereopsis.[300]

Computers and video tapes have been adapted to provide a variety of vergence training methods.[288,301,302] These devices provide a good means of maintaining interest while presenting a controlled target.

Reviews of the success of vergence training are available.[303,304] These conclude that there is a wide array of evidence supporting its efficacy in a variety of situations.

Mechanism for Vergence Training

Fatigue (which can be caused by tracking a monocular accommodative ramp stimulus, e.g., monocular push-up training) is responsible for changes in the binocular system as a result of training.[165] When the accommodative system is affected in this manner, strong increases in the AC/A ratio and decreases in the CA/C ratio occur concomitantly (reverse changes, decreases in AC/A, and increases in CA/C are also possible). Changes in the interlinkage of accommodation and vergence seem to happen because the fatigue causes increased sensitivity to blur and a consequent increase in accommodative convergence for a given stimulus.

A step stimulus can also change the adaptability of the accommodative and vergence systems, with fatigue again being primarily responsible for the effects.[165,285]

Indications for Vergence Training

Vergence training should be considered when there are reliable, visually-associated subjective problems, such as asthenopia, headache, drawing or pulling sensations, blur, or diplopia. Ordinarily, vergence training should be considered when there are objective deficits, such as decreased performance, head tilts or turns, loss of stereopsis, suppression, reduced accommodative ability, strabismus, significant vertical or horizontal phorias, or reduced vergence amplitudes. In children, training is sometimes undertaken entirely on objective grounds, with no symptoms. Further, the problem should be one that is amenable to vergence training, such as a deficit of the binocular oculomotor system or associated with accommodative ability. Finally, vergence training should be selected in view of other possible treatments. Vergence training is contraindicated if other modes of treatment are better.

Considerations in Using Vergence Training

There are several problems with vergence training, including acceptance of the length of time and effort necessary.[305] Vergence training works best if the patient is young and depends somewhat on the patient's abilities.[306] More than one technique is usually necessary. Vergence training works best on positive vergences, less well on negative vergences, and even less well on vertical vergences or cyclovergences. Similar to accommodative training, a key factor in vergence training is patient management. Its important to choose an activity that the patient can understand. Training that is successful should be continued; unsuccessful training should be altered.

 CLINICAL PEARL

> Vergence training works best on positive vergences, less well on negative vergences, and even less well on vertical vergences or cyclovergences.

Vergence Training Techniques

Shorter, more frequent sessions of vergence training are more efficient than drawn-out casual sessions.[307] Slow (0.75 PD/sec) rather than fast (5 PD/sec) vergence rates are most efficient at training vergences.[288]

Many techniques have been used to train vergences (Table 6-11). Techniques selected for individuals with severe problems should be those that have the largest, most detailed stimuli.[25,86,174] Computerized techniques

TABLE 6-11 TYPES OF VERGENCE TECHNIQUES IN VARIOUS CLASSES OF TRAINING

Class	Technique
Computerized	Computer Orthopter*
Vectographic	Vectograms, minivectograms (polachrome orthopter), B & L Orthofuser
Anaglyphic	Tranaglyph, minitranaglyph
Chiastopic (chiatopic, orthopic)	Eccentric circles, lifesaver cards, aperture rule
Stereoscopes	Variable mirror stereoscope-cheiroscope, Keystone hand-held stereoscope, Keystone Telebinocular, Titmus Biopter, synoptophore
Other	Push-up training, flip lenses, flip prisms

*Teletherapy, Inc., Indianapolis, Ind.

have the advantage in that they can be controlled, and training can be easily documented. These are largely in-office techniques. Vectographic devices have good image quality and are easy to understand, although patients sometimes have difficulty understanding what their eyes are supposed to do (Fig. 6-20). Tranaglyphic devices are cheaper, although lighting demands are more stringent (Fig. 6-21). Chiastopic techniques (Fig. 6-22) are effective but difficult for patients and are usually given toward the end of the treatment regimen.[308] Stereoscopes are somewhat cumbersome to use. Push-up training is a standard method of vergence training, especially for convergence insufficiency (Fig. 6-23). Push-up training has the advantage, because it is easy and it is clearly evident that the eyes must converge to complete the training. Unfortunately, push-up training often causes a significant degree of eyestrain and can become boring quickly. In most cases, we commence training using either vectograms or tranaglyphs, proceed to the aperture rule (Fig. 6-24), and end with chiastopic techniques, such as eccentric circles or life-saver cards.

Conditions in Which Vergence Training is Prescribed

Vergence training may be useful in a wide variety of situations (Table 6-12). The most common situations in which vergence training is used are convergence insufficiency and other exodeviation problems (phoria or intermittent tropia).[309] Simple vergence training is not generally appropriate for constant strabismus unless fusion potential is demonstrated when the angle of deviation is compensated for with the synoptophore or prism. Compliance is the most significant problem associated with fusional vergence training.

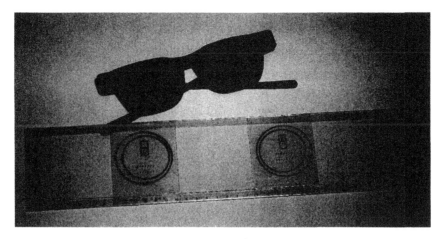

FIG. 6-20 Minivectograms are a very common method of training vergences. (Bernell Corporation, South Bend, Ind.)

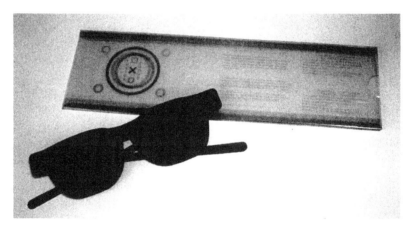

FIG. 6-21 Tranaglyphs can be used to train vergence ranges. (Bernell Corporation, South Bend, Ind.)

PRESCRIBING LENSES AND PRISMS
Effects of Added Lenses and Prisms

Lenses alter the accommodative demand. They do not change the vergence demand. Prisms change the vergence demand without altering the accommodative demand. Table 6-13 illustrates the effects of changing lenses and/or prisms on a patient with an interpupillary distance of 60 mm, an orthophoria at the near point, and an AC/A ratio of 6 PD/D. The clinician must use the AC/A ratio, phorias, and so on to calculate the demands and the resultant phoria.

Indications for Added Lenses and Prisms

Optical means should be used when other modes of treatment are not better for solving the problem(s). Other modes of treatment include orthoptics/vision therapy, ergonomics, and changes in the task or in the approach to the task or surgery.

TABLE 6-12 CONDITIONS IN WHICH VERGENCE TRAINING IS APPLIED

Type of Training	Condition
Base-out or positive vergence	Convergence insufficiency, intermittent exotropia, divergence excess, basic exophoria, constant exotropia if there is good fusion potential, A and V deviations if exo in a significant field of gaze
Base-in or negative vergence	Nonrefractive accommodative esotropia, convergence excess: if the patient is motivated and the deviation is small
	V deviations if eso in down gaze: if the patient is motivated and the deviation is small
	Basic (equal) esodeviations (tropia or phoria): if the problem is small and only if the patient is motivated

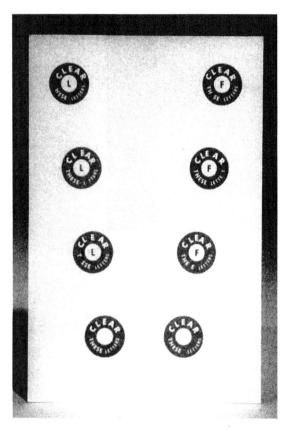

FIG. 6-22 Chiastopic fusion cards can be used to train positive vergences.

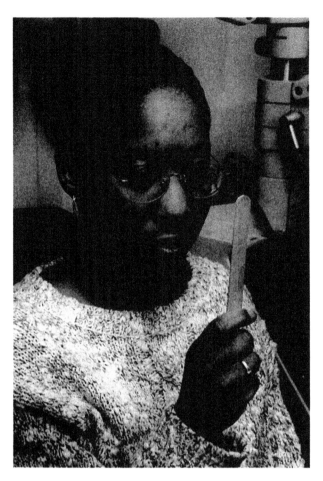

FIG. 6-23 Push-up training is a convenient method of doing positive vergence training.

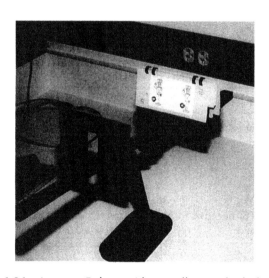

FIG. 6-24 Aperture Rule provides excellent method of training quality of fusional vergences. (Bernell Corporation, South Bend, Ind.)

Considerations in Using Added Lenses and Prisms

Lenses and/or prisms should be used as judiciously as possible. If feasible, the additions should be used on a trial basis, particularly if the effect is questionable. The use of a clip-on or a Fresnel prism on a trial basis is helpful in finding the appropriate prism.[126] Trial lenses or prisms, although time consuming, may be an effective way to deal with the problem of prism adaptation, should it become a problem. The vergence system frequently adapts to prisms prescribed to alleviate the deviation; however, those with impaired binocularity adapt less than those with good binocular vision.[250,310] The patient should understand that there is no guarantee that the additional lenses or prisms will solve the problem(s) to their expectations, and they should realize that more than one trial may be necessary.

Criteria Used In Prescribing Lenses and Prisms

Several criteria are used to prescribe added lenses or prisms. These include Sheard's criterion, Percival's criterion, the associated phoria or other techniques us-

TABLE 6-13 EXERCISE CALCULATING THE EFFECTS OF PRISMS AND LENSES ON ACCOMMODATIVE AND VERGENCE DEMAND AND THE PHORIA

Distance (cm)	Added Prisms (PD)	Added Lenses (D)	Accommodative Demand (D)	Vergence Demand (PD)	Phoria at This Distance (PD)
40	0	0	2.5	15	0
40	0	+1.00	1.5	15	6 XP
40	0	−2.00	4.5	15	12 EP
25	0	+2.00	0.5	15	12 XP
40	5 BI	0	2.5	10	6 EP
40	10 BO	0	2.5	25	10 XP
40	6 BI	+2.00	0.5	9	6 XP
100	5 BO	−1.00	3.5	20	1 EP
100	15 BO	0	2.5	30	15 XP
33	15 BI	0	2.5	0	15 EP
33	0	+0.50	2	15	3 XP
10	20 BO	+3.00	0 (blur 0.5)	35	35 XP
67	10 BI	−1.50	4	5	19 EP
67	0	−1.00	3.5	15	6 EP
50	0	+3.00	0 (blur 0.5)	15	15 XP
50	5 BO	+4.00	0 (1.5 blur)	20	20 XP

ing fixation disparity, flip prism, equalizing the fusional vergence ranges, and arbitrary selection methods. A common technique is the associated phoria or arbitrary method. There is little evidence demonstrating the superiority of one technique over others.

Associated Phoria

The associated phoria is one of the most common methods of prescribing either vertical or lateral prism. Various projected (AO vectograph) or other methods (Borish or Wesson card, the Disparometer) can be used at either distance or near. Prescribing the associated phoria is a reliable method of prescribing prism.[74,251,272]

Fixation Disparity Techniques

Individuals with poor prism adaptation have steep slopes on their fixation disparity curves, and prisms can be used to move the demand into an area that is relatively flat. Prescribing the minimum amount of prism to shift the fixation disparity curve so that the flat portion of the fixation disparity curve is just at the Y axis is a good method of prescribing prism.[74] A relationship exists between the slope of the vertical fixation disparity curve and the amount of prism adaptation; flatter fixation disparity curves are related to greater prism adaptation.[243,252,269,275,276]

Arbitrary Selection Methods

Many experienced clinicians arbitrarily select prism for prescription. Generally, the amount of prism is around one quarter to one half of the deviation. If a deviation is small, it is more likely that nearly the entire deviation will be prescribed.

Sheard's Criterion

Although primarily used for the diagnosis of vergence anomalies (particularly exophoria), Sheard's criterion can also be used for prescribing lateral prism.[116] The amount of prism is calculated so that the opposing vergence is twice the phoria (demand). Consider an example in which the patient is 6-PD esophoric with negative vergences of x/10/8 and positive vergences of x/6/4. The clinician should use the opposing vergence (negative) to calculate the amount of prism necessary to allow the criterion to be met. In this case, 1 PD BO gives a phoria of 5 PD EP, and an opposing BI vergence of 11 PD to break. Sheard's criterion may suggest fairly large amounts of prism. For example, for a patient with a 15-PD esophoria, BI vergence of x/10/8, and BO vergence of x/6/4, 7 PD BO is suggested.

Percival's Criterion

Percival's criterion is also used for the diagnosis of vergence-related problems, especially esophoria, and for prescribing lateral prism. The amount of prism is calculated to place the demand in the middle third of the vergence range (see Criteria for Normal Binocular Vision). The prism to be prescribed is independent of the phoria. For example, in a patient with a 6-PD esophoria with a negative vergence of x/10/8 and a positive vergence of x/6/4, if one vergence range is large, as sometimes happens with positive vergences, the amount of prism suggested may be quite sizable.

TABLE 6-14 CONDITIONS IN WHICH LENSES AND/OR PRISMS ARE USED IN TREATMENT

Appliance	Conditions
Lenses: plus adds	Accommodative dysfunction (including presbyopia); non-refractive accommodative esotropia; convergence excess esophoria; V deviations if eso in down gaze; esodeviations (tropia or phoria) if problem is primarily at the nearpoint
Lenses: minus additions, overminus	Intermittent exotropia; divergence excess; congenital nystagmus if deviation causes convergence that damps the nystagmus
Prisms: base-out	Basic esophoria; constant esotropia if there is good fusion potential; intermittent esotropia if the deviation is about the same at distance and near; convergence that damps the nystagmus
Prisms: base-in	Basic exophoria; intermittent exotropia if deviation is about the same at distance and near, particularly if accommodation is defective so that overminus cannot be used; constant exotropia if there is good fusion potential
Prisms: base vertical	Vertical phorias
Prisms: yoked (bases in the same direction)	Incomitancies to move lines of sight away from the field of difficulty (e.g., bilateral base-down prisms in V pattern eso or A pattern exodeviations; A and V deviations to move lines of sight away from the area of greatest difficulty

Equalizing Fusional Vergence Ranges

The method of equalizing fusional vergence ranges is primarily useful for vertical deviations. In this technique, the clinician prescribes the amount of prism necessary to equalize the base-up and base-down vertical ranges. For example, if the base-up range is 6/2 and the base-down range is 2/1, then 2 PD BU would provide equal up and down ranges.

Limits in Prescribing Added Prisms and Lenses

Practical limits for prescribing added lenses are relatively few, although a near add generally should not exceed 2.5 to 3 D. An overminus addition generally should not exceed −2.5 D, unless it is clear that the patient's accommodative system can function adequately with the additional accommodative demand. Dynamic retinoscopy can be used to check the ability of the accommodative system to respond. If a normal lag is maintained over the added lens, accommodation is adapting well.

Limits for the use of prisms are more stringent. Except on rare occasions, no more than 5 to 6 PD should be used in each lens. The degradation of the optical quality and the weight and thickness imbalance become significant when this limit is exceeded. Fresnel prisms can be prescribed up to 40 PD per lens. Visual acuity is somewhat degraded with these prisms.

Conditions in Which Lenses and/or Prisms Are Prescribed

Lenses or prisms alone or in combination are appropriate in many situations. Table 6-14 lists the most significant occasions.

Problems Associated with the Use of Prisms and Lenses

The problems associated with the use of prisms and lenses are several, and there is no foolproof method of selecting the right corrective means. The patient should understand that more than one trial is sometimes necessary. The tentative lens or prism should be evaluated on a trial basis using dynamic retinoscopy (if a lens) and by letting the patient do a few minutes of reading in the office, if possible. The accommodative and prismatic demands change when going from spectacles to contact lenses and vice versa and should be considered.[311] For example, spectacle lenses provide prism whenever the patient does not view through the optical center of the correction. Accommodative demand changes when going from spectacles to contact lenses (individuals with myopia must accommodate more). The cosmesis of the correction is important. High-index materials can dramatically reduce edge thickness. Variable-focus lenses are important in eliminating the detrimental effects of cosmesis in prescribing plus adds.

The stability of a correction achieved with prisms is a concern. The tendency to adapt to a prism may completely negate the beneficial effects of the device. The prism adaptation test can be used to evaluate the possibility of prism adaptation, but selection of a sufficient time interval is difficult.[312] Prism adaptation occurs to a lesser extent in patients with binocular vision problems and can result in a re-creation of the deviation through the added prism.[250,313,314] A major proportion of prism adaptation occurs in several minutes to an added prism; however, complete adaptation to prism continues for a much longer period after the phoria has returned to its baseline.[315,316,317] This helps in dealing with changing demands in new spectacle prescriptions.[316] Adaptation can also occur to spectacle lens anisometropia, but it occurs to a lesser extent and less often.[318] Patients have been shown to adapt to 3 D of induced anisometropia within a two-and-a-half-hour period.

Evaluating Prisms and Lenses

Lens and prism efficacy can be evaluated both subjectively and objectively. This task is sometimes difficult because of the many confounding variables. Objectively, clinicians should check to see if a normal lag is being maintained and if prism adaptation has occurred to a significant extent. Carefully questioning the patient about the effects of the treatment is important in subjective evaluation of the condition.

REFERENCES

1. Cooper J and others: Reduction of asthenopia in patients with convergence insufficiency after fusional vergence training, *Am J Optom Physiol Opt* 60:982, 1983.
2. Sheedy JE and others: Task performance with base-in and base-out prism, *Am J Optom Physiol Opt* 65:65, 1988.
3. Eskridge JB: A specific procedure for the cover test, *J Am Optom Assoc* 33:53, 1961.
4. Eskridge JB: The cover test, *Optom Today* 2:2, 1972.
5. Eskridge JB: The complete cover test, *J Am Optom Assoc* 44:602, 1973.
6. Peli E, McCormack G: Dynamics of cover test eye movements, *Am J Optom Physiol Opt* 60:712, 1983.
7. Daum KM: Heterophoria and heterotropia. In Eskridge JB, Amos JF, Bartlett JD, editors: *Clinical procedures in optometry*, Philadelphia, 1991, JB Lippincott.
8. Wesson MD: Normalization of prism bar vergences, *Am J Optom Physiol Opt* 59:628, 1982.
9. Vaegan, Pye D: Independence of convergence and divergence: norms, age trends and potentiation in mechanized prism tests, *Am J Optom Physiol Opt* 56:143, 1979.
10. Boltz RL and others: Vertical fusional vergence ranges of the Rhesus monkey, *Vision Res* 20:83, 1980.
11. Houtman WA, Roze JH, Scheper W: Vertical vergence movements, *Doc Ophthalmol* 51:199, 1981.
12. Jones R, Kerr KE: Motor responses to conflicting asymmetrical vergence stimulus information, *Am J Optom Arch Am Acad Optom* 48:989, 1971.
13. Kertesz AE: The effect of stimulus complexity on human cyclofusional response, *Vision Res* 12:699, 1972.
14. Kertesz AE, Jones RW: Human cyclofusional response, *Vision Res* 10:891, 1970.
15. Kertesz AE, Sullivan MJ: The effect of stimulus size on human cyclofusional response, *Vision Res* 18:567, 1978.
16. Sullivan MJ, Kertesz AE: Peripheral stimulation and human cyclofusional response, *Invest Ophthalmol Vis Sci* 18:1287, 1979.
17. Nauheim JS: A preliminary investigation of retinal locus as a factor in fusion, *AMA Arch Ophthalmol* 58: 122, 1957.
18. Wesson MD, Amos JF: Norms for hand-held rotary prism vergences, *Am J Optom Physiol Opt* 62:88, 1985.
19. Morgan MW: The clinical aspects of accommodation and convergence, *Am J Optom Arch Am Acad Optom* 21:301, 1944.
20. Morgan MW: Analysis of clinical data, *Am J Optom Arch Am Acad Optom* 21:477, 1944.
21. Sheni DD, Remole A: A new method of measuring vergence limits: the rotatory grid technique, *Am J Optom Physiol Opt* 59:240, 1982.
22. Feldman JM and others: Comparison of fusional ranges measured by Risley prisms, vectograms and Computer Orthopter, *Optom Vis Sci* 66:375, 1989.
23. Hardesty HH: Management of intermittent exotropia, *Binoc Vis Eye Muscle Surg* 5:145, 1990.

24. Hampton DR, Kertesz AE: Human response to cyclofusional stimuli containing depth cues, *Am J Optom Physiol Opt* 59:21, 1982.
25. Kertesz AE: Effect of stimulus size on fusion and vergence, *J Opt Soc Am* 71:289, 1981.
26. Boman DK, Kertesz AE: Effect of stimulus parameters on fusional and stereoscopic performance, *Am J Optom Physiol Opt* 62:222, 1985.
27. Fowler MS, Riddell PM, Stein JF: The effect of varying vergence speed and target size on the amplitude of vergence eye movements, *Brit Orthopt J* 45:49, 1988.
28. Cooper J, Feldman J, Eichler R: Relative strength of central and peripheral fusion as a function of stimulus parameters, *Optom Vis Sci* 69:966, 1992.
29. Wick B: Clinical factors in proximal vergence, *Am J Optom Physiol Opt* 62:1, 1985.
30. Wick B, Bedell HE: Magnitude and velocity of proximal vergence, *Invest Ophthalmol Vis Sci* 30:755, 1989.
31. Gray LS and others: Objective concurrent measures of open-loop accommodation and vergence under photopic conditions, *Invest Ophthalmol Vis Sci* 34:2996, 1993.
32. Stephens GL, Jones R: Horizontal fusional amplitudes after adaptation to prism, *Ophthalmic Physiol Opt* 10:25, 1990.
33. Eskridge JB: Heterophoria and fusional vergence amplitude, *Refract Lett* 19:2, 1975.
34. Grisham JD: Treatment of binocular dysfunctions. In Schor CM, Ciuffreda KJ, editors: *Basic and clinical aspects of vergence eye movements*, Boston, 1983, Butterworth-Heinemann.
35. Griffin JR, Grisham JD: *Binocular anomalies, diagnosis and vision therapy*, Boston, 1995, Butterworths-Heinemann.
36. Buzzelli AR: Vergence facility: developmental trends in a school-age population, *Am J Optom Physiol Opt* 63:351, 1986.
37. Ogle KN, Martens TG, Dyer JA: *Oculomotor imbalance in binocular vision and fixation disparity*, Philadelphia, 1969, Lea and Febiger.
38. Sheedy JE, Saladin JJ: Exophoria at near in presbyopia, *Am J Optom Physiol Opt* 52:474, 1975.
39. Sheedy JE, Saladin JJ: Phoria, vergence, and fixation disparity in oculomotor problems, *Am J Optom Physiol Opt* 54:474, 1977.
40. Sheedy JE, Saladin JJ: Association of symptoms with measures of oculomotor deficiencies, *Am J Optom Physiol Opt* 55:670, 1978.
41. Sheedy JE: Fixation disparity analysis of oculomotor imbalance, *Am J Optom Physiol Opt* 57:632, 1980.
42. Sheedy JE: Actual measurement of fixation disparity and its use in diagnosis and treatment, *J Am Optom Assoc* 51:1079, 1980.
43. Crone R, Hardjowijoto S: What is normal binocular vision? *Doc Ophthalmol* 47:163, 1979.
44. Goss DA: Ocular accommodation, convergence, and fixation disparity: a manual of clinical analysis, New York, 1986, Professional.
45. Yeager MD, Boltz RL: Computerized fixation disparity measurements, *Am J Optom Physiol Opt* 63:654, 1986.

46. Pickwell LD, Jenkins TCA, Yetka AA: Fixation disparity in binocular stress, *Ophthalmic Physiol Opt* 7:37, 1987.

47. Garzia RP, Dyer G: Effect of nearpoint stress on the horizontal forced vergence fixation disparity curve, *Am J Optom Physiol Opt* 63:901, 1986.

48. Brownlee GA, Goss DA: Comparisons of commercially available devices for the measurement of fixation disparity and associated phorias, *J Am Optom Assoc* 59:451, 1988.

49. Rutstein RP, Godio LB: Zone of zero-associated phoria in patients with convergence insufficiency, *Am J Optom Physiol Opt* 60:582, 1985.

50. Duwaer AL: New measures of fixation disparity in the diagnosis of binocular oculomotor deficiencies, *Am J Optom Physiol Opt* 60:586, 1983.

51. London R, Wick B: Relationship between fixation disparity curves and symptoms in monofixators, *J Am Optom Assoc* 53:881, 1982.

52. Hung GK, Ciuffreda KJ, Semmlow JL: Static vergence and accommodation: population norms and orthoptics/vision therapy effects, *Doc Ophthalmol* 62:165, 1986.

53. Schor CM, Ciuffreda KJ, editors: *Basic and clinical aspects of vergence eye movements,* St Louis, 1983, Butterworth-Heinemann.

54. Saladin JJ: Convergence insufficiency, fixation disparity, and control systems analysis, *Am J Optom Physiol Opt* 63:645, 1986.

55. Saladin JJ, Carr LW: Fusion lock diameter and the forced vergence fixation disparity curve, *Am J Optom Physiol Opt* 60:933, 1983.

56. Mitchell AM, Ellerbrock VJ: Fixation disparity and the maintenance of fusion in the horizontal meridian, *Am J Optom* 32:520, 1955.

57. Carter DB: Studies in fixation disparity. III. The apparent uniocular components of fixation disparity, *Am J Optom Arch Am Acad Optom* 37:408, 1960.

58. Schor C: The influence of rapid prism adaptation upon fixation disparity, *Vision Res* 19:757, 1979.

59. Debysingh SJ, Orzech PL, Sheedy JE: Effect of a central fusion stimulus on fixation disparity, *Am J Optom Physiol Opt* 63:277, 1986.

60. Sheedy JE: Should a central fusion stimulus be used on the Disparometer? *Am J Optom Physiol Opt* 63:627, 1986.

61. Remole A: Fixation disparity vs. binocular fixation misalignment, *Am J Optom Physiol Opt* 62:25, 1985.

62. Irving EL, Robertson KM: Monocular components of the fixation disparity curve, *Optom Vis Sci* 68:117, 1991.

63. Reading RW: Vergence errors: some hitherto unreported aspects of fixation disparity, *Optom Vis Sci* 69:538, 1992.

64. Hebbard FW: Foveal fixation disparity measurements and their use in determining the relationship between accommodative convergence and accommodation, *Am J Optom* 37:3, 1960.

65. Hebbard FW: Effect of blur on fixation disparity, *Am J Optom* 41:540, 1964.

66. Mitchell D: A review of the concept of "Panum's fusional areas," *Am J Optom* 43:387, 1966.

67. Frantz KA, Scharre JE: Comparison of Disparometer fixation disparity curves as measured with and without the phoropter, *Optom Vis Sci* 67:117, 1990.

68. Wesson MD, Koenig R: A new clinical method for direct measurement of fixation disparity, *South J Optom* 1:48, 1983.

69. Van Haeringen R, McClurg P, Cameron KD: Comparison of Wesson and modified Sheedy fixation disparity tests. Do fixation disparity measures relate to normal binocular status? *Ophthalmic Physiol Opt* 6:397, 1986.

70. Goss DA, Patel J: Comparison of fixation disparity curve variables measured with the Sheedy Disparometer and the Wesson fixation disparity card, *Optom Vis Sci* 72:580, 1995.

71. Dowley D: Fixation disparity, *Optom Vis Sci* 66:98, 1989.

72. Scheiman M, Wick B: *Clinical management of binocular vision: heterophoric, accommodative, and eye movement disorders,* Philadelphia, 1994, JB Lippincott.

73. Schor CM, Narayan V: Graphical analysis of prism adaptation, convergence accommodation, and accommodative convergence, *Am J Optom Physiol Opt* 59:774, 1982.

74. Wick B, London R: Analysis of binocular visual function using tests made under binocular conditions, *Am J Optom Physiol Opt* 64:227, 1987.

75. Cooper J, Feldman J: Operant conditioning of fusional convergence ranges using random dot stereograms, *Am J Optom Physiol Opt* 57:205, 1980.

76. Cooper J, Feldman J: Operant conditioning and assessment of stereopsis in young children, *Am J Optom Physiol Opt* 55:532, 1978.

77. Duane A: A new classification of the motor anomalies of the eyes based on physiological principles, together with their symptoms, diagnosis, and treatment, *Ann Ophthalmol Otolaryngol* 6:84, 1897.

78. Duane A: *A new classification of motor anomalies of the eye,* New York, 1897, JH Vail.

79. Michaels D: *Visual optics and refraction,* ed 2, St Louis, 1980, Mosby.

80. Burian H, Spivey B: The surgical management of exodeviations, *Am J Ophthalmol* 59:603, 1959.

81. Norn MS: Convergence insufficiency: incidence in ophthalmic practice—results of orthoptic treatment, *Acta Ophthalmol (Kbl)* 44:132, 1966.

82. Duke-Elder S, Wybar K: Ocular motility and strabismus. In: Duke-Elder S, editor: *System of ophthalmology,* vol 6, St Louis, 1973, Mosby.

83. Grisham JD: Visual therapy results for convergence insufficiency: a literature review, *Am J Optom Physiol Opt* 65:448, 1988.

84. Passmore JW, MacLean F: Convergence insufficiency and its management, *Am J Ophthalmol* 43:448, 1957.

85. Cushman B, Burri C: Convergence insufficiency, *Am J Ophthalmol* 24:1044, 1941.

86. Kertesz AE: The effectiveness of wide-angle fusional stimulation in the treatment of convergence insufficiency, *Invest Ophthalmol Vis Sci* 22:690, 1982.

87. Hirsch MJ: A study of forty-eight cases of convergence insufficiency at the near point, *Am J Optom Arch Am Acad Optom* 20:52, 1943.

88. Mahto RS: Eye strain from convergence insufficiency, *Br Med J* 2:564, 1972.

89. Daum KM: Convergence insufficiency, *Am J Optom Physiol Opt* 61:16, 1984.

90. Cooper J, Duckman R: Convergence insufficiency: incidence, diagnosis, and treatment, *J Am Optom Assoc* 49:673, 1978.

91. Kent PR, Steeve JH: Convergence insufficiency: incidence among military personnel and relief by orthoptic methods, *Milit Surgeon* 112:202, 1953.

92. Kratka Z, Kratka WH: Convergence insufficiency: its frequency and importance, *Am Orthopt J* 6:72, 1956.

93. Mayou S: The treatment of convergence deficiency, *Br Orthopt J* 3:72, 1945.

94. Mould WL: Recognition and management of atypical convergence insufficiency, *J Pediatr Ophthalmol* 7:212, 1970.

95. White J, Brown H: Occurrence of vertical anomalies associated with convergent and divergent anomalies: a clinical study, *Arch Ophthalmol* 21:999, 1939.

96. Smith A: Convergence deficiency: an occupational study, *Br Orthopt J* 8:56, 1951.

97. Burian HM: Third Symposium on Strabismus, New Orleans, 1970. In Jampolsky A, editor: *Transactions of the New Orleans Academy of Ophthalmology,* St Louis, 1971, Mosby.

98. Mellick A: Convergence deficiency: an investigation into the results of treatment, *Br J Ophthalmol* 34:41, 1950.
99. Mann I: Convergence deficiency, *Br J Ophthalmol* 24:373, 1940.
100. Mann I: Convergence deficiency: the condition, its occurrence in private practice and the results of treatment, *Br Med J* 1:208, 1940.
101. Fink WH: Symposium: convergence insufficiency— pathophysiology, *Am Orthopt J* 3:5, 1953.
102. Nawratzki I, Avrouskine M: Psychogenic factors of ocular muscle balance, *Acta Med Orient* 16:94. 1957.
103. Daum KM: Characteristics of convergence insufficiency, *Am J Optom Physiol Opt* 65:426, 1988.
104. Daum KM: Characteristics of exodeviations. I. A comparison of three classes, *Am J Optom Physiol Opt* 63:237, 1986.
105. Hung GK: Reduced vergence response velocities in dyslexics: a preliminary report, *Ophthalmic Physiol Opt* 9:420, 1989.
106. Cinotti A and others: Diplopia in the aged: etiology and management, *J Am Geriatr Soc* 28:84, 1980.
107. Capobianco NM: Incidence and diagnosis, *Am Orthopt J* 3:13, 1953.
108. Hermann JS: Surgical therapy for convergence insufficiency, *J Pediatr Ophthalmol Strab* 18:28, 1981.
109. Davies CE: Orthoptic treatment in convergence insufficiency, *Can M A J* 55:47, 1946.
110. Shippman S and others: Convergence insufficiency with normal parameters, *J Pediatr Ophthalmol Strab* 20:158, 1983.
111. Simpson GV: Medical management, *Am Orthopt J* 3:18, 1953.
112. Krohel GB and others: Post-traumatic convergence insufficiency, *Ann Ophthalmol* 18:101, 1986.
113. Wilmer WH, Berens CV: The effect of altitude on ocular functions, *JAMA* 71:1394, 1918.
114. Bugola J: Hypoaccommodation and convergence insufficiency, *Am Orthopt J* 27:85, 1977.
115. Mazow ML: The convergence insufficiency syndrome, *J Pediatr Ophthalmol Strab* 8:243, 1971.
116. Sheard C: Zones of ocular comfort, *Am J Optom* 7:9, 1930.
117. Schwyzer EB: Aspects of the treatment of convergence insufficiency, *Br Orthopt J* 35:28, 1978.
118. LeTourneau JE, Lapierrre N, Lamont A: The relationship between convergence insufficiency and school achievement, *Am J Optom Physiol Opt* 56:18, 1979.
119. Pickwell LD, Stephens LC: Inadequate convergence, *Br J Physiol Opt* 30:34, 1975.
120. Brinkley JR, Walonker F: Convergence amplitude insufficiency, *Ann Ophthalmol* 15:826, 1983.
121. Michaels DD: A clinical study of convergence insufficiency, *Am J Optom Arch Am Acad Optom* 30:65, 1953.
122. Pickwell LD, Hampshire R: The significance of inadequate convergence, *Ophthalmic Physiol Opt* 1:13, 1981.
123. Pickwell LD, Hampshire R: Jump-convergence test in strabismus, *Ophthalmic Physiol Opt* 1:123, 1981.
124. Hokoda SC: General binocular dysfunctions in an urban optometry clinic, *J Am Optom Assoc* 56:560, 1982.
125. Prakash P, Agarwal LP, Nag SG: Accommodational weakness and convergence insufficiency, *Orient Arch Ophthal* 10:261, 1972.
126. Berens C, Connolly PT, Kern D: Certain motor anomalies of the eye in relation to prescribing lenses, *Am J Ophthalmol* 16:199, 1933.
127. von Noorden GK, Brown DJ, Parks M: Associated convergence and accommodative insufficiency, *Doc Ophthalmol* 34:393, 1973.
128. Raskind R: Problems at the reading distance, *Am Orthopt J* 26:53, 1976.
129. Stark L and others: Accommodative disfacility presenting as intermittent exotropia, *Ophthalmic Physiol Opt* 4:233, 1984.
130. Davies CE: Etiology and management of convergence insufficiency, *Am Orthopt J* 6:124, 1956.
131. Rosenfeld J: Convergence insufficiency in children and adults, *Am Orthopt J* 17:93, 1967.
132. Pickwell LD, Hampshire R: Convergence insufficiency in patients taking medicines, *Ophthalmic Physiol Opt* 4:151, 1984.
133. Morgan OG: Convergence weakness, *Br J Ophthalmol* 24:564, 1940.
134. von Noorden GK: Resection of both medial rectus muscles in organic convergence insufficiency, *Am J Ophthalmol* 81:223, 1976.
135. Haldi BA: Surgical management of convergence insufficiency, *Am Orthopt J* 28:106, 1978.
136. Dalziel CC: Effect of vision training on patients who fail Sheard's criterion, *Am J Optom Physiol Opt* 58:21, 1981.
137. Carroll R, Seaber JH: Acute loss of fusional convergence following head trauma, *Am Orthopt J* 24:57, 1974.
138. Anderson M: Orthoptic treatment of loss of convergence and accommodation caused by road accidents ("whiplash" injury), *Br Orthopt J* 18:117, 1961.
139. Burian HM: Symposium: convergence insufficiency—summary, *Am Orthopt J* 3:26, 1953.
140. Bennett GR, Blondin M, Ruskiewicz J: Incidence and prevalence of selected visual conditions, *J Am Optom Assoc* 53:647, 1982.
141. Gordon YJ, Mokete M: Screening of pre-school and school children for ocular anomalies in Lesotho, *J Trop Med Hyg* 85:135, 1982.
142. Morris CW: A theory concerning adaptation to accommodative impairment, *Optom Wkly* 50:255, 1959.
143. Duthie OM: Convergence deficiency, *Br Orthopt J* 2:38, 1944.
144. Grieve J, Archibald DH: Some facts and figures relating to heterophoria in symptom-free individuals, *Trans Ophthalmol Soc U K* 62:285, 1942.
145. Manson N: Anaemia as an etiological factor in convergence insufficiency, *Br J Ophthalmol* 46:674, 1962.
146. Benton CD: Management of dyslexias associated with binocular control anomalies. In Keeney AH, Kennedy VT, editors: *Dyslexia: diagnosis and treatment of reading disorders,* St Louis, 1968, Mosby.
147. Eames TH: Comparison of eye conditions among 1000 reading failures, 500 ophthalmic patients and 150 unselected children, *Am J Ophthalmol* 31:713, 1948.
148. Cohen AH, Sodden R: Effectiveness of visual therapy for convergence insufficiencies for an adult population, *J Am Optom Assoc* 55:491, 1984.
149. Daum KM: Accommodative insufficiency, *Am J Optom Physiol Opt* 60:352, 1983.
150. Liepmann ME: Accommodative and convergence insufficiency after decompression sickness, *Arch Ophthalmol* 99:453, 1981.
151. Shearer RV: Eye findings in children with reading difficulties, *J Pediatr Ophthalmol Strab* 3:47, 1966.
152. Norn MS, Rindziunski E, Skysgaard H: Ophthalmologic and orthoptic examinations of dyslectics, *Acta Ophthalmol (Kbh)* 47:147, 1969.
153. Atzmon D: Positive effect of improving relative fusional vergence on reading and learning disabilities, *Binoc Vis Eye Muscle Surg* 1:39, 1985.
154. Cohen RL, Moore S: Strabismus in the aphakic patient, *Am Orthopt J* 86:2101, 1979.
155. Ohtsuka K and others: Accommodation and convergence insufficiency with left middle cerebral artery occlusion, *Am J Ophthalmol* 106:60, 1988.
156. Cogan D: *Neurology of the ocular muscles,* ed 2, Springfield, Ill, 1956, CC Thomas.
157. Zorn M, Sajban T: Convergence insufficiency masks a growing tumor, *Optometry* p 96, Oct 1986 (review).

158. Tassinari J: Methyldopa-related convergence insufficiency, *J Am Optom Assoc* 60:311, 1990.

159. Cohen M and others: Convergence insufficiency in brain-injured patients, *Brain Injury* 3:187, 1989.

160. Potaznick W, Kozol N: Ocular manifestations of chronic fatigue and immune dysfunction syndrome, *Optom Vis Sci* 69:811, 1992.

161. Sasaki JDI: Exophoria and accommodative convergence insufficiency, *Optom Wkly* 47:811, 1956.

162. Sasaki JD: Convergence-accommodative dysfunction due to anoxia, *Optom Wkly* 42:2044, 1952.

163. Brown B: The convergence insufficiency masquerade, *Am Orthopt J* 40:94, 1990.

164. Kokmen E and others: Neurological manifestations of aging, *J Geront* 32:411, 1977.

165. Schor CM: The Glenn A Fry Award Lecture: Adaptive regulation of accommodative vergence and vergence accommodation, *Am J Optom Physiol Opt* 63:587, 1986.

166. Jampolsky A: Ocular divergence mechanisms, *Trans Amer Ophthalmol Soc* 68:730, 1971.

167. Sheedy JE, Saladin JJ: Validity of diagnostic criteria and case analysis in binocular vision disorders. In Schor CM, Ciuffreda KJ, editors: *Vergence eye movements: basic and clinical aspects*, Boston, 1983, Butterworth-Heinemann.

168. Hammerberg E, Norn MS: Defective dissociation of accommodation and convergence in dyslectic children, *Acta Ophthalmol (Kbh)* 50:651, 1972.

169. Wick B: Vision training for presbyopic nonstrabismic patients, *Am J Optom Physiol Opt* 54:244, 1977.

170. Anderson EC: Treatment of convergence insufficiency: a review, *Am Orthopt J* 19:72, 1969.

171. Appleman LF: Prism exercises for functional insufficiency of the ocular muscles, *Arch Ophthalmol* 13:1118, 1935.

172. Healy E: Orthoptic treatment, *Am Orthopt J* 3:23, 1953.

173. Lyle TK, Jackson S: *Practical orthoptics/vision therapy*, ed 2, Philadelphia, 1941, Blakiston & Son.

174. Kertesz AE, Kertesz J: Wide-field fusional stimulation in strabismus, *Am J Optom Physiol Opt* 63:217, 1986.

175. Cason HA: Convergence insufficiency and foveal fusion, *Am Orthopt J* 10:80, 1960.

176. Manas L: The effect of visual training upon the AC/A ratio, *Am J Optom Arch Am Acad Optom* 35:428, 1958.

177. Flom MC: On the relationship between accommodation and accommodative convergence. III. Effects of orthoptics/vision therapy, *Am J Opt Arch Am Acad Optom* 37:619, 1960.

178. Judge SJ: Optically-induced changes in tonic vergence and AC/A ratio in normal monkeys and monkeys with lesions of the flocculus and ventral paraflocculus, *Exp Brain Res* 66:1, 1987.

179. Miles FA, Judge SJ, Optican LM: Optically induced changes in the couplings between vergence and accommodation, *J Neurosci* 7:2576, 1987.

180. Grisham JD and others: Vergence orthoptics/vision therapy: validity and persistence of training effect, *Optom Vision Sci* 68:441, 1991.

181. Pantano F: Orthoptic treatment of convergence insufficiency: a two year follow-up report, *Am Orthopt J* 32:73, 1982.

182. Flax N, Selenow A: Results of surgical treatment of intermittent divergent strabismus, *Am J Optom Physiol Opt* 62:100, 1985.

183. Daum KM: Equal exodeviations: characteristics and results of treatment with orthoptics/vision therapy, *Aust J Optom* 67:53, 1984.

184. Romano PE, Wilson ME, Robinson D: In this issue: preview and comment, *Binoc Vis Eye Muscle Surg* 8:127, 1993.

185. Berard P: Prisms: their therapeutic use in the child—instrumentation, indications and management, *J Pediatr Ophthalmol Strab* 5:53, 1968.

186. Sanfilippo S, Clahane A: Effectiveness of orthoptics/vision therapy alone in selected cases of exodeviation: the immediate results and several years later, *Am Orthopt J* 20:104, 1970.

187. Keech RV, Stewart SA: The surgical overcorrection of intermittent exotropia, *J Pediatr Ophthalmol Strab* 27:218, 1990.

188. Daum KM: A model for predicting the results of orthoptics/vision therapy in patients with equal exodeviations, *Aust J Optom* 67:171, 1984.

189. Rutstein RP, Marsh-Tootle W, London R: Changes in refractive error for exotropes treated with overminus lenses, *Optom Vis Sci* 66:487, 1989.

190. Cooper J: Intermittent exotropia of the divergence excess type, *J Am Optom Assoc* 48:1261, 1977.

191. Burian H: Exodeviations: their classifications, diagnosis, and treatment, *Am J Ophthal* 62:1161, 1966.

192. Cooper J, Medow N: Major review: intermittent exotropia—basic and divergence excess type, *Binoc Vis Eye Muscle Surg* 8:185, 1993.

193. Daum KM: Divergence excess: characteristics and results of treatment with orthoptics/vision therapy, *Ophthalmic Physiol Opt* 4:15, 1984.

194. Dunnington J: Divergence excess: its diagnosis and treatment, *Arch Ophthalmol* 56:344, 1927.

195. Kran BS, Duckman R: Divergence excess exotropia, *J Am Optom Assoc* 58:921, 1987.

196. Wang FM, Chryssanthou G: Monocular eye closure in intermittent exotropia, *Arch Ophthalmol* 106:941, 1988.

197. Jampolsky A: Differential diagnostic characteristics of intermittent exotropia and true exophoria, *Am Orthopt J* 4:48, 1954.

198. Ogle KN, Dyer JA: Some observations on intermittent exotropia, *Arch Ophthalmol* 73:58, 1965.

199. Larson WL: A technique to measure accommodative convergence, heterophoria, and the AC/A during single binocular vision, *Am J Optom Physiol Opt* 59:111, 1982.

200. Dunlap E, Gaffney R: Surgical management of intermittent exotropia, *Am Orthopt J* 13:20, 1963.

201. von Noorden GK: Divergence excess and simulated divergence excess: diagnosis and surgical managemen, *Ophthalmologica* 26:719, 1969.

202. Cooper J, Ciuffreda KJ, Kruger PB: Stimulus and response AC/A ratios in intermittent exotropia of the divergence-excess type, *Brit J Ophthalmol* 66:398, 1982.

203. Parks MM: Comitant exodeviations in children. In Haik GM, editor: *Strabismus: Symposium of the New Orleans Academy of Ophthalmology*, St Louis, 1962, Mosby.

204. Cooper EL: Surgical management of secondary exotropia, *Trans Am Acad Ophthalmol Otolaryngol* 65:595, 1961.

205. Costenbader FD: The physiology and management of divergent strabismus. In Allen JH, editor: *Strabismus: ophthalmic symposium*, St Louis, 1950, Mosby.

206. Ciancia A, Melka N: A new treatment for anomalous retinal correspondence in intermittent exotropia. In Fells P, editor: *First Congress of the International Strabismological Association*, St Louis, 1971, Mosby.

207. Pickwell L: Prevalence and management of divergence excess, *Am J Optom Physiol Opt* 56:78, 1979.

208. Bruce GM: Ocular divergence: its physiology and pathology, *Arch Ophthalmol* 13:639, 1935.

209. Jampolsky A: Physiology of intermittent exotropia, *Am Orthopt J* 13:5, 1963.

210. Posner A: Divergence excess considered as an anomaly of the postural tonus of the muscular apparatus, *Am J Ophthalmol* 27:1136, 1944.

211. Binion W: The surgical treatment of intermittent exotropia, *Am J Ophthalmol* 61:869, 1966.

212. Knapp P: Intermittent exotropia: evaluation and therapy, *Am Orthopt J* 3:27, 1953.

213. Mann D: The role of orthoptic treatment, *Brit Orthopt J* 4:30, 1947.

214. Daum KM: Modeling the results of the orthoptic treatment of divergence excess, *Ophthalmic Physiol Opt* 4:25, 1984b.

215. Caltrider N, Jampolsky A: Overcorrecting minus lens therapy for treatment of intermittent exotropia, *Ophthalmology* 90:1160, 1983.

216. Frantz KA: The importance of multiple treatment modalities in a case of divergence excess, *J Am Optom Assoc* 61:457, 1990.

217. Durran F: Orthoptic treatment of intermittent divergent strabismus of the divergent excess type, *Br Orthopt J* 18:110, 1961.

218. Goldrich SG: Optometric therapy of divergence excess strabismus, *Am J Optom Physiol Opt* 57:7, 1980.

219. Rowe FJ: Treatment of intermittent distance exotropia, *Brit Orthopt J* 47:90, 1990.

220. Moore S. Orthoptic treatment for intermittent exotropia. *Am Orthopt J* 3:14, 1963.

221. Ludlam W: The orthoptic treatment of strabismus, *Am Optom Arch Am Acad Optom* 38:369, 1961.

222. Fry GA: Fundamental variables in the relationship between accommodation and convergence, *Optom Wkly* 34:153, 1943.

223. Ludlam W, Kleinham B: The long range results of orthoptic treatment of strabismus, *Am J Optom Arch Am Acad Optom* 42:647, 1965.

224. Hill RV: The accommodative effort syndrome, *Am J Ophthalmol* 34:423, 1951.

225. Moore S: The accommodative effort syndrome, *Am Orthopt J* 7:5, 1967.

226. von Noorden GK, Avilla CW: Accommodative convergence in hypermetropia, *Am J Ophthalmol* 110:287, 1990.

227. Raab EL, Spierer A: Persisting accommodative esotropia, *Arch Ophthalmol* 104:1777, 1986.

228. Jacob JL, Beaulieu Y, Brunet E: Progressive addition lenses in the management of esotropia with a high accommodation/convergence ratio, *Can J Ophthalmol* 15:166, 1980.

229. Valentino JA: Clinical use of progressive addition lenses on non-presbyopic patients, *Optom Mnthly* 73:1, 1982.

230. Goss DA, Grosvenor T: Rates of childhood myopia progression with bifocals as a function of nearpoint phoria: consistency of three studies, *Optom Vis Sci* 67:637, 1990.

231. Repka MX and others: Changes in refractive error of 94 spectacle-treated patients with acquired accommodative esotropia, *Binoc Vis Eye Muscle Surg* 4:15, 1989.

232. Smith JB: Progressive-addition lenses in the treatment of accommodative esotropia, *Am J Ophthalmol* 99:56, 1985.

233. Libassi DP, Barron CL, London R: Soft bifocal contact lenses for patients with nearpoint asthenopia, *J Am Optom Assoc* 56(11):866, 1985.

234. Wick B: Accommodative esotropia: efficacy of therapy, *J Am Optom Assoc* 58:562, 1987.

235. Kushner BJ, Preslan MW, Morton GV: Treatment of partly accommodative esotropia with a high accommodative convergence-accommodation ratio, *Arch Ophthalmol* 105:815, 1987.

236. Scheiman M, Ciner E: Surgical success rates in acquired, comitant, partially accommodative and non-accommodative esotropia, *J Am Optom Assoc* 58:556, 1987.

237. Hiatt RL, Ringer C, Cope-Troupe C: Miotics vs. glasses in esodeviation, *J Pediatr Ophthalmol Strab* 16:213, 1979.

238. Scheiman M, Gallaway M, Ciner E: Divergence insufficiency: characteristics, diagnosis, and treatment, *Am J Optom Physiol Opt* 63:425, 1986.

239. Reinecke RD: Management of acquired intermittent esotropia, *South Med J* 69:1588, 1976.

240. Rutstein RP, Eskridge JB: Clinical evaluation of vertical fixation disparity, *Am J Optom Physiol Opt* 60:688, 1983.

241. Scobee RG, Bennett EA: Hyperphoria, a statistical study, *Arch Ophthalmol* 43:458, 1950.

242. Amos J: Vertical deviations. In Amos J, editor: *Diagnosis and management in vision care,* Boston, 1987, Butterworth-Heinemann.

243. Carter DB: Effects of prolonged wearing of prism, *Am J Optom Arch Am Acad Optom* 40:265, 1963.

244. Carter DB: Notes on fixation disparity, *J Am Optom Assoc* 39:1103, 1968.

245. Duwaer AL, van den Brink G: Diplopia thresholds and the initiation of vergence eye-movements, *Vision Res* 21:1727, 1981.

246. Ellerbrock VJ: Experimental investigation of vertical fusion, *Am J Optom Arch Am Acad Optom* 26:388, 1949.

247. Cooper J: Orthoptic treatment of vertical deviations, *J Am Optom Assoc* 59:463, 1988.

248. Walsh R: The measurement and correction of hyperphoria in refractive cases, *Am J Optom Physiol Opt* 23:373, 1946.

249. Sucher DF, Stewart J: Vertical fixation disparity in learning disabled, *Optom Vision Sci* 70:1038, 1993.

250. Slavin ML, Potash SD, Rubin SE: Asymptomatic physiologic hyperdeviation in peripheral gaze, *Ophthalmology* 95:778, 1988.

251. Lightholder PA, Phillips LJ: Evaluation of the binocularity of 147 unilateral and bilateral pseudophakic patients, *Am J Optom Physiol Opt* 56:451, 1979.

252. Rutstein RP, Eskridge JB: Studies in vertical fixation disparity, *Am J Optom Physiol Opt* 63:639, 1986.

253. Robertson KW, Kuhn L: Case report: successful visual training for alternating sursumduction, *J Am Optom Assoc* 55:911, 1984.

254. Robertson KW, Kuhn L: Effect of visual training on the vertical vergence amplitude, *Am J Optom Physiol Opt* 62:568, 1985.

255. Ogle KN, Prager A: Observations on vertical divergences and hyperphorias, *Arch Ophthalmol* 49:313, 1953.

256. Owens DA, Wolf-Kelly KL: Near work, visual fatigue, and variations in oculomotor tonus, *Invest Ophthalmol Vis Sci* 16:743, 1987.

257. Wick B: Forced vergence fixation disparity curves at distance and near in an asymptomatic young adult population, *Am J Optom Physiol Opt* 62:591, 1985.

258. Purcell LR and others: The cost effectiveness of selected optometric procedures, *J Am Optom Assoc* 54:643, 1983.

259. Stein JF, Riddell PM, Fowler S: Disordered vergence control in dyslexic children, *Brit J Ophthalmol* 72:162, 1988.

260. Jackson TW, Goss DA: Variation and correlation of standard clinical phoropter tests of phorias, vergence ranges, and relative accommodation in a sample of school-age children, *J Am Optom Assoc* 62:540, 1991.

261. Flom MC: The use of the accommodative convergence relationship in prescribing orthoptics/vision therapy, *Penn Optometrist* 14:3, 1954.

262. Schapero M: The characteristics of ten basic visual training problems, *Am J Optom Arch Am Acad Optom* 32:333, 1955.

263. Semmlow JL, Heerema D: The role of accommodative convergence at the limits of fusional convergence, *Invest Ophthalmol Vis Sci* 18:970, 1979.

264. Daum KM and others: Evaluation of a new criterion of binocularity, *Optom Vis Sci* 66:218, 1989.

265. Schor CM. Fixation disparity: a steady-state error of disparity-induced vergence, *Am J Optom Physiol Opt* 57:618, 1980.

266. Schor C, Robertson KM, Wesson M: Disparity vergence dynamics and fixation disparity, *Am J Optom Physiol Opt* 63:611, 1986.

267. Press LJ: The clinical calculation of fixation disparity, *J Am Optom Assoc* 52:877, 1981.

268. Cooper J and others: Reliability of fixation disparity curves, *Am J Optom Physiol Opt* 58:960, 1981.

269. Eskridge JB, Rutstein RP: Clinical evaluation of vertical fixation disparity. III. Adaptation to vertical prism, *Am J Optom Physiol* 62:585, 1985.

270. Yekta AA, Pickwell LD, Jenkins TCA: Binocular vision without stress, *Optom Vis Sci* 66(12):815, 1989.

271. Daum KM: The stability of the fixation disparity curve, *Ophthalmic Physiol Opt* 3:13, 1983.

272. Payne CJ, Grisham JD, Thomas KL: A clinical evaluation of fixation disparity, *Am J Optom Physiol Opt* 51:88, 1974.

273. Wick B: Forced vergence fixation disparity curves in presbyopia, *Am J Optom Physiol Opt* 63:895, 1986.

274. Schor CM: The relationship between fusional vergence eye movements and fixation disparity, *Vision Res* 19:1359, 1979.

275. Eskridge JB, Rutstein RP: Clinical evaluation of vertical fixation disparity. II. Reliability, stability, and association with refractive status, stereoacuity, and vertical heterophoria, *Am J Optom Physiol* 62:579, 1986.

276. Eskridge JB, Rutstein RP: Clinical evaluation of vertical fixation disparity. Part IV. Slope and adaptation to vertical prism of vertical heterophoria patients, *Am J Optom Physiol* 63:662, 1986.

277. Carroll JP: Control theory approach to accommodation and vergence, *Am J Optom Physiol Opt* 59:658, 1982.

278. Schor CM, Kotulak JC: Dynamic interactions between accommodation and convergence are velocity sensitive, *Vision Res* 26:927, 1986.

279. Semmlow JL, Hung G: Accommodative and fusional components of fixation disparity, *Invest Ophthalmol Vis Sci* 18:1082, 1979.

280. Semmlow JL, Hung GK: Experimental evidence for separate mechanisms mediating accommodative vergence and vergence accommodation, *Doc Ophthalmol* 51:209, 1981.

281. Semmlow JL, Hung GK: The near response: theories of control. In Schor CM, Ciuffreda KJ, editors: *Vergence eye movements: basic and clinical aspects,* Boston, 1984, Butterworths-Heinemann.

282. Krishnan VV, Stark L: A heuristic model for the human vergence eye movement system, *IEEE Trans Biomed Eng* 24:44, 1977.

283. Semmlow JL, Hung GK, Ciuffreda KJ: Quantitative assessment of disparity vergence components, *Invest Ophthalmol Vis Sci* 27:558, 1986.

284. Schor CM: Analysis of tonic and accommodative vergence disorders of binocular vision, *Am J Optom Physiol* 60:1, 1983.

285. Schor CM, Tseutaki TK: Fatigue of accommodation and vergence modifies their mutual interactions, *Invest Ophthalmol Vision Sci* 28:1250, 1987.

286. Balliet R, Nakayama K: Training of voluntary torsion, *Invest Ophthalmol Vis Sci* 17:303, 1978.

287. Manny RE: Monocular vergence movements produced by external visual feedback, *Am J Optom Physiol Opt* 57:236, 1980.

288. Daum KM, Rutstein RP, Eskridge JB: Efficacy of computerized vergence therapy, *Am J Optom Physiol Opt* 64:83, 1987.

289. Daum KM: Characteristics of exodeviations. II. Changes with treatment with orthoptics/vision therapy, *Am J Optom Physiol Opt* 63:244, 1986.

290. North RV, Henson DB: Effect of orthoptics/vision therapy upon the ability of patients to adapt to prism-induced heterophoria, *Am J Optom Physiol Opt* 59:983, 1982.

291. Dowley D: Heterophoria and monocular occlusion, *Ophthalmic Physiol Opt* 10:29, 1990.

292. Mannen DL, Bannon MJ, Septon RD: Effects of base-out training on proximal convergence, *Am J Optom Physiol Opt* 58:1187, 1981.

293. Griffin JR, Hattan MA, Hertkney RL: Vision therapy with stereoscopic motion pictures: a comparative evaluation, *Am J Optom Physiol Opt* 59:890, 1982.

294. Daum KM: Horizontal and vertical vergence training and its effect on vergences and fixation disparity curves. I. Horizontal data. *Am J Optom Physiol Opt* 65:1-7, 1988.

295. Daum KM: Negative vergence training in humans, *Am J Optom Physiol Opt* 63:487, 1986.

296. Goldrich SG: Oculomotor biofeedback therapy for exotropia, *Am J Optom Physiol Opt* 59:306, 1982.

297. Letourneau JE, Giroux R: Using biofeedback in an exotropic aphake, *J Am Optom Assoc* 55:909, 1984.

298. Afanador AJ: Auditory biofeedback and intermittent exotropia, *J Am Optom Assoc* 53:481, 1982.

299. Scheiman MM, Peli E, Libassi D: Auditory biofeedback used to enhance convergence insufficiency therapy, *J Am Optom Assoc* 54:1001, 1983.

300. Goodson PA, Rahe AJ: Visual training effects on normal vision, *Am J Optom Physiol Opt* 58:787, 1981.

301. Cooper J, Citron M: Microcomputer produced anaglyphs for evaluation and therapy of binocular anomalies, *J Am Optom Assoc* 54:785, 1983.

302. Somers WW, Happel AW, Phillips JD: Use of personal microcomputer for orthoptic therapy, *J Am Optom Assoc* 55:262, 1984.

303. Griffin JR: Efficacy of vision therapy for non-strabismic vergence anomalies, *Am J Optom Physiol Opt* 64:411, 1987.

304. Suchoff IB, Petito GT: The efficacy of vision therapy: accommodative disorders and non-strabismic anomalies of binocular vision, *J Am Optom Assoc* 57:119, 1986.

305. Eger MJ: Vision therapy: optometry's wallflower, *J Am Optom Assoc* 54:591, 1983.

306. Feldman J: Behavior modification in vision training: facilitating prerequisite behaviors and skills, *J Am Optom Assoc* 52:329, 1981.

307. Daum KM: Double-blind placebo-controlled examination of timing effects in the training of positive vergences, *Am J Optom Physiol Opt* 63:807, 1986.

308. Laird K: Monitoring the home training of fusional reserves, *Aust J Optom* 63:232, 1980.

309. Vaegan: Convergence and divergence show large and sustained improvement after short isometric exercise, *Am J Optom Physiol Opt* 56:23, 1979.

310. Sethi B, North RV: Vergence adaptive changes with varying magnitudes of prism-induced disparities and fusional amplitudes, *Am J Optom Physiol Opt* 64:263, 1987.

311. Colasanti A and others: The AC/A ratio and convergence in hypermetropia corrected with spectacles or contact lenses, *Am J Optom Physiol Opt* 59:51, 1982.

312. Griffin JR: *Binocular anomalies: procedures for vision therapy,* ed 2, Chicago, 1982, Professional.

313. North RV, Henson DB: Adaptation to prism-induced heterophoria in subjects with abnormal binocular vision or asthenopia, *Am J Optom Physiol Opt* 58:746, 1981.

314. Birnbaum MH: Adverse response to prism therapy in strabismus, *J Am Optom Assoc* 47:1195, 1976.

315. Larson WL, Faubert J: An investigation of prism adaptation latency, *Optom Vis Sci* 71:38, 1994.

316. Henson DB, North R: Adaptation to prism-induced heterophoria, *Am J Optom Physiol Opt* 57:129, 1980.

317. North RV, Sethi B, Henson DB: Effects of prolonged forced vergence upon the adaptation system, *Ophthalmic Physiol Opt* 6:391, 1986.

318. Henson DB, Dharamshi BG: Oculomotor adaptation to induced heterophoria and anisometropia, *Invest Ophthalmol Vis Sci* 22:234, 1982.

Strabismus, from the Greek word *strabismós,* meaning to squint or look obliquely at, is a manifest deviation of the visual axes of the eye of 1 PD or more. The lines of sight of the two eyes are not directed toward the same fixation point either constantly or intermittently when the patient is fixating on the object. The image of the fixation point is thus not formed on the fovea of the strabismic eye. Also known as *heterotropia, squint,* and *tropia,* strabismus results in the failure to maintain bifoveal fixation under normal viewing conditions. Unlike heterophoria, fusional vergence is poor or absent and cannot compensate for the tendency toward deviation, which then becomes manifest.

PREVALENCE

According to American and European studies, strabismus exists in 2% to 6% of the general population.[1,2] It has been estimated that strabismus is present in 3% to 4% of the preschool population in the United States.[1] In a country of 250,000,000 inhabitants, approximately 9 million individuals will have strabismus, a figure greater than many common ocular diseases.

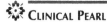 CLINICAL PEARL
Strabismus exists in 2% to 6% of the general population.

Overall, strabismus does not show racial, social class, or gender preference, although some studies have reported a slightly higher prevalence in males.[2] On the other hand, certain types of strabismus, such as Duane's

syndrome and thyroid myopathy, are more likely in females. There are also indications that esotropia may be more common in whites than in blacks and exotropia more common in Orientals.[3] The incidence of strabismus increases significantly for patients with multiple handicaps.[4-15] The association, for example, between overt brain damage, birth trauma, and low birth weight and prematurity to strabismus is well known (Table 7-1). In addition, recent evidence indicates that maternal cigarette smoking during pregnancy increases the risk of strabismus for offspring, with the risk increasing with the number of cigarettes smoked per day.[3,16] Increasing age of the mother has also been identified as a risk factor for esotropia.[3]

Although it may occur at any age, strabismus is more frequently diagnosed during early childhood. Excluding deviations that are paretic or mechanically restrictive and associated with systemic or neurologic disease, most strabismic deviations (90%) commence before age 6 (Fig. 7-1). The age of onset is highest during the third year of life, with a median age of onset of 29 months.[17] Esotropia appears to be more prevalent than exotropia. In a series of 1110 consecutive cases, for example, 61.5% had esotropia, whereas only 20.4% had exotropia.[18] The number of patients with exotropia may be underestimated because it presents mostly as an intermittent strabismus.

 CLINICAL PEARL
Most strabismic deviations commence before age 6.

Despite the fact that strabismus is a disease of childhood, functional signs provoked by a decompen-

TABLE 7-1 **PREVALENCE OF STRABISMUS**

Associated Condition	Prevalence (Percent)
Neurologically normal	3.5
Prematurity	18
Birth trauma	45
Down syndrome	50
Meningomyelocele	53
Cerebral palsy	44
Hydrocephalus and meningomyelocele	74
Craniofacial dysostosis	90

From Harcourt B: Strabismus affecting children with multiple handicaps, *B J Ophthalmol* 58:224,1974.
See also references 5-15.

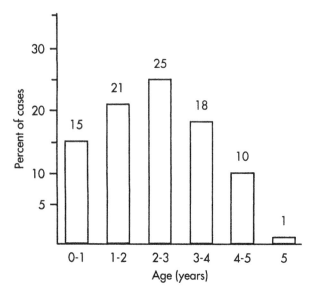

FIG. 7-1 Age of onset for 3243 cases of strabismus. (Modified from Adelstein AM, Scully J: Epidemiological aspects of squint, *Br Med J* 3:334, 1967.)

TABLE 7-2 FREQUENCY OF STRABISMUS AMONG SIBLINGS OF AFFECTED INDIVIDUALS ACCORDING TO PARENTAL STATUS

Parental Status	Percent of Offspring Affected
Neither parent has strabismus	14-30%
One parent has strabismus	30%
Both parents have strabismus	30-50%

From Cross HE: The heritability of strabismus, *Am Orthopt J* 11, 1975.

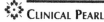 **CLINICAL PEARL**

An increased incidence of strabismus exists among brothers and sisters in families with members who are strabismic.

Genetics in strabismus is evident in twin studies.[27-32] Strabismus in twins strongly supports a hereditary influence when present in both twins and when the strabismus is similar (concordant). Conversely, environmental factors or incomplete genetic penetration likely contribute to the presence of strabismus when only one monozygotic twin is affected or when the strabismus affecting each twin is dissimilar (discordant). The strabismus concordance rate was shown to be 81.2% in identical twins, compared with 8.9% in fraternal twins.[27-32] This is compatible with polygenetic or multifactorial inheritance.

As certain as we are that strabismus has a hereditary tendency, the definite mode of inheritance is not yet established. No specific defect has been identified. Multiple questions remain as to the exact mode of transmission. Is strabismus a polygenetic trait, a Mendelian trait, or a nongenetic disorder? Various inheritance patterns have been described, but it appears likely that in many instances multiple genes are involved. Some authors have reported that strabismus is recessively transmitted, whereas other authors have reported a dominant mode of transmission.[25] It has even been suggested that the tendency to develop strabismus is probably more environmental than genetic. A certain degree of interaction among the various factors involved may be necessary to produce strabismus. Whether the strabismus itself is inherited or whether the conditions underlying the strabismus are inherited and, depending on circumstances, may or may not lead to strabismus is also unclear. Apparently, no good predictions are yet available to precisely quantitate the risks to subsequent family members.

As an approach to the understanding of familial tendency for strabismus, Griffin and others[33] reported on the families of four patients with infantile esotropia. Available family members were evaluated for strabismus and other vision disorders. Increased prevalence of

sation of a heterophoria may occur at any age but are more common in older patients. For example, in adolescence and early adulthood, uncorrected hyperopia associated with esophoria may produce intermittent diplopia with esotropia, because a greater accommodative effort is necessary to see clearly. In presbyopia a reduction in accommodation leads to less accommodative convergence, shifting an exophoria to an exotropia. Also, congenital superior oblique paresis may change from hyperphoria in childhood to hypertropia in adulthood.

HEREDITY

Heredity is a likely factor in the etiology of strabismus that is not associated with an obvious traumatic paresis, an ocular or systemic disease, or a well-recognized syndrome, such as Crouzon's disease. A familial tendency for strabismus was proposed as early as Hippocrates, who stated that "the children of parents having disturbed eyes squint also for the most part."[19]

Clinically, an increased incidence of strabismus exists among brothers and sisters in families with members who are strabismic. Children with strabismus are more likely to have a parent or first-order relative with strabismus.[20,21] Likewise, offspring of two affected parents have a greater risk of developing strabismus than offspring of either two normal parents or one affected parent (Table 7-2). Several strabismic types and syndromes have been noted to have familial dispositions.[19,22,23] The prevalence of strabismus in affected families ranges from 23% to 70%, compared with the 2% to 6% in the general population.[23-26]

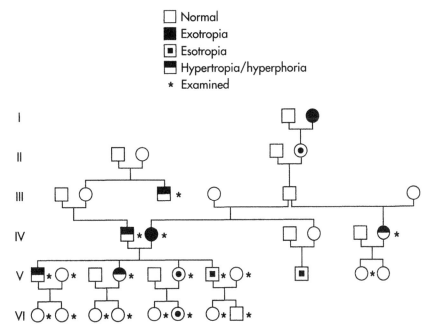

□ Normal
■ Exotropia
▣ Esotropia
▤ Hypertropia/hyperphoria
* Examined

FIG. 7-2 Pedigree of one family showing high prevalence of strabismus. (Courtesy G. Thomas Rader, OD.)

infantile esotropia (7%) was found among the family members as compared with the general population (1%), but with no consistent pattern of single gene inheritance. These findings are consistent with a polygenetic and environmental interaction model. Interestingly, the presence of a high accommodative convergence-to-accommodation ratio (AC/A ratio) was common for those family members examined who were not strabismic. Others have also suggested the possibility of an abnormal AC/A ratio being inherited.[34,35]

Cantolino and von Noorden[36] evaluated the motor and sensory status of parents and siblings of 20 patients with microtropia, an ultrasmall angle of strabismus. They found an uncommonly high incidence of oensomo tor and refractive anomalies in the families of these patients. These anomalies included heterotropias, anisometropia, and various sensory and motor deficits, such as diminished fusional amplitudes, eccentric fixation, anomalous correspondence, and reduced stereopsis. Cantolino and von Noorden[36] concluded that microtropia is not a primary congenital defect inherited in any simple Mendelian manner but rather is caused by multiple and independent sensory and motor anomalies. Microtropia results from the cumulative effect of these genetically determined binocular vision anomalies.

Deficient sensory fusion may be inherited and, in some cases, lead to strabismus. Helveston[37] examined parents of children with infantile esotropia. In spite of having at least 20/20 vision in each eye and no heterophoria greater than 2 PD, these patients had a 16% incidence of reduced stereopsis of 80 seconds or less in contrast with a control group of parents who had only

a 2% incidence of reduced stereopsis. Parker and others[38] measured the stereopsis with the TNO stereotest for 36 parents of children with infantile esotropia and compared these findings to 36 age-matched adults. All 72 subjects had normal binocular vision. The parents of the children with infantile esotropia performed significantly worse than the other adults. Scott and others[39] also reported an increased prevalence of reduced stereopsis in parents of children with infantile esotropia compared with the general population. These separate studies suggest that reduced stereopsis may represent a subthreshold effect on the gene or genes that cause infantile esotropia and may lead to strabismus under appropriate circumstances. Both genetic and environmental factors are likely implicated in the etiology of strabismus.

Fig. 7-2 illustrates the pedigree for one family in our clinic. Of the 37 family members, 19 were examined. Medical records and photographs were used to determine if strabismus existed in the other family members. In 12 of the 37 family members (32.4%), strabismus was present. The type of strabismus did not take the same form (esotropia, exotropia, hypertropia) throughout the family.

The type of strabismus appears not in the strict sense to be directly inherited.[30] The strabismic deviation appears to be a facultative complication of factors such as ametropia, an abnormal AC/A ratio, reduced fusional amplitudes, unusual configuration of the face, large interpupillary distance, reduced stereopsis, and, possibly, the readiness to suppress. Further studies involving clinical and psychophysical measurements (i.e., retinal rivalry, fusional amplitudes, and stereopsis) on the nonstrabismic family members may be quite helpful in detecting minor manifestations of the gene. The consensus is that strabismus is multifactorial, with a probable genetic component. Strabismus might be explained as being the result of the unfortunate coincidence of several independently inherited genetic factors occurring in one individual. Nevertheless, the common occurrence of sensorimotor anomalies in the pedigrees of strabismic probands obliges the clinician to evaluate all siblings of a child with strabismus to rule out the presence of neurosensory anomalies of the eyes.

 CLINICAL PEARL

> The strabismic deviation appears to be a facultative complication of factors such as ametropia, an abnormal AC/A ratio, reduced fusional amplitudes, unusual configuration of the face, large interpupillary distance, reduced stereopsis, and, possibly, the readiness to suppress.

CLASSIFICATION

Strabismus can be classified according to its (1) nature, (2) direction and magnitude, (3) laterality, (4) frequency, (5) distance-near relationship, and (6) time of onset.

NATURE

Strabismus can be either comitant or incomitant. A comitant or concomitant strabismus exists when the angle of deviation is within physiologic limits, with each eye fixating in turn and for a specific fixation distance, the same in all positions of gaze. The extraocular muscles show neither underaction nor overaction. A patient with a 20-PD esophoria in upgaze and a 20-PD esotropia in downgaze is still considered to have a comitant deviation, because the size did not vary; only the fusional control varied. Comitant deviations are supranuclear in origin.

An incomitant or noncomitant strabismus exists when the angle of deviation changes by more than 5 PD for a specific fixation distance either in the different directions of gaze or with each eye fixating in turn. Usually, one or more extraocular muscles shows underaction or overaction. When strabismus is incomitant, it is frequently the result of damage to either the oculomotor, trochlear, and abducens nerves or nuclei that innervate the extraocular muscles. However, lesion sites causing incomitancy can occur anywhere from the nuclear level to the extraocular muscle itself.

DIRECTION AND MAGNITUDE

A strabismus may be horizontal, vertical, torsional, or a combination of these. If the visual axes converge so that the cornea is rotated nasally, the con-

dition is esotropia (Fig. 7-3). If the visual axes diverge so that the cornea is rotated temporally, the condition is exotropia (Fig. 7-4).

A vertical deviation exists when one visual axis either is higher or lower than the other. When the visual axis is higher, it is a hypertropia and when it is lower, it is a hypotropia. According to Hering's law of equal innervation, when one eye is hypertropic, the contralateral eye becomes hypotropic when the hypertropic eye fixates. The deviation is described according to which eye is fixating. Left hypertropia indicates right eye fixation (Fig. 7-5), whereas right hypotropia indicates left eye fixation. Vertical strabismus can be isolated or coexist with an esotropia or exotropia. Most vertical deviations are incomitant.

A torsional deviation, or cyclodeviation, exists when there is a misalignment of one or both eyes around the sagittal axis, producing clockwise or counterclockwise rotations of the globe. Cyclodeviations are diagnosed mainly with special tests, such as the double Maddox rod test. Cyclodeviations are frequently associated with vertical deviations, particularly those related to oblique muscle disorders, and rarely exist alone. A clockwise rotation of the right eye indicates an incyclodeviation, or intorsion, (Fig. 7-6, *A*), whereas a counterclockwise movement of the right eye indicates an excyclodeviation, or extorsion, (Fig. 7-6, *B*). The reverse is true for the left eye. With incyclodeviation or intorsion the superior portion of the vertical meridian of the eye is torted nasally, and the inferior portion of the vertical meridian is torted temporally. With excyclodeviation or extorsion the superior portion of the vertical meridian is torted temporally, and the inferior portion of the vertical meridian is torted nasally.

 CLINICAL PEARL

> Cyclodeviations are frequently associated with vertical deviations, particularly those related to oblique muscle disorders, and rarely exist alone.

The magnitude of strabismus can be classified as either being small, intermediate, or large. Generally, small deviations measure 10 PD or less; intermediate or moderate deviations measure 11 PD to 30 PD; and large deviations exceed 30 PD. Esotropias can range from small to large, whereas exotropias are rarely small. Vertical deviations exceeding 20 PD in the primary position are uncommon.

The alternate cover test with prisms is the best method to measure strabismus. However, for patients who cannot maintain accurate fixation for a long enough time, the Hirschberg or Krimsky test can be used. With the Hirschberg test the patient fixates on a penlight at near while the clinician records any difference between the two corneal reflections in 0.5-mm in-

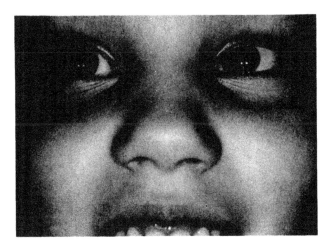

FIG. 7-3 Left esotropia.

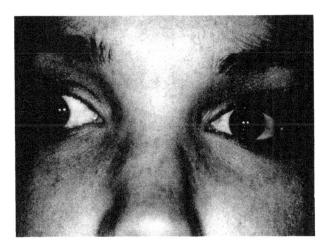

FIG. 7-4 Right exotropia.

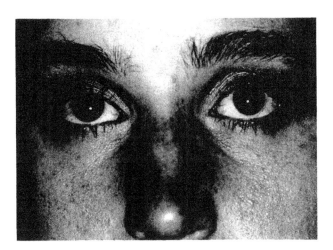

FIG. 7-5 Left hypertropia.

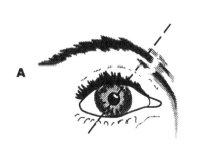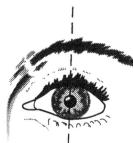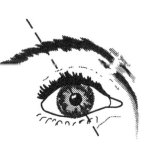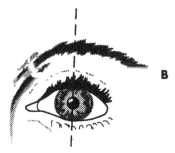

FIG. 7-6 Cyclodeviation. **A,** Right incyclodeviation. **B,** Right excyclodeviation.

crements. Esotropia exists if the deviating eye's corneal reflection is displaced temporally, and exotropia exists if the deviating eye's corneal reflection is displaced nasally. This is transferred into prism diopters (1 mm difference = 22 PD of strabismus). The Krimsky test is more accurate. A prism to partially compensate for the strabismus is placed in front of the fixating eye while the patient views a penlight at near. The fixating eye turns to maintain fixation. By Hering's law, the strabis-

mic eye makes a simultaneous and equal movement. Larger prisms are placed before the fixating eye until the corneal reflection is centered in the strabismic eye. For example, if 20 PD-base-out before the fixating eye is necessary to center the corneal reflection in the deviating eye, then the patient has a 20-PD esotropia.

As far as appearance is concerned, 15 PD is usually enough to make an esotropia apparent by casual observation, whereas 20 PD is enough for an exotropia. Hy-

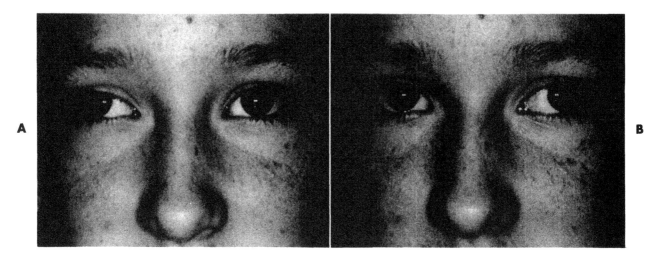

FIG. 7-7 Alternating strabismus. **A,** Right exotropia. **B,** Left exotropia.

pertropias and hypotropias exceeding 10 PD are usually noticeable, although many exceptions occur.

LATERALITY

A strabismus may be either unilateral or alternating. With a monocular, or unilateral, strabismus, there is definite preference for fixation with one eye (see Figs. 7-3 and 7-4). When the preferred eye is covered and the patient picks up fixation with the deviated eye, there is an immediate return to the original fixation status after removal of the occluder. This condition is amblyopiagenic in young children having constant strabismus.

With an alternating strabismus, there is either spontaneous alternation of fixation from one eye to the other or, by the cover test, the patient maintains fixation with either eye. For example, at times a right exotropia is noted, and at other times a left exotropia is noted (Fig. 7-7). Alternate fixation ability prevents the development of amblyopia in young children with constant strabismus.

 CLINICAL PEARL

Alternate fixation ability prevents the development of amblyopia in young children with constant strabismus.

FREQUENCY

Strabismus is either constant or intermittent. With constant strabismus, the eyes are always misaligned and fusion never occurs. The fusion mechanism is inadequate to keep the eyes properly aligned under any circumstance. If there is evidence that the patient is able to demonstrate bifoveal fusion without the use of lenses or compensatory prisms, the diagnosis of constant strabismus is incorrect; the deviation is intermittent. Most esotropias are constant.

For intermittent strabismus, the eyes may or may not be aligned at different times (Fig. 7-8). The fusion

mechanism functions well in some but not all circumstances. The strabismus may appear only when the patient is tired, under stress, or in particular test situations. Most exotropias are intermittent.

 CLINICAL PEARL

Most esotropias are constant. Most exotropias are intermittent.

In some cases the deviation will become manifest only when the individual is viewing in a certain position of gaze, such as with incomitant deviations or only when viewing at a particular fixation distance. Binocular vision will be displayed under all other circumstances. This is known as a *periodic strabismus*. The strabismus is quite predictable and will become manifest only under these specific circumstances.

DISTANCE-NEAR RELATIONSHIP

Similar to heterophoria, a strabismus is also classified according to the magnitude that is measured with the alternate prism cover test at distance and near. This is based on the role of accommodative convergence in determining the relative positions of the visual axes. If the measurements of the deviation at distance and near are similar, the deviation is a basic esotropia or exotropia.

Generally, if the deviation for esodeviations is larger by 10 PD or more at distance, a divergence insufficiency is present, and when the esodeviation is larger at near by 10 PD or more, a convergence excess is present. For exodeviations, if the strabismus is greater by 10 PD or more for distance, a divergence excess exists, and when the exodeviation at near exceeds the exodeviation at distance by 10 PD or more, a convergence insufficiency exists.

In rare instances a patient may present with strabismic types dependent on fixation distance.

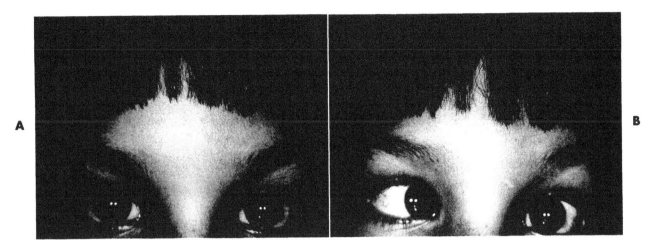

FIG. 7-8   Intermittent strabismus. Orthophoria **(A)** changes to esotropia **(B).**

AGE OF ONSET

Strabismus can be congenital or acquired. Congenital indicates that the strabismus was documented at birth or in the first months of life. Because of the difficulty in documenting strabismus at birth, the term *infantile* is preferred and indicates that the strabismus commenced at or before 6 months of age.[40]

An acquired strabismus is any strabismus that began after 6 months of age. Some of these may have a sudden onset, particularly in older individuals.

Classification based on the exact age of onset should be approached with caution, especially in children. Parents, for example, frequently report that the child was born with esotropia. What they are referring to in many cases is the prominent epicanthal folds (Fig. 7-9) that mimic or exaggerate an esotropia. Because of the high prevalence of epicanthal folds in children, it has been our policy to put more emphasis on what the parents say regarding the onset of exotropia rather than esotropia.

ETIOLOGY

A key to understanding strabismus starts with its etiology. The cause of strabismus is by no means fully understood. Too little is known about the etiology of strabismus, except in certain specific instances, to make it the basis of classification of all strabismus.[41,42] It is likely that the etiology can be determined with reasonable certainty in only 50% of all cases. For many patients, it is presumed to be related to abnormal development of the oculomotor control center. Support for this theory is provided by studies showing that strabismus is frequently associated with systemic and neurologic abnormalities (Table 7-1). For other patients the etiology remains unknown. Furthermore, multiple etiologies may exist for one patient, each of which, if acting alone, would not cause strabismus.

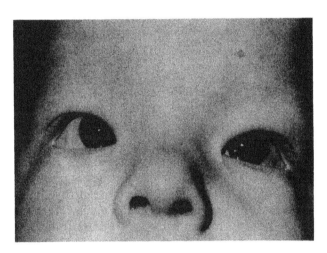

FIG. 7-9   Prominent epicanthal folds.

> ❊ **CLINICAL PEARL**
>
> The etiology of strabismus can be determined with reasonable certainty in only 50% of all cases.

A patient is vulnerable to developing strabismus when (1) the images seen by both eyes are blurred or not equivalent and do not reach the brain normally (refractive or sensory causes); (2) the motor apparatus of the eyes is not intact, thus preventing the corresponding retinal points from receiving impressions of constantly fixed objects (anatomic and motor causes); or (3) the brain is unable to transpose these sensations into a single percept (central and innervational causes).

REFRACTIVE CAUSES

High refractive errors, through their effect on accommodation, are one of the leading causes of strabismus. The relationship between hyperopia and esotropia has been known since 1864.[43] Hyperopia is more commonly associated etiologically with esotropia than is myopia with exotropia. With uncorrected hyperopia, an excessive amount of accommodation is required to clear the retinal images at a given fixation distance. For example, if a patient has 3 D of uncorrected hyperopia, a 3-D accommodative effort is required to see clearly for distance viewing and a 5.50-D accommodative effort is required to see clearly at 40 cm. Dependent on the patient's AC/A ratio and fusional divergence amplitudes, an esophoria or an esotropia may result. More than 30% of children with hyperopia exceeding 4 D develop esotropia by age 3.[44] There is no correlation between the amount of hyperopia and size of the esotropia.

Up to one third of all patients with comitant esotropia, with hyperopic correction, may obtain ocular alignment, whereas another one third obtain significant reduction but not complete elimination of the esotropia.[45] For the remaining patients, correcting the hyperopia does not alter the esotropia. It must be kept in mind that patients with esotropia can be emmetropic and even myopic. Similarly, patients with exotropia can be hyperopic.

Refractive anomalies such as anisometropia and aniseikonia result in the formation of corresponding retinal images so blurred and dissimilar that they cannot be fused. If this remains uncorrected in early childhood, the likelihood of strabismus is high.

Anisometropia has been associated with a unique form of small-angle strabismus. In these cases the anisometropia, not having been corrected in time, gives rise to a central suppression region of minor extent and causes noncentral fixation by some point in the parafoveal area, which both binocularly and monocularly, has replaced the fovea.[46]

ORGANIC AND SENSORY CAUSES

Development and maintenance of ocular alignment requires binocular sensory feedback to the controlling motor mechanisms. Any disease of the globe, retina, or optic nerve may provoke a strabismus if it lasts long enough, if it reaches a stage of irreversibility, and if it is unilateral or asymmetric. Because of a sensory obstacle to fusion the fusion reflex innervation becomes suspended, and the visually impaired eye changes its position relative to that of the fixating eye, and esotropia or exotropia develops. This is known as *sensory strabismus* (Fig. 7-10). A bilateral intraocular disease with marked visual acuity reduction will usually cause a sensory nystagmus and, rarely, strabismus.

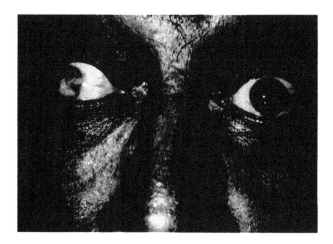

FIG. 7-10   Sensory strabismus.

The direction of the strabismus depends on the age at which the visual impairment occurred. Because of the extremely powerful convergence tonus that exists in early childhood, esotropia is predicted with unilateral visual loss in very young patients, whereas exotropia is predicted with unilateral visual loss in adolescents and adults. However, in a series of 121 patients with various causes of unilateral visual loss, including anisometropic amblyopia, in patients in whom the onset of visual impairment occurred at age 5 or younger the chances of developing esotropia or exotropia were similar, whereas exotropia predominated in older children and adults.[47] Exotropia was the only deviation encountered when vision was lost after age 15. The less forceful convergence tonus in adults may explain the prevalence of exotropia for the older patients.

ANATOMIC AND MOTOR CAUSES

Abnormalities in the anatomic structures, including orientation, size, and shape of the orbits and globes; volume and viscosity of the retrobulbar tissue; functioning of the extraocular muscles as determined by their insertion, length, elasticity, and structure; and the anatomic arrangement and condition of fascia and ligaments of the orbits can all cause strabismus.

A high incidence of strabismus, as much as 90%, exists with craniofacial dysostosis such as Apert's syndrome and Crouzon's disease.[48-52] The skull defects in patients with these anomalies involve premature closure of one or more suture lines in the developing cranium. This causes a misshapen skull with a shallow orbit. The resulting abnormal extraocular muscle vectors of action, altered orbital distances, and angulation and cranial nerve involvement all contribute to strabismus. Patients with craniofacial dysostosis demonstrate a variety of deviations in the primary position, although exotropia is more frequent (Fig. 7-11). The most consistent finding usually is a marked V pattern, most fre-

---

❖ **CLINICAL PEARL**

Any disease of the globe, retina, or optic nerve may provoke a strabismus if it lasts long enough, if it reaches a stage of irreversibility, and if it is unilateral or asymmetric.

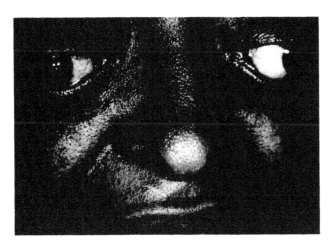

FIG. 7-11 Strabismus with Crouzon's syndrome.

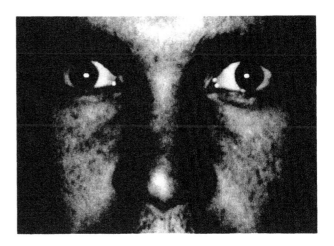

FIG. 7-12 Pseudoexotropia.

quently with a large exotropia in upgaze, moderate exotropia in primary position, and a small exotropia, orthophoria, or esotropia in downgaze. Oblique muscle dysfunctions are common. Congenital absence of one or more recti muscles may occur. Other ocular manifestations may include exophthalmos, obliquity of the palpebral fissures, ptosis, hypertelorism, unusual and asymmetric refractive errors, nystagmus, iridic and choroidal coloboma, optic atrophy, and cataract. Many of these factors also contribute to the high incidence of strabismus. Also contributing to strabismus is mental retardation that may occur as a primary finding or secondary to increased intracranial pressure. It seems logical therefore to postulate a multifactorial etiology for the strabismus in craniofacial dysostosis, the mechanical factors apparently being more severe than the sensory and innervational factors.

Certain anatomic abnormalities, such as abnormal interpupillary distance, facial asymmetry, abnormal globe position, and abnormal palpebral fissures can mimic strabismus. Patients with hypertelorism, an increased separation often exceeding 80 mm between the two bony orbits, appear to be exotropic (Fig. 7-12). The unilateral cover test and Hirschberg test allow the clinician to distinguish pseudostrabismus from true strabismus. If there is no movement of either eye with the unilateral cover test and if the reflected images from the two corneas appear centered, assume the eyes are properly aligned. Pseudoexotropia may also be caused by exophthalmos, a large positive-angle kappa (corneal light reflex is displaced nasally), or an ectopic macula. In ectopic macula the macula is dragged temporally as a result of the contraction of choroid and retinal lesions in choroiditis or in retinopathy of prematurity. The dragging of the retina either unilaterally or bilaterally causes the fovea to be located temporal to its normal position, thus changing the relationship between the visual line and pupillary axis.[53] This re-

sults in a large positive-angle kappa. Visual acuity is usually reduced but may remain normal or near normal despite retinal distortion. In rare cases, ectopic macula can make an esotropic patient appear exotropic. When occluding the fixating eye, a slight abduction movement occurs in the uncovered eye to center the object of regard on the fovea.

> ### ✿ CLINICAL PEARL
>
> Certain anatomic abnormalities, such as abnormal interpupillary distance, facial asymmetry, abnormal globe position, and abnormal palpebral fissures can mimic strabismus.

Pseudoesotropia occurs more frequently than pseudoexotropia. Pseudoesotropia is the appearance of having esotropia when actually no convergent misalignment of the visual axis exists. Infants and very young children often have wide, flat, and broad nasal bridges, with prominent medial epicanthal folds, a reduced interpupillary distance, and, occasionally, a large negative-angle kappa (see Fig. 7-9). The epicanthus varies considerably in width and may approach and obscure the inner canthus. These findings may cause these children to appear esotropic. In one study, nearly half of all children evaluated for esotropia were pseudoesotropic and orthophoric.[54] This demonstrates the frequent unreliability of parental observation with esotropia and is a major reason for requiring optometric verification of the diagnosis. The parents may give the history of an intermittent crossing that is more noticeable when the child looks to either the right or left side. This is a result of the covering of usually the entire nasal bulbar conjunctiva of the left eye by the epicanthal skin fold when the child looks to the right and the nasal bulbar conjunctiva of the right eye when the child looks to the left. The parents must be convinced that their child's eyes are not crossed. Careful inspection with the unilateral cover test and Hirschberg test will reveal ocular alignment. Demonstration to the parents of the centered pupillary reflexes with the muscle light and pulling the skin forward over the bridge of the nose to show the "straightening" effect of exposing the medial conjunctiva eliminates their concern. Epicanthal folds frequently coexist with esotropia and accentuate the appearance of the strabismus.

The esotropic appearance of children with pseudoesotropia eventually disappears partially or totally. With maturation of the face as the child grows, the bridge of the nose becomes more prominent and displaces the epicanthal folds, so that the sclera medially becomes proportional to the amount visible on the lateral side. The eyes gradually appear to be aligned properly, when in fact they always have been. Total disappearance of the epicanthal folds is more likely in whites than in other races.

It must be remembered that even though a young child may have pseudoesotropia, true esotropia may subsequently develop. Parents must be told of this possibility and cautioned that reassessment is necessary if the apparent deviation does not improve or gets worse. Unfortunately, with the onset of true esotropia, some parents are reluctant to return for fear of being "wrong" once again.

Abnormalities in the extraocular muscles and their adjacent structures, including hypoplasia or absence of the muscles and abnormal check ligaments or other fibrous bands connecting the muscles and the orbital walls, lead to strabismus that is incomitant. Anomalies of the lateral and/or medial rectus insertion have been associated with A or V patterns. Fibrosis, or enlargement of the extraocular muscles, particularly the inferior rectus, is frequently a part of thyroid myopathy, whereas fibrosis of the lateral rectus has been associated with Duane's syndrome.

Paresis of either the oculomotor, trochlear, or abducens cranial nerve leads to incomitant strabismus. Some of these cases can evolve as comitant deviations if complete remission does not occur. Thus there is a tendency to presume that some cases of childhood strabismus without causative refractive error or apparent anatomic abnormalities are paretic in origin. This is probably overestimated. Nevertheless, cases have been reported in which patients with incomitant esotropia as a result of lateral rectus paresis, for example, develop comitant esotropia with time.

INNERVATIONAL CAUSES

Innervational causes of strabismus are the most complex and the least understood. They involve all nervous impulses that reach the eye. Included are comovements of the extraocular muscles with intrinsic muscles; psycho-optic reflexes (fixation reflex and fusional impulses); influences of the static apparatus on

the extraocular muscles and their tonus (endolymph, vestibular system, reflexes from neck muscles); and influences of the several nuclear and supranuclear areas that govern ocular motility.[55]

Innervational disorders usually include (1) abnormal accommodative convergence, (2) weak fusion ability, (3) excessive or insufficient tonic innervation to the extraocular muscles, and (4) inadequate or excessive central coordination from the brain.

An abnormal accommodation-convergence relationship is a frequent cause of strabismus.[34,35] The amount of deviation induced by accommodation depends on the AC/A ratio. The AC/A ratio for patients with strabismus can be estimated by comparing the alternate prism cover test measurements at distance and near. If the measurements are equal or nearly equal, the AC/A ratio is said to be normal. A difference exceeding 10 PD usually indicates an abnormal AC/A ratio. Other methods of determining the AC/A ratio, such as by calculation or the gradient method, are more precise and are discussed in Chapter 6.

 CLINICAL PEARL

An abnormal accommodative convergence relationship is a frequent cause of strabismus.

Differences in the accommodative convergence relationship may explain why young patients with essentially similar degrees of uncorrected hyperopia may or may not develop esotropia. This is most intriguing, particularly when found in siblings. (See Cases 1 to 4.)

CASE 1

JD, a 4-year-old boy, was first examined in January, 1984. His parents reported that his eye began to cross approximately 6 months earlier. The patient was in excellent health and had not suffered any trauma or injury.

Visual acuity was 20/30 for each eye with the Broken Wheel test. With the cover test, while viewing an accommodative target the patient was 2-PD esophoric at distance and 15-PD esotropic at near. Versions were normal. Cycloplegic refraction revealed OD $+7.50 -1.00 \times 180$ and OS $+7.00$ sphere. With spectacle correction the patient fused at all distances. Follow-up visits continued to show fusion with the glasses and esotropia at near without the glasses.

CASE 2

KD, the younger sister of JD, was examined in January, 1988, when she was also 4 years old. The parents had not noticed any eye turn. However, they did report that she sat very close when viewing television.

Visual acuity was OD 20/60 and OS 20/60 with the Broken Wheel test. Cover testing while viewing an accommodative target revealed a 4-PD esophoria at distance and near. Cycloplegic refraction was OD $+7.75 -1.75 \times 15$ and OS $+8.25 -1.75 \times 5$. The patient was prescribed the above, as well as amblyopia treatment. Visual acuity improved to 20/30. Over a period of 5 years, she never manifested an esotropia, even when she was without her glasses.

CASE 3

VP, a 3-year-old boy, was examined in March, 1991. His parents claimed to have noticed his eyes crossing occasionally. With the Broken Wheel test, 20/40 vision was measured for each eye. The patient was orthophoric by cover test at distance and near while viewing an accommodative target. Cycloplegic refraction revealed OD +5.00 − 1.00 × 180 and OS +4.00 sphere.

CASE 4

DP, the 5-year-old brother of VP, was examined on the same day as VP. At age 2, DP was prescribed glasses by another practitioner. He recently lost his glasses, and, according to his parents, his eyes are always crossed.

Our examination revealed 20/40 vision for each eye. With the cover test while viewing an accommodative target, a 25-PD esotropia at distance and a 35-PD esotropia at near were measured. Cycloplegic refraction revealed OD +6.50 sphere and OS +6.50 − 1.00 × 180. The esotropia could not be elicited while DP was wearing the glasses.

From these cases, it can be surmised that possibly an intrinsically low AC/A ratio may protect certain children with uncorrected hyperopia from developing esotropia.[56] For KD and VP, small esophoria or orthophoria occurred without glasses, despite the excessive accommodation required to recognize the fixation target used during measurement of the near deviation.

Some cases of strabismus have been explained by a weak or absent fusion mechanism. Whether this weakness is innate has been debated for years. Motor and sensory components of binocular vision, such as visual acuity, fixation, contrast sensitivity, stereopsis, ocular motility, and vergences, are incompletely developed in newborns.[57-59] Does the child who ultimately develops strabismus start life with the potential for normal binocular vision and lose it because of acquired motor-induced factors, or does the child begin life with an inborn lack of binocularity? Worth,[60] making no distinction between motor and sensory fusion, proposes the latter and reports that some infants have a congenitally weak or absent fusion mechanism. He theorizes that this puts the eyes in a state of unstable equilibrium, ready to become strabismic with slight provocation. Provoking factors may be uncorrected hyperopia, anisometropia, physical or mental illness, injury during birth, motor anomalies, hereditary factors, and iatrogenic causes, such as occlusion. Worth[60] came to this conclusion after attempting to establish fusion with several patients with constant, alternating esotropia without either significant hyperopia or muscle paresis.

No amount of treatment could render the deficient fusion faculty normal. As already noted, deficient stereopsis may be innate and lead to strabismus under certain circumstances.

The idea that fusion is congenitally absent or weak was rejected by Chavasse,[61] who claimed that the fusion mechanism is intact at birth for all neurologically normal infants but must be used to develop. Weak fusion results from disuse. Chavasse[61] considered fusion to be a conditioned reflex, with a limited period in which it can develop. Strabismus could be provoked by pathology either in the motor component of the reflexes innervating the extraocular muscles or by anatomic abnormalities within the muscles and their surrounding tissue. According to Chavasse,[61] a defective peripheral motor eye muscle component causes strabismus on a reflex basis initially and then produces a secondary fusion loss. A functional cure with establishment of normal binocular vision was possible if the strabismus was treated at an early enough age.

Recent studies on the ocular alignment status of infants shed more light on whether or not poor fusion ability is innate.[62-65] In the past, disorders of ocular motility that present in the first months of life were rarely diagnosed in the neonatal period. This was because of the difficulty of performing a motility examination and also because of the shortage of precise guidelines as to what constituted normal ocular motility in the neonate. Nixon and others[62] reported the ocular alignment status for 1219 3-day-old neurologically normal newborns. Of these, 593 (48.6%) were orthophoric, 398 (32.7%) had exotropia, 40 (3.2%) had esotropia (mostly intermittent and variable), and 188 (15.4%) were not sufficiently alert to permit classification. No newborn exhibited the large, constant deviation associated with infantile esotropia.

Archer, Sondhi, and Helveston[63] evaluated the ocular alignment of neurologically normal newborns examined at 1 or 2 days of age. Several infants were followed until 23 months of age. The findings confirmed the unstable ocular alignment during the first few weeks of life and showed a higher incidence of exotropia (66.5%) than did previous findings. A steady progression toward more frequent periods of straight eyes occurred during the first 6 months, with the alignment status at birth and 1 month being similar (Fig. 7-13).

From these and other studies on ocular motility in newborns, it can be concluded that normal infants and infants who are destined to develop strabismus during infancy or early childhood are indistinguishable in the first few months by usual clinical measures. The critical period for the development of binocular vision appears to begin at 2 to 3 months after birth. The infants in the study who subsequently developed the large deviation of infantile esotropia were initially either orthophoric or exotropic. The majority of newborns have an unsta-

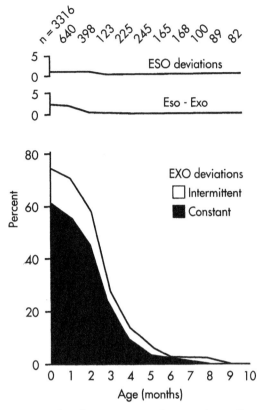

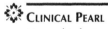

FIG. 7-13 Ocular alignment status for neurologically normal infants during first 10 months of life. (Modified from Archer SM, Sondhi N, Helveston EM: Strabismus in infancy, *Ophthalmology* 96:133, 1989.)

ble ocular alignment biased toward exotropia. Prolonged strabismus in the first weeks or even months does not necessarily preclude normal binocular vision.

❖ CLINICAL PEARL

Normal infants and infants who are destined to develop strabismus during infancy or early childhood are indistinguishable in the first few months by usual clinical measures.

Apparently, all normal newborns have an "anomalous" and weak binocular sensory experience during the first few months of life. This is the result of incompletely developed visual acuity, retinal disparity sensitivity, contrast sensitivity, and stereopsis. The absence of a strong vergence control mechanism in the presence of weak sensory input explains the high prevalence of transient strabismus in newborns that later develop binocular vision.[37] With maturation of motor fusion, stabilization of ocular alignment occurs for most infants. If development of motor fusion is delayed or if the vergence system is defective, a persisting strabismus may develop as a result of excessive tonic convergence, hyperopia, anisometropia, or other factors. What may

be innate and genetically determined, therefore, is the inability of the sensory and motor systems to adequately interact with each other and sustain binocular vision.[37]

A disturbance in the balance of tonic innervation from anomalies of the subcortical centers and pathways for convergence and divergence is the usual explanation for certain types of horizontal strabismus in which refractive error or muscle paresis is absent. Tonic innervation is the factor that causes convergence other than accommodative and fusional convergence. The roles of tonic innervation and strabismus have merit, because many patients with strabismus tend to diverge when under general anesthesia, providing there are no associated mechanical factors restricting passive adduction or abduction.[66] In many cases the large angle of deviation associated with infantile esotropia (40 PD to 60 PD) disappears entirely under surgical plane anesthesia. Patients with exotropia diverge considerably less (10.9 PD) on average than do patients with esotropia (44.5 PD).[67] An increase in tonic convergence to the extraocular muscles may also account for the increasing esodeviation associated with fatigue, illness, and emotional disturbances.

Patients with brain damage have a much higher incidence of strabismus, suggesting that brain asymmetry or anomalous wiring of the visual system may be the cause of strabismus.[6,15] In addition, motor retardation, either exogenous or endogenous, a sign of early brain damage, has been found in some patients with strabismus.

With Down syndrome, the most common chromosome abnormality, as many as 50% of the patients manifest strabismus (Fig. 7-14).[12,13,68,69] A high incidence of epicanthal folds, oblique and shortened palpebral fissure, cataract, high refractive error, nystagmus, and keratoconus has also been reported with Down syndrome.[68] Esotropia is much more likely than exotropia, the latter rarely occurring. Because high refractive errors are frequent, many esotropias might initially appear to be the result of uncorrected hyperopia. However, high myopia occurs just as frequently for patients with Down syndrome who have esotropia. The esotropia in Down syndrome is more likely attributed to decreased fusional or visual resolution capacity or a failure to develop an adequate accommodative convergence mechanism.[70]

With cerebral palsy, the incidence of strabismus ranges from 15% to 68%, averaging 44%.[5,71,72] Similar to Down syndrome, esotropia occurs more frequently than exotropia. The incidence of incomitancy, mostly A and V patterns, is about 25%.[71] Some cerebral palsy patients manifest a peculiar fluctuation between esotropia and exotropia (Fig. 7-15) that is pathognomonic for cerebral palsy and is absent in the neurologically normal population. This variable and nonstabilizing strabismus, known as *dyskinetic strabismus,* exists in approximately 30% of patients with cerebral palsy who have strabismus.[72] Dyskinetic strabismus can actually precede the other clinical signs of cerebral palsy and its identification can facilitate earlier referral and treatment.

When a patient with dyskinetic strabismus is asked to fixate on a given accommodative target, the clinician may see one or both eyes slowly converge. Then with no change in attention or accommodation the eyes may straighten or diverge. Various degrees of supravergence may also occur. The variable movement resembles a slow, tonic vergence. Alternation of fixation is common, whether the eye is esotropic or exotropic. Ocular movements are usually full. The constant changing of the strabismus makes accurate quantification with the alternate prism cover test impossible. The extreme variability associated with dyskinetic strabismus must be taken into consideration when planning treatment.

Brain injuries acquired during late childhood, adolescence, and adulthood may affect the centers for motor control. In that regard, there exists a type of strabismus that is associated with intractable diplopia. Disruption of fusion can occur in adults with previous normal binocular vision, following central nervous system insult, whether it be mechanical, vascular, or inflammatory.[73-77] These patients become incapable of single binocular vision on examination, and fusional amplitudes are severely reduced or absent altogether. Prolonged monocular vision deprivation, such as occurs when an acquired cataract is left in situ, or uncorrected monocular aphakia can also result in a similar disruption of fusion with resulting intractable diplopia.[78] Unlike patients with horror fusionis (see Chapter 5), these patients frequently exhibit fleeting sensory fusion when evaluated with the synoptophore or with prisms. After momentary superimposition or fusion, the eyes will begin to drift into a position of small-angle strabismus, and diplopia will occur. Attempts to eliminate the diplopia with prisms are met with failure because of the disruption of fusional amplitudes. Frequently, these patients have suffered head trauma followed by periods of unconsciousness, suggesting a midbrain center for fusional disruption, as shown in the following case.

CASE 5

A 66-year-old man was examined in September, 1986. His ocular history was significant for diplopia coincident with severe head trauma that he had suffered 3 years earlier following a motor vehicle accident. His medical history was significant for malaria, of which he had numerous recurrences. Other practitioners were unsuccessful in eliminating the diplopia. The patient reported also a vertical "bobbing" of the diplopic image.

Examination revealed corrected vision of 20/20 for each eye with OD +1.50 −0.75 × 75 and OS +2.25 −0.75 ×

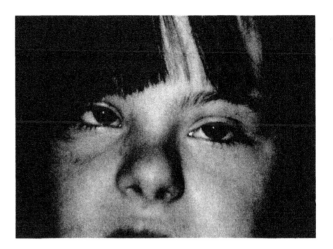

FIG. 7-14 Strabismus with Down syndrome.

90. The patient showed by cover test a 3-PD left hypertropia that was comitant. With the Randot stereotest, momentary fusion (50 seconds of arc) was demonstrated with compensating prisms. A 3-degree excyclodeviation for the left eye was measured with the double Maddox rod test. There was no sign of a superior oblique paresis or aniseikonia.

Prisms (2-PD base-down OS) were given to the patient. A week later, he returned and reported no improvement in the diplopia. Further examination with the synoptophore showed only momentary sensory fusion. Attempts to measure motor fusion amplitudes in both the vertical and horizontal directions resulted in immediate diplopia.

Excessive excitability and innervation from the brain influences the conditioned reflexes forming binocular vision. The action of the superior centers may increase a small strabismic deviation caused by other factors. For example, an older child or adult with an acquired esotropia unable to suppress usually will be less bothered by the diplopia if the images are farther apart. The exaggerated innervation from the superior centers deliberately increases the size of the deviation, so that the retinal zone stimulated in the deviating eye has a weaker visual potential and ignoring of the diplopic image is facilitated. In some cases, this may cause the diplopic image to become situated on the optic disc.[79,80] Similarly, in paretic deviations the paretic eye can be used for fixation, thus increasing the separation of the diplopia images to make the diplopia more tolerable.

Psychogenic or emotional disorders rarely lead to strabismus. Usually, in these instances, strabismus can only develop if an additional predisposing factor exists, such as high refractive error or excessive heterophoria. An exception is the strabismus associated with spasm of the near reflex.[81,82] Young patients with this condition present with a varying and intermittent esotropia (Fig. 7-16). The visual symptoms include diplopia, blurred vision, headaches, photophobia, and ocular

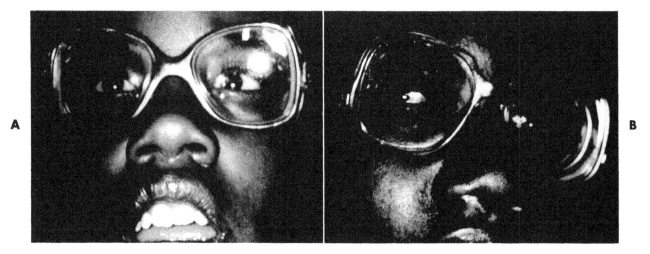

FIG. 7-15   Dyskinetic strabismus in a patient with cerebral palsy. Left esotropia **(A)** is spontaneously replaced by right exotropia **(B).**

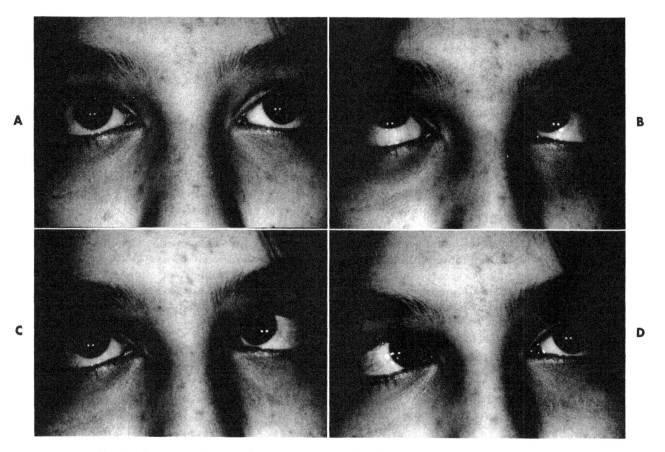

FIG. 7-16   Spasm of near reflex. **A,** Patient is orthophoric when viewing at distance. **B,** When viewing target in upgaze, an accommodative convergence spasm with esotropia occurs. During episode, limited motility is noted in right eye **(C)** when looking to right and in left eye **(D)** when looking to left with version testing.

pain. The limited ocular motility that accompanies the spasm mimics a bilateral lateral rectus paresis. The case history frequently reveals some stressful situations, such as death in the family, divorce, or school problems. Refractive errors are not excessive, and rarely does a large heterophoria exist when the patient is not manifesting the episode. As mentioned in Chapter 3, the esotropia is attributed solely to accommodative spasm. It is imperative to monitor accommodation with dynamic retinoscopy when measuring ocular deviations.

CASE 6

A 9-year-old girl had been experiencing intermittent diplopia, headaches, and blurred vision for the previous few months. The visual symptoms commenced at approximately the time the patient's parents divorced. The patient was in excellent health and not taking any medications. There had been no history of trauma.

The examination revealed 20/20 vision for each eye. Orthophoria existed at distance and near. However, when viewing a 20/30 letter at near, she began to become variably "esotropic." Both eyes converged. Pupillary miosis and limited abduction bilaterally accompanied the episode. Dynamic retinoscopy at this time revealed a large lead of accommodation, indicating an accommodative spasm. Visual fields with the tangent screen were constricted and tubular, confirming a psychogenic etiology. Ocular health findings were normal.

Plus-reading lenses to inhibit the accommodation spasm were given, and the patient was referred for psychologic evaluation.

SUMMARY

Many views exist on the etiology of strabismus. In some cases the etiology is obvious, whereas in other cases it remains speculative or unknown. We see many children with hyperopia who are esotropic and probably an equal number of children with hyperopia who are not esotropic. We also see multiple etiologies combining to produce strabismus. For example, although many patients with esotropia are hyperopic, prescribing the refractive correction does not always eliminate the strabismus. Other factors, such as excessive tonic convergence, weak fusion, or abnormal extraocular muscles must also be involved. Despite the unclear etiology in many of these cases, therapy should not be postponed.

REFERENCES

1. Friedman L and others: Screening for refractive errors, strabismus, and other anomalies from age 6 months to 3 years, *J Pediatr Ophthalmol Strab* 14:315, 1977.
2. Graham PA: Epidemiology of strabismus, *Br J Ophthalmol* 58:224, 1974.
3. Chew E and others: Risk factors for esotropia and exotropia, *Arch Ophthalmol* 112:1349, 1994.
4. Harcourt B: Strabismus affecting children with multiple handicaps, *Br J Ophthalmol* 58:272, 1974.
5. Lossef S: Ocular findings in cerebral palsy, *Am J Ophthalmol* 54:1114, 1962.
6. Bankes JLK: Eye defects of mentally handicapped children, *Br Med J* 2:533, 1974.
7. Gallo JE, Lennerstrand G: A population-based study of ocular abnormalities in premature children aged 5 to 10 years, *Am J Ophthalmol* 111:539, 1991.
8. Kushner BJ: Strabismus and amblyopia associated with regressed retinopathy of prematurity, *Arch Ophthalmol* 100:256, 1982.
9. Alberman E, Benson J, Evans S: Visual defects in children of low birth weight, *Arch Dis Child* 57:818, 1982.
10. Hammer HM and others: Ophthalmic findings in very low birth weight children, *Trans Ophthalmol Soc U K* 104:329, 1985.
11. Rutstein RP and others: Visual parameters in infants with intrauterine growth retardation, *Am J Optom Physiol Op* 63:697, 1986.
12. Eissler R, Longenecker JP: The common eye findings in mongolism, *Am J Ophthalmol* 54:398, 1962.
13. Falls HF: Ocular changes in mongolism, *Ann N Y Acad Sci* 171:627, 1970.
14. Walker J: Squint in the dysmorphic child, *Br Orthopt J* 46:93, 1989.
15. Bothe N, Lieb B, Schaffer D: Development of impaired vision in mentally handicapped children, *Klin Monatsbl Augenheilkd* 198:509, 1991.
16. Hakim RB, Tielsch JM: Maternal cigarette smoking during pregnancy: a risk factor for childhood strabismus, *Arch Ophthalmol* 110:1459, 1992.
17. Adelstein AM, Scully J: Epidemiological aspects of squint, *Br Med J* 3:334, 1967.
18. Fletcher MC, Silverman SJ: Strabismus. I. A summary of 1110 consecutive cases, *Am J Ophthalmol* 61:86, 1966.
19. Paul TO, Hardage LK: The heritability of strabismus, *Ophthalmic Genet* 15:1, 1994.
20. Brodsky MC, Fritz KJ: Hereditary congenital exotropia: a report of three cases, *Bin Vis Eye Muscle Surg* 8:133, 1993.
21. Cross HE: The heritability of strabismus, *Am Orthopt J* 25:11, 1975.
22. Tong PY, Parks MM: Inheritance of strabismus: esotropia and exotropia, *Invest Ophthalmol Vis Sci* 36:5953, 1995.
23. Maumenee IH and others: Inheritance of congenital esotropia. *Trans Am Ophthalmol Soc* 84:85, 1986.
24. Scholssman A, Priestly BE: Role of heredity in etiology and treatment of strabismus, *Arch Ophthalmol* 47:1, 1952.
25. Grutzner P, Yazawa K, Spivey BE: Heredity and strabismus, *Surv Ophthalmol* 14:441, 1970.
26. Norbis AL, Malbran E: Concomitant esotropia of late onset: pathological report in four cases in siblings, *Br J Ophthalmol* 40:373, 1956.
27. Bucci FA, Catalano RA, Simon JW: Discordance of accommodative esotropia in monozygotic twins, *Am J Ophthalmol* 107:84, 1989.
28. Shippman S and others: Unusual ocular findings in identical twins, *J Pediatr Ophthalmol Strab* 25:298, 1988.

29. Lang J: Strabismus in monozygotic twins, *Klin Monatsbl Augenheilkd* 196:275, 1990.

30. Trew DR, Ainslie CE: Prematurely born triplets displaying different types of esodeviation, *Br Orthopt J* 47:76, 1990.

31. Ahmed S, Young JDH: Late onset esotropia in monozygous twins, *Br J Ophthalmol* 77:189, 1993.

32. Smith K: An evaluation of identical twins with strabismus, *Am Orthopt J* 44:92, 1994.

33. Griffin JR and others: Heredity in congenital esotropia, *J Am Optom Assoc* 50:1237, 1979.

34. Hofstetter HW: Accommodative convergence in identical twins, *Am J Optom Arch Am Acad Optom* 25:480, 1948.

35. Franceschetti AT, Burian AM: Gradient accommodative convergence accommodative ratio in families with and without esotropia, *Am J Ophthalmol* 70:558, 1970.

36. Cantolino SJ, von Noorden GK: Heredity in microtropia, *Arch Ophthalmol* 81:753, 1969.

37. Helveston EM: *Surgical management of strabismus: an atlas of strabismus surgery,* St Louis, 1993, Mosby.

38. Parker L and others: Monocular OKN asymmetry and defective stereopsis in parents of children with infantile esotropia, *Am Orthopt J* 43:71, 1993.

39. Scott MH and others: Prevalence of primary monofixation syndrome in parents of children with congenital esotropia, *J Pediatr Ophthalmol Strab* 31:298, 1994.

40. Parks MM: Congential esotropia vs. infantile esotropia, *Graefes Arch Clin Exp Ophthalmol* 266:106, 1988.

41. Plenty JV: The aetiology of squint, *Br Orthopt J* 47:94, 1990.

42. Hugonnier R, Hugonnier S: *Strabismus, heterophoria, ocular mator paralysis,* St Louis, 1969, Mosby.

43. Donders FC: *On the anomalies of accommodation and refraction of the eye.* London, 1864, The New Sydenham Society (Translated by WD Moore).

44. Dobson V, Sebris SL: Longitudinal study of acuity and stereopsis in infants with or at risk for esotropia, *Invest Ophthalmol Vis Sci* 30:1146, 1989.

45. Adler FH: Pathologic physiology of convergence strabismus. Motor aspects of the non-accommodational type, *Arch Ophthalmol* 33:362, 1945.

46. Helveston EM, von Noorden GK: Microtropia: a newly defined entity, *Arch Ophthalmol* 78:272, 1968.

47. Sidikaro Y, von Noorden GK: Observations in sensory heterotropia, *J Pediatr Ophthalmol Strab* 19:12, 1982.

48. Carruthers JDA: Strabismus in craniofacial dysostosis, *Graefes Arch Clin Exp Ophthalmol* 226:230, 1988.

49. Caputo AR, Lingua RW: Aberrant muscle insertions in Crouzon's disease, *J Pediatr Ophthalmol Strab* 17:239, 1980.

50. Miller M, Folk E: Strabismus associated with craniofacial anomalies, *Am Orthopt J* 25:27, 1975.

51. Spir M, Gilad E, Ben-Sira I: An unusual extraocular muscle anomaly in a patient with Crouzon's disease, *Br J Ophthalmol* 66:253, 1982.

52. Pollard ZE: Bilateral superior oblique palsy associated with Apert's syndrome, *Am J Ophthalmol* 106:337, 1988.

53. Scheiman M, Gallaway M, McKewicz L: Heterotopia of the macula (ectopic macula): an unusual presentation, *Am J Optom Phys Opt* 63:567, 1986.

54. Manley DR: Classification of esodeviation. In Manley RD, editor: *Symposium on horizontal ocular deviations,* St Louis, 1971, Mosby.

55. von Noorden GK: *Binocular vision and ocular motility: theory and management of strabismus,* ed 4, St Louis, 1996, Mosby.

56. von Noorden GK, Avilla CW: Accommodative convergence in hypermetropia, *Am J Ophthalmol* 110:287, 1991.

57. Held R, Birch EE, Gwiazada J: Stereoacuity of human infants, *Proc Natl Acad Sci U S A* 77:5572, 1980.

58. Manny RE, Klein SA: The development of vernier acuity in infants, *Curr Eye Res* 3:453, 1984.

59. Atkinson J, Braddick O: Stereoscopic discrimination in infants, *Perception* 5:29, 1976.

60. Worth C: *Squint: its causes, pathology and treatment,* ed 6, London, 1929, Bailliére, Tindall and Cox.

61. Chavasse FB: *Worth's squint: on the binocular reflexes and the treatment of strabismus,* ed 7, Philadelphia, 1939, Blakiston & Sons.

62. Nixon RB and others: Incidence of strabismus in neonates, *Am J Ophthalmol* 100:798, 1985.

63. Archer SM, Sondhi N, Helveston EM: Strabismus in infancy, *Ophthalmology* 96:133, 1989.

64. Sondhi N, Archer SM, Helveston EM: Development of normal ocular alignment, *J Pediatr Ophthalmol Strab* 25:210, 1988.

65. Rennie AGR: Some syndromes affecting the eyes seen in the neonatal period, *Br Orthopt J* 46:88, 1989.

66. Apt L, Isenberg S: Eye position of strabismus patients under general anesthesia, *Am J Ophthalmol* 84:574, 1977.

67. de Molina AC, Munoz LG: Ocular alignment under general anesthesia in congenital esotropia, *J Pediatr Ophthalmol Strab* 28:278, 1991.

68. Pueschel SM, Rynders JE, editors: *Down syndrome: advances in biomedicine and the behavioral sciences,* Cambridge, Mass, 1982, Ware.

69. Perez-Carpinell J, de Fez MD, Climent V: Vision evaluation in people with Down's syndrome, *Opthalmic Physiol Opt* 14:115, 1994.

70. Catalono RA: Down syndrome, *Surv Ophthalmol* 34:385, 1990.

71. Seaber JH, Chandler AC: A five-year study of patients with cerebral palsy and strabismus. In Moore S, Mein J, Stockbridge L, editors: *Orthoptics: past, present, and future,* New York, 1976, Stratton Intercontinental.

72. Buckley E, Seaber JH: Dyskinetic strabismus as a sign of cerebral palsy, *Am J Ophthalmol* 91:652, 1981.

73. Pratt-Johnson JA: Central disruption of fusional amplitudes, *Br J Ophthalmol* 57:347, 1973.

74. Pratt-Johnson JA, Tillson G: Acquired central disruption of fusional amplitude, *Ophthalmology* 86:2140, 1979.

75. London R, Scott SH: Sensory fusion disruption syndrome, *J Am Optom Assoc* 58:544, 1987.

76. Pratt-Johnson JA: Fusion and suppression: development and loss, *J Pediatr Ophthalmol Strab* 29:4, 1992.

77. Kushner B: Unsuspected cyclotropia simulating disruption of fusion, *Arch Ophthalmol* 110:1415, 1992.

78. Sharkey J, Sellar W: Acquired central fusion disruption following cataract extraction, *J Pediatr Ophthalmol Strab* 31:391, 1994.

79. Rutstein RP, Levi DM: Blindspot syndrome, *J Am Optom Assoc* 50:1387, 1979.

80. Olivier P, von Noorden GK: The blindspot syndrome: does it exist? *J Pediatr Ophthalmol Strab* 18:20, 1981.

81. Rutstein RP, Galkin K: Convergence spasm, *J Am Optom Assoc* 55:495, 1984.

82. Rutstein RP, Daum KM, Amos JF: Accommodative spasm: a study of 17 patients, *J Am Optom Assoc* 59:527, 1988.

Esotropia

Esotropia occurs when the visual axes cross in front of the point of fixation, resulting in an inward, or convergent, misalignment of the eyes. There is nasal displacement of the object of regard on the retina of the deviating eye. Unlike esophoria, esotropia is a manifest deviation that is not controlled by fusional divergence. If fusional divergence amplitudes are only occasionally inadequate, an intermittent esotropia occurs. The unilateral cover-uncover test differentiates whether the deviation is an esophoria or esotropia.

PREVALENCE

Esotropia is the most commonly found type of strabismic deviation, occurring in 2% to 4% of the general population.[1,2] Some investigators have reported a higher incidence of esotropia in Caucasian versus other races, but this has not been our experience.[3] Esotropia has no gender preference and is found to occur much more frequently than exotropia. The prevalence ratio of esotropia to exotropia ranges from 2/1 to 4/1.[4]

  CLINICAL PEARL

Esotropia is the most common type of strabismic deviation.

AGE OF ONSET

The clinical picture, and especially the prognosis, depend considerably on the age of onset. Most esotropias commence during early life. It is most frequently diagnosed in children between ages 1 and 3. It begins less frequently between the ages of 3 and 4 and even less between ages 4 and 5. Esotropias that develop in late childhood, adolescence, or adulthood are frequently associated with lateral rectus paresis or other underlying neurologic or systemic disorders.

The very early age of onset is attributed mostly to the narrow interpupillary distance and the exuberance of convergence that exist in young children. Any strabismogenic factor would be more likely to cause esotropia than exotropia. However, as indicated earlier, with sensory strabismus, such as that caused by unilateral cataract, optic atrophy, or macular lesion, the incidences of esotropia and exotropia are similar when the time of onset of the unilateral visual loss occurs before age 5.[5] Esotropia will not develop when the unilateral organic visual loss commences on or after the age of 15.

GENERAL CLINICAL FEATURES

Despite the differences that exist among the various types of esotropias, the following clinical features should come to mind when examining a patient with esotropia:
- Most esotropias are stable and constant. A variable, or intermittent, angle of esotropia occurs either in neurologically impaired children, divergence insufficiency, the nystagmus blockage syndrome, cyclic esotropia, abducens nerve palsy, spasm of the near reflex, and accommodative esotropia.[6] If left untreated, some accommodative esotropias that start out being intermittent become constant. The high degree of constancy makes esotropia detrimental to establishing and/or maintaining normal binocular vision in the pediatric patient.

- Most esotropias are unilateral. As many as 80% of patients demonstrate a fixation preference, whereas 20% exhibit an alternating fixation pattern.[7] The high degree of fixation preference makes pediatric patients with esotropia vulnerable to developing amblyopia. Alternating fixation with esotropia generally precludes strabismic amblyopia.
- The refractive error for many esotropias can be either totally or partly causative. The incidence of hyperopia is larger than in the nonstrabismic population. One third of children with hyperopia exceeding 4 D develop esotropia by age 3.[8] A cycloplegic refraction is mandatory for all children with esotropia.
- Differences in the angle of esotropia in the different gaze positions of less than 5 PD are consistent with the diagnosis of comitant esotropia. However, as many as 25% of all esotropic deviations are truly incomitant. Nearly 50% have an associated vertical component.[7] The latter may result in vertical incomitancies in lateral gaze secondary to overaction of the oblique muscles.[9] Horizontal incomitancies in vertical directions of gaze, (i.e., A and V patterns) are commonly seen with esotropia.
- An esotropia is frequently larger at near than at distance fixation because of the effect of accommodative and proximal convergence.

CLASSIFICATION

An adequate classification of the many types of esotropia is difficult because knowledge of the cause of many of them is uncertain. As well as differences in etiology, variable clinical features include the state of comitance, fusion ability, age of the patient at the onset, the magnitude of the strabismus, and the laterality of the strabismus. A useful clinical classification of the recognizable types of esotropia is given below.

1. Infantile, or congenital, esotropia
2. Accommodative esotropia
   a. Refractive
   b. Nonrefractive
   c. Partly
3. Nonaccommodative esotropia
   a. Early onset
   b. Acute onset
      (1) Acute acquired comitant esotropia
      (2) Divergence insufficiency
4. Secondary esotropia
   a. Sensory
   b. Consecutive
5. Microtropia
6. Blind-spot esotropia
7. Cyclic esotropia
8. Mechanically restrictive or paretic esotropia
   a. Duane's syndrome types I and III
   b. Thyroid myopathy

   c. Fibrosis of the medial rectus muscles
   d. Traumatically induced esotropia
   e. Abducens nerve palsy (lateral rectus paresis)

The incomitant esotropias that are mechanically restrictive or paretic in origin are discussed in Chapter 10.

INFANTILE ESOTROPIA

Infantile, or congenital, esotropia is a common type of esotropia, accounting for 28% to 54% of all esotropias, with having an incidence of 1% of the general population.[10-13] It is characterized as a large and stable angle esotropia in an otherwise neurologically normal child, whose onset is documented during the first 6 months of life by a reliable observer. Several forms of esotropia with a different pathophysiology that meet the criterion of commencing at the same time must be differentiated from infantile esotropia. The differential diagnosis includes (1) pseudoesotropia, (2) Duane's syndrome, (3) congenital abducens nerve palsy, (4) early-onset accommodative esotropia, (5) sensory esotropia, and (6) esotropia in the neurologically impaired child.

 CLINICAL PEARL

Infantile, or congenital, esotropia is characterized as a large and stable angle esotropia in an otherwise neurologically normal child, whose onset is documented during the first 6 months of life by a reliable observer.

Although the vast majority of children with infantile esotropia do not have clinically overt neurologic or developmental disorders and are normal in all other respects, an increased incidence occurs in children with neurologic impairment. Frequent neurologic disorders associated with infantile esotropia include prematurity, hydrocephalus, mental retardation, cerebral palsy, meningomyelocele, intraventricular hemorrhages, and seizures.[14] A high prevalence of infantile esotropia in Williams syndrome has also been reported.[15] Abnormal computed tomographic findings, such as midline anomalies, cortical atrophy, ventricular dilatation, brain stem atrophy, and cerebellar atrophy for 44 of 100 patients with infantile esotropia were described by Lo.[16] Unlike neurologically normal children, children with brain injuries who have infantile esotropia manifest an angle of strabismus that is variable, frequently diminishing with age. Some may eventually become exotropic.

Special examination techniques in otherwise normal children with infantile esotropia may reveal subtle or temporary abnormalities that have been sufficient to disrupt binocular functions at the height of the sensitive period. Some patients with infantile esotropia show moderate or severe reduction in the vestibulo-ocular response, suggesting possible evidence of brain stem dysfunction.[17] Apparently, infantile esotropia can develop from widely disparate anatomic abnormalities in the developing human brain.

Most children with infantile esotropia are reported by their parents to have crossed eyes since birth or shortly thereafter. However, esotropias characteristic of infantile esotropia are rarely present at birth, and the labels *infantile esotropia or essential infantile esotropia* rather than congenital esotropia are preferred by some. Archer, Sondhi, and Helveston[18] report only a 0.7% incidence of esotropia during the first few days of life for 2917 neurologically normal infants. All esotropias were small and unimpressive, and 70% were intermittent. Follow-up was obtained on every infant who had esotropia as a neonate, and none developed infantile esotropia. Of the 3 infants examined by Archer, Sondhi, and Helveston[18] who did develop the clinical features of infantile esotropia, the ages of onset were documented as being 3 months, 4 months, and 6 months, respectively. Two of the infants were previously diagnosed as having exotropia. Thus, infantile esotropia commences at about ages 3 to 4 months, and, because of the oculomotor instability of almost all infants, it is extremely difficult to diagnose before this age. The eyes of children who develop infantile esotropia are becoming crossed at a time when the eyes of nonstrabismic infants are becoming orthophoric.

It is common to find a history of infantile esotropia in the parents or siblings of affected patients. Transmission in many families seems to be as an irregular autosomal dominant trait; in others, it may be recessive. A 7% prevalence of infantile esotropia has been reported in family members of affected patients.[19] Various inheritance patterns of infantile esotropia have been described, but it seems likely that in many instances multiple genes are involved. Different genes may affect sensory and motor phenomena, and the phenotype recognized as infantile esotropia is likely the result of an interplay between both types of genetic influences and the child's environment.

ETIOLOGY

Present understanding of the cause of infantile esotropia is fragmentary at best. The label *essential* infantile esotropia emphasizes the obscure etiology of the condition. Infantile esotropia has been attributed in the past to innervational factors. The innervational disturbance consists of a poorly understood imbalance between tonic convergence and tonic divergence. With the child under general surgical plane anesthesia, the esotropia either reduces considerably or disappears entirely, providing no peripheral mechanical factors restrict passive abduction; therefore excessive tonic convergence has been cited as the cause in many cases.[20]

Worth,[21] as discussed in Chapter 7, emphasizes an innate deficient fusion as being the major factor in the cause of infantile esotropia. If this is the case, restoring binocularity is considered hopeless, because there is no way to provide this innate absent neural function. However, fusion can be achieved following appropriately timed therapy for many patients with infantile esotropia. This concurs more with the views of Chavasse,[22] who reports that the infant's eyes crossed on a reflex basis under the influence of muscular forces. Some binocular vision is obtainable if the eyes are aligned at an early enough age. Lack of bifoveal fusion and high-grade stereopsis in patients with treated infantile esotropia does not discount the theory of Worth, however.

Current investigators have emphasized delayed development of a congenitally defective motor fusion as being causative with infantile esotropia.[23,24] Strabismogenic factors such as excessive tonic convergence, abnormal accommodative-convergence relationship, uncorrected hyperopia and anisometropia, genetic components, and unknown factors impinge on a sensorially normal but immature and functionally imperfect infantile visual system. A normally functioning vergence system is capable of overcoming these forces and maintains ocular alignment. Delayed development or a defect in the vergence system results in infantile esotropia. Infantile esotropia likely results from a failure of cortical motor fusion to stabilize ocular alignment during the critical developmental period between 3 and 4 months of age.[23]

CLINICAL FEATURES

Infantile esotropia represents a cluster of findings that include a constant large-angle esotropia that is commonly associated with overaction of the inferior oblique muscles, nystagmus, dissociated vertical deviations, amblyopia, and limited potential for normal binocular vision.

Size of Deviation

The magnitude of infantile esotropia in most cases is considerably larger than most other forms of esotropia (Fig. 8-1). The angle of deviation ranges on the average from 40 PD to 60 PD. Nearly 50% of the patients with infantile esotropia have a deviation larger than 50 PD, with some measuring 80 PD or more.[25] Rarely is the angle less than 30 PD. The esotropia is constant and usually equal in magnitude at distance and near. The angle of deviation remains stable in neurologically normal infants if there is no superimposed accommodative esodeviation. However, one report did document three cases of infantile esotropia that all resolved to less than 10 PD without treatment over a minimum period of 37 months. [26]

Because of the difficulty in getting the very young child to fixate at distance, the distance measurement is usually approximated. To measure the near deviation

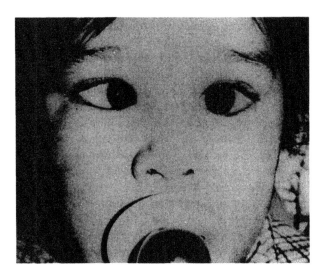

FIG. 8-1 Infantile esotropia.

when the alternate cover test with prisms is not possible, the Krimsky or Hirschberg tests can be used while the child fixates a muscle light. Because of the large magnitude of the strabismus, when performing the Krimsky test it may be necessary to hold the base-out prisms before both eyes simultaneously to center the corneal reflections.

Refractive Error

Most patients with infantile esotropia have low-to-moderate levels of hyperopia by the usual amount for their chronologic age. Costenbader[27] refracted 500 patients with infantile esotropia and found that 5.6% were myopic, 46.4% had refractive errors ranging from emmetropia to 2 D of hyperopia, 41.8% were hyperopic from 2 to 5 D, and 6.4% had hyperopia exceeding 5 D. In a later evaluation on 408 patients with infantile esotropia, a similar distribution of refractive errors was found.[23] These findings contrast markedly with the degree of hyperopia associated with refractive accommodative esotropia.

Despite the lack of a relationship between the refractive error and size of the deviation, the refractive errors for those with infantile esotropia differ from the refractive errors of other children. Whereas only 11% of orthophoric 1 year olds have hyperopia exceeding 2 D, nearly 50% of all infants with infantile esotropia have greater than 2 D of hyperopia.[23,27,28] More significant is that with infantile esotropia there is persistence of the strabismus in spite of correcting the hyperopia.

Amblyopia

Between 35% and 70% of infants with infantile esotropia will have amblyopia.[23,27,29] Determining whether an infant prefers fixation with one eye or the other can be challenging. Amblyopia would not be ex-

pected in infants with infantile esotropia who cross-fixate and use the left eye to view targets in the field of right gaze and the right eye to view targets in the field of left gaze (Fig. 8-2). Nevertheless, amblyopia has been diagnosed in as many as 50% of those who cross-fixate.[30] The point at which alternation of fixation occurs is a more reliable means of detecting a difference in visual acuity between the eyes. The change of fixation can be seen as the patient follows a target moving horizontally. If there is equal visual acuity, alternation of fixation will occur at the midline of each eye. If amblyopia exists, the sound eye will continue to follow the target beyond midline into abduction, before the poorer eye picks up fixation.

Amblyopia may develop several months following the onset of a nonalternating infantile esotropia. Steger and Birch[31,32] examined 100 infants with esotropia by preferential looking (PL) techniques. PL visual acuities of those who freely alternated fixation and of the preferred eyes of patients with unilateral esotropia were not significantly different from monocular acuity of age-matched normal infants. PL acuity of the nonpreferred eye of patients with unilateral esotropia was normal during months 3 to 5 but became abnormal during months 6 to 14. Less than half of the infants with esotropia who were judged amblyopic by fixation preference were found amblyopic by PL. Most discrepancies between PL and fixation preference occurred when clinically amblyopic infants under 8 months were found not amblyopic by PL.

Ocular Motility

Several ocular motility disorders exist with infantile esotropia. Although these may occur more frequently with infantile esotropia, they are not pathognomonic for infantile esotropia.

Because of the large angle of strabismus, many infants with infantile esotropia will cross-fixate and view with the right eye for left gaze and view with the left eye for right gaze (see Fig. 8-2). Cross-fixation must be differentiated from other conditions causing defective abduction, such as bilateral abducens nerve palsy and bilateral Duane's syndrome. It is virtually impossible to evaluate ductions in infants because they usually object strongly to having one eye covered. Using the doll's-head maneuver, in which the clinician turns the infants's head in one direction as the eyes shift in the opposite direction, the clinician looks for abduction of either eye caused by the maneuver. Brief periods of alternating occlusion should improve the apparent abduction deficit secondary to cross-fixation but not the abduction deficit associated with bilateral Duane's syndrome or bilateral abducens nerve palsy. Abducens nerve palsy is extremely rare in infancy, and, when it does occur, is often transient and without further sequelae. Also, rarely in Duane's syndrome does a large

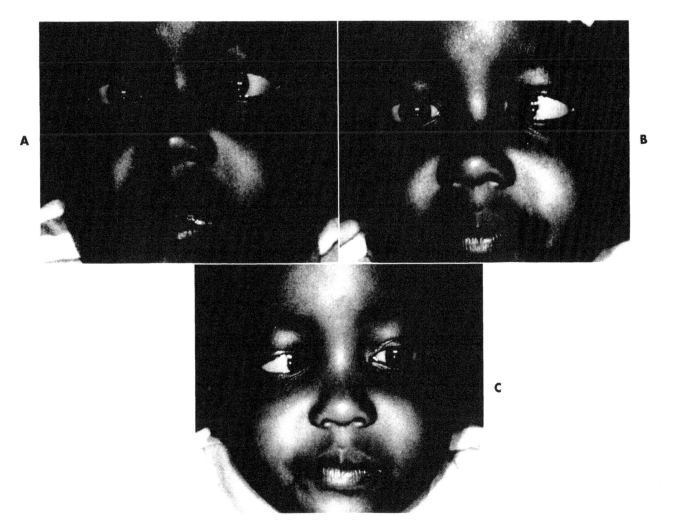

FIG. 8-2 Cross-fixation with infantile esotropia. **A,** Left esotropia in primary position. **B,** In right gaze, patient fixates with left eye and there is limited abduction in the right eye. **C,** In left gaze, patient fixates with right eye and there is limited abduction in the left eye. (From Rutstein RP: Incomitant deviations in children, In Scheiman MM, editor: *Problems in optometry,* Philadelphia, 1990, JB Lippincott.)

esotropia exist in primary position, as is the case in infantile esotropia.

Inferior oblique overaction has been estimated to occur in as many as 78% of all cases of infantile esotropia.[33] It can be unilateral or bilateral and is commonly associated with a V-pattern esotropia in downgaze. The age of onset of the inferior oblique overaction is usually later, averaging 3.6 years.[9] It is rarely found in children with infantile esotropia under 1 year of age and may not be apparent until after treatment for the large-angle esotropia is completed. Early treatment of the esotropia does not prevent the later development of inferior oblique overaction.

Between 50% and 90% of patients with infantile esotropia also have a dissociated vertical deviation.[33,34] It may be latent (detected only when the involved eye is covered) or manifest and may occur intermittently or constantly. In relation to infantile esotropia, dissociated vertical deviation is a time-related phenomenon whose onset is greatest during the second year of life. In some cases, dissociated vertical deviation may develop years after treatment of the infantile esotropia. Dissociated vertical deviation is easier to detect following reduction in the large angle of esotropia.

Because of the association of dissociated vertical deviation and infantile esotropia, when evaluating for the first time an older patient with dissociated vertical deviation, we presume a history of infantile esotropia even in the presence of exotropia. For these patients, dissociated vertical deviations may occur simply as a response to long-standing defective binocularity. (See Case 1.)

CASE 1

A 10-year-old boy was brought to the clinic by his school nurse. His ocular history was significant for strabismus surgery at 14 months of age and therapy for amblyopia from ages 4 to 5. Glasses were prescribed at age 3. At the time of examination, the nurse noticed that the child's left eye occasionally looked up and out.

Our examination revealed corrected vision of 20/30 for the right eye and 20/20 for the left eye, with OD +3.50 −1.00 × 155 and OS +0.50 sphere. The patient manifested a 12-PD constant right exotropia at distance and near with a dissociated vertical deviation that was greater for the left eye. Bilateral inferior oblique overactions and bilateral superior oblique overactions were apparent with versions, which caused an X-pattern exodeviation, with the exotropia measuring 20 PD in upgaze and 50 PD in downgaze. With the synoptophore, normal correspondence existed, without evidence of second-degree sensory or motor fusion. The patient, when tested with the Bagolini striated lens test, showed suppression when fixating with the left eye and harmonious anomalous correspondence when fixating with the right eye. Stereopsis was not present with the Randot stereotest without or with compensatory prisms.

Because of the early age of extraocular muscle surgery, we suspect that the patient had an infantile esotropia. On a subsequent visit, his parents brought previous medical records and baby photographs that confirmed the presence of a large esotropia.

An additional feature of infantile esotropia is nystagmus. As many as 30% of patients may exhibit a rotary nystagmus, which tends to diminish during the first decade of life.[33] It is always bilateral and rhythmic, with a high frequency and low amplitude. More common is the presence of latent nystagmus, which occurs in approximately 50% of patients with infantile esotropia.[35] Latent nystagmus is a horizontal jerk nystagmus elicited by occluding either eye. When one eye is occluded, nystagmus develops in both eyes, with the fast component directed toward the uncovered eye. Latent nystagmus rarely exists without dissociated vertical deviation.

In patients without strabismus the optokinetic response elicited by a rotating nystagmus drum consists of a smooth pursuit movement in the direction of the moving stripes or pictures, followed by a corrective saccade in the opposite direction. The pursuit movement occurs with equal facility, regardless of whether the stripes move in a nasal-to-temporal or temporal-to-nasal direction. In infantile esotropia, the monocularly elicited optokinetic nystagmus (OKN) is asymmetric.[36-42] When the OKN target is rotated from the temporal to the nasal direction, the elicited slow phase or pursuit movement is normal, whereas when the target is rotated from the nasal to the temporal direction, the pursuit movement is poor. OKN-elicited asymmetry has been used by some clinicians to distinguish between infantile esotropia and esotropia of later onset. Adults who had infantile esotropia show the same movement asymmetry. It has been suggested that its persistence even after treatment in infantile esotropia may be of etiologic significance, reflecting an imbalance in brain stem ocular alignment factors. OKN-elicited asymmetry has also been observed in nonstrabismic patients with other causes of deficient binocular input, such as anisometropic amblyopia and monocular congenital cataracts.[38,40]

The association of a distinct subgroup of patients with infantile esotropia with a jerky horizontal nystagmus and a face turn was first described by Ciancia.[43] The nystagmus increased in abduction and was absent in adduction. This supposedly occurred in several patients with infantile esotropia. Adelstein and Cüppers[44] suggest that these patients make a continuous effort to maintain both eyes in adduction through the use of convergence. The convergence mechanism augments adduction of the fixating eye. An inverse relationship exists between the angle of esotropia and the amplitude of nystagmus. As the fixating eye follows a target moving laterally toward the primary position and then into abduction, the nystagmus increases and the angle of esotropia decreases. Characteristically, when one eye is occluded, a face turn by the patient develops in the direction of the uncovered eye to have it remain in the adducted position. According to Adelstein and Cüppers, the sustained convergence over time causes hypertonicity of the medial rectus muscles and esotropia. This is known as the *nystagmus blockage syndrome* and may exist in up to 12% of all individuals with infantile esotropia.[44] It likely is much less common, and the esotropia may be the primary defect and nystagmus secondary.[45]

Compared with other patients with infantile esotropia, those with nystagmus blockage syndrome have (1) a variable and frequently smaller esotropia, with both eyes being convergent; (2) nystagmus in the primary position; (3) nystagmus that is dampened by convergence; (4) limited abduction of either eye, with increased nystagmus on attempted abduction; (5) a compensatory head posture, predominantly a face turn to the side of the fixating eye to bring about adduction; (6) a lower incidence of inferior oblique overaction and dissociated vertical deviation; (7) a much higher incidence of neurologic abnormalities, such as Down syndrome, hydrocephalus, and cerebral palsy; and (8) different and quite unpredictable results following treatment.[46]

Limited Potential for Normal Binocular Vision

Patients with infantile esotropia apparently lack potential for normal binocular vision.[25,47-50] Even with perfect ocular alignment following treatment, most pa-

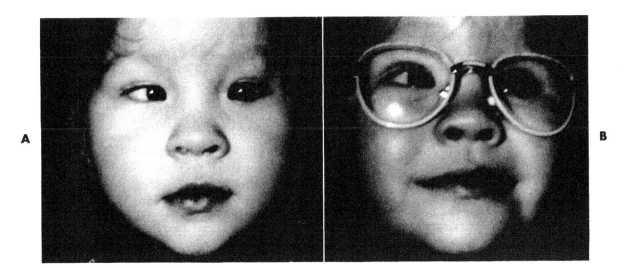

FIG. 8-3 Hyperopic glasses for infantile esotropia reduces deviation slightly.

tients achieve at best only peripheral fusion. Treated infantile esotropia is a leading cause of microtropia. Because of the lack of bifoveal fusion, achieving high-grade stereopsis is unexpected, although isolated case reports have shown otherwise.[42,51,52] Random-dot stereopsis may occur when the deviation is either corrected with prisms or very early surgery.[31,51-54] Mohindra and others[55] report that children corrected with prisms equal in size to the deviation showed some degree of binocularity up to at least 2½ years, as measured by a Polaroid bar stereogram procedure with 1800 seconds of arc disparity. Approximately 35% of patients showed stereopsis with random-dot stereograms. Older children failed to appreciate any stereopsis. Possibly, infantile esotropia does not cause loss of good stereopsis potential until near the second birthday.

Because of the young age of the patient, extensive sensory testing cannot be performed before treatment in many cases. In older patients in whom sensory testing is possible, the absence of normal binocular vision potential is the invariable finding. We rarely encounter an adult with untreated infantile esotropia (see Case 8-2).

TREATMENT

Although as clinicians we tend to place greatest emphasis on good visual acuity and fusion, parents usually place the most emphasis on the child's appearance. The improved appearance enhances the child's psychologic acceptance by the parents. This is instrumental in normal development of parent-child relationship. Some parents report improvement in their child's fine motor development and visual function after the eyes are straightened, even when our testing indicates no improvement in sensory function.[56-58] Parents often

ask the question "How early should my child be examined?" Because of the high incidence of transient strabismus in neurologically normal infants, a child suspected of having infantile esotropia need not be examined before 3 months of age, unless some organic lesion or additional ocular finding (i.e., cataract) is suspected.[18,48,59,60] Once the diagnosis has been made, treatment consists of the following:

1. *Correction of clinically significant refractive errors.* Because the degree of refractive error does not correlate with the large angle of esotropia, the question arises whether correction of a hyperopic refractive error is indicated at all. Patients with infantile esotropia have refractive errors skewed more toward hyperopia than do nonstrabismic infants, and, for some, giving the glasses reduces the size of the esotropia. Furthermore, accommodative esotropia, although usually beginning later, may occur in infants and respond to optical correction. We therefore prescribe glasses for all infants with esotropia whose hyperopic refraction exceeds 2.50 D. The child wears the glasses for 1 month and is rechecked. In most cases a large esotropia remains, confirming that the angle of infantile esotropia is not consistent with the excess of accommodation required to overcome the hyperopia (Fig. 8-3). Repeat refractions are done, but rarely uncover significantly more hyperopia. We do not prescribe overcorrecting hyperopic lenses for these patients.

✿ CLINICAL PEARL

It is best to prescribe glasses for all esotropic infants whose hyperopic refraction exceeds 2.50 D.

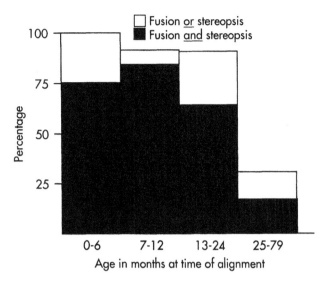

FIG. 8-4 Binocular vision status for 106 patients with infantile esotropia treated surgically. (From Ing MR: Early surgical alignment for congenital esotropia, *Ophthalmology* 90:135, 1983.)

2. *Therapy for amblyopia.* Treatment for amblyopia with infantile esotropia consists mainly of occlusion therapy. During periods of occlusion, small toys can be shown to the child to stimulate monocular fixation and accommodation.

We rely on fixation preference in determining the success of treatment. The acquisition of an alternating fixation pattern signals elimination of amblyopia, and maintenance of alternation should prevent any regression.[61] Maintenance therapy may be required for children who revert to their original fixation pattern.

3. *Obtaining ocular alignment.* Following correction of the refractive error and treatment of amblyopia, the esotropia persists. Prism therapy can be attempted. Because prisms have been somewhat successful in creating stereopsis at least in laboratory studies, some clinicians advocate their use, with hopes of establishing better fusion.[55,62] In a 10-year retrospective study of patients with infantile esotropia treated initially with prisms, there was a significantly better alignment and sensorial improvement than for patients not treated with prisms.[63] Because of the large esotropia and parental concern about the child's appearance, we feel that surgical treatment of the esotropia at this time should be strongly considered.

Disagreement regarding the best age for surgery is common. Some ophthalmic surgeons prefer operating at 6 months of age or earlier. They feel the earlier that ocular alignment is obtained, the better the chance to establish some binocular vision. Surgical treatment has

been performed as early as 3 months of age.[52,64] Others prefer to do surgery from 6 to 18 months or at age 2 or older. Postponing surgery till a later age supposedly allows for more precise measurements of the deviation. Other reasons given for not performing surgery at a very early age include (1) the infant's eye is too small, (2) anesthesia may be too risky for the very young patient, (3) unwanted and necessary scar tissue is more likely in younger infants, and (4) the creation of anomalous correspondence prevents the likelihood of good surgical results. The most reasonable approach seems to be having surgery done as soon as an accurate and consistent determination can be made of the deviation and its associated characteristics and only after attention has been directed to any refractive component, amblyopia treatment, and other nonsurgical intervention, such as prisms. Most ophthalmic surgeons prefer to intervene by 18 months of age, if possible (see Chapter 11).

Numerous studies report on the efficacy of surgery for infantile esotropia. Many of these studies also include some type of assessment for fusion.[23,45,65-69] Scheiman, Ciner, and Gallaway[65] performed a literature search and found the success rate overall for achieving some level of binocular vision was 22% in 1286 patients and the overall cosmetic success rate was 63% in 2113 patients. The need for multiple surgery was common.

With regard to the optimal age for surgery and achieving fusion, Ing,[66,67] in a frequently referenced study, evaluated retrospectively the binocular vision of 106 patients with infantile esotropia who had extraocular muscle surgery. All patients were aligned within plus or minus 10 PD of the ortho position when evaluated. Approximately 47% required two or more operations to obtain this status. The sensory tests used were the Bagolini striated lens test, with fixation at 1/3 m, the Worth four dot test at 1/3 m, and the Titmus stereotest. "Binocularity" was said to be present in these patients if they were able to appreciate any stereopsis at all with the Titmus stereotest and/or fuse the near Worth four dot test and Bagolini striated lens test. The results (Fig. 8-4) showed that the fusion ability for those adequately aligned by the age of 6 months versus 12 months versus 24 months was not statistically different, whereas the fusion ability for the children aligned within plus or minus 10 PD after 24 months was significantly less. One half to two thirds of the patients also required glasses to maintain an acceptable cosmetic appearance.

The most extensive evaluation is reported by von Noorden.[23,45] He describes four sensory outcomes encountered in 358 patients with surgically treated infantile esotropia (Table 8-1). The optimal treatment result is subnormal binocular vision. These patients are orthophoric or minimally heterophoric by cover testing

TABLE 8-1 STATUS OF BINOCULAR VISION FOLLOWING SURGERY FOR INFANTILE ESOTROPIA

	Subnormal Binocular Vision	Microtropia	Small Angle	Large Angle
Cover test	Orthophoria or asymptomatic heterophoria	Flick (2-3 PD) on unilateral cover test	≥4-20 PD esotropia/exotropia	>20 PD esotropia/exotropia
Visual acuity	No amblyopia	Amblyopia may exist	Amblyopia may exist	Amblyopia may exist
Motor fusion*	Yes	Yes (based on anomalous correspondence)	On anomalous correspondence basis only	No
Retinal correspondence†	Normal	Anomalous	Anomalous	Usually suppression
Stereopsis	Reduced (<120 sec on random-dot test)	Reduced or absent	Gross or stereoblind	Stereoblind
Course	Stable alignment	Some stability of alignment	Less stability of alignment	Unstable
Treatment result	Optimal	Desirable	Acceptable	Undesirable

From von Noorden GK: Infantile esotropia: a continuing riddle, *Am Orthopt J* 34:52, 1984.
*Demonstrated using rotary prism or a synoptophore.
†As determined by the Bagolini striated lens test.

following strabismus surgery. Despite the perfect ocular alignment, a unilateral foveal suppression persists under binocular conditions and prevents high-grade stereopsis. Subnormal binocular vision occurred in 71 of 358 patients (20%). A more frequent outcome was the categories of microtropia and small-angle strabismus (46%). These categories are similar sensorially, except for the magnitude of the residual strabismus. The small-angle category also shows less stability in ocular alignment over the years. An undesirable result is any residual strabismus exceeding 20 PD (large-angle category). These patients have no demonstrable fusion. Concurring with earlier reports, von Noorden found that as the age of the patient at completion of surgery became greater, the probability of achieving the optimal outcome, subnormal binocular vision, decreased. Nevertheless, many patients still achieved the status of microtropia or small-angle strabismus, even when surgery was done well beyond age 4. Persistence of amblyopia, dissociated vertical deviation, inferior oblique overaction, and nystagmus were more frequently associated with the occurrence of less satisfactory fusion outcomes.[68-70]

From these reports and our clinical experience, we believe it matters little sensorially whether surgery is performed at 6 months or 2 years. We are content to see an esotropia of 10 PD or less after surgery, with no amblyopia, and some fusion as demonstrated with either the Worth four-dot test at near, the Bagolini striated lens test, or stereopsis testing. It should be emphasized that a fusion response in the presence of constant strabismus indicates fusion based on anomalous correspondence; therefore prism compensation does not improve the fusion.

 CLINICAL PEARL

A fusion response in the presence of constant strabismus indicates fusion based on anomalous correspondence.

With regard to achieving fusion, the final ocular alignment status and its stability may be the key factors and not necessarily the age of the patient when undergoing surgery. Some untreated adults who have surgery for infantile esotropia have been reported to develop fusion if aligned within 10 PD of orthophoria.[71-74] In one study, 60 of 74 adults (81%) with a known or suspected history of infantile esotropia developed fusion as measured with the Bagolini striated lens test postsurgically.[72] Morris, Scott, and Dickey report on 24 adults with esotropia, four of whom had untreated infantile esotropia. Despite the late age of surgery, all four patients fused the Worth four dot test at near and also achieved some degree of stereopsis with the Titmus stereotest (Table 8-2).[73]

We have also seen adults with untreated infantile esotropia achieve some level of fusion, as indicated by the following Case:

CASE 2

A 28-year-old man was examined in our clinic in March, 1990. He had an esotropia since infancy. Occlusion therapy for amblyopia was performed when the patient was 3 years old. There had been no other treatment except for glasses and contact lenses.

Our examination revealed 20/25 vision in the right eye and 20/30 vision in the left eye, with a refractive correction of OD −6.00 D and OS −9.00 D. The patient manifested a 50-PD constant alternating esotropia at distance and near.

TABLE 8-2   FUSION STATUS AFTER SURGICAL ALIGNMENT OF INFANTILE ESOTROPIA IN ADULTS

Patient	Age (Years)	Preoperative Deviation (Prism Diopters)	Postoperative Deviation (Prism Diopters)	Stereopsis (Seconds of Arc)	Worth Four-Dot (6 Meters and 1/3 Meter)
1	20	30 ET* (Distance and near)	2 ET* (Distance and near)	400	Suppression/fusion
2	19	45 ET (Distance and near)	Ortho (Distance and near)	140	Suppression/fusion
3	16	30 ET (Distance and near)	8 XT (Distance and near)	100	Suppression/fusion
4	12	40 ET (Distance and near)	4 ET (Distance and near)	400	Suppression/fusion

From Morris RJ, Scott WE, Dickey CF: *Ophthalmology* 100:135, 1993.
*ET, esotropia; XT, exotropia.

There was also a dissociated vertical deviation. Versions revealed limited abduction secondary to cross-fixation.

With both the Worth four dot and Bagolini striated lens tests, alternating suppression was shown at all viewing distances. Stereopsis was not present with the Randot stereotest with compensating prisms. Synoptophore evaluation showed an objective angle of 50 PD base-out and a subjective angle of 18 PD base-out, indicating unharmonious anomalous correspondence. The patient alternately suppressed with the Hering-Bielschowsky afterimage test.

The diagnosis was presumed to be infantile esotropia. The patient desired extraocular muscle surgery. Based on our sensory testing, we believed there was little hope for achieving any form of fusion.

Three months following recession of both medial rectus muscles, the patient manifested a 12-PD constant alternating exotropia at distance and near. He denied any diplopia. The dissociated vertical deviation persisted. He fused the Worth 4 dot test at near and suppressed with the left eye at distance. With the Bagolini striated lenses an X was perceived, indicating fusion based on harmonious anomalous correspondence. With the synoptophore the objective angle was 8 PD base-in and the subjective angle was 10 PD base-in, indicating normal correspondence. There was only superimposition without evidence of second degree sensory or motor fusion.

The mechanism for this "fusion" is unclear, but it is possible that in early infancy some fusional development may occur before the onset of esotropia, allowing the development of at least some binocular neurons in the visual cortex. Because infantile esotropia is not congenital, some patients having straight eyes during the critical period of binocular vision development, or the first few months of life, have an advantage over those with a constant esotropia since the first or second month of life. This concurs with the acquisition of stereopsis in isolated cases following prism therapy and very early surgery.[52,54,55] In addition, almost all patients with infantile esotropia, regardless of the age when treated, experience an expansion of their binocular vi-

sual field if their eyes are satisfactorily aligned.[75,76] The developmental gains that are reported by parents in children undergoing surgery for infantile esotropia may very well be the result of this expanded binocular field.[58]

Instead of conventional incisional surgery for patients with infantile esotropia, some have used botulinum toxin type A injections into the medial rectus.[77-79] The dose-related but temporary paralysis of the medial rectus muscle leads to a change in position of the eye, which is followed by some degree of contracture of the opposing lateral rectus muscle. This supposedly results in long-lasting and permanent changes in ocular alignment. Of 12 patients with infantile esotropia, 6 demonstrated alignment to within 10 PD of orthophoria.[77] A minimum of 1 month after the botulinum injection was necessary to establish this alignment. Only 3 of the 6 aligned patients could both fuse and demonstrate some stereopsis. Transient ptosis and vertical deviations developed in some cases. The use of bilateral simultaneous medial rectus botulinum injection may prove more effective.[79] At this time, alignment by botulinum appears to be less effective than conventional incisional surgery in the treatment of infantile esotropia. It has been used much more effectively in adults with acquired lateral rectus paresis (see Chapter 11).

CLINICAL COURSE

Early ocular alignment resulting in straight or nearly straight eyes does not ensure long-term stability. Some investigators have emphasized the instability of ocular alignment in patients treated for infantile esotropia and the need for repeated evaluations throughout the first decade of life.[33,34,70,80-82] The possibility of recurring strabismus, a superimposed accommodative esotropia, amblyopia, increasing dissociated vertical deviation, and inferior oblique overaction exist.

Consecutive exotropia may develop several years

after treatment. Caputo and others[80,81] followed 142 patients with infantile esotropia. All patients had alignment within plus or minus 10 PD of orthophoria 6 months after surgery. Four years after surgery, 27 patients (19%) developed consecutive exotropia. Of the 82 patients followed for 6 years, 21 patients (26%) developed consecutive exotropia.

Achieving perfectly straight eyes may ensure better ocular alignment stability. Shauly, Prager, and Mazow[70] followed 103 patients with treated infantile esotropia an average of 8.7 years. All patients were categorized according to the classification in Table 8-1. The eyes of all 28 patients in the subnormal binocular vision group remained aligned after an average follow-up of 8 years. The eyes of 6 of 30 patients (20%) in the microtropia group and 11 of 43 (26%) in the small-angle deviation group lost the stability of horizontal alignment. Stability of ocular alignment is more likely in small-angle esotropia than in small-angle exotropia.[83]

Because hyperopia increases during the first few years of life, accommodative esotropia can follow surgery for infantile esotropia. Hiles, Watson, and Biglan[33] reported that 65% of patients with surgically corrected infantile esotropia required spectacle correction of hyperopia to control the esotropia at some time postoperatively. Baker and DeYoung-Smith[84] followed 101 patients for a minimum of 3 years following surgery. Of these patients, 52 (51%) developed an accommodative esotropia, 25 within 3 months of surgery, and 27 from 3 to 60 months after surgery. Freely, Nelson, and Calhoun[85] found that 28% of 83 patients with infantile esotropia who had been surgically aligned by 18 months of age subsequently redeveloped esotropia. In 78% of these patients, the esotropia was corrected with a hyperopic correction of as little as 1.5 D. All these authors found no clues during infancy as to which children would eventually need glasses for accommodative esotropia.

As many as 40% of patients with surgically treated infantile esotropia may subsequently develop amblyopia.[33,67,84] This is likely attributed to a large, alternating esotropia being changed to a small-angle unilateral esotropia. Apparently, it is easier for the child with esotropia to maintain alternate fixation in the presence of a larger deviation than in the presence of a smaller deviation. Because the parents are frequently satisfied with the child's appearance following surgery, they may neglect further care, not realizing the risk of amblyopia. Fixation preference must be evaluated at each examination, until the visual acuity can be measured. This may be difficult when the residual angle of deviation is less than 10 PD.

Dissociated vertical deviation and inferior oblique overaction may become more apparent following surgical reduction of the large-angle esotropia. With few exceptions, patients with dissociated vertical deviation have deep suppression and do not experience diplopia and other related visual symptoms. The parents may be bothered by the upturning eye. If the disorder is entirely latent and detected only by the clinician on cover testing, no further treatment is indicated. Our clinical impression is that dissociated vertical deviation occurs less frequently in adults than in children. Dissociated vertical deviations that are manifest and cosmetically displeasing and persisting inferior oblique overactions graded +3 or +4 are treated with additional surgery. (See Cases 3 and 4.)

CASE 3

A 2½-year-old girl was examined in July, 1985. According to her parents, the child's eyes had turned in since birth. The patient was in excellent health. At 10 months of age, another clinician diagnosed strabismus and recommended occlusion therapy, but it was not performed. Glasses were not prescribed. The father had undergone 3 surgeries as a child for infantile esotropia.

With the Broken Wheel test, visual acuity was 20/40 for the right eye and 20/80 for the left eye. A 60-PD constant left esotropia was measured at distance and near (Fig. 8-5, *A*). There was a dissociated vertical deviation, more in the left eye, causing a hypertropia. Version testing revealed inferior oblique overactions, underaction of the lateral rectus muscles and overaction of the medial rectus muscles. Cycloplegic refraction was OD +2.75 and OS +3.50 −0.50 × 180. Funduscopic examination was normal.

The diagnosis was probable infantile esotropia and amblyopia. The cycloplegic refractive findings were given with occlusion therapy. An alternating occlusion regimen was used (the right eye was patched for 3 days, the left eye was patched for 1 day, and so on). The child was also given drawing exercises to stimulate fixation and accommodation.

After 2 months, the visual acuity for the right and left eyes was 20/25 and 20/40, respectively. With the glasses the esotropia measured 50 PD. Occlusion therapy was continued.

In October, 1985, the visual acuity was unchanged, as was the cycloplegic refraction. At this time, a surgical referral was made to reduce the magnitude of the esotropia. The patient was to continue with occlusion therapy.

In December, 1985, extraocular muscle surgery was performed and consisted of bilateral medial rectus muscle recessions 5 mm OU and bilateral inferior oblique myectomies.

In January, 1986, visual acuities were 20/25 for each eye with the Broken Wheel test. A 10-PD left esotropia was measured with the cover test (Fig. 8-5, *B*). The dissociated vertical deviation and inferior oblique overaction were less apparent.

A month later the deviation was stable. However, the visual acuity in the left eye had regressed to 20/40. Occlusion of the right eye for 6 hours a day was prescribed.

In July, 1986 the visual acuities were again equal (20/25) for each eye. The parents mentioned that they now saw the left eye turn again. The patient denied any diplopia. Our findings indicated that the dissociated vertical deviation for the left eye

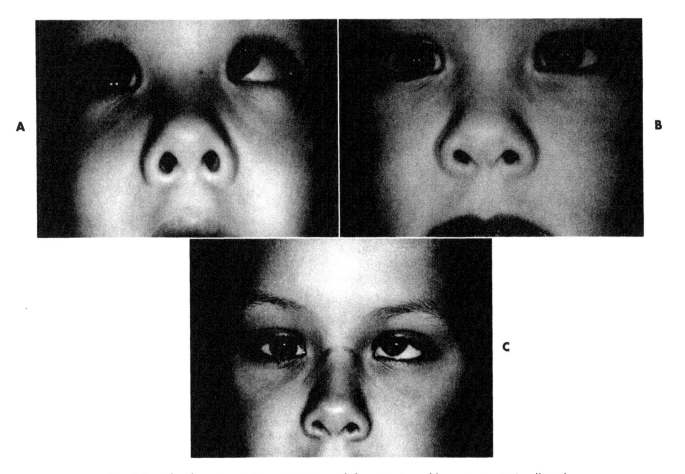

FIG. 8-5   Infantile esotropia (Case 3). **A,** Large left esotropia and hypertropia. **B,** Small-angle esotropia after treatment. **C,** Increasing dissociated vertical deviation with time.

was becoming more apparent (Fig. 8-5, *C*). The esotropia also had increased to 25 PD. Cycloplegic refraction revealed OD +4.00 −1.50 × 180 and OS +4.50 −2.50 × 10, which was prescribed.

In September, 1987 the nearly 5-year-old girl with glasses manifested a 10-PD constant left esotropia at distance and near with a dissociated vertical deviation. There was no amblyopia. With the Worth four dot test, the patient suppressed the left eye at all distances and could not perceive any stereopsis with the Randot or TNO stereotests. With prisms compensating for the strabismus, fusion could not be elicited. The patient eventually moved away from the area and was therefore unavailable for further evaluation and treatment.

Comment

This case of infantile esotropia confirms the necessity of careful follow-up after surgery. A superimposed accommodative esotropia, recurring amblyopia, and an increasing dissociated vertical deviation occurred for this patient. The lack of any fusion ability in all likelihood was the result of the instability of the angle of strabismus over time.

CASE 4

A 22-year-old man was examined for the first time in our clinic. His ocular history was significant for strabismus surgery performed at the age of 6 months. Photography and previous records confirmed a large-angle esotropia in infancy. No other treatment had been given, except glasses that were prescribed at age 3. The patient wore contact lenses and has no visually related symptoms.

Our examination revealed 20/20 corrected vision for each eye, with OD −3.75 −0.50 × 170 and OS −2.00 −0.50 × 40. The patient manifested a 12-PD constant left esotropia at distance and near. There was also a dissociated vertical deviation, occurring more in the left eye. Versions were normal.

With the Worth four dot test, fusion existed as long as the flashlight was held within 3 feet of the patient. Beyond that distance, he suppressed the left eye. The Bagolini striated lens test indicated harmonious anomalous correspondence. With the synoptophore and Hering-Bielschowsky afterimage test, normal retinal correspondence existed. Because of suppression, second-degree sensory and motor fusion could not be demonstrated either with the synoptophore or with compensatory prisms.

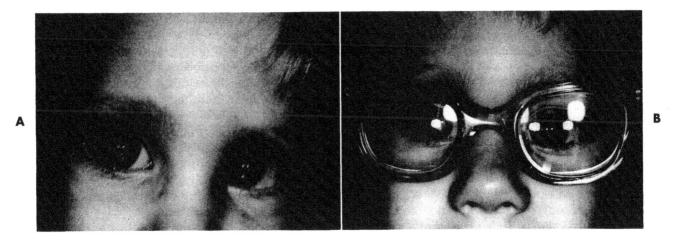

FIG. 8-6 Infant with refractive accommodative esotropia (Case 5).

Comment

This is an acceptable sensory outcome for a patient with infantile esotropia (see Table 8-1). There is absence of amblyopia and the residual deviation is small. Rudimentary binocular vision, albeit anomalous, exists for this patient. In addition, there is an absence of symptoms.

ACCOMMODATIVE ESOTROPIA

Accommodative esotropia is an acquired convergent deviation of the eyes associated with activation of the accommodation reflex.[86] This was reported as early as 1864 by Donders, who found significant amounts of hyperopia in 133 of 172 (77%) patients with esotropia.[87] Donders reasoned that these individuals must accommodate more to overcome the hyperopia to clear the retinal image. When this happens the associated accommodative convergence causes esotropia. Accommodation was confirmed to be the causative factor, because the esotropia lessened considerably or was eliminated completely when the refractive error was neutralized with glasses. Thus, Donders provided the first rational approach to the evaluation and treatment of accommodative esotropia. There is no other form of strabismus whose mechanism is better understood.

Accommodative esotropia is common. Early investigators estimated that as many as one third of all patients with comitant esotropia obtain ocular alignment when given their hyperopic correction, whereas another one third obtain reduction but not complete elimination of their esotropia.[88] In a more recent survey on 1760 strabismic patients, 17% were classified as fully accommodative and 30% as partly accommodative.[89] Thus, approximately 50% of all esotropias can be attributed either entirely or partly to accommodation.

Accommodative esotropia begins later than infantile esotropia. The average age of onset is 2½ years, with a range between 6 months and 7 to 8 years. The esotropia occurs at a time when a child becomes interested in viewing near objects. It is most often seen by the parents when the child is tired or unwell, and the onset may be precipitated by a febrile illness. The onset may be delayed and can develop in older children following either illness or ocular or head trauma.[90] Prolonged occlusion or ptosis in a teenager with hyperopia may also provoke accommodative esotropia.[91] Although accommodative esotropia is rare in infancy, it must be differentiated from infantile esotropia; we have diagnosed and treated it in children younger than 1 year of age. (See Case 5.)

CASE 5

A 9-month-old girl was examined in February, 1981. The child had been hospitalized a month earlier with an ear infection, and the parents had since noticed an increasing eye turn, mostly when she was playing with her toys.

Our examination revealed a 35- to 40-PD intermittent left esotropia at distance and near (Fig. 8-6). Version testing showed no abnormalities. Cycloplegic retinoscopy was OD +4.00 −1.00 × 90 and OS +4.00 sphere. Ophthalmoscopy was normal. The cycloplegic findings were prescribed.

A month later the patient returned, and there was no esotropia while wearing the refractive correction. Removal of the glasses resulted in esotropia.

The patient was followed for 7 years. During that time, because of a high AC/A ratio, a bifocal lens was given. Treatment also included orthoptics/vision therapy. At the last visit, with the correction OD +4.25 −1.50 × 90 and OS +4.25 −1.50 × 80 with a +2.00 D add OU, the patient was 4-PD esophoric at distance and near. She fused the Worth four dot test at all distances and had 25 seconds of arc with the Randot stereotest.

Comment

The intermittency and size of the deviation, the magnitude of hyperopia, and that the esotropia was eliminated with hyperopic glasses were the clinical features distinguishing this early-onset accommodative esotropia from infantile esotropia. Interestingly, the parents later indicated that the youngster was strabismic since birth, with the esotropia becoming much more apparent following the ear infection.

Accommodative esotropia beginning in infancy may differ in some aspects from the accommodative esotropia that begins later. Baker and Parks[92] treated 21 infants with accommodative esotropia. Either the esotropia was present only for near fixation or it was manifest for distance and near but increased for near. In all cases the esotropia was eliminated initially with either glasses or pharmacologic treatment. The age of onset, according to the parents, varied from birth to 11 months, with an average age of 4.6 months. The esotropia was intermittent on initial examination in 15 cases and constant in 6 cases. Only one infant had an esotropia that exceeded 40 PD. The amount of hyperopia was less for the infants with higher AC/A ratios. Only 11 of the 21 infants continued to be aligned with glasses after several months of follow-up. None achieved bifoveal fusion and high-grade stereopsis. Two children developed a dissociated vertical deviation, and 13 required amblyopia therapy.

Accommodative esotropia can be classified as either being (1) refractive, (2) nonrefractive, or (3) partly, or mixed. The latter refers to an esotropia present without hyperopic correction and a significantly reduced but not totally eliminated esotropia with hyperopic correction.

REFRACTIVE ACCOMMODATIVE ESOTROPIA

Refractive accommodative esotropia exists when the esotropia is completely eliminated at distance and near fixation when the patient wears the full hyperopic correction. The esotropia may be present mostly for near fixation, because there is a greater need for accommodation at near.

 CLINICAL PEARL

Refractive accommodative esotropia exists when the esotropia is completely eliminated at distance and near fixation when the patient wears the full hyperopic correction.

The significance of hyperopia in the esotropic process is unquestioned. The mechanism for refractive accommodative esotropia, however, is not limited to hyperopia. The majority of patients with uncorrected hyperopia do not become esotropic. Whether esotropia develops depends not only on the degree of hyperopia

but also on the amount of fusional divergence amplitudes in reserve and the AC/A ratio. If fusional divergence ability is sufficient to overcome the excessive convergence innervation, esophoria is likely, whereas if fusional divergence ability is insufficient, esotropia is likely. The AC/A ratio must also be normal or larger than normal to produce enough accommodative convergence to cause esotropia. The larger the AC/A ratio, the greater the chance for esotropia, whereas the smaller the AC/A ratio, the less the chance for esotropia. As mentioned in Chapter 7, an intrinsically low AC/A ratio protects some children with high hyperopia from developing esotropia.[93]

Clinical Features
Size of the Deviation

The magnitude of refractive accommodative esotropia varies considerably. Of 131 patients with refractive accommodative esotropia, 30% had a deviation of 10 PD or less without glasses, 70% had a deviation between 11 and 45 PD, and none had a deviation exceeding 45 PD.[94] Dependent on the AC/A ratio, the esotropia may be larger at near than at distance (high AC/A) or similar at both distances (normal AC/A).

Refractive Error

The refractive error for patients with refractive accommodative esotropia generally ranges from 2 to 6 D of hyperopia, with most in the higher part of this range. Higher refractive errors are unlikely, because with larger degrees of uncorrected hyperopia the effort to accommodate may be too great and the patient may prefer blurred but single vision rather than the constant effort required to maintain focus. In these cases the eyes will be orthophoric, but the patients will likely develop isoametropic amblyopia because of the bilaterally blurred foveal images.

There does not appear to be a relationship between the amount of hyperopia and the size of the esotropia. However, the amount of hyperopia causing refractive accommodative esotropia is inversely related to the size of the AC/A ratio. For patients with normal ratios (similar distance and near deviations) the average amount of hyperopia is 4.75 D; whereas for patients with high AC/A ratios (near deviation exceeds distance deviation by 10 PD or more), the average hyperopic refractive error is only 2.25 D.[95]

Variation in the Angle of Strabismus

Unlike most other esotropias, refractive accommodative esotropia usually begins as an intermittent and variable deviation. Clinicians examining a neurologically normal child with an intermittent esotropia should presume an accommodative esotropia until it is proven otherwise.

CLINICAL PEARL

Clinicians examining a neurologically normal child with an intermittent esotropia should presume an accommodative esotropia until it is proven otherwise.

The intermittency of the strabismus is explained by the fluctuating status of accommodation. A child with 4 D of uncorrected hyperopia when accommodating may develop esotropia and diplopia. The child's reaction to the diplopia will be manifested by fretfulness and irritability and possibly by closing one eye. Eventually, suppression will develop. In the meantime the child may underaccommodate and see singly, although blurred. The blurred vision stimulates accommodation particularly when viewing at near, and esotropia returns.

Because of the unstable accommodation during the initial stage, a nonaccommodative target such as a fixation light is not suitable for detecting and measuring the esotropia because it does not stimulate and, more importantly, control accommodation. A fixation light looks the same whether it is in focus or out of focus. A child with refractive accommodative esotropia may have straight eyes when viewing a fixation light and, a moment later, esotropia when presented with a small target with letters or pictures requiring accurate accommodation.

The length of the intermittent phase, whether all individuals with refractive accommodative esotropia pass through an intermittent phase, and the number od cases that progress to constant esotropia are unknown. It would be expected that if treatment is delayed, the esotropia would become constant. However, we have examined older children and even teenagers with untreated refractive accommodative esotropia who still maintained intermittency at the time of examination. On the other hand, we have diagnosed 2 year olds with refractive accommodative esotropia who were never observed as having intermittent esotropia. Apparently, refractive accommodative esotropia tends to remain intermittent for long periods in some patients and yet progress rapidly to constant esotropia in others.

Amblyopia

Amblyopia is rarely present with refractive accommodative esotropia as long as the deviation remains intermittent. The cases with amblyopia are associated either with anisometropia or esotropia that has become constant and unilateral. Rarely is the amblyopia deep and it is usually very treatable.

Suppression and Retinal Correspondence

Symptoms of diplopia occur at the onset of the strabismus but are quickly eliminated because the young patient usually develops a facultative suppression zone on the nasal hemiretina of the strabismic eye.

Retinal correspondence, when evaluated with the synoptophore, is typically normal for patients with refractive accommodative esotropia. The normal correspondence can be attributed to the initial intermittency and variability of the esotropia. Unequivocal anomalous correspondence likely does not represent a pure refractive accommodative esotropia.[96] Usually, such cases are only partly accommodative or represent refractive accommodative esotropias that have deteriorated.

Ocular Motility

Ocular motility disorders, including limited abduction, dissociated vertical deviation, and inferior oblique overactions, are not as common as with infantile esotropia. We have not seen dissociated vertical deviations with refractive accommodative esotropia, although it has been reported in cases that begin during the first year of life.[92] Approximately 35% of patients with accommodative esotropia develop inferior oblique overaction by an average age of 5.2 years.[9] A large vertical deviation in primary position coexisting with refractive accommodative esotropia most likely indicates a concurrent cyclovertical paretic muscle. This is confirmed by careful evaluation of versions and the three-step test. This can prevent achieving normal fusion in some cases. (See Case 6.)

CASE 6

A 2½-year-old girl was examined in September, 1991. The parents reported that the youngster's left eye turned in and upward occasionally during the past year. The patient's general health was excellent. No recent illness or head trauma had occurred. She was a twin. The twin had spina bifida and was not strabismic.

Our examination revealed visual acuities of OD 20/30 and OS 20/100 with the Broken Wheel test. There was no compensatory head posture. A 35-PD constant left esotropia with a 15-PD left hypertropia were present at distance and near. Versions revealed left inferior oblique overaction and left superior oblique underaction. The hyperdeviation increased on dextroversion and with left head tilt. Refraction was OD +5.00 −1.00 × 180 and OS +6.00 D sphere.

The diagnosis was refractive accommodative esotropia with a probable congenital left superior oblique paresis.

Over a period of 4 years the amblyopia was successfully treated, as was the esotropia, with refractive correction and bifocals. The hyperdeviation remained, and normal binocular vision could not be achieved, despite treatment with prisms, orthoptics/vision therapy, and surgery.

Treatment

The treatment for refractive accommodative esotropia is straightforward. The basic treatment involves curbing accommodation. Extraocular muscle surgery should not be considered for these patients.[97]

The hyperopic refractive error as determined by cycloplegic retinoscopy is prescribed for continuous wear.[98] We rarely reduce the amount of hyperopia for young children. If there is intolerance with acceptance of the glasses, it is usually caused by an error with the refraction or the fit of the glasses.

 CLINICAL PEARL

The hyperopic refractive error as determined by cycloplegic retinoscopy is prescribed for continuous wear.

Discussion exists as to whether near noncycloplegic retinoscopy is as effective as cycloplegic refraction for determining the refractive correction for these patients.[99] Velasco-Cruz, Sampaio, and Vargos[100] compared the refractive values obtained by near retinoscopy and by cycloplegia, as measured by two examiners, for patients with refractive accommodative esotropia. The interobserver variability was the same for the two techniques for the refractive values of the horizontal and vertical meridians and spheric equivalent. For the astigmatism, there was greater variability for near retinoscopy. The correlation between the two methods was good, but the variability of the differences was high. Therefore near retinoscopy should be employed only as a noninvasive method for screening refractive errors and not for prescribing for refractive accommodative esotropia.

Whether 1% atropine sulfate is more effective than 1% cyclopentolate hydrochloride in uncovering the hyperopia has also been discussed. Atropine is usually given to a child one drop a day, 3 days before the refraction. Side effects, such as flushing and photophobia, may accompany atropine use. Cyclopentolate is given to the child only on the day of the refraction. Unlike atropine, cyclopentolate rarely causes side effects. Most studies have indicated that the dioptric difference between the use of atropine and cyclopentolate averages about 0.50 D to 0.75 D, with atropine uncovering the greater amount of hyperopia.[101-106] Such a difference would be clinically insignificant for most patients. When there is doubt about the effectivity of cyclopentolate, atropine can be used.

Therapy for amblyopia is restricted to the child who manifests a constant unilateral esotropia or is significantly anisometropic at the time of diagnosis. In some cases, we begin amblyopia therapy a few days before the glasses are given. The reason for this is that parents tend to associate success with ocular alignment. If the child's eyes appear straight with the glasses, the vision is good according to the parents. A 2 year old with a 20-PD constant left esotropia and 4 D of uncorrected hyperopia may appear "cured" with the glasses, and the parents may see no need to have the youngster return until 1 or 2 years later. At that time,

we find a residual esotropia and amblyopia. This can be avoided by initiating amblyopia therapy a few days before giving the glasses and emphasizing to the parents the need to improve both visual acuity and binocular vision. Because the amblyopia in these cases is usually mild, the period for treatment will usually be short.

Parents should be warned that the esotropia may become more noticeable after the child begins treatment. We have been confronted by parents who are displeased because the esotropia is now always present and much more obvious when the child removes the glasses and takes a bath, whereas before, the esotropia was smaller and only intermittent. The parents tend to blame this increased deviation on the glasses and describe a dependence on glasses produced by the prescription. An explanation to the parents should be given before beginning therapy. The more noticeable esotropia can be explained on the basis of the child using the proper amount of accommodative effort after the glasses have been prescribed. Before treatment, the child vacillated between blurred vision when not accommodating and fusing and clear vision with diplopia or suppression. With the glasses, the child now recognizes how things should look. When the glasses are removed, there is a desire for clear vision; therefore the child accommodates, resulting in an esotropia that will remain as long as the child continues to accommodate.

With totally refractive accommodative esotropia, no esotropia should remain at distance and near after the patient is optically corrected. If esotropia still exists at distance and near, a partly accommodative esotropia is present, whereas if esotropia remains only at near, refractive accommodative esotropia with a high AC/A ratio is likely indicated. For the latter, a bifocal lens is given. The bifocal will permit fusion at near. The power of the bifocal ranges from approximately +1.00 to +3.00 D. To determine the appropriate power, we have the child fixate an accommodative target at near while wearing full hyperopic correction. Plus lenses, starting with 1.00 D, are added in 0.50 D increments until fusion is maintained, as determined by the unilateral cover test. The minimum power of bifocal to achieve this is prescribed. Ideally, a small esophoria (3 to 4 PD) at near should remain to allow the child to continually exercise fusional divergence. The ultimate goal is to attempt to titrate the power of the bifocal over time, until the child can maintain comfortable fusion without it. This occurs as fusional divergence ranges increase. In many cases, phasing out of the bifocal is a long process and may take several years.

Bifocals are an effective form of treatment, provided they are well fitted and used correctly by the child. Too many times, viewing with the bifocal is avoided by the child (Fig. 8-7). For these cases, the bi-

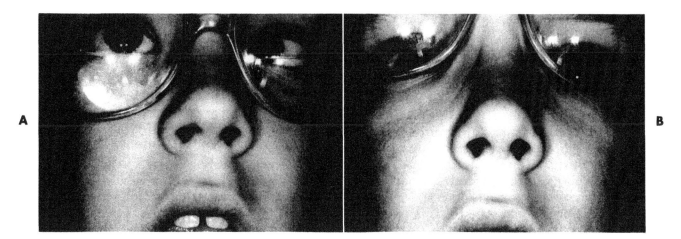

FIG. 8-7   Effect of bifocal lens in a child with refractive accommodative esotropia with a high AC/A ratio. **A,** Child views above bifocal and remains esotropic at near. **B,** While viewing with bifocal, ocular alignment occurs.

focal segment may be too low or too small. The bifocal must be set higher for children than for adults. For patients age 5 and younger, we prescribe a wide-segment bifocal, either on executive type or D-35, and instruct the optician to either bisect the pupil or set it just below the lower pupil margin. The top of the segment is ideally 3 mm above the 6-o'clock limbus position when the eyes are in the primary position. For older children, we set the bifocal to the lower lid margin and usually prescribe more cosmetically appealing bifocals. Fresnel press-on lenses can be used temporarily to determine the efficacy of the bifocal. A month's trial is usually sufficient. Ideally, it is desirable to prescribe the bifocals at the first visit, thus obviating the need to repurchase glasses following the second visit. For some patients, such as the child who has an esotropia at near that is 15 PD larger than the esotropia at distance, the need for bifocals at the first visit is obvious. This is especially true if the refractive error is less than 2.50-D hyperopia. With other patients, this may not be the case. Accordingly, we inform the parents that the glasses may have to be changed in a short time. Most parents accept this.

Progressive-addition lenses have been used in the treatment of refractive accommodative esotropia as an alternative to conventional bifocals.[107,108] This variable-power bifocal is generally fit higher when treating a child than an adult with presbyopia. The beginning of the optic blur produced by the variable-power add is placed at the pupillary axis. This places the optical center of the add slightly below where it usually occurs in the executive bifocal but higher than with the usual fitting of a progressive add. Advocates of progressive-addition lenses claim that this treatment offers a more useful add for near and intermediate distances and that

the glasses are better for sports. The most obvious advantage is that the child does not have to worry about the cosmetic problem imposed by the visible line of the bifocal.

Smith[108] treated 32 children, ages 18 months to 16 years, who had refractive accommodative esotropia, using the Varilux 2 lenses. More difficulty in correctly fitting the lenses existed with the younger children because of the large size of the lenses required. Many younger children were too small to wear frames that accepted the Varilux 2 lenses. However, none of the children or parents were willing to return to conventional bifocals after having worn the progressive-addition lenses.

We recommend progressive-addition lenses to patients who still require a bifocal in their adolescent and teenage years to achieve fusion. The high cost of the lenses, the frequency with which younger children either lose or break their glasses, and the difficulty in determining the proper height of the progressive-lenses, causes us to avoid this form of treatment in younger patients.

Contact lenses have been used as an alternative form of treatment for refractive accommodative esotropia.[109,110] The hyperopic child wearing contact lenses requires less accommodation per unit distance than when wearing glasses. Thus the child with a high AC/A ratio may perform better using contact lenses than glasses and not require bifocals. Calcutt[110] treated 22 of these children with contact lenses instead of glasses for the correction of the refractive error. Initially, the contact lenses prescribed were of the same strength as the patient's glasses. If the esotropia persisted, the power of the contact lenses was increased by 1 D. According to Calcutt, the children did as well with contact lenses as with glasses when the deviation was controlled with glasses. The deviation became latent in the majority of cases, reducing the angle of deviation by as much as 15 PD and resulting in binocular vision. On the other hand, contact lenses deprive the patient of the base-out prism effect at near that occurs when using high plus glasses. This may cause difficulty with near vision tasks, in spite of full correction in the contact lenses. Bifocal contact lenses have also been used in these cases.[111] When using contact lenses, other factors, including socioeconomic status, standard of hygiene, absence of recurrent eye infection, and good compliance and motivation must also be considered. More extensive studies are needed to determine whether contact lenses are better than glasses for refractive accommodative esotropia. We feel that for some patients contact lenses may provide another useful form of treatment.

Orthoptics/vision therapy for refractive accommodative esotropia involves the use of procedures that emphasize developing and enhancing normal sensory and motor fusion. Examples of the former include procedures such as anaglyphic and cheiroscopic tracings, bar reader, TV trainer, and recognition of physiologic diplopia. The latter includes the use of stereoscopes, vectograms, tranaglyphs and/or prism flippers. Because of the sophistication of many of these procedures, they are frequently reserved for children age 5 or older.

Pharmacologic agents, specifically cholinesterase-inhibiting miotics such as echothiophate iodide (Phospholine Iodide) or isoflurophate (Floropryl) have also been used to treat refractive accommodative esotropia.[106,112,113] Unlike treatment with glasses, this therapy should not be used over long periods. These drugs allow sufficient accommodation to take place for clear vision without the associated convergence. The recommended procedure and dosage are described in Chapter 11. The mechanism permits accumulation of excessive acetylcholine at the myoneural junction. This results in a decrease in the nerve impulses required for accommodation. The child's accommodative effort is lessened, thereby decreasing the associated accommodative-convergence.

Pharmacologic treatment is an alternative for children who cannot wear glasses because of facial deformities, as well as hyperactive children who continually remove, lose, or break their glasses. It may also provide the child some relief for periods when glasses are not worn, such as swimming or other physical activities in which glasses may be a hinderance. Pharmacologic treatment should not be used in cases in which normal binocular vision cannot be achieved. Adverse effects, both systemic and local, have been associated with prolonged use of cholinesterase-inhibiting agents in treating accommodative esotropia (see Chapter 11).

 CLINICAL PEARL

Pharmacologic treatment is an alternative for children who cannot wear glasses because of facial deformities, as well as hyperactive children who continually remove, lose, or break their glasses.

Prognosis and Clinical Course

The prognosis for achieving normal single binocular vision with refractive accommodative esotropia is excellent if treatment is provided immediately. Over 90% of all patients are capable of achieving bifixation and high-grade stereopsis.[114] If the esotrophia remains untreated, a nonaccommodative esodeviation may develop secondary to changes in the medial recti muscles associated with their increased and more frequent contraction. Sensory anomalies such as amblyopia and anomalous correspondence frequently accompany the nonaccommodative deviation. Glasses, bifocals, prisms, and orthoptics/vision therapy may not be successful in totally eliminating the angle of esotropia. It is unfortunate to examine an older child with an apparently untreated and neglected refractive accommodative esotropia, as in Case 7.

CASE 7

A 9-year-old boy was referred to the clinic from a school screening. The parents reported that the child's eyes began to cross occasionally at about age 2½. The crossing of the eyes occurred mostly when the child was doing near tasks. The parents thought the eye turn would go away and did not seek treatment. Now the eyes were reported to cross all of the time.

Visual acuities were 20/20 in the right eye and 20/50 in the left eye. The patient manifested a constant left esotropia of 20 PD at distance and 25 PD at near and suppressed the left eye at distance and near with the Worth four dot test. Synoptophore evaluation revealed anomalous correspondence, as did the Bagolini striated lenses. Cycloplegic refraction was +4.00 D sphere for each eye.

Although amblyopia therapy was successful, a constant esotropia of 10 PD remained with full hyperopic correction. Attempts to establish normal single binocular vision with prisms and orthoptics/vision therapy were unsuccessful.

Comment

It was presumed that the esotropia was at first totally accommodative because of (1) the initial intermittency, (2) the age of onset, (3) the amount of hyperopic refractive error, and (4) the larger esotropia at near. Lack of timely treatment likely led to a superimposed nonaccommodative esotropia with amblyopia and anomalous correspondence, which prevented the establishment of normal binocular vision.

Some patients with refractive accommodative esotropia who at first achieve ocular alignment and normal binocular vision later develop additional esotropia and risk losing normal binocular vision. Such deterioration can begin anywhere from 3 months to several years after treatment and has been associated with (1) an esotropia presenting before age 1, (2) prolonged delay between the onset of esotropia and the initiation of treatment, (3) large increases in hyperopia, and (4) incomplete treatment, such as less-than-full hyperopic correction or part-time wearing of the glasses.[115,116]

The causative factor for deterioration has also been related to a high AC/A ratio.[116-118] Ludwig and others[117] followed 119 patients whose vision was aligned while wearing their glasses. Deterioration, which was characterized by a nonaccommodative component of esotropia greater than 10 PD superimposed on the accommodative esotropia, occurred in 7.9% of patients with normal AC/A ratios (near deviation within 10 PD of distance deviation) and 40.7% of the patients with high AC/A ratios (near deviation 10 PD or more greater than distance deviation). Other factors, including time to deterioration, delay in treatment, age of onset of the esotropia, and amblyopia, were not significantly related to the rate of deterioration.

Whether the esotropia is intermittent or constant when treatment begins may also be a factor as to which patients deteriorate and which patients do not. Patients presenting with intermittent esotropia are 2.7 times more likely not to deteriorate over time than patients presenting with constant esotropia.[114]

Although the actual mechanisms and the prevalence for deterioration in refractive accommodative esotropia are unclear, all patients should be followed with the clinician keeping this undesirable sequela in mind. We have seen deterioration almost exclusively in children who are without their glasses for extended periods, as in the following case.

CASE 8

A 3-year-old boy was referred from a school screening in April, 1987. The parents had noticed an occasional left eye turn beginning during the last year. This was the youngster's first eye examination. He was in excellent health.

Visual acuities were 20/25 for each eye with the Broken Wheel test. A 20-PD intermittent esotropia at distance and a 30-PD intermittent esotropia at near were measured. Versions were full. With the Titmus stereotest, the patient had 100 seconds of arc. Cycloplegic refraction was +2.50 D sphere OU. This was was prescribed, along with +2.00 D add. Orthoptics/vision therapy procedures to help enhance fusion were done at home.

Over a period of 1½ years, progress exams indicated ocular alignment and normal fusion with the glasses.

In April, 1989 the patient presented without his glasses, reporting he had lost them 4 months earlier. He now manifested a 40-PD constant alternating esotropia at distance and near. The refractive findings were unchanged. Glasses with bifocals were again prescribed.

A month later, while wearing the glasses the patient manifested a 20-PD constant alternating esotropia at distance and near. With the Worth four dot test, he suppressed the right eye at distance and near. He showed no stereopsis with the Randot or Titmus stereotests. When evaluated with the synoptophore, normal correspondence and fusion occurred. Prisms (9-PD base-out for each lens) were given to compensate for the nonaccommodative esotropia.

In October, 1989, while wearing the prism glasses the patient was 10-PD constantly esotropic at distance and 10-PD intermittently esotropic at near. With the Randot stereotest, he had 70 seconds of arc. Cycloplegic retinoscopy did not disclose more hyperopia. Because of the large amount of prism necessary to maintain fusion, surgical treatment was recommended. Following recession of both medial recti, the patient was esophoric (2 PD) with the hyperopic correction and maintained good stereopsis.

Comment

This patient was doing well until he lost his glasses and was without them for 4 months. A refractive accommodative esotropia with a high AC/A ratio deteriorated and subsequently required prisms and surgery.

Most studies on refractive accommodative esotropia have been concerned primarily with its management in childhood. There is little information on its course into adulthood and of the ultimate results of treatment.[119] We rarely see refractive accommodative esotropia in adult patients (Fig. 8-8). Convergence requirements for near vision increase with widening of the interpupillary distance as patients get older. Lessened esodeviation or greater exodeviation in near deviation may occur for older patients, commensurate with broadening of their facial features. Also, myopia increases and hyperopia usually decreases during rapid bodily growth in the second decade of life. For these reasons, it has been suggested that many cases of refractive accommodative esotropia resolve by ages 10 to 12.[116,120] However, the refractive shift, or emmetropization, that typically occurs in children without strabismus may not necessarily occur with patients with accommodative esotropia.[121] We have heard from parents that they were told by other clinicians that their child would eventually "outgrow" the need for glasses by the early teenage years. It has been our experience that relatively few children actually undergo a large reduction in hyperopia and are able to be taken completely out of glasses.

> **CLINICAL PEARL**
> Relatively few children actually undergo a large reduction in hyperopia and are able to be taken completely out of glasses.

Raab and Spierer[120] document the course for 202 patients with refractive accommodative esotropia. The

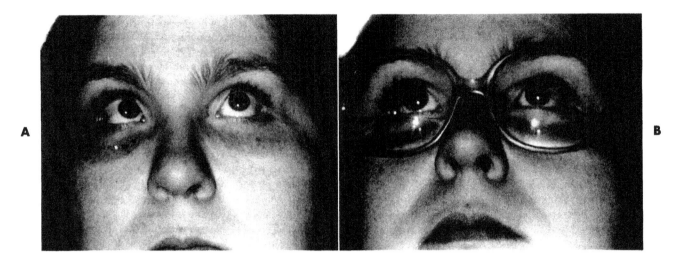

FIG. 8-8 Adult with refractive accommodative esotropia.

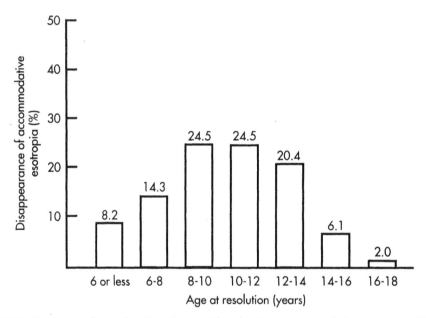

FIG. 8-9 Age at resolution for 49 patients with refractive accommodative esotropia. (From Raab EL, Spierer A: Persisting accommodative esotropia, *Arch Ophthalmol* 104:1777, 1986.)

mean follow-up was 4.1 years. Of the 202 patients, only 49 (24.4%) resolved at a mean age of 10.2 years (Fig. 8-9). Twenty-six cases (53.1%) persisted beyond age 10, and 14 cases (28.6%) persisted beyond age 12. According to these authors, the esotropia was to have resolved if it decreased to 8 PD or less without the need for glasses. This is not an acceptable result for patients who are generally capable of achieving bifoveal fusion and high-grade stereopsis with glasses.

Swan[122] reported on the course and current status of 39 adults (ages 23 to 46) who underwent treatment for refractive accommodative esotropia in childhood and had been reexamined for 20 years or more. Of 39 adults, 38 continued to wear glasses full-time to control their esotropia and maintain fusion. Apparently, many patients with refractive accommodative esotropia will continue to need optical correction, whether it be glasses or contact lenses.[123]

We do attempt to wean the bifocal from patients by the time they are teenagers. If the patient is fusing readily, we remeasure the near deviation with 0.50-D to 1-D reduction in the add. If the cover test reveals exophoria, orthophoria, or a small esophoria (4 PD or less), the bifocal is changed. As mentioned earlier, the existence of esophoria requires the patient to continually exert fusional divergence and serves as an effective orthoptics/vision therapy procedure. If with the proposed bifocal reduction the patient becomes either highly esophoric or intermittently esotropic, the bifocal is not changed. In 37% to 60% of cases, the bifocal can either be removed totally or reduced in power.[124,125] For the remaining patients, either total dependence on the bifocals with fusional control persists or deterioration of binocular fusion occurs while being treated with bifocals. For those patients who still require a bifocal during the teenage years, progressive-addition lenses or contact lenses can be used. (See Cases 9, 10, and 11.)

CASE 9

An 18-month-old girl was examined in September, 1986. The parents reported that the child had fallen 10 days earlier. One week before examination the right eye began turning. The medical history was unremarkable.

The patient manifested a 15- to 20-PD intermittent right esotropia at distance and near. Versions were normal. Cycloplegic retinoscopy revealed +4.50 D sphere OU. Funduscopic findings were normal.

The diagnosis was refractive accommodative esotropia. The patient was treated with full cycloplegic findings. Follow-up examination 1 month later revealed absence of the esotropia with glasses.

The patient was seen every 4 months until October, 1989, at which time the family moved. On her last visit, vision for each eye was 20/20, and a 4-PD esophoria was measured at distance and near. The patient fused the Worth four dot test at distance and near and had 50 seconds of arc with the Randot stereotest.

Comment

This is an example of an uneventful refractive accommodative esotropia with a relatively early onset. The esotropia was apparently provoked by the fall suffered. Amblyopia was never suspected because of the intermittency of the deviation and the lack of anisometropia.

CASE 10

A 4-year-old healthy girl was seen in the clinic in August, 1980. Two years earlier, the parents began noticing the left eye turning inward. An examination by another clinician at that time had diagnosed intermittent esotropia but no treatment was given. The parents believe the eye turn is now much more frequent.

Our examination revealed a constant 30-PD left esotropia at distance and near (Fig. 8-10). Visual acuities were OD 20/25 and OS 20/40 with the Broken Wheel test. Version testing showed bilateral inferior oblique overactions with a V pattern; the esotropia was 35 PD in downgaze and 20 PD in upgaze.

The patient suppressed the left eye with the Worth four dot test at distance and near. Stereopsis was not present.

Cycloplegic retinoscopy was OD +3.00 −1.00 × 180 and OS +3.50 −1.00 × 180. Ophthalmoscopy was normal.

The diagnosis was probable refractive accommodative esotropia and amblyopia. The full refractive findings were prescribed, along with occlusion therapy for the amblyopia (the right eye was occluded for 4 days, the left eye was occluded for 1 day, and so on).

On follow-up examination a month later, the visual acuity was 20/25 for each eye. With the glasses a 15-PD alternating esotropia at distance and near was measured. Ocular alignment at near could apparently be obtained with +2.00-D add. A Fresnel press-on bifocal was given, as well as orthoptics/vision therapy (anaglyphic tracings and the TV trainer) to enhance binocular vision at distance and near.

Over a period of 2 years, the refraction showed increased hyperopia (1 D each eye), and a regular bifocal was given. During the evaluation in July, 1982, the patient was 3-PD esophoric at distance and near, fused the Worth four dot test at all distances, and had 100 seconds of arc with the Randot stereotest.

Comment

This case represents a likely sequelae of a refractive accommodative esotropia that should have received earlier treatment. When the patient was 2 years old, the parents detected an eye turn but treatment was not given. The intermittent esotropia apparently converted to a constant unilateral esotropia with amblyopia. The amblyopia was mild and responded readily to treatment. A bifocal was necessary, even though the distance and near deviations were similar in magnitude.

CASE 11

A 19-year-old man was referred for a second opinion. The patient had recently had his eyes examined and an esotropia was found. The patient was a college student and developed "eye aches" when reading for long periods. He denied any diplopia. There was no history of trauma or systemic disease.

Visual acuity was 20/20 for each eye. A constant alternating esotropia of 20 PD at distance and 15 PD at near was measured with the cover test. The esotropia was hardly noticeable by casual observation. Versions were full, and the esotropia measured the same in extreme right and extreme left gazes. Sensory testing with the Worth four dot test showed homonymous diplopia at near and alternating suppression at distance. Anomalous correspondence was present with the Bagolini striated lens test. The patient did not perceive stereopsis with the Randot stereotest. With the synoptophore, he demonstrated normal correspondence, second-degree sensory fusion, and a limited range of motor fusion.

Manifest refraction was OD +0.75 and OS +0.50, whereas cycloplegic retinoscopy was OD +3.50 and OS +4.00. Funduscopic examination and all other ocular health evaluations were normal.

Because of the patient's age, the full cycloplegic refraction was reduced arbitrarily for each eye by +1.25 D and prescribed. The patient was to return after 1 month but failed to do so. Attempts to reschedule were unsuccessful.

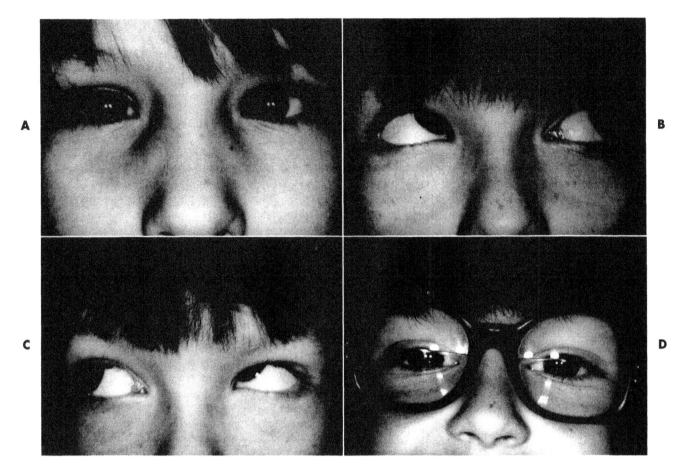

FIG. 8-10   Refractive accommodative esotropia (Case 10). **A,** Left esotropia. **B,** Right inferior oblique overaction during left gaze. **C,** Left inferior oblique overaction during right gaze. **D,** Final correction, with bifocal giving ocular alignment and normal fusion (patient is viewing at near).

Comment

This case, in all likelihood, represents a late-onset refractive accommodative esotropia. The finding of a slightly larger esodeviation at distance was ominous, but no lateral rectus paresis was found, and medical tests done by the patient's physician were normal. The large degree of hyperopia uncovered with cycloplegia supports an accommodative etiology.

Although minimal sensory adaptations were present, fusion ability could be demonstrated with the synoptophore. Because the cycloplegic finding had to be reduced, compensating base-out prisms, gradually increasing the hyperopic correction over time, and orthoptics/vision therapy to establish fusion were future therapy options for this patient.

NONREFRACTIVE ACCOMMODATIVE ESOTROPIA

Nonrefractive accommodative esotropia (near esotropia, or convergence excess esotropia) is an accommodative esotropia characterized by little or no esotropia at distance fixation and a significantly larger esotropic deviation (usually 10 PD or more) at near fixation. Some of these patients are orthophoric or esophoric at distance. Unlike refractive accommodative esotropia, the refractive error need not be hyperopic and can be emmetropic or even myopic.[126,127] Characteristically, 1 D or less of hyperopic refractive error is found. About 5% of all esotropias show nonrefractive accommodative esotropia.

Nonrefractive accommodative esotropia has many of the features of refractive accommodative esotropia. The onset occurs at a time when a young individual becomes interested in viewing near objects. The peak age at onset is between ages 2 and 5, occasionally earlier, and frequently there is a history of the parents having seen the eyes crossing at the dinner table and not during automobile trips. The deviation angle is initially small and intermittent. Rarely does it exceed 30 PD. As with refractive accommodative esotropia, the child must fixate on an accommodative target and not a fixation light to make the correct diagnosis. Suppression occurs early during the intermittent stage.[128] Until then, the child may periodically close one eye to avoid diplopia. Most of the children do not develop amblyopia because they fuse at distance and rarely have associated vertical deviations. If amblyopia exists, it is associated with anisometropia.

The causative factor for nonrefractive accommodative esotropia is innervational and attributed to a high AC/A ratio. An abnormal synkinesis exists between accommodation and accommodative convergence. For these patients, an excessive amount of accommodative convergence occurs with each diopter of accommodation and causes the near esotropia. For example, suppose a 5 year old who is emmetropic has an AC/A ratio of 12/1. Assuming an interpupillary distance of 55 mm and a near viewing distance of 33 cm, the amount of convergence required to maintain fusion at near is 16.5 PD. Because of the high AC/A ratio, however, the child will converge much more than this. To clear the image at near, 3 D of accommodation is required, resulting in 36 PD of accommodative-convergence. The result is approximately 20-PD esodeviation. Depending on the magnitude of fusional divergence amplitude in reserve, either esophoria or esotropia will occur.

Nonrefractive accommodative esotropia must be differentiated from V-pattern esotropia (see Chapter 10). Careful examination of ocular motility and measurement of the esotropia in the different positions of gaze should clearly distinguish these two conditions. With a V pattern the esodeviation increases in downgaze and decreases in upgaze. Unilateral or bilateral inferior oblique overactions are often present. With nonrefractive accommodative esotropia the esodeviation increases only at near fixation in the primary position and is the same magnitude when viewing up, down, or straight ahead. Inferior oblique overactions need not be present.

Nonrefractive accommodative esotropia must also be differentiated from spasm of the near reflex (see Chapter 3). This differential diagnosis is made by evaluating the patient's accommodative response. With spasm of the near reflex, a lead of accommodation, as detected with dynamic retinoscopy, occurs during the esotropic phase. Limited abduction, blurred vision, and diplopia are also part of spasm of the near reflex. With nonrefractive accommodative esotropia, a normal accommodative response usually exists during the esotropic phase. Abduction is full, vision is clear, and diplopia may or may not be present. A high lag of accommodation can occur during the phoric phase.

An atypical form of nonrefractive accommodative esotropia that is etiologically associated with accommodative dysfunction has been described.[129] In these cases a child is found to be emmetropic or has hyperopia normal for the age, but the accommodation is inadequate. An extremely remote near point of accommodation exists. Supposedly, the accommodative impulses sent by the brain are exaggerated to compensate for the accommodative insufficiency, and overconvergence with near-point esotropia results. Such an observation can sometimes be induced pharmacologically. After instillation of a cycloplegic agent, some children who are esophoric become esotropic. This is because with cycloplegia a change in stimulus to accommodation results in a stronger impulse to the ciliary muscle than without cycloplegia, and consequently the stimulus to the extraocular muscles is also stronger. A more or less unsuccessful effort by the child is made to clear the retinal image, resulting in the near-point esotropia.

Treatment

Patients with nonrefractive accommodative esotropia are ideal candidates for bifocals. As occurs with refractive accommodative esotropia, bifoveal fusion with high-grade stereopsis is the expected functional result, although some may achieve only gross stereopsis. Reduction of and/or elimination of the bifocal entirely by the teenage years with the maintenance of fusion is a reasonable goal for therapy. The latter is more readily obtained with supportive orthoptics/vision therapy.[124] As with refractive accommodative esotropia, presence of a superimposed nonaccommodative esodeviation may develop over time. Increasing the bifocal power does not eliminate the esotropia, and base-out prisms may be needed.

 CLINICAL PEARL
Patients with nonrefractive accommodative esotropia are ideal candidates for bifocals.

Concluding from the finding of larger esodeviation at near that a patient has a high AC/A ratio is not always justified. Some patients who have a large-angle esotropia at near fixation in the presence of orthophoria or a small-angle esotropia or esophoria at distance fixation do not show reduction in the near esodeviation when bifocals are given. Factors other than accommodative convergence, such as proximal and tonic convergence, are involved. von Noorden and Avilla[130] describe these patients as having "nonaccommodative convergence excess" esotropia. Similar to nonrefractive accommodative esotropia, the esotropia is acquired during early childhood and is preceded by a period of intermittency. The AC/A ratio, determined with the gradient method, however, is normal or abnormally low, and consequently relaxation of accommodation with bifocals causes little decrease in the angle of strabismus. Supposedly, excessive tonic convergence plays

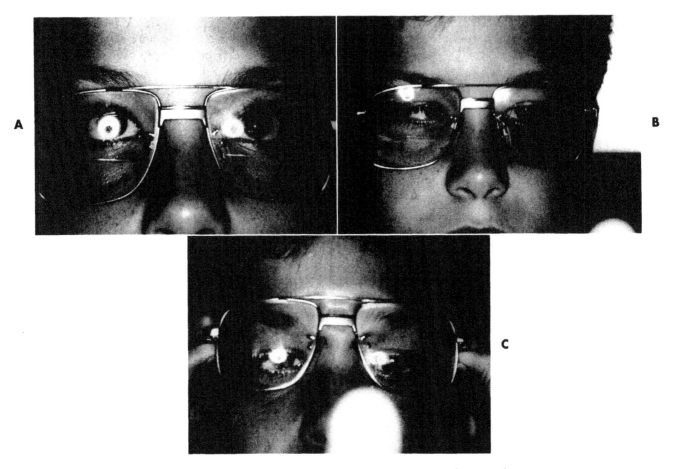

FIG. 8-11   Nonrefractive accommodative esotropia (Case 12). **A,** Absence of esotropia at distance. **B,** Esotropia when viewing at near. **C,** Absence of esotropia when viewing at near with bifocal lens.

a major role in the development of nonaccommodative convergence excess esotropia and not a high AC/A ratio. von Noorden and Avilla treated these patients surgically, performing bilateral medial rectus recessions. Only 4 of 24 patients (16.6%) obtained 60 seconds or better of arc of stereopsis. Prism therapy and orthoptics/vision therapy may provide better functional results for nonaccommodative convergence excess esotropia. In our experience, this type of esotropia is very rare. (See Cases 12 and 13.)

CASE 12

A 6-year-old boy was first examined in the clinic in July, 1982. The parents had noticed the right eye turning inward, which supposedly began the previous year. The patient was having academic difficulties in school. Two years earlier, he had head trauma and suffered a concussion. There were no other health problems. Four months previously, an examination by another clinician indicated hyperopia, for which the patient was given glasses. The patient does not complain of diplopia.

Our examination revealed 20/25 vision for the right and left eyes. The cover test showed an 8-PD esophoria at distance and a 35-PD intermittent right esotropia at near (Fig. 8-11). The esotropia could be significantly reduced at near with added plus lenses. Versions were normal. With the Worth four dot test the patient fused at distance and had homonymous diplopia at near. With the Randot stereotest, 200 seconds of arc was perceived. The amplitude of accommodation was 15 D for each eye. Noncycloplegic and cycloplegic refractions were similar, +0.75 D for each eye. Biomicroscopy and ophthalmoscopy were normal.

The diagnosis was nonrefractive accommodative esotropia. The patient was treated with the refractive correction and a +2.50 D add.

The patient returned a month after beginning treatment and measured 4-PD esophoria at distance and 4-PD esophoria at near while viewing with the bifocal. The Randot stereotest revealed 60 seconds of arc. Supplementary orthoptics/vision therapy to develop vergence ranges and vergence facility was also given. The goal was to titrate and possibly wean the bifocal entirely.

In October, 1985 the patient continued to fuse at near

with the bifocal. Compensatory fusional vergences at near were 14/12 (base-in) and 40/35 (base-out). The bifocal was reduced to +1.75 D.

In October, 1987 the patient stated that he had been without his glasses, which he had lost, for 3 months. He showed by cover test 2-PD esophoria at distance and 40-PD constant right esotropia at near. The bifocal was increased to +2.50 D and orthoptics/vision therapy was resumed.

In October, 1988 the patient was esophoric through the bifocal lenses and had 20 seconds of arc with the Randot stereotest. Any lessening of the bifocal power caused esotropia.

Comment

This patient with nonrefractive accommodative esotropia responded well to bifocals and orthoptics/vision therapy. Unfortunately, he lost his glasses (not uncommon with children), and some therapy gains had to be achieved again. The bifocal power could only be reduced 0.75 D over a 3-year period, and after the glasses were lost could not be reduced at all.

CASE 13

An 8-year-old boy was referred for treatment for esotropia. Specifically, the referring clinician wanted to know if further treatment, that is, bifocals, prisms, orthoptics/vision therapy, or surgery, would be beneficial for achieving normal binocular vision. The patient had undergone extraocular muscle surgery 2 years previously for an esotropia that the parents said began when the patient was 4 years old. Past therapy had also included occlusion for amblyopia and glasses.

With his present glasses (+1.50 −1.00 × 180, OU), the patient had 20/42 OD and 20/32 OS, as measured with Psychometric visual acuity cards. A constant 10-PD right esotropia at distance and a constant 20-PD right esotropia at near were measured by cover test. Added plus lenses at near did not reduce the esotropia significantly. Versions showed slight inferior oblique overactions in each eye. There was no V pattern. Refractive measurements were similar to the glasses.

The patient suppressed the right eye at distance and near with the Worth four dot test. Stereopsis was not present. Anomalous correspondence was diagnosed with the Bagolini striated lens test, the synoptophore, and the Hering-Bielschowsky afterimage test. With the Bagolini filter bar, diplopia could not be elicited with the denser filters. The patient was sent back to the referring clinician with the recommendation of no further treatment for the esotropia.

Comment

A residual, postsurgical esotropia simulating nonrefractive accommodative esotropia existed for this patient. Added plus lenses did not alter the near esotropia. Deep sensory adaptations precluding normal fusion were found, which are not characteristic of nonrefractive accommodative esotropia. Using bifocals, prisms, orthoptics/vision therapy, or surgery would not likely reverse these sensory adaptations and allow better fusion. The esotropia was not noticeable at distance

and only rarely noticed by the parents at near. Based on these findings, no further treatment was recommended.

PARTLY ACCOMMODATIVE ESOTROPIA

Refractive or nonrefractive accommodative esotropias do not always occur in their pure form. Approximately one third of esotropic patients experience reduction but not total elimination of the strabismic deviation when wearing full hyperopic correction.[88] When residual esotropia persists while the patient wears full hyperopic refractive correction and bifocals, a partly accommodative esotropia, or mixed esotropia, exists. The finding in a patient with 4-D hyperopia of 40-PD constant esotropia without glasses and 25-PD constant esotropia with glasses implies that 15 PD of the esotropia is the result of hyperopic refractive error and is accommodative and 25 PD is nonaccommodative.

 CLINICAL PEARL

When residual esotropia persists while the patient wears full hyperopic refractive correction and bifocals, a partly accommodative esotropia, or mixed esotropia, exists.

The onset of partly accommodative esotropia can be earlier than the onset of refractive and nonrefractive accommodative esotropia. It is often insidious and frequently not observed or is described to be intermittent by the parents until the deviation increases in size.[131] For all partly accommodative esotropias, repeat cycloplegic retinoscopy should be performed, because additional hyperopia may be uncovered.

The cause of the nonaccommodative portion of the esotropia is speculative. Traditionally, it has been attributed to either increased convergence tonus or mechanical factors, such as contracture or hypertrophy of the medial rectus muscles, conjunctiva, or Tenon's capsule. In some cases it likely represents a refractive accommodative esotropia in which a nonaccommodative element develops following alignment of the eyes with glasses or bifocal lenses. The fact that deterioration of refractive accommodative esotropia can occur has been mentioned.

Another possibility is that these patients had infantile esotropia and developed a superimposed accommodative esotropia at ages 2 to 3. As mentioned earlier, some individuals with infantile esotropia reveal more hyperopia and larger esotropia as they get older.

Partly accommodative esotropia is a constant and mostly unilateral deviation. Amblyopia is common, as are suppression and anomalous correspondence. The size of the deviation is usually less than 40 PD at distance and may be greater for near viewing. Moderate-to-high amounts of hyperopia are usually present, as are anisometropia and astigmatism. Hyperopia greater

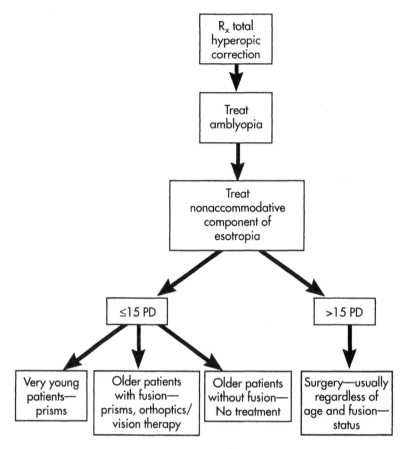

FIG. 8-12   Treatment sequence for partly accommodative esotropia.

than 4.50 D presents a risk of consecutive exotropia for these patients.

The patient's binocular vision status depends on the age of onset and time of treatment. Normal binocular vision potential is found in a minority of patients. Associated vertical deviations are common, usually manifesting as either an overaction of the oblique muscles or, rarely, as a dissociated vertical deviation.

Treatment

Consistent with the other types of accommodative esotropias, the full hyperopic refractive error, as determined by cycloplegic retinoscopy, is prescribed in young children. Bifocal lenses are usually not given, because the deviation is not eliminated entirely and fusion is not provided.

When treating amblyopia, we also attempt to establish alternate fixation but in many cases cannot because of the older age at the initiation of treatment and/or the presence of significant anisometropia.[61]

The type of treatment for the nonaccommodative component of the esotropia depends on its magnitude, the age of the patient, and the potential for normal fusion (Fig 8-12). The latter is determined best with the

synoptophore or other stereoscopes. Performing sensory tests, such as the Worth four dot, Bagolini striated lens tests, and stereopsis tests, without prisms and then with prisms equivalent to the angle of deviation serves a similar purpose. If normal binocular vision occurs with the prisms, fusion potential exists, whereas if the compensatory prisms have no effect, normal fusion ability is usually not present. When using plastic prisms with polarizing glasses, it is best to place the prisms behind the glasses to avoid any birefringence effect. Holding plastic prisms interposed between the polarizing glasses and the stereotest can give erroneous results.[132] These techniques are restricted to mature and coherent patients, even though we have been able to perform them occasionally in patients as young as age 3.

Prisms can be given to children when the nonaccommodative esotropia is 15 PD or less, assuming normal sensory fusion. For older patients with a nonaccommodative esotropia of 15 PD or less and potential for normal binocular vision, we also give prisms as well as orthoptics/vision therapy. If after careful examination it is determined that no potential exists for normal binocular vision and the nonaccommodative esotropia is 15 PD or less, no further treatment for the strabismus is recommended.

Some patients with partly accommodative esotropia or other esotropias, when given prisms, will manifest a substantial angle buildup.[133-137] The period during which this increase of the deviation occurs ranges from minutes to hours, days, or weeks after prisms are worn. Further addition of prism may even cause a greater increase in the deviation. Originally associated only with patients with poor fusion ability as a result of anomalous correspondence (see Chapter 5), this angle buildup or "prism adaptation" can also occur in patients with bifoveal fusion and high-grade stereopsis.[133] Apparently, prism adaptation uncovers a larger latent angle of esotropia that substantially exceeds that found in the initial measurement. Removal of the prisms usually allows the patient to return to the original angle of esotropia within a few days.

Regardless of the patient's age and the binocular vision status, when the nonaccommodative esotropic component exceeds 15 PD and is cosmetically displeasing, surgical treatment is an option. Surgery is performed to reduce or eliminate the nonaccommodative component, not the accommodative component, of the esotropia. The child must wear glasses continually for the accommodative component. In a review from the literature on the efficacy of surgical treatment for partly accommodative and nonaccommodative esotropias, Scheiman and Ciner[134] found a 15% functional success rate in 1170 cases and a 43% cosmetic success rate in 1473 cases. The category of functional success included any patient who following surgery demonstrated little or no strabismus at any distance and had demonstrable sensory and motor fusion. Sensory fusion ranged from stereopsis to fusion with the synoptophore. Motor fusion indicated that ranges could be measured either by prism or the synoptophore. Cosmetic success included patients who following surgery demonstrated a residual strabismus, esotropia, or exotropia of 10 PD or less. The presence of functional binocularity was not necessary. Scheiman and Ciner[134] report a reoperation rate ranging from 26% to 41% and a prevalence of consecutive exotropia from 4% to 20%. Unsuccessful surgery was frequently associated with factors such as associated vertical deviations, untreated amblyopia, underestimation of the accommodative component, high hyperopia, and lack of attention by the clinician to the status of retinal correspondence.

Prism adaptation has been advocated as a method of improving the results of surgery for partly accommodative esotropia and other types of nonaccommodative esotropia. Fresnel press-on prisms are prescribed in increasing amounts until there is no or little remaining esotropia. The patient wears the prisms for a month or so, and the prisms are adjusted weekly if necessary to maintain alignment. Surgical success rates have been reported to be significantly higher (89%) when the amount of surgery is based on the prism-adapted angle of deviation rather than the initial, or entry, angle of deviation (72%).[135-139] Surgery that does not take into account this increased angle supposedly results more frequently in undercorrection and less chance of achieving some fusion. (See Cases 14, 15, 16, and 17.)

CASE 14

A 5-year-old girl was examined in May, 1981. The parents reported that the youngster had a head turn and sometimes used just one eye. They were unsure of the onset. The patient was in excellent health. This was the first eye examination.

Visual acuities were 20/40 OD and 20/25 OS. A constant right esotropia of 30 PD at distance and near was measured with the cover test (Fig. 8-13). Versions were normal. Refraction without cycloplegia was +0.75 OU. The patient suppressed the right eye at distance and near with the Worth four dot test. Stereopsis of 400 seconds of arc was measured with the Titmus stereotest. Cycloplegic retinoscopy revealed OD +4.50 D and OS +3.50 −0.50 × 90. Ophthalmoscopy was normal.

The patient was prescribed the cycloplegic findings and occlusion therapy for the amblyopia.

During the progress evaluation a month later, visual acuity was 20/25 OD and 20/25 OS. A 15-PD constant right esotropia with the glasses persisted at distance and near. The synoptophore showed normal correspondence and suppression of the right eye, which prevented second-degree sensory and motor fusion.

The patient was given Fresnel prisms, 5-PD base-out for the right eye and 10-PD base-out for the left eye, to compensate for the nonaccommodative esodeviation. Orthoptics/vision therapy included anaglyphic tracings and the TV trainer.

Three months later, the patient was 6-PD esophoric at distance and near and had 80 seconds of arc with the Randot stereotest. Orthoptics/vision therapy procedures were altered to improve motor fusion (vectograms and tranaglyphs) and so that the prisms required for fusion could be reduced.

The last examination was performed in September, 1984. The patient had 20/20 vision for each eye. A 5-PD esophoria at distance and near was present while wearing glasses with a total of 6-PD base-out. Compensatory base-in vergence amplitudes were 8/6 (break/recovery) at distance and 30/10 for near. The patient fused the Worth four dot test at distance and near and had 25 seconds of arc with the Randot stereotest.

Comment

This is an example of a partly accommodative esotropia that achieved bifoveal fusion with occlusion, prisms, and orthoptics/vision therapy. The large difference between the noncycloplegic and cycloplegic refractions for this patient confirms the necessity of always doing the latter. The patient still requires prisms to maintain fusion.

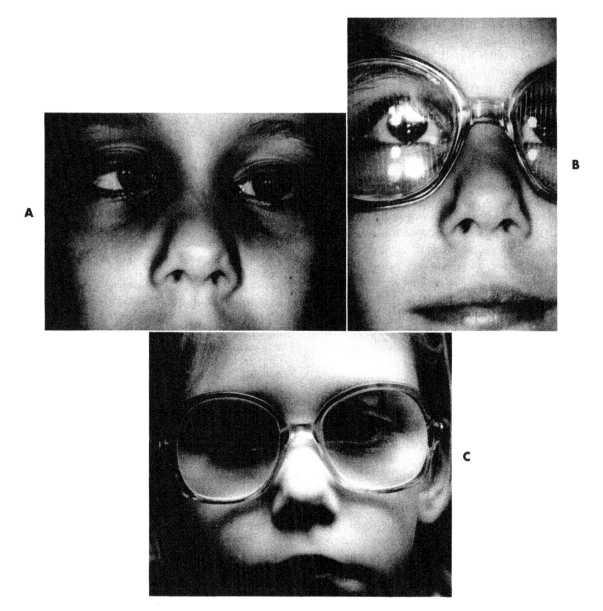

FIG. 8-13 Partly accommodative esotropia (Case 14). **A,** Right esotropia. **B,** Fresnel press-on prisms given for nonaccommodative component of esotropia. **C,** Final alignment status includes glasses with ground-in prism.

CASE 15

A 5-year-old girl was referred in August, 1991. The patient was treated for esotropia with glasses with bifocals. The parents reported that the child's eyes turned, even while wearing the glasses. According to the parents, the strabismus began a year previously.

The patient had corrected visual acuity of 20/20 for each eye. With glasses she manifested a 35-PD constant right esotropia at distance, which increased to 45 PD at near. The esotropia measured 35 PD while viewing at near with the bifocal. A 60-PD esotropia existed at distance and near without the glasses. Versions showed mild lateral rectus underactions for each eye. The patient alternately suppressed with the Worth four dot test at distance and near. The synoptophore showed normal correspondence, without any evidence of sec-

ond-degree fusion. Cycloplegic refraction revealed +4.75 D OU, which was 3 D more than what the patient had been prescribed previously. The ocular health was normal. The cycloplegic findings were prescribed.

The patient returned 2 months later and manifested 25-PD esotropia at distance and 35-PD esotropia at near with the glasses. Corrected visual acuity was 20/20 for each eye. Added plus lenses did not change the deviation at near. The synoptophore again showed normal correspondence, with no second-degree fusion. With prisms compensating for the nonaccommodative esodeviation, the patient continued to suppress with both the Worth four dot test and Randot stereotest. Cycloplegic refraction was repeated and revealed findings identical to those of the previous examination.

The diagnosis was partly accommodative esotropia. Because of the large nonaccommodative esotropia and the apparent lack of fusion, a surgical referral was made.

A month after surgery the patient was 3-PD esophoric at distance and near with her glasses. She fused the Worth four dot test at distance and near and had 60 seconds of arc with the Randot stereotest. Without the glasses, 35-PD esotropia existed at distance and near.

Comment

This is an example of an unusually large partly accommodative esotropia with nearly equal accommodative and nonaccommodative components. The bifocal, although reducing the esotropia slightly, was not warranted because it did not provide fusion. Prisms were not used because of the large size of the nonaccommodative esotropia. Despite showing normal correspondence without second-degree fusion before surgery, the patient achieved bifoveal fusion following surgery. This concurs with the parent's observation that the esotropia began 1 year previously. The surgeon operated only on the nonaccommodative portion of the esotropia. It is important when discussing the case with the parents to emphasize the fact that the child must continue wearing glasses following surgery.

CASE 16

In October, 1986 a 7-year-old boy presented for his first eye examination. His mother had noticed the child holding reading material very close. There was no mention of strabismus. The patient denied any visual symptoms, such as diplopia.

Our examination revealed equal vision (20/25) for each eye. The patient manifested a constant left esotropia of 25 PD at distance and near. Version testing was normal. No fusion was evident with either the Worth four dot test or the Randot stereotest. The synoptophore showed normal correspondence with limited second-degree sensory and motor fusion. With the Bagolini filter bar, the patient was made diplopic with a minimally dense filter. Cycloplegic refraction was +2.50 D for each eye. Ophthalmoscopy revealed normal findings.

Treatment consisted of giving the cycloplegic refraction with bifocal lenses (+2.00 D) and base-out prisms (3.5 PD each eye).

Two months later a 15-PD constant esotropia persisted at distance and near with the glasses. The patient continued to show fusion ability with the synoptophore. Orthoptics/vision therapy with the variable mirror stereoscope/cheiroscope and the synoptophore to enhance sensory and motor fusion was undertaken.

In May, 1987 the patient continued to manifest a 15-PD esotropia. Without glasses, the esotropia measured 30 PD. Cycloplegic retinoscopy was identical to that measured during the first examination. Fresnel prisms (10-PD base-out OD, 5-PD base-out OS) were given to compensate for the nonaccommodative esotropia. Orthoptics/vision therapy was continued.

In August, 1987 the patient manifested 12-PD esotropia despite the added prisms. Without glasses the esotropia was still 30 PD. Because of the inability to develop adequate fusion with lenses, prisms, and orthoptics/vision therapy, surgical therapy was recommended.

One month later, a bimedial rectus recession was performed. The amount of surgery performed was based on the prism-adapted angle. After surgery and while wearing hyperopic glasses without prisms, the patient demonstrated a 2-PD esophoria at distance and a 4-PD esophoria at near. The patient fused the Worth four dot test at distance and near and had 400 seconds of arc with the Randot stereotest. When the glasses were removed a 15-PD esotropia became manifest.

Comment

Because of the fusion ability demonstrated with the synoptophore and the minimal sensory adaptations, the esotropia probably began later, possibly after age 5. Indeed, at the initial visit, there was no mention of an eye turn by the parents.

We treated the patient aggressively with bifocals, prisms, and orthoptics/vision therapy. Despite having fusion potential, the patient had an angle buildup with the prisms. Surgical therapy converted the esotropia to an esophoria, but bifoveal fusion was not achieved, as indicated by the reduced stereopsis. Additional orthoptics/vision therapy did not change this.

CASE 17

In April, 1987 an 8-year-old girl came to the clinic. The patient was diagnosed at 12 months of age as having esotropia. Through the years the patient has been treated with glasses, bifocals, and occlusion. Surgery was recommended at one time but never performed. The patient was presently wearing +4.50-D glasses with a +3.00-D bifocal.

Visual acuity was 20/40 and 20/20 OS. A 30-PD constant right esotropia was measured at distance and near. The near deviation was reduced to a 15-PD constant esotropia while viewing with the bifocal. Without correction the esotropia increased to 35 PD at distance and 60 PD at near. Version testing showed bilateral superior oblique overactions with an A pattern, with 40-PD esotropia in upgaze and 20-PD esotropia in downgaze.

The patient suppressed the right eye at distance and near when tested with the Worth four dot and Bagolini striated lens tests. Anomalous correspondence was diagnosed with the synoptophore. The patient was not aware of diplopia with the Bagolini filter bar. Stereopsis was absent with the Randot stereotest.

Cycloplegic refraction was identical to the patient's present glasses. Ophthalmoscopy was normal.

The diagnosis was partly accommodative incomitant esotropia. The parents and patient refused any additional amblyopia treatment. Because of the large nonaccommodative esotropia and the lack of fusion ability, surgery was recommended. For financial reasons, the surgery was not performed until 3 years later, at which time a recession and supraplacement of the right medial rectus was undertaken.

On the most recent examination, the patient manifested an 8-PD esotropia at distance and near with the hyperopic glasses. Visual acuity was unchanged. Version testing revealed similar amounts of esotropia in up and downgaze. She fused the Worth four dot test at 40 cm and suppressed the right eye at further distances. With the Bagolini striated lens test, she perceived an X, indicating harmonious anomalous correspondence. The synoptophore showed an objective angle of 14 BO and a subjective angle of 1 BO, also indicating harmonious anomalous correspondence. Stereopsis was not present with the Randot and Lang stereotests with compensatory prisms. No further treatment was recommended.

Comment

This case is more representative, at least functionally, of partly accommodative esotropia. Amblyopia, well-established suppression, and anomalous correspondence prevented normal fusion for the patient. Peripheral fusion, albeit anomalous, was achieved following surgery. The presence of an early-onset esotropia possibly suggests that this patient had an infantile esotropia and as she got older developed accommodative esotropia with a high AC/A ratio. Normal fusion was not a realistic possibility for the patient.

NONACCOMMODATIVE ESOTROPIA

Esotropias that are nonaccommodative are not affected by the glasses when a hyperopic refractive error is corrected or when a bifocal is given. Some may occur suddenly.

EARLY-ONSET NONACCOMMODATIVE ESOTROPIA

Patients with early-onset nonaccommodative esotropia that is not infantile comprise a small group among patients with acquired esotropia. The onset is often variable, occurring after 6 months but mostly before 2 years. Occasionally, it may develop later. Some children with nonaccommodative esotropia occurring between ages 2 and 6 have diplopia and do not develop sensory adaptations; they may close or cover one eye. Many of these children have normal binocular vision development up to a certain age before the esotropia develops. The prognosis for normalization of binocular function is better than in those with infantile esotropia.

The etiology for early-onset nonaccommodative esotropia is likely innervational and is thought to be excessive tonic convergence normally controlled by negative relative vergence. This agrees with the findings that the eyes usually straighten out or become divergent under general anesthesia, as is the case with infantile esotropia, provided there are no associated mechanical factors restricting passive adduction or abduction.[20,140] In some instances, early-onset nonaccommodative esotropia may be a manifestation of an intraocular disease process.[141] Although a rare condition, retinoblastoma can present as a strabismus, and the possibility of this serious condition should be investigated in young children with nonaccommodative esotropia. Ellsworth[142] reports early-onset nonaccommodative esotropia as the presenting sign in 11% of children with retinoblastomas. Some of these children unfortunately receive treatment for the esotropia be-

fore the correct diagnosis is made. If the esotropia is caused by a fundus lesion, the lesion will necessarily involve the posterior pole. A purely peripheral lesion will generally not cause strabismus unless it is so extensive that it disrupts peripheral fusion.

With the exception of the time of onset, many clinical findings for early-onset nonaccommodative esotropia are similar to those for infantile esotropia. Clinical features usually include (1) onset that is either sudden or insidious, starting in early childhood; (2) the presence of amblyopia if the deviation is unilateral; (3) a constant, comitant deviation generally ranging in magnitude from 30 PD to 70 PD; (4) similar magnitudes of esotropia at distance and near; (5) a refractive error similar to that occurring in nonstrabismic children of the same age; (6) absence of an accommodative factor; (7) frequently a family history of strabismus; and (8) normal neurologic findings. The incidence of inferior oblique overaction, dissociated vertical deviation, and nystagmus is less than with infantile esotropia. Treatment is similar to that for infantile esotropia. However, because of its later onset, the use of prisms and orthoptics/vision therapy to achieve normal binocular vision may be more helpful than with infantile esotropia.

ACUTE-ONSET ESOTROPIA

When a convergent strabismus develops suddenly in a patient with previously normal binocular vision, it is called *acute-onset esotropia*. Acute-onset esotropia is always a disturbing experience to the patient, who, because of diplopia, promptly seeks attention. Its onset can often be traced to a precise hour of a particular day. It can present as decompensated esophoria, late-onset refractive accommodative esotropia, divergence insufficiency or divergence paralysis esotropia, acute acquired comitant esotropia, or lateral rectus paresis (Table 8-3).

Acute Acquired Comitant Esotropia

This is characterized by a moderate-to-large angle of deviation at distance and near, absence of signs of extraocular muscle paresis, and good potential for normal binocular vision. It can be provoked by chronic illness, emotional stress, injury, or prolonged occlusion of one eye.[143-146] Fusional divergence amplitudes may rapidly deteriorate after disruption of binocular vision by wearing a patch. An esophoria may become an esotropia when the patch is removed. Acute acquired comitant esotropia can be idiopathic. It appears to be an age-related phenomenon occurring most commonly in children over age 5 and rarely in adults. Four young siblings with acute comitant esotropia have been reported.[143]

An especially careful ocular motility analysis is essential to rule out a paretic deviation. As discussed in

TABLE 8-3 CLINICAL PRESENTATIONS OF ACUTE-ONSET ESOTROPIA

Condition	Deviation in Primary Position	Motility	Refraction	Diplopia	Fusion	Underlying Disease
Decompensated esophoria	$10\text{-}20^\Delta$ at distance and near	Full	Similar to nonstrabismic population	Yes, at distance and near	Yes	No
Late onset refractive accommodative esotropia	$10\text{-}40^\Delta$, which may be larger at near	Full	2-6 D of hyperopia	Yes	Yes	No
Lateral rectus paresis	$20\text{-}40^\Delta$, which may be larger at distance	Restricted abduction in one or both eyes	Similar to nonstrabismic population	Yes, more at distance	Yes	Frequent
Divergence insufficiency or paralysis	$8\text{-}30^\Delta$ at distance, $4\text{-}18^\Delta$ at near	Full	Similar to nonstrabismic population	Yes, but only at distance	Yes	Possibly
Acute acquired comitant esotropia	$20\text{-}75^\Delta$ at distance and near	Full	Similar to nonstrabismic population	Yes	Most of the time	Possibly

From American Optometric Association: *Optometric Clinical Practice Guidelines: Strabismus—esotropia and exotropia,* St Louis, 1995, American Optometric Association.

Chapter 10, lateral rectus paresis causes an acute and incomitant esotropia that may over time become less incomitant. Acute nonaccommodative esotropia without evidence of either lateral rectus paresis or divergence insufficiency/paralysis and with normal ophthalmoscopic findings has been considered mostly to have a benign cause and can develop without any preceding disruption of fusion.[147-150]

Clark and associates[150] report on six children ages 5 to 11 with acute acquired comitant esotropia. The esotropia ranged from 20 PD to 55 PD. The full cycloplegic refraction was prescribed for all patients, with no change in the deviation noted. Neurologic examination in each child gave normal results. All six patients underwent a bilateral medial rectus recession an average of 8 months after initial presentation. Five of the six patients were orthophoric following surgery and achieved 40 seconds of arc stereoacuity.

The possibility of serious underlying neurologic disorders and intracranial disease exists with acute acquired comitant esotropia (see Chapter 13, Case 4). Williams and Hoyt[151] describe six children who developed acute comitant esotropia and were found to have tumors of the brain stem or cerebellum. In each case the esotropia was the initial sign of the intracranial disease, and in no case did the esotropia become incomitant. Additional neuro-ophthalmologic signs, such as torsional and upbeating nystagmus, occurred in three patients. Ophthalmoscopic findings for all patients were normal. Interestingly, in none of these children could fusion be achieved with prisms, the synoptophore, or extraocular muscle surgery. Other investigators have reported neurologic disorders in patients with acute acquired comitant esotropia.[141,152,153] There-

fore we require neurologic evaluations for all patients, even in the absence of signs and symptoms that can be associated with intracranial disease, such as headache, nausea, vomiting, ataxia, nystagmus, pupillary abnormalities, and papilledema.

Optometric treatment involves maintenance of fusion with prisms and orthoptics/vision therapy to expand fusional vergence ranges. Some patients can be eventually weaned from the prisms.[146] If the esotropia exceeds 15 PD and remains unchanged over a period of usually 6 to 8 months, extraocular muscle surgery can be considered as possible treatment. The refractive error in acute acquired comitant esotropia can be hyperopic in some cases and mimic late-onset refractive accommodative esotropia. (See Case 18.)

Case 18

An 8 year-old girl was referred because of recent-onset diplopia and strabismus.[154] The patient was in excellent health. There had not been any recent illness or physical or emotional trauma. The patient and parents were specific that the diplopia and strabismus began 8 days earlier. Past ocular history was unremarkable. An examination by another clinician at age 4 had shown 2-D hyperopia, orthophoria, and 20/30 vision.

Our examination revealed visual acuity of 20/20 OD and 20/30 OS. A constant left esotropia of 30 PD at distance and 25 PD at near was present. Ductions and versions were full, and the size of the deviation did not change in left or right gaze. With the Worth four dot test, homonymous diplopia was reported at distance and near. Examination with the synoptophore indicated normal correspondence. Sensory and motor fusion existed with the synoptophore, and stereopsis occurred when the deviation was compensated with prisms equivalent to the angle of deviation. Cycloplegic

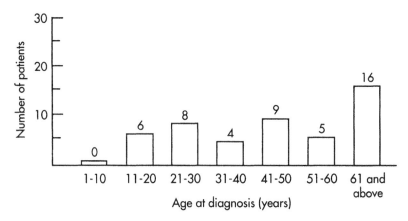

FIG. 8-14 Age distribution for 48 patients diagnosed with divergence insufficiency esotropia.

refraction revealed OD +3.75 and OS +4.50. Ophthalmoscopy indicated normal findings.

It was suspected that the patient had late-onset refractive accommodative esotropia. However, no change in the magnitude of the esotropia occurred while wearing the glasses. Prisms (25-PD base-out) were given to allow fusion. Because the hyperopia was unrelated to the esotropia and the evaluation 4 years earlier indicated orthophoria, a neurologic evaluation was requested. All findings were normal.

After 8 months, the esotropia remained unchanged. With the refractive findings and 25-PD base-out, the patient continued to fuse. Subsequent extraocular muscle surgery made the patient slightly esophoric.

Divergence Insufficiency (Distance Esotropia)

This is a type of nonaccommodative esotropia that can also develop suddenly. It may persist as an esophoria for a considerable time before becoming an esotropia. Its clinical features include (1) intermittent or constant esotropia at distance fixation but not at near fixation, (2) comitance, (3) refractive errors similar to the nonstrabismic population, (4) reduced negative fusional vergence amplitudes, and (5) lack of sensory adaptations with diplopia.[155] Unlike acute acquired comitant esotropia, divergence insufficiency appears to occur mostly in older patients and rarely in young children. We have not diagnosed divergence insufficiency esotropia in patients younger than age 10 (Fig. 8-14).

The angle of deviation is greater for distance fixation than near fixation. The amount of esodeviation at distance usually ranges from 8 to 30 PD, with an average of 16 PD.[156] At near, the deviation ranges from 4 to 18 PD.[156] According to some authorities, a 10-PD difference from one distance to another is essential for the diagnosis.[155] A patient with divergence insufficiency, however, may have an esodeviation only 5 PD larger at distance than at near, yet the deviation at distance might be an esotropia and the deviation at near an esophoria.

Divergence insufficiency is associated with a low AC/A ratio. The low ratio is based on comparing the magnitudes of the distance and near deviations and not on the gradient method. The low AC/A ratio can be an important consideration when treatment is given.

Divergence insufficiency is a comitant deviation.[157] The esotropia as measured with the alternate prism cover test in primary position remains the same amount in both extreme right and extreme left gazes, as well as with each fixating in turn. Ductions and versions are unrestricted in all positions of gaze. When performing diplopia fields with the red-lens test, the separation between the diplopic images at distance, as perceived by the patient, is homonymous and remains the same when viewing to the extreme right and extreme left. Because of the comitance, a compensatory head posture is not used by the patient.

Patients with divergence insufficiency have refractive errors that are unrelated to the deviation. In studies that document the refractive error, myopia occurred in 21% and 68%, and hyperopia occurred in 70% and 3%.[156,158] The prevalence of hyperopia does not appear to be any greater in divergence insufficiency than in the general population.

Fusional divergence amplitudes at distance are markedly reduced or absent. The divergence power is usually reduced proportionally to the degree of esotropia. Fusional amplitudes are best measured in space, with either prism bars or rotary prisms for intermittent esotropia. With constant esotropia, amplitudes are measured from the angle of deviation, either with compensatory prisms or with the synoptophore. Fusional divergence amplitudes may also be reduced at near fixation.

Amblyopia, suppression, and anomalous correspondence are uncommon with divergence insufficiency. This is attributed to its later onset relative to the other esotropias. The maintenance of a phoric status at near also preserves bifoveal fusion and high-grade stereopsis.

The most frequent symptom is diplopia that increases with viewing distance. A fixation light held 3 m in front of the patient elicits uncrossed diplopia. As the light is brought closer to the patient, the images become closer and the patient usually fuses them at 50 or 60 cm.

Any esotropia or esophoria that is greater at distance than at near fixation should alert the examiner to search for neurologic cause. As with acute acquired comitant esotropia, the differential diagnosis for divergence insufficiency includes lateral rectus paresis. Both conditions present with larger esodeviation at distance. Unlike divergence insufficiency, with acquired lateral rectus paresis the angle of deviation changes in right and/or left gaze, primary and secondary angles of deviation exist, and there is restricted abduction either unilaterally or bilaterally.

CLINICAL PEARL

Any esotropia or esophoria that is greater at distance than at near fixation should alert the examiner to search for neurologic cause.

Nevertheless, it has been suggested that divergence insufficiency esotropia is not a distinct clinical entity from lateral rectus paresis.[159-161] Minimal interference of abducens cranial nerve function by raised intracranial pressure may produce the clinical features of divergence insufficiency esotropia without other evidence of lateral rectus paresis.[161] Some patients with divergence insufficiency, although having apparently full ductions and versions, have electro-oculographically determined saccadic velocities of the eye that are significantly reduced in abduction, confirming lateral rectus weakness.[161] The difference in abduction versus adduction velocity may be too subtle for detection by gross observation. As mentioned in Chapter 10, we have examined patients with lateral rectus paresis whose clinical sequelae was divergence insufficiency esotropia (Chapter 10, Case 11). Apparently, for these patients there was a spread of comitance over time. We have also examined patients with divergence insufficiency esotropia that evolved into frank lateral rectus paresis (Chapter 10, Case 12). This observation has been documented by other investigators.[162] Scheiman, Gallaway, and Ciner[155] emphasized that the differentiation between divergence insufficiency and lateral rectus paresis depends mostly on the patient's symptoms. Patients with divergence insufficiency present with a longer history of diplopia. The diplopia associated with lateral rectus paresis always occurs suddenly. Scheiman, Gallaway, and Ciner[155] also stressed that endpoint nystagmus and other neurologic signs and symptoms usually accompany lateral rectus paresis but not divergence insufficiency. In that regard the condition of divergence paralysis esotropia has been differentiated from diver-

gence insufficiency esotropia. In divergence paralysis the comitant esotropia at distance is associated with a history of head trauma or other apparent neurologic problem. An organic lesion involving the divergence center or pathways of divergence innervation must be considered. In divergence insufficiency esotropia, possibly a preexisting esophoria has become manifest. Thus clinically it may not be easy to differentiate the benign from the not so benign. We request neurologic evaluations for all patients with divergence insufficiency esotropia where there is no apparent cause.

Treatment involves providing glasses with base-out prisms in the amount required to give the patient single vision at distance. The least amount of prism is prescribed, that is, the amount of the associated phoria. Fresnel press-on prisms can be bisected and applied to the upper portion of the glasses. If this is successful, we usually prescribe ground prisms into the patient's glasses. Although the prisms may not be indicated for near vision, they rarely cause problems. Supplementary orthoptics/vision therapy to expand fusional divergence amplitudes may be helpful. Rarely do these patients require extraocular muscle surgery. We have not found divergence insufficiency esotropia to be self-limiting, and continued binocular vision care is necessary.

SECONDARY ESOTROPIA

An esotropia that results from either a primary sensory deficit or from surgical correction of exotropia is classified as a *secondary esotropia*. Secondary esotropia can be sensory or consecutive.

SENSORY ESOTROPIA

Sensory esotropia is a convergent strabismus that develops following loss of visual function or marked reduction in visual function in one eye. An anomaly that prevents development of sight in an infant or decreased vision in a young child after the sight has developed can be associated with esotropia. Congenital or early-acquired monocular organic lesions, such as cataract, corneal scarring, optic atrophy, macular lesion, ptosis, or prolonged blurred or distorted retinal images as a result of uncorrected anisometropia may cause an esotropia, supposedly because of the excessive tonic convergence that exists in childhood. Congenital or traumatic unilateral cataracts account for nearly 30% of all cases. As reported earlier, sensory esotropia and sensory exotropia occur with approximately the same frequency when unilateral visual impairment occurs at birth, during the first year of life, and between the ages of 1 and 5.[5] When the monocular visual impairment begins in older children and adulthood, sensory exotropia is more likely. The degree of visual impairment causing sensory esotropia extends from 20/60 to light perception. Functional amblyopia may become superimposed on the organically caused sensory esotropia.[163,164]

The magnitude of sensory esotropia ranges between 10 and 45 PD, with the deviation usually being the same at distance and near. The esotropia gradually increases but usually does not increase to equal the large angle found in patients with infantile esotropia. Because of the poor visual acuity in the deviating eye, the Krimsky test with prisms is more appropriate than the cover test for quantifying the deviation.

Sensory esotropia can be comitant or incomitant. Incomitance may be the result of restrictions caused by hypertrophy of the medial rectus muscle or contracture of Tenon's capsule and the conjunctiva. This results in limited abduction and excessive adduction. The poorly sighted eye often develops an associated hypertropia that is accompanied by oblique muscle disorders. Sensory esotropia is frequently associated with overaction of the inferior or superior oblique muscles.[5] The overacting oblique muscle usually occurs in the visually impaired eye and rarely exists in the sound eye, although it may be bilateral in some cases. A high prevalence of dissociated vertical deviation has also been reported with sensory esotropia.[165]

Because the cause of sensory esotropia may be untreatable, normal single binocular vision is not usually a realistic goal of treatment. Treatment is usually directed toward the cosmetic appearance, and this is handled surgically if warranted by the magnitude of the deviation. Infants with cataracts and sensory esotropia are treated aggressively within the first weeks of life. Strabismus surgery is usually done subsequently. In only rare cases can normal binocular vision be achieved.[166,167]

CONSECUTIVE ESOTROPIA

An esotropia is consecutive if it develops following an exotropia. Consecutive esotropia results iatrogenically from exogenous mechanical factors or occurs spontaneously. A spontaneous change from exotropia to esotropia in the absence of exogenous mechanical factors or an acquired lateral rectus paresis is rare. Cases that have occurred spontaneously involved changes from infantile exotropia to infantile esotropia.[168] Consecutive esotropia is more likely to result from the surgical correction of an exotropia. Consecutive accommodative esotropia has been reported in children following surgical correction of intermittent exotropia.[169] In these instances, all patients had high AC/A ratios before surgery.

Overcorrecting an intermittent exotropia with the anticipation of a postoperative drift toward orthophoria is a common objective for many ophthalmic surgeons (see Chapters 9 and 11). Persistent esotropia in the absence of a postoperative drift becomes a problem for the very young child or older patient.[170,171] In the

child who is visually immature, it bears the risk of causing amblyopia and loss of bifoveal fusion and high-grade stereopsis. For the older patient, it causes diplopia, because the extrafoveal image is now placed on the unsuppressed nasal hemiretina. An increasing esotropia to place the diplopic image coincident with the optic nerve may result.[172] Occlusion, glasses with full hyperopic correction, bifocals, prisms, and orthoptics/vision therapy can be used for patients with consecutive esotropia. Bifocals may be used in patients with high AC/A ratios. Only if all the above approaches have been exhausted is additional surgery considered. (See Case 19.)

CASE 19

In 1985 an 11-year-old girl was referred for an evaluation of esotropia. The patient had diplopia that was longstanding. The patient underwent extraocular muscle surgery for exotropia at age 4½. For 1 year following surgery, she had occlusion therapy. She was also given glasses for hyperopia (+2.75 −0.50 × 180, OU).

The patient had corrected visual acuities of 20/20 for each eye. The cover test showed a 12-PD constant left esotropia at distance and a 20-PD constant left esotropia at near. The esotropia measured the same in left and right gazes. Versions showed inferior oblique overactions that gave a mild V pattern, with more esodeviation in downgaze.

Sensory testing with the Worth four dot test and Bagolini striated lens test showed homonymous diplopia at distance and near. With a +2.00-D add and 8-PD base-out, the patient could fuse the Bagolini striated lenses at near. The synoptophore showed normal correspondence and fusion. No stereopsis was perceived with the Randot stereotest. Refraction was similar to what the patient was presently wearing. Biomicroscopy and ophthalmoscopy were normal.

The diagnosis was iatrogenically induced consecutive esotropia. Treatment consisted of the refractive correction, a +2.00-D bifocal, and 8-PD base-out (4 PD each lens).

One month later, the diplopia was intermittent and limited to distance. The patient manifested a residual 6-PD intermittent esotropia at distance and 3-PD esophoria at near when viewing with the bifocal. She fused the Worth four dot test at near and had homonymous diplopia at distance. With the Randot stereotest, 100 seconds of arc was present. Motor fusion ranges were restricted. Orthoptics/vision therapy was given to increase vergence ranges and facility.

Over the years, the esotropia remained well controlled and the patient did not experience diplopia. The bifocal was eventually eliminated, and the magnitude of prisms necessary for fusion was decreased.

In 1991 the patient reported less dependence on the glasses and felt they were now too strong. She wears them only when she gets tired. Without correction, a 12-PD intermittent esotropia at distance and 4-PD esophoria at near were measured. Versions continued to show a V pattern. The patient fused the Worth four dot test at near and had intermittent diplopia at distance. Refraction was +0.75 D OU. Prism bar vergences at near were base-in 8/6 (break/recovery) and base-out 25/20. The glasses were changed to +0.75 D, with 2-PD base-out in each lens. The patient is seen annually.

TABLE 8-4   DIFFERENTIAL DIAGNOSIS: NORMAL BINOCULAR VISION VERSUS MICROTROPIA

	Normal Binocular Vision	Microtropia
Cover/uncover test	No manifest deviation.	Constant esotropia of 10 PD or less; rarely exotropia. In some cases, the deviation increases with the alternate cover test.
Visual acuity	No amblyopia.	Frequently amblyopia.
Refractive error	Usually equal between eyes, if present.	High incidence of anisometropia.
Fixation	Central.	May be eccentric.
Worth four dot test	Fusion at distance and near.	Fusion at near; suppression at distance.
4-PD base-out prism test	Biphasic movement (version/vergence) of the eye without the prism, indicating absence of suppression.	Absence of eye movement of either eye when prism is placed before microtropic eye, indicating suppression.
Bagolini striated lens test	No gap is seen around lines radiating from fixation light.	Gap is seen around lines radiating from fixation light, indicating suppression zone in microtropic eye.
Stereopsis	60 sec of arc or better with contour stereotests.	Less than 60 sec of arc with contour stereotests.

Comment

This case illustrates consecutive esotropia in an older child, accompanied by diplopia, in which glasses, bifocals, prisms, and orthoptics/vision therapy were used. An apparently high AC/A esodeviation over time became a divergence insufficiency esodeviation with a supposedly low AC/A ratio. The hyperopic refractive error over a 6-year period decreased by 2 D. Although the esotropia remains at distance, it is smaller and intermittent and can be controlled with minimal prisms.

MICROTROPIA

Microtropia refers to small angles of esotropia that may escape diagnosis by conventional methods and are easily overlooked. It occurs in patients with childhood-onset esotropia and appears to develop in most cases before age 3. The esotropia is constant, usually unilateral, and 10 PD or smaller. Other labels for microtropia include *flick, microesotropia, microsquint, microstrabismus, small-angle deviation, minitropia, and monofixation syndrome*. Microexotropia, a constant small-angle exotropic deviation, is very rare.

 CLINICAL PEARL

Microtropia refers to small angles of esotropia that may escape diagnosis by conventional methods and are easily overlooked.

The clinical features for patients with microtropia include (1) a favorable cosmetic appearance despite the esotropia, (2) a suppression zone at the fovea and/or the fixation point of the deviated eye during binocular vision, (3) peripheral fusion, and (4) poor stereopsis. Patients with microtropia have demonstrable binocular vision (Table 8-4).

Many of these patients manifest amblyopia of two lines or more (rarely deeper than 20/100), eccentric fixation, anisometropia, anomalous correspondence, and a larger deviation with the alternate prism cover test than with the unilateral cover test. Some patients may show no discernible movement with the unilateral cover test.

The most common etiology for microtropia is treated strabismus. Microtropia can be the residual deviation resulting from treating a larger esotropia either by glasses, orthoptics/vision therapy, pharmacologic agents, or extraocular muscle surgery. As mentioned earlier, microtropia is a desirable end-stage of treatment for infantile esotropia. On the other hand, microtropia is an undesirable end-stage of treatment for refractive and nonrefractive accommodative esotropia and intermittent exotropia.

Anisometropia can be causative for microtropia. Helveston and von Noorden[173] described a unique form of microtropia that they classified as "microtropia of identity." For these patients, the unilateral cover test revealed no shift. All patients had amblyopia, suppression, anisometropia, and deficient stereopsis. Visuoscopy in the amblyopic eye revealed eccentric fixation. The eccentric area of the deviating eye replaced the fovea for binocular vision, as well as monocular vision, and no refixation movement was required by the amblyopic eye when the other eye was covered. Supposedly, the anisometropia not corrected at an earlier age gave rise to foveal suppression, leading to nonfoveal fixation in the interest of achieving better visual acuity. Absence of a shift on the cover test in the presence of eccentric fixation can be interpreted as an identity between the degree of eccentric fixation, the angle of anomaly, and the angle of strabismus. Unlike other strabismic deviations in which suppression results from strabismus, in "microtropia of identity" suppression precedes strabismus. Therefore a negative cover test does not automatically indicate bifoveal fusion.

CLINICAL PEARL

> A negative cover test does not automatically indicate bifoveal fusion.

Rarely do we encounter "microtropia of identity." In the majority of cases in which eccentric fixation exists, its amount is not identical either to the angle of anomaly or the angle of esotropia, giving a discernible shift with the unilateral cover test.[174,175]

Some patients with microtropia do not have a history of treated strabismus or anisometropia. These cases are classified as being primary or idiopathic. If the esotropia is so small, the obvious cause may not be determined for the associated amblyopia and poor stereopsis. In a review by Hahn, Cadera, and Orton[176] on 398 patients with microtropia, 104 patients (26%) failed to manifest a tropia shift of the nonpreferred eye when the preferred eye was covered. For these patients the magnitude of the esotropia was 2 PD or smaller, which is the limit of the accuracy of the cover test, and/or the strabismus was concealed by eccentric fixation. The correct diagnosis for these patients will spare needless diagnostic evaluation, as indicated by the following case example.

CASE 20

A 6-year-old boy presented with a history of reduced vision in the right eye. Because no apparent cause had been determined by a previous clinician, extensive neurologic testing was scheduled. The parents wanted a second opinion. The youngster was in excellent health and not taking any medications. There was no history of trauma or previous vision disorders.

Visual acuities were 20/40 for the right eye and 20/20 for the left eye. The patient manifested with cover test a 2-PD constant right esotropia at distance and near. The deviation increased to 6 PD with the alternate cover test. Versions were full and smooth. Visuoscopy for the right eye indicated parafoveal-to-central fixation. The patient suppressed the right eye at distance and showed fusion at near with the Worth four dot test. The 4-PD base-out prism test was positive for the right eye. Stereopsis was not present with either the Random-dot E or TNO stereotests. Cycloplegic refraction was +0.50 D for both eyes. Dilated ophthalmoscopy revealed normal findings.

The diagnosis was amblyopia secondary to microtropia. The patient was treated for the amblyopia. After 2 months the visual acuity had improved to 20/30, and gross stereopsis was present with both the TNO stereotest (480 seconds of arc) and the Frisby stereotest (340 seconds of arc).

When quantifying the deviation with the alternate cover test and prisms, the deviation may become larger than what was determined first with the unilateral cover test, in some cases by as much as 10 to 15 PD. Such patients can be mistaken for having intermittent esotropia. The lack of high-grade stereopsis and the presence of amblyopia are inconsistent with intermittent esotropia. Apparently, for these patients there exists both a manifest strabismic and a latent phoric component to the deviation.[177] The phoric component is the difference in magnitude between the unilateral and alternate cover tests and represents the fusional divergence amplitudes of the patient. The phoric deviation remains latent because of the strength of the peripheral fusion mechanism but may become manifest when the patient is tired or the eyes are dissociated for any length of time. When recording the magnitude of the deviation, a distinction should be made between the esodeviation determined by the unilateral cover test and the esodeviation measured with the alternate cover test. For practical purposes, an estimation of the strabismic portion of the deviation may be sufficient. Occluding the preferred eye and simultaneously placing base-out prisms in front of the nonpreferred eye until no movement occurs allows a more accurate quantification of the strabismic portion.

The majority of patients with microtropia demonstrate stereopsis.[178,179] Factors such as the type of stereotest used affect the degree of stereopsis. We prefer random-dot stereotests like the Randot, TNO, Lang, and Frisby, because contour or non–random-dot stereotests have the disadvantage of providing monocular clues. Nearly 70% will demonstrate some stereopsis with the Titmus stereotest, whereas a significantly smaller percentage will demonstrate stereopsis with stereotests using computer-generated random-dot stereograms.[178,179] Patients with deviations smaller than 5 PD, superfical anomalous correspondence, and a nonsurgical history tend to have better stereopsis.[178]

The actual mechanism for the fusion and stereopsis demonstrated in microtropia has been the subject of much discussion. It has been attributed either to an enlarged Panum's area with persistence of normal correspondence in the periphery or to anomalous correspondence.[180,181] The very small strabismus may permit these patients to still maintain normal correspondence. Because peripheral fusion occurs simultaneously with a shift on the unilateral cover test, anomalous correspondence seems to be the more likely mechanism.

Microtropia is a fully adapted strabismus and rarely gives rise to visual symptoms.[182] Treatment typically consists of correcting significant refractive errors and any amblyopia. We rarely use prisms or orthoptics/vision therapy to attempt to establish bifoveal fusion and accept the rudimentary fusion that occurs with microtropia as a final treatment status. Wick[183] proposes an orthoptics/vision therapy technique using the synoptophore. This therapy assumes that patients with microtropia can be taught to diverge their eyes as the tubes of the synoptophore are moved. Stereoscopic

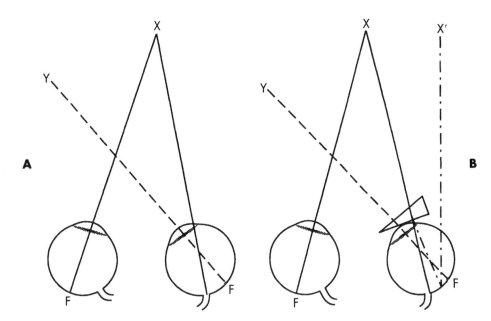

FIG. 8-15 Blind-spot esotropia. **A,** Object of regard *(x)* is imaged on fovea of fixating eye and blind-spot (optic disc) of deviating eye, thus preventing diplopia. Subtle suppression at fovea of deviating eye prevents visual confusion. **B,** A 15-PD base-out prism places object of regard *(x)* outside of blind-spot of deviating eye on nonsuppressed retina, thus producing homonymous diplopia *(x¹)*. (From Rutstein RP, Levi DM: The blind-spot syndrome, *J Am Optom Assoc* 50:1388, 1979.)

slides with suppression checks are used. Divergence must be slow, approximately 1 PD or less per minute. When the patient makes the necessary eye movement (difference between the objective and subjective angles) the anomalous correspondence covaries and changes to normal correspondence, resulting in intermittent esotropia. Suppression and vergence training procedures are then given, as are prisms. To our knowledge the efficacy of this approach on a group of patients has not been reported.

BLIND-SPOT ESOTROPIA

A unique and somewhat controversial esodeviation is blind-spot esotropia. This esotropia was described initially by Swan in 1948 as the *blind-spot syndrome*.[172] These patients use the optic nerve of the deviated eye as a suppression zone and eliminate the need at the zero measure point to adapt to diplopia (Fig. 8-15, *A*). Supposedly, they not only lack suppression but also other sensory adaptations, such as anomalous correspondence and amblyopia. Subtle foveal suppression of the deviating eye still occurs to prevent visual confusion. Unlike other nonaccommodative esotropias with an early-childhood onset, the potential for normal binocular vision persists despite the constancy of the deviation. Clinically, it is probably seen most frequently in surgically overcorrected exotropia but may also occur after the undercorrection of esotropia with

glasses.[172] According to Swan,[172] these cases are usually accompanied by hyperopic anisometropia.

 CLINICAL PEARL

Unlike other nonaccommodative esotropias with an early-childhood onset, the potential for normal binocular vision persists despite the constancy of the deviation.

The clinical features and signs for blind-spot esotropia usually include (1) a constant, comitant esotropia of 20 to 35 PD at distance and near, with the blind-spot of the deviating eye overlying the fixation area; (2) normal visual acuity in each eye; (3) normal correspondence; (4) fusion potential with some amplitudes of convergence and divergence as measured with the synoptophore; and (5) diplopia when the extrafoveal image is placed out of the blind-spot with prisms onto the adjacent retina (Fig. 8-15, *B*), necessitating a continuous motor readjustment on the part of the patient.

Rutstein and Levi[185] report on 4 patients with presumed blind-spot esotropia. Fusion with stereopsis was achieved for 2 patients following treatment. (See Case 21.)

CASE 21

A 12-year-old boy was referred to the clinic for an evaluation of an esotropia, which the parents claimed began during the first year of life.[185] Previous treatment had not been given. The esotropia was not cosmetically displeasing, and no diplopia or other visual symptoms were reported by the patient.

Our evaluation revealed a constant esotropia of 25 PD at distance and near. Best corrected vision was OD 20/20 and OS 20/25. Versions were full.

Sensory testing with the Worth four dot test and Bagolini striated lens test showed homonymous diplopia, possibly resulting from placing the extrafoveal image out of the blind-spot. Compensation for the esotropia with prisms equivalent to the angle of deviation produced fusion, indicating normal correspondence. Synoptophore evaluation also revealed normal correspondence, fusion ranges, and stereopsis. With the synoptophore placed at the zero setting and while viewing superimposition targets, the patient suppressed the image before the deviating eye. Movement of the targets of approximately 3 PD elicited diplopia. Placing 15-PD base-out before the left eye also produced diplopia of the fixation light.

The diagnosis was blind-spot esotropia. Based on sensory testing, the prognosis for establishing normal binocular vision was excellent. Because extraocular muscle surgery was rejected by the parents, prisms (18 PD) that permitted fusion were given along with orthoptics/vision therapy to increase vergence ranges and facility.

The magnitude of prisms necessary to maintain fusion was eventually reduced (14 PD). Despite continued therapy, further prism reduction resulted in esotropia and diplopia. The patient was told to continue wearing the prism lenses and return in 6 months.

The patient returned 8 months later. He had lost his glasses and had been without them for 2 months. Diplopia began immediately after loss of the glasses and lasted for 2 days. Examination findings at this time were consistent with those of the earlier examination. Again, prisms (14 PD) and orthoptics/vision therapy were given. At the last visit and while wearing the prism glasses, the patient was orthophoric at distance and near, fused the Worth four dot test at distance and near, and had 100 seconds of arc with the Titmus stereotest.

Comment

This patient fulfilled the criteria for blind-spot esotropia by showing absence of sensory adaptations, despite manifesting an esotropia of 25 PD to 35 PD at distance and near. By treating the motor aspect only, sensory and motor fusion could be achieved, despite the very early onset and constancy of the deviation.

Blind-spot esotropia has been refuted by investigators who have claimed that the small size of the optic disc and variations of the angle of deviation at different positions of gaze and fixation distances make it implausible that the blind-spot is the mechanism by which diplopia is relieved.[186] Furthermore, there is no known mechanism for continuous oculomotor readjustment with the purpose of locking a retinal image onto the optic nerve head. According to these investi-

gators, a superficial anomalous correspondence and not the optic disc is more likely the mechanism that prevents diplopia for these patients.[186]

Esotropic deviations of 20 to 35 PD that are not totally accommodative have a high incidence, yet most of these patients have poor fusion potential when the onset of the deviation is in early childhood. Patients with suppression, anomalous correspondence, and amblyopia may also use the blind-spot, but these sensory adaptations preclude the establishment of normal binocular vision with prisms. Thorough sensory testing should always be undertaken to determine whether blind-spot esotropia is present.

CYCLIC ESOTROPIA

Cyclic (hyperkinetic, or circadian) esotropia is a rare and poorly understood deviation, with an estimated incidence of 1 in 3000 to 1 in 5000 strabismic cases.[187] It mostly occurs in association with childhood strabismus and depends on a clock mechanism. The esotropia follows a circadian rhythm. Aids to diagnosis include a strong suspicion and a log of the strabismus periods kept by the parents. It is present temporarily and alternates with single binocular vision typically on a 48-hour cycle (alternate-day esotropia). A 24-hour period of normal binocular vision is followed by 24 hours of manifest esotropia. Cyclic exotropia, cyclic vertical deviations, and cyclic oculomotor nerve palsies have also been reported.[188,189] The periodicity is not always so precise, and the duration of the esotropia may be variable and sometimes more prolonged. Cycles of 72 hours and 96 hours have been documented. Many cases become constant with time. During the esotropic phase the deviation is usually large (30 to 70 PD), unilateral, and without diplopia awareness because of suppression and anomalous correspondence. During the nonesotropic phase, there is no manifest deviation, a small esophoria may be present, and fusion and stereopsis are normal, as are fusional amplitudes. Some patients may not be completely aligned on alternating days and do not manifest normal binocular vision.[187] The age of onset is generally between ages 3 and 4, although several adult-onset cases have been documented.[190-194] Despite the sensory adaptations with the strabismus and the unilateral nature of the deviation, amblyopia does not develop. Undoubtedly this is because both eyes are stimulated during the nonesotropic day.

Cyclic esotropia is not a form of intermittent esotropia. Unlike intermittent esotropia, on normal days there is no large latent deviation and the deviation does not become manifest during conditions of either fatigue, illness, accommodative stress, or prolonged occlusion.

The etiology of cyclic esotropia is unknown. It can

be idiopathic and appear spontaneously. It can also be precipitated by central nervous system abnormalities involving the hypothalamus, oculomotor nuclei, and superior colliculus and by peripheral factors, such as strabismus surgery, retinal detachment surgery, and ocular trauma.[190,192,193] High AC/A ratios, moderate hyperopia, and V-pattern esodeviations have also been documented with these cases. It occurs more frequently in association with acquired nonaccommodative esotropia but may also occur in association with accommodative, infantile, or consecutive esotropia.[191,192] Some have suggested that cyclic esotropia may actually represent deteriorated accommodative esotropia and, if followed up for a sufficiently long time, develops constant strabismus.

Some cases have been attributed to psychogenic disorders; its periodicity suggests the biologic clock mechanism that is sometimes apparent in the alternate-day behavior of psychotic patients. It may be associated with anxiety, depression, phobia, or compulsive behavior that may be cyclic. No systemic medication has been found that influences the disorder, and psychotherapy is without benefit. Seldom does the deviation cease spontaneously.

Treatment is contraindicated until the deviation has become constant or nearly constant. Surgery, both conventional and nonincisional with botulinum toxin injections, is usually the treatment of choice. This is based on the full amount of esotropia that occurs on the strabismic days and has been successful in bringing the condition to a halt and in restoring normal binocular functions.[191,194] Consecutive exotropia, interestingly, has not been reported for these patients.

REFERENCES

1. Fletcher MC, Silverman S: Strabismus. I. A summary of 1110 cases, *Am J Ophthalmol* 61:86, 1966.
2. Adelstein AM, Scully J: Epidemiological aspects of squint, *Br Med J* 3(561):334, 1967.
3. Chew E and others: Risk factors for esotropia and exotropia, *Arch Ophthalmol* 112:1349, 1994.
4. Nordlow W: Squint: the frequency of onset of different ages and the incidence of some defects in a Swedish population, *Acta Ophthalmol* 42:1015, 1964.
5. Sidikaro Y, von Noorden GK: Observations in sensory heterotropia, *J Pediatr Ophthalmol Strab* 19:12, 1982.
6. Goldstein JH: Non-accommodative intermittent esotropia, *Am Orthopt J* 32:117, 1982.
7. Hugonnier R, Hugonnier S: *Strabismus, heterophoria, ocular motor paralysis,* St Louis, 1969, Mosby.
8. Dobson V, Sebris SL: Longitudinal study of acuity and stereopsis in infants with or at risk for esotropia, *Invest Ophthalmol Vis Sci* 30:1146, 1989.
9. Wilson ME, Parks MM: Primary inferior oblique overaction in congenital esotropia, accommodative esotropia, and intermittent exotropia, *Ophthalmology* 96:950, 1989.
10. Nordlow W: Age distribution of onset of esotropia, *Br J Ophthalmol* 37:593, 1953.
11. Scobee RG: Esotropia: incidence, etiology, and results of therapy, *Am J Ophthalmol* 34:817, 1951.
12. Friedman Z and others: Ophthalmic screening of 38,000 children age 1 to 2½ years, in child welfare clinics, *J Pediatr Ophthalmol Strab* 17:261, 1980.
13. Scheiman MM, Wick B: Optometric management of infantile esotropia. In Scheiman MM, editor: *Problems in optometry,* Philadelphia, 1990, JB Lippincott.
14. Holman RE, Merritt JC: Infantile esotropia: results in the neurologic impaired and "normal" child at NCMH (six years), *J Pediatr Ophthalmol Strab* 23:41, 1986.
15. Kapp ME, von Noorden GK, Jenkins, R: Strabismus in Williams syndrome, *Am J Ophthalmol* 119:355, 1995.
16. Lo CY: Brain computed tomographic evaluation of concomitant strabismus and congenital nystagmus. In Hendkin P, editor: *ACTA Twenty-third International Congress of Ophthalmology,* vol 2, Philadelphia, 1983, JB Lippincott.
17. Hoyt CS: Abnormalities of the vestibulo-ocular response in congenital esotropia, *Am J Ophthalmol* 93:704, 1982.
18. Archer SM, Sondhi N, Helveston EM: Strabismus in infancy, *Ophthalmology* 96:133, 1989.
19. Griffin JR and others: Heredity in congenital esotropia, *J Am Optom Assoc* 50:1237, 1979.
20. de Molina AC, Munoz LG: Ocular alignment under general anesthesia in congenital esotropia, *J Pediatr Ophthlmol Strab* 28:278, 1991.
21. Worth C: *Squint: its cause, pathology, and treatment,* ed 6, London, 1929, Balliére, Tindall and Cox.
22. Chavasse FB: *Worth's squint on the binocular reflexes and the treatment of strabismus,* ed 7, Philadelphia, 1939, Blakiston & Sons.
23. von Noorden GK: A reassessment of infantile esotropia, *Am J Ophthalmol* 105:1, 1988.
24. Helveston EM: The origins of congenital esotropia, *J Pediatr Ophthalmol Strab* 30:215, 1993.
25. Nelson LB and others: Congenital esotropia, *Surv Ophthalmol* p 363, 1987.
26. Clark WN, Noel LP: Vanishing infantile esotropia, *Can J Ophthalmol* 17:100, 1982.
27. Costenbader FD: Infantile esotropia, *Trans Am Ophthalmol Soc* 59:397, 1961.
28. Ingram RM, Barr A: Changes in refraction between the ages of 1 and 3½ years, *Br J Ophthalmol* 63:339, 1979.
29. Robb RM, Rodier DW: The broad clinical spectrum of early infantile esotropia, *Trans Am Ophthalmol Soc* 84:103, 1986.
30. Dickey CF and others: The diagnosis of amblyopia in cross-fixation, *J Pediatr Ophthalmol Strab* 28:171, 1991.
31. Steger DR, Birch EE: Preferential-looking acuity and stereopsis in infantile esotropia, *J Pediatr Ophthalmol Strab* 23:160, 1986.
32. Birch EE, Steger DR: Monocular acuity and stereopsis in infantile esotropia, *Invest Ophthalmol Vis Sci* 26:1624, 1985.
33. Hiles DA, Watson A, Biglan AW: Characteristic of infantile esotropia following early bimedial rectus recession, *Arch Ophthalmol* 98:697, 1980.
34. Helveston EM: Dissociated vertical deviation: a clinical and laboratory study, *Trans Am Ophthalmol Soc* 78:734, 1981.
35. Lang J: Der kongenitale order fruhkindliche Strabismus, *Ophthalmologica* 154:201, 1967.

36. Tyschen L, Hurtig RR, Scott WE: Pursuit is impaired but the vestibulo-ocular reflex is normal in infantile strabismus, *Arch Ophthalmol* 103:536, 1985.

37. Demer JL, von Noorden GK: Optokinetic asymmetry in esotropia, *J Pediatr Ophthalmol Strab* 25:286, 1988.

38. Parker L and others: Monocular OKN asymmetry and defective stereopsis in parents of children with infantile esotropia, *Am Orthopt J* 43:71, 1993.

39. Schor CM, Levi DM: Disturbances of small field horizontal and vertical optokinetic nystagmus in amblyopia, *Invest Ophthalmol Vis Sci* 19:668, 1980.

40. Duin Hof-van Van J: Early and permanent effects of monocular deprivation on pattern discrimination and visiomotor behavior in cats, *Brain Res* 111:261, 1976.

41. Lewis TL, Maurer D, and Brent HP: Optokinetic nystagmus in children treated for bilateral cataracts. In Groner R, McConkie GW, Menz C, editors: *Eye movements and human information processing*, Amsterdam, 1985, Elsevier.

42. Aiello A, Wright KW, Borchert M: Independence of optokinetic nystagmus asymmetry and binocularity in infantile esotropia, *Arch Ophthalmol* 112:1580, 1994.

43. Ciancia AO: La esotropia con limitacion bilateral de la abduccion en el lacante, *Arch Ophthalmol (Buenos Aries)* 27:207, 1962.

44. Adelstein F, Cüppers C: Zum Problem der echten und der scheinbaren Abducens Iahmung (das sogenannte Blockierung Ssyndrom), *Büch Augenarzt,* 46:271, 1966.

45. von Noorden GK: Infantile esotropia: a continuing riddle, *Am Orthopt J* 34:52, 1984.

46. von Noorden GK, Wong SY: Surgical results in nystagmus blockage syndrome, *Ophthalmology* 93:1028, 1986.

47. Helveston EM: Esotropia in the first year of life. In *Transactions of the New Orleans Academy of Ophthalmologists*, New York, 1986, Raven.

48. Archer SM and others: Stereopsis in normal infants and infants with congenital esotropia, *Am J Ophthalmol* 101:591, 1986.

49. Pratt-Johnson JA, Tillson G: Sensory results following treatment of infantile esotropia, *Can J Ophthalmol* 18:175, 1983.

50. Botet RV, Calhoun JH, Harley RD: Development of monofixation syndrome in congenital esotropia, *J Pediatr Ophthalmol Strab* 18:49, 1981.

51. Parks MM: Congenital esotropia with a bifixation result: report of a case, *Doc Ophthalmol* 58:109, 1984.

52. Wright KW and others: High-grade stereoacuity after early surgery for congenital esotropia, *Arch Ophthalmol* 112:913, 1994.

53. Birch EE, Stager DR, Berry P, Everett ME: Prospective assessment of acuity and stereopsis in amblyopic infantile esotropes following early surgery, *Invest Ophthalmol* 31:758, 1990.

54. Birch EE, Stager DR, Everett ME: Random dot stereoacuity following surgical corection of infantile esotropia, *J Pediatr Ophthalmol Strab* 32:231, 1995.

55. Mohindra I and others: Development of acuity and stereopsis in infants with esotropia, *Ophthalmology* 92:691, 1985.

56. Eustis S, Smith DR: Parental understanding of strabismus, *J Pediatr Ophthalmol Strab* 24:232, 1987.

57. Satterfield D, Keltner JL, Morrison TL: Psychological aspects of strabismus study, *Arch Ophthalmol* 111:1100, 1993.

58. Rogers GL and others: Strabismus surgery and its effect upon infant development in congenital strabismus, *Ophthalmology* 89:479, 1982.

59. Nixon RB and others: Incidence of strabismus in neonates, *Am J Ophthalmol* 100:798, 1985.

60. Sondhi N, Archer SM, Helveston EM: Development of normal ocular alignment, *J Pediatr Ophthalmol Strab* 25:210, 1988.

61. Campos EC, Gulli R: Lack of alternation in patients treated for strabismic amblyopia, *Am J Ophthalmol* 99:63, 1985.

62. Christenson GN, Rouse MW: Management of a young esotrope using vision therapy and prismatic prescription, *J Am Optom Assoc* 58:592, 1987.

63. Zehetmayer M, Stangler-Zuschrott, Schemper M: Prolonged preoperative prism treatment in alternating convergent squint, *Acta Ophthalmol* 72:103, 1994.

64. Helveston EM and others: Early surgery for essential infantile esotropia, *J Pediatr Ophthalmol Strab* 27:115, 1990.

65. Scheiman M, Ciner E, Gallaway M: Surgical success rates in infantile esotropia, *J Am Optom Assoc* 60:22, 1989.

66. Ing MR: Early surgical alignment for congenital esotropia, *J Pediatr Ophthalmol Strab* 20:11, 1983.

67. Ing MR: Early surgical alignment for congenital esotropia, *Ophthalmology* 90:132, 1983.

68. Zak TA, Morin D: Early surgery for infantile esotropia: results and influence of age upon results, *Can J Ophthalmol* 17:213, 1982.

69. Pratt-Johnson JA, Tillson G: Results of treatment in congenital infantile esotropia. In: *Strabismus II,* New York, 1984, Grune and Stratton.

70. Shauly Y, Prager TL, Mazow ML: Clinical characteristics and long-term postoperative results of infantile esotropia, *Am J Ophthalmol* 117:183, 1994.

71. Kushner BJ: Postoperative binocularity in adults with long-standing strabismus: is surgery cosmetic only? *Am Orthopt J* 40:64, 1990.

72. Kushner BJ, Morton GV: Postoperative binocularity in adults with long-standing strabismus, *Ophthalmology* 99:316, 1992.

73. Morris RJ, Scott WE, Dickey CF: Fusion after surgical alignment for long-standing strabismus in adults, *Ophthalmology* 100:135, 1993.

74. Ball A, Drummond GT, Pearce WG: Unexpected stereoacuity following surgical correction of long-standing horizontal strabismus, *Can J Ophthalmol* 28:217, 1993.

75. Wortham EV, Greenwald MJ: Expanded binocular peripheral visual fields following surgery for esotropia, *J Pediatr Ophthalmol Strab* 26:109, 1989.

76. Kushner BJ: Binocular field expansion in adults after surgery for esotropia, *Arch Ophthalmol* 112:639, 1994.

77. Ing MR: Botulinum alignment for congenital esotropia, *Ophthalmology* 100:318, 1993.

78. Magoon E, Scott AB: Botulinum toxin chemodenervation in infants and children: an alternative to incisional strabismus surgery, *J Pediatr Ophthalmol Strab* 110:719, 1987.

79. McNeer KW, Spencer RF, Tucker MG: Observations on bilateral simultaneous botulinum toxin injection in infantile esotropia, *J Pediatr Ophthalmol Strab* 31:214, 1994.

80. Caputo AR and others: Preferred postoperative alignment after congenital esotropia surgery, *Ann Ophthalmol* 22:269, 1990.

81. Caputo AR and others: Long-term follow-up of extraocular muscle surgery for congenital esotropia, *Am Orthopt J* 41:67, 1991.

82. Infield D and others: The long-term results of surgical correction of childhood esotropia, *Aust N Z J Ophthalmol* 21:23, 1993.

83. Kushner BJ, Fisher M: Is alignment within 8 prism diopters of orthotropia a successful outcome for infantile esotropia surgery? *Arch Ophthalmol* 114:176, 1996.

84. Baker JD, Smith-DeYounge M: Accommodative esotropia following surgical correction of congenital esotropia: frequency and characteristics, *Graefes Arch Clin Exp Ophthalmol* 226:175, 1988.

85. Freely DA, Nelson LB, Calhoun JH: Recurrent esotropia following early successful surgical correction in congenital esotropia, *J Pediatr Ophthalmol Strab* 20:68, 1983.

86. Burian HM: Hypermetropia and esotropia, *J Pediatr Ophthalmol Strab* 9:135, 1972.

87. Donders FC: On the anomalies of accommodation and refraction of the eye, London, 1864, The New Sydenham Society (Translated by WD Moore).

88. Adler FH: Pathologic physiology of convergent strabismus: motor aspects of the non-accommodational type, *Arch Ophthalmol* 33:362, 1945.

89. Stidwell D: *Orthoptic assessment and management,* Oxford, 1990, Blackwell.

90. Pollard ZF: Accommodative esotropia after ocular and head injury, *Am J Ophthalmol* 109:195, 1990.

91. Swan KC: Esotropia following occlusion, *Arch Ophthalmol* 37:444, 1947.

92. Baker JD, Parks MM: Early onset accommodative esotropia, *Am J Ophthalmol* 90:11, 1980.

93. von Noorden GK, Avilla CW: Accommodative convergence in hypermetropia, *Am J Ophthalmol* 110:287, 1991.

94. Nakagawa T, Kii T, Mori S: Outcome of accommodative esotropia. In Campos EC, editor: *Strabismus and ocular motility disorders,* Indianapolis, Ind, 1990, MacMillian.

95. Parks MM: Abnormal accommodative convergence in squint, *Arch Ophthalmol* 59:364, 1958.

96. Inatomi A: Retinal correspondence in typical accommodative esotropia, *Graefes Arch Clin Exp Ophthalmol* 226:165, 1988.

97. von Noorden GK, Avilla CW: Refractive accommodative esotropia: a surgical problem? *Int Ophthalmol* 16:45, 1992.

98. Wick B: Accommodative esotropia: efficacy of treatment, *J Am Optom Assoc* 58:562, 1987.

99. Mohindra I, Molinari JF: Near retinoscopy and cycloplegic retinoscopy in early primary grade school children, *Am J Optom Phys Opt* 56:34, 1979.

100. Velasco-Cruz AA, Sampaio NM, Vargos JA: Near retinoscopy in accommodative esotropia, *J Pediatr Ophthalmol Strab* 27:245, 1990.

101. Auffarth G, Hunold W: Cycloplegic refraction in children: single-dose atropinization versus three-day atropinization, *Doc Ophthalmol* 80:353, 1992.

102. Rosenbaum L, Bateman JB, Bremer DL: Cycloplegic refraction in esotropic children, *Ophthalmology* 88:1031, 1981.

103. Ingram RM, Barr A: Refraction of 1-year-old children after cycloplegic with 1% cyclopentolate: comparison with findings after atropinization, *Br J Ophthalmol* 63:348, 1979.

104. Robb RM, Peterson RA: Cycloplegic refraction in children, *J Pediatr Ophthalmol Strab* 5:110, 1968.

105. Stolovitch C: The use of cyclopentolate versus atropine cycloplegia in esotropic caucasion children, *Binoc Vis Eye Muscle Surg* 7:93, 1992.

106. Amos DM: Pharmacologic management of strabismus. In Bartlett JD and Jaanus SD, editors: *Clinical ocular pharmacology,* ed 2, Boston, 1989, Butterworth-Heinemann.

107. Jacob JL, Beaulieu OC, Brunet E: Progressive-addition lenses in the management of esotropia with a high accommodative/convergence ratio, *Can J Ophthalmol* 15:166, 1980.

108. Smith JB: Progressive-addition lenses in the treatment of accommodative esotropia, *Am J Ophthalmol* 99:56, 1985.

109. Baker JD: Contact lenses in accommodative esotropia, *Am Orthopt J* 35:13, 1987.

110. Calcutt C: Contact lenses in accommodative esotropia therapy, *Br Orthopt J* 46:59, 1989.

111. Rich LS, Glusman M: Tangent streak RGP bifocal contact lenses in the treatment of accommodative esotropia with high AC/A ratio, *CLAO J* 18:56, 1992.

112. Hiatt RL, Ringer C, Cope-Troupe C: Miotics vs glasses in esodeviation, *J Pediatr Ophthalmol Strab* 16:213, 1979.

113. Goldstein JH: The role of miotics in the Rx of strabismus, *Can J Ophthalmol* 2:107, 1967.

114. Wilson ME, Bluestein EC, Parks MM: Binocularity in accommodative esotropia, *J Pediatr Ophthalmol Strab* 30:233, 1993.

115. Dickey CF, Scott WE: The deterioration of accommodative esotropia: frequency, characteristics, and predictive factors, *J Pediatr Ophthalmol Strab* 25:172, 1988.

116. Raab EL: Etiologic factors in accommodative esodeviation, *Trans Am Ophthalmol Soc* 80:657, 1982.

117. Ludwig IH and others: Rate of deterioration in accommodative esotropia correlated to the AC/A relationship, *J Pediatr Ophthalmol Strab* 25:8, 1988.

118. Stewart SA, Scott WE: Prognosis for accommodative esotropia treated with bifocals, *Am Orthopt J* 43:77, 1993.

119. Shippman S, Weseley AC, Cohen KR: Accommodative esotropia in adults, *J Pediatr Ophthalmol Strab* 30:368, 1993.

120. Raab EL, Spierer A: Persisting accommodative esotropia, *Arch Ophthalmol* 104:1777, 1986.

121. Repka MX and others: Changes in the refractive error of 94 spectacle-treated patients with acquired accommodative esotropia, *Binoc Vis Eye Muscle Surg* 4:15, 1989.

122. Swan KC: Accommodative esotropia: long range follow-up, *Ophthalmology* 90:1141, 1983.

123. Taylor RH, Armitage IM, Burke JP: Fully accommodative esotropia in adolescence, *Br Orthopt J* 52:25, 1995.

124. von Nooren GK, Morris J, Edelman P: Efficacy of bifocals in the treatment of accommodative esotropia, *Am J Ophthalmol* 85:830, 1978.

125. Ludwig IH, Parks MM, Getson PR: Long-term results of bifocal therapy for accommodative esotropia, *J Pediatr Ophthalmol Strab* 26:264, 1989.

126. Luttenbacher L, Weaver RG: Esotropia with high AC/A ratio and myopic refractive error, *Am Orthopt J* 44:80, 1994.

127. Jenkins PF: Myopic accommodative esotropia, *Am Orthopt J* 39:79, 1989.

128. Pratt-Johnson JA, Tillson B: Sensory outcome with nonsurgical management of esotropia with convergence excess (a high accommodative-convergence/accommodation ratio), *Can J Ophthalmol* 19:220, 1984.

129. Costenbader FD: Clinical course and management of esotropia. In Allen JH, editor: *Strabismus ophthalmic symposium II,* St Louis, 1958, Mosby.

130. von Noorden GK, Avilla CW: Nonaccommodative convergence excess, *Am J Ophthalmol* 101:70, 1986.

131. Raab EL: The accommodative portion of mixed esotropia, *J Pediatr Ophthalmol Strab* 28(2):73, 1991.

132. Frantz KA and others: Erroneous findings in polarized testing caused by plastic prisms, *J Pediatr Ophthalmol Strab* 27:259, 1990.

133. Bagolini B: Sesorio-motorial anomalies in strabismus (anomalous movements). II, *Doc Ophthalmol* 41:23, 1976.

134. Scheiman M, Ciner E: Surgical success rates in acquired comitant, partially accommodative and nonaccommodative esotropia, *J Am Optom Assoc* 58:556, 1987.

135. Prism Adaptation Study Research Group: Efficacy of prism adaptation in the surgical management of acquired esotropia, *Arch Ophthalmol* 108:1248, 1990.

136. Giangiacomo J: Efficacy of prism adaptation in the management of acquired esotropia, *Arch Ophthalmol* 109:765, 1991 (letter).

137. Delisle P, Strasfeld M, Pelletier D: The prism adaptation test in the preoperative evaluation of esodeviations, *Can J Ophthalmol* 23:208, 1988.

138. Scott WE, Thalacker JA: Preoperative prism adaption in acquired esotropia, *Ophthalmologica* 189:49, 1984.

139. Repka MX, Wentworth D: Prism Adaptation Study Research Group, *J Pediatr Ophthalmol Strab* 28:202, 1991.

140. Apt L, Isenberg S: Eye position of strabismus patients under general anesthesia, *Am J Ophthalmol* 84:574, 1977.

141. DeYoung-Smith M, Baker JD: Esotropia as the presenting sign of brain tumor, *Am Orthopt J* 40:72, 1990.

142. Elsworth RM: The practical management of retinoblastoma, *Trans Am Ophthalmol Soc* 78:462, 1969.

143. Norbis AL, Malbran E: Concomitant esotropia of late onset: pathological report of four cases in siblings, *Br J Ophthalmol* 40:373, 1956.

144. Burian HM: Motility clinic: sudden onset of comitant convergence strabismus, *Am J Ophthalmol* 28:407, 1945.

145. Burian HM, Miller JE: Comitant convergence strabismus with acute onset, *Am J Ophthalmol* 45:55, 1958.

146. Elhatton K, Repka MX: Prism treatment of acute esotropia following interruption of fusion, *Am Orthopt J* 44:76, 1994.

147. Goldstein JH, Wolintz AH, Stein SC: Concomitant strabismus as a sign of intracranial disease, *Ann Ophthalmol* 15:53, 1983.

148. Anderson WD, Lubow M: Astrocytoma of the corpus callosum presenting as acute concomitant esotropia, *Am J Ophthalmol* 69:594, 1970.

149. Goldman HD, Nelson LB: Acute acquired comitant esotropia, *Ann Ophthalmol* 17:777, 1985.

150. Clark AC and others: Acute acquired comitant esotropia, *Br J Ophthalmol* 73:636, 1989.

151. Williams AS, Hoyt CS: Acute comitant esotropia in chiildren with brain tumors, *Arch Ophthalmol* 107:376, 1989.

152. Mickatavage RC: Neuro-ophthalmologic disease presenting as orthoptic problems, *Am Orthopt J* 11:44, 1972.

153. Astle WF, Miller SJ: Acute comitant esotropia: a sign of intracranial disease, *Can J Ophthalmol* 29:151, 1994.

154. Rutstein RP: Acute acquired comitant esotropia simulating late onset accommodative esotropia, *J Am Optom Assoc* 59:446, 1988.

155. Scheiman M, Gallaway M, Ciner E: Divergence insufficiency: characteristics, diagnosis, and treatment, *Am J Optom Physiol Opt* 63:425, 1986.

156. Moore S, Harbison JW, Stockbridge L: Divergence insufficiency, *Am Orthopt J* 21:59, 1971.

157. Barresi BJ, editor: *Ocular assessment: the manual of diagnosis for office practice,* Boston, 1984, Butterworth-Heinemann.

158. Prangen AH, Koch FL: Divergence insufficiency: a clinical study, *Am J Ophthalmol* 21:510, 1938.

159. Jampolsky A: Ocular divergence mechanism, *Trans Am Ophthalmol Soc* 68:730, 1979.

160. Bedrossian EH: Bilateral sixth nerve paresis simulating divergence paralysis, *Am J Ophthalmol* 45:417, 1958.

161. Kirkham TH, Bird AC, Sanders MD: Divergence paralysis with raised intracranial pressure: an electro-oculographic study, *Br J Ophthalmol* 56:776, 1972.

162. Curran RE: True and simulated divergence paresis as a precursor of benign sixth nerve palsy, *Binoc Vis Eye Muscle Surg* 4:125, 1989.

163. Kushner BJ: Functional amblyopia associated with organic ocular disease, *Am J Ophthalmol* 91:39, 1981.

164. Kushner BJ: Functional amblyopia associated with abnormalities of the optic nerve, *Arch Ophthalmol* 102:683, 1984.

165. Kutluk S, Avilla CW, von Noorden GK: The prevalence of dissociated vertical deviation in patients with sensory heterotropia, *Am J Ophthalmol* 119:744, 1995.

166. Beller R and others: Good visual function after neonatal surgery for congenital monocular cataracts, *Am J Ophthalmol* 91:559, 1981.

167. Robb RM, Mayer DL, Moore BD: Results of early treatment of unilateral congenital cataracts, *J Pediatr Ophthalmol Strab* 24:178, 1987.

168. Fitton MH, Jampolsky A: A case report of spontaneous consecutive esotropia, *Am Orthopt J* 14:144, 1964.

169. Raab EL: Consecutive accommodative esotropia, *J Pediatr Ophthalmol Strab* 22:58, 1985.

170. Pratt-Johnson JA, Barlow JM, Tillson G: Early surgery in intermittent exotropia, *Am J Ophthalmol* 84:689, 1977.

171. Edelman PM and others: Consecutive esodeviation...then what? *Am Orthopt J* 38:111, 1988.

172. Swan K: The blindspot syndrome, *Arch Ophthalmol* 40:371, 1948.

173. Helveston EM, von Noorden GK: Microtropia: a newly defined entity, *Arch Ophthalmol* 78:272, 1968.

174. Lang J: Management of microtropia, *Br J Ophthalmol* 58:281, 1974.

175. Palimeris G and others: Some clinical aspects of microtropia, *Ann Ophthalmol* 7:1343, 1975.

176. Hahn E, Cadera W, Orton RB: Factors associated binocular single vision in microtropia/monofixation syndrome, *Can J Ophthalmol* 26:12, 1991.

177. Clarke WN, Noel LP: Amblyopia and the monofixation syndrome, *Can J Ophthalmol* 14:239, 1979.

178. Rutstein RP, Eskridge JB: Stereopsis in small-angle strabismus, *Am J Optom Physiol Opt* 61:491, 1984.

179. Clark WN, Noel LP: Stereoacuity in the monofixation syndrome, *J Pediatr Ophthalmol Strab* 27:161, 1990.

180. Jampolsky A: Retinal correspondence in patients with small-degree strabismus, *Arch Ophthalmol* 45:18, 1951.

181. Parks MM: The monofixation syndrome, *Trans Am Ophthalmol Soc* 67:609, 1969.

182. Arthur BW, Smith JT, Scott WE: Long-term stability of alignment in the monofixation syndrome, *J Pediatr Ophthalmol Strab* 26:224, 1989.

183. Wick B: Visual therapy for small-angle esotropia, *Am J Optom Physiol Opt* 51:490, 1974.

184. Deleted in galleys.

185. Rutstein RP, Levi DM: The blindspot syndrome, *J Am Optom Assoc* 50:1387, 1979.

186. Olivier P, von Noorden GK: The blindspot syndrome: does it exist? *J Pediatr Ophthalmol Strab* 18:20, 1981.

187. Riordan-Eva P and others: Cyclic strabismus without binocular function, *J Pediatr Ophthalmol Strab* 30:106, 1993.

188. Costenbader FD, Mousel DK: Cyclic esotropia, *Arch Ophthalmol* 71:88, 1964.

189. Clarke WN, Scott WE: Cyclic third nerve palsy, *J Pediatr Ophthalmol Strab* 12:94, 1975.

190. Troost BT and others: Acquired cyclic esotropia in an adult, *Am J Ophthalmol* 91:8, 1981.

191. Helveston EM: Cyclic strabismus, *Am Orthopt J* 23:48, 1973.

192. Muchnick RS, Sanfilippo S, Dunlap EA: Cyclic esotropia developing after strabismus surgery, *Arch Ophthalmol* 94:459, 1976.

193. Pillai P, Dhand UK: Cyclic esotropia with central nervous system diseases: report of two cases, *J Pediatr Ophthalmol Strab* 24:237 1987.

194. Metz HS, Bigelow C: Changes in the cycle of circadian strabismus, *Am J Ophthalmol* 120:124, 1995.

Exotropia exists when the visual axes cross beyond the point of fixation, resulting in an outward, or divergent, misalignment of the eyes. There is temporal displacement of the object of regard on the retina of the deviating eye. Unlike exophoria, exotropia is a manifest deviation that is not controlled by fusional convergence. If fusional convergence amplitudes are only occasionally inadequate, an intermittent exotropia occurs. Here, the exodeviation vacillates between a heterophoria and a heterotropia. The majority of exotropias are intermittent.

PREVALENCE

Exotropia occurs less frequently than esotropia. Occurrence in children is approximately one case of exotropia for every three to five cases of esotropia, whereas in adults, occurrence is one case of exotropia for every two cases of esotropia.[1,2] Exotropia occurs more frequently in females than males.[3] Approximately two thirds of patients with exotropia are females.[4] The reason for this is unknown. Exotropia also supposedly occurs more frequently in Asians and blacks than in Caucasians.[5]

 CLINICAL PEARL
Exotropia occurs less frequently than esotropia.

The prevalence of exotropia varies in different parts of the world. It is more common in regions that are closer to the equator, such as the Middle East, the Orient, and Africa, and less common in countries farther from the equator.[5] Whereas 54% of all individuals with strabismus in Japan and 76% in Nepal are exotropic, only 30% of those with strabismus in the United States and 10% in Germany are exotropic.[5]

Intensity of sunlight probably has some effect on exotropia. A common observation is that closure of one eye and light sensitivity occurs in bright sunlight.[6,7] Exotropia has also been reported to be more frequent in societies and cultures that are less involved in prolonged near work.[5]

AGE OF ONSET

The onset of exotropia has traditionally been reported as being later than esotropia, which begins at age 7 or 8.[1] However, the age of onset for most exodeviations is considerably earlier. Clinically significant exotropia can be seen in infancy. In one series of 412 patients, for example, exotropia was present at birth in (43%) 204 cases, appeared in 16 cases (3%) at 6 months of age and in 72 cases (15%) between 6 and 12 months of age.[8] In only 24 cases (5%), did the exotropia develop after age 5. In two other studies, 9% and 14% of the exotropias began after age 5.[9,10] Thus between 35% and 70% of all exotropias begin within the first 2 years of life, with a mean age of onset of 18 to 36 months. Some exotropias beginning later probably start as exophoria. The deterioration from exophoria to exotropia in older patients may be related to the decrease in tonic convergence, the gradual lessening of accommodation, and the increased divergence of the orbits with age.

When considering the age of onset of exotropia in the young child, it is important to remember that transient exotropia is common during the first few months of life. An exotropia may exist sometime during a motility examination in as many as 66% of all neurologically normal newborns.[11-13] The exotropia is seen

TABLE 9-1   COMPARISON OF THE FEATURES OF EXOTROPIA AND ESOTROPIA

	Exotropia	Esotropia
Age of onset	First years of life	First years of life
Prevalence	Less common	More common
Constancy/intermittency	Most are intermittent	Most are constant
Amblyopia	Rare	Frequent
Refractive error	Unusually noncausative. Similar to nonstrabismic population	Frequently causative totally or partly; skewed toward hyperopia
Magnitude	On the average, larger; rarely microtropia	On the average, smaller; frequently microtropia
Vertical component	16% - 52%	As many as 50%
Prognosis for normal binocular vision	Good in most cases	Poor in many cases that are nonaccommodative
Systemic disease	Rare	More common
Sexual bias	More in females	None
Consecutive strabismus	Frequent; either spontaneous or iatrogenic	Rare; always iatrogenic

in fewer cases as examinations are done on older infants at monthly intervals. This pattern of development makes it difficult to make a firm diagnosis of exotropia in the infant. Most transient exotropias disappear by 6 months of age.

 CLINICAL PEARL

> When considering the age of onset of exotropia in the young child, it is important to remember that transient exotropia is common during the first few months of life.

Unlike esotropia, the parental report of exotropia is usually accurate and we rarely find pseudoexotropia. However, it is difficult for parents to describe the deviation. They state that their child "does not look at me" or the eyes "don't look right." At other times, parents have said that they have seen their child's eyes turn inward. After careful questioning, it becomes clear that they are actually describing the recovery movement from the exotropia to the straight position in cases of intermittent exotropia, thus the turning inward.

GENERAL CLINICAL FEATURES

Despite the differences that exist clinically among the various types of exotropias, certain clinical features differing from esotropia should come to mind when examining a patient with exotropia (Table 9-1).

INTERMITTENCY

As many as 85% of all exotropias are intermittent.[14] The power of convergence, being much greater than that of divergence, counteracts the tendency toward divergence for a period and explains the intermittence. To determine how a patient copes with an exodeviation, repeated examinations at different

times of the day are generally required. A patient may exhibit an exophoria early in the morning and an intermittent exotropia later in the day. With exotropia the percentage of time the eyes are exotropic should be determined. This is frequently more important than the size of the deviation. An intermittent exotropia of 30 PD that is manifest only 5% of the time may be less clinically significant than an intermittent exotropia of 20 PD that is manifest 80% of the time.

With many patients the pattern of the exodeviation over time can be characterized by a steady progression of increasing periods of strabismus. For an adult with alternating exotropia, the deviation may appear to be constant, but often a scrupulously well-conducted examination reveals normal binocular vision potential and fleeting control. To elicit the binocularity, appropriate diagnostic means must be employed. The fusion ability in exotropia can best be demonstrated when measuring stereopsis, as shown in Case 1.

CASE 1

A 33-year-old man presented with a history of childhood-onset exotropia that had never been treated (Fig. 9-1). He had been told by other clinicians that he had no ability to use both eyes together, and any treatment would be for cosmesis and not function.

Our examination indicated visual acuity of 20/20 for each eye with a slight myopic correction. Cover test showed a 50-PD constant alternating exotropia at distance and near. Versions revealed bilateral inferior oblique overactions resulting in a V pattern.

With both Worth four dot and Bagolini striated lens tests, alternating suppression was present. Examination with the synoptophore showed suppression and anomalous correspondence. It was about to be concluded that there was no binocular vision ability. However, with the Randot stereotest, the patient's eyes suddenly became aligned and he had 25 seconds of arc.

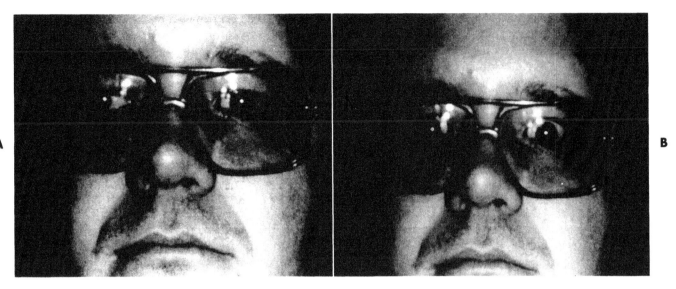

FIG. 9-1 Patient with an apparently constant exotropia (Case 1). **A,** Large-angle exotropia. **B,** Fusion.

Comment

Patients with large exotropias sometimes pull straight and have perfect fusion during stereotesting. For the remainder of the examination, as with everyday seeing conditions, they have a "constant" exotropia, suppression, and no fusion. It is difficult to hold together dissimilar images either in a synoptophore or in a stereoscope, and most patients with exotropia suppress alternately. When evaluating a patient with a long-standing and apparently constant exotropia, stereopsis testing is essential. This was apparent with this patient, who despite having a large deviation, showed bifoveal fusion potential with stereoscopic targets and not by any other method.

AMBLYOPIA

Functional amblyopia rarely accompanies exotropia and, when present, generally does not pose a very difficult problem. Of the 15% of patients who are exotropic and are constant, 6% fixate unilaterally and 9% have alternating fixation patterns, supposedly with normal vision in each eye.[14,15] Deep amblyopia with eccentric fixation is rare and is restricted to constant and unilateral deviations beginning in very early childhood. Some of these cases are likely consecutive exotropia. Amblyopia can develop when clinically significant anisometropia coexists with intermittent exotropia. Organic causes should be considered with amblyopia in exotropia without either anisometropia or history of esotropia.

REFRACTIVE ERROR

The refractive error generally plays a relatively unimportant etiologic role with exotropia. Although earlier investigators reported that myopia was a major factor, its role is much less prominent than that of hyperopia with esotropia.[16-20] The distribution of refractive errors in exotropia resembles that in the nonstrabismic population.[17] Most patients have a refractive error nearer emmetropia or slightly on the myopic side, with or without moderate astigmatism. Low-to-moderate amounts of hyperopia are likely not as common, at least with intermittent exotropia, because they are usually accompanied by accommodation to provide a clear image. This would involve accommodative convergence with elimination or reduction of the deviation. We occasionally see patients in whom correction of the refractive error, particularly in cases of anisomyopia and/or anisoastigmatism, either reduces or eliminates the exotropia entirely.

VERTICAL DEVIATIONS AND INCOMITANCY

Vertical deviations are present in 16% to 52% of patients with exotropia.[21-24] The vertical deviation may be more frequent in distance testing than near testing, particularly in intermittent exotropia. Overaction of the inferior oblique muscles may occur by age 5 in nearly one third of the patients with intermittent exotropia.[23] Overaction of the superior oblique muscles occurs in large-angle sensory exotropia with uncommon frequency. Because of the overacting oblique muscles, the angle of exotropia changes in upward and downward gazes, resulting in **A** and **V** patterns.[24] Other vertical deviations can be the result of dissociated vertical deviation or palsy of a cyclovertical muscle. Dissociated vertical deviations are unlikely with intermittent exotropia with good sensory fusion. In some cases there may be no definable cause for the vertical deviation. Many of these are very small comitant hyperdeviations. In these cases the vertical deviation can usually be ignored, because it typically disappears after treatment of the exotropia.

The prevalence of lateral gaze incomitance in exotropia has been estimated to be as high as 24%.[22,25] These patients demonstrate a smaller exodeviation when the alternate cover test with prisms is performed in lateral gaze to either side, in spite of having full ocular motility. Lateral gaze incomitance is clinically significant when the exotropia measures at least 20% less to each side than it does in the primary position. Supposedly, patients with lateral incomitance have a greater risk of being overcorrected if treated surgically.[25-27] Lateral gaze incomitance may be more a result of measurement artifacts induced by improperly positioned prisms than mechanical and innervational factors.[28] It may also be a measure of the patient's convergence response to the unnatural exercise of fixation in extremes of lateral gaze maintained during prism and cover testing.

SYSTEMIC AND NEUROLOGIC DISEASE

Exotropia associated with systemic or neurologic abnormalities is rare.[29,30] Exotropia presenting in the context of general or pediatric practice probably represents, for the most part, benign comitant strabismus. The birth and general medical histories of children with exotropia are usually unremarkable, with no overrepresentation of prematurity with intraventricular hemorrhage, birth trauma, or chromosomal disorder. Of the exodeviations, infantile or congenital exotropia is more likely to be associated with neurologic defects and craniofacial anomalies.[31-33] With the exception of acquired oculomotor nerve paresis, acute-onset exotropia, unlike acute-onset esotropia, is not a well-defined clinical entity. The acquisition of an incomitant exotropia at any age usually represents a manifestation of an underlying systemic or neurologic disease.[34]

ETIOLOGY

The cause of exotropia in many cases is speculative. Genetic factors do not seem to be important. The percentage of family-related exotropia may be higher, because many intermittent exotropic cases go unreported because of the infrequency of the strabismic phase. Sensory, motor, anatomic, and innervational factors may contribute to the development of an exotropia. Sensory causes, such as marked decrease in monocular visual acuity or change in the visual field, may induce an exotropia over time. Motor causes include adduction deficits, muscular restriction, paresis of an eye muscle, convergence or accommodation dysfunction, and conjugate gaze weakness.

Whether exotropias are caused mostly by an abnormal position of rest as a result of anatomic factors within the orbit or mostly by innervational abnormalities has been the subject of discussion. The fact that exotropia is common in patients with craniofacial dysostosis, such as Apert's and Crouzon's syndromes, in which shallow and laterally directed orbits are prominent clinical features and the interpupillary distance is very large, gives credence to anatomic factors.[32,35] A high incidence of exotropia secondary to abnormal orbital anatomy, connective tissue laxity, and looser tendinous attachments has also been reported in Marfan syndrome.[36]

In the vast majority of cases, however, anatomic factors contribute minimally, and the underlying pathophysiology is presumed to be innervational. Innervational factors include an imbalance between tonic divergence and tonic convergence, with exotropia resulting from either excessive tonic divergence or too little convergence innervation. Electromyographic studies have indicated that divergence is an active physiologic process and not merely a result of passive inhibition of convergence.[37] When exotropia begins to manifest, the lateral rectus muscle of the deviating eye begins to fire. The lateral rectus continues to fire while the eye is divergent, having its maximum potential during divergence.[38] Active divergence is also supported by the fact that the angle of deviation is outside the fusional divergence range.[39]

Exotropia can result from a combination of anatomic and innervational factors, as indicated by the following case.

CASE 2

A 20-year-old man sustained trauma to his left eye and subsequently developed a dense unilateral cataract. An examination 4 years earlier had shown orthophoria, 20/20 vision in each eye, and 40 seconds of arc of stereopsis. The cataract reduced the vision to 20/200. An exotropia gradually developed in the cataractous eye, and the size of the deviation increased from 15 PD to 40 PD over a period of 2 years. Limited adduction of the left eye, likely caused by contracture of the lateral rectus and shortening of the temporal conjunctiva and Tenon's capsule, was eventually detected with the forced duction test.

Comment

For this patient the cataract resulted in loss of binocular vision. Tonic divergence prevailed over tonic convergence, which led to exotropia. The increase in the angle of exotropia over time was caused by the anatomic changes in the extraocular muscles and surrounding tissues.

CLASSIFICATION

The classification of exotropia is not as complex as that of esotropia. Exotropias are classified according to whether they are constant or intermittent. The intermittent exotropias are further classified according to differences between the size of the deviation at distance and the size of the deviation at near fixation.

The types of exotropia encountered are shown in Box 9-1.

Mechanically restrictive and paretic exodeviations, such as those caused by oculomotor nerve paresis and isolated medial rectus paresis, ocular myasthenia, thyroid myopathy, trauma, and Duane's syndrome type II are discussed in Chapter 10.

Intermittent exotropia can deteriorate and become constant exotropia, but this appears to be the exception, occurring in just 4% of the cases.[40] Exotropia that is neither infantile, secondary, nor associated with paresis or mechanical restriction of an extraocular muscle in an otherwise healthy patient should be considered intermittent until proven otherwise.

 CLINICAL PEARL

> Exotropia that is neither infantile, secondary, nor associated with paresis or mechanical restriction of an extraocular muscle in an otherwise healthy patient should be considered intermittent until proven otherwise.

INFANTILE EXOTROPIA

The development of a constant exotropia in an otherwise normal full-term infant without craniofacial or neurologic defects is extremely rare, occurring in only 1 per 30,000 patients.[41-46] Infantile, or congenital, exotropia is an idiopathic large-angle deviation that occurs within the first year of life. Clinical data from retrospective reviews suggest that infantile exotropia is mostly a sporadic disorder.[41-43] In rare cases the findings of infantile exotropia in members of an extended family suggest the pattern of inheritance as being either autosomal dominant transmission or a multiple factor mode of inheritance.[44]

Except for the direction of the deviation, patients with infantile exotropia have findings similar to those with infantile esotropia.[45-49] Infantile exotropia develops during the first year of life, more precisely during the first 6 months. It involves a constant, large-angle deviation, represents a barrier to the development of normal single binocular vision, and can also present with neurologic and other ocular abnormalities. Unlike infantile esotropia, latent or other forms of nystagmus are uncommon.

 CLINICAL PEARL

> Patients with infantile exotropia have findings similar to those with infantile esotropia.

Infantile exotropia must be differentiated from the transient exotropias seen during the first months of life.[11-13] It must also be differentiated from the exotropias in infancy caused by poor vision related to diseases such as retinal detachment, vitreous/retinal hemorrhage, and congenital cataract and the exotropia associated with craniofacial anomalies.

Conditions Associated with Infantile Exotropia
Constant Angle of Exotropia
A constant angle of exotropia ranging from 30 to 80 PD can be associated with infantile exotropia. The average size is 50 PD at distance and near. The magnitude may increase over time.[42,44]

Infrequency of amblyopia
Amblyopia is not likely in the presence of alternating fixation, which exists for many of these patients. Our impression is that less than 5% of patients with infantile exotropia have significant amblyopia. Amblyopia was present in only 1 of 34 cases reported in the literature, and this was likely iatrogenically induced.[42-46] That patient was found to have a 75- to 80-PD constant exotropia at 2½ months of age and subsequently underwent extraocular muscle surgery.[45] The patient was orthophoric until age 2½ years and then developed consecutive esotropia with amblyopia.

Ocular Motility Disorders
Unlike infantile esotropia, in which limited abduction as a result of cross-fixation may occur, patients with infantile exotropia may show limited adduction. Because of the large-angle exotropia, individuals with infantile exotropia may use their abducting eye to fixate and not adduct either eye. When viewing to the right, limited adduction in the left eye may occur, and, when viewing to the left, limited adduction in the right eye may occur. Momentarily occluding the opposite eye or using the doll's-head maneuver (the oculocephalic reflex) improves adduction. In adult patients with untreated infantile exotropia the motility deficiency can be the result of structural changes secondary

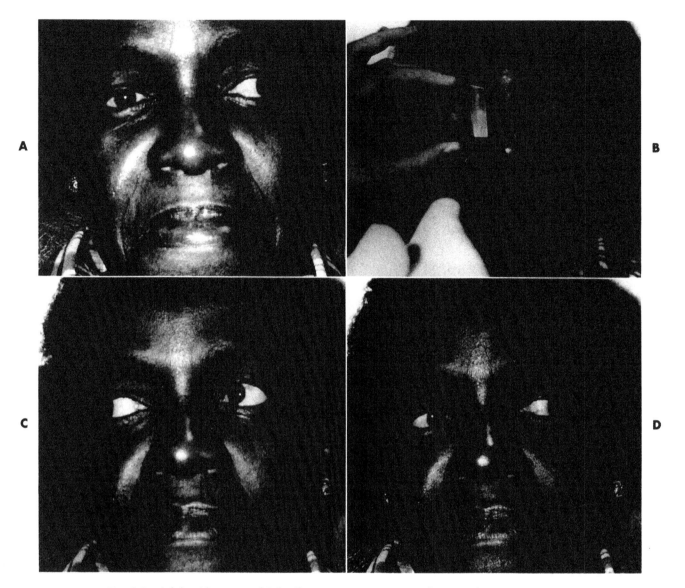

FIG. 9-2   Adult with untreated infantile exotropia. **A,** Constant large-angle exotropia is present (patient can alternately fixate and has 20/30 in each eye). **B,** Measurement of deviation with Krimsky test. **C,** Versions show limited adduction in left and **(D)** right eye.

to long-standing strabismus (Fig. 9-2). Forced duction tests reveal restriction of passive adduction, a finding that must be interpreted as either evidence for contracture or tightening of the lateral rectus muscle and/or the temporal conjunctiva and Tenon's capsule.

Oblique muscle disorders and dissociated vertical deviations occur frequently with infantile exotropia. In one series, 9 of 10 patients had or eventually developed a dissociated vertical deviation.[41] The presence of dissociated vertical deviation confirms the early onset of the deviation. The high prevalence of inferior and/or superior oblique overactions requires checking for A and V patterns. Large-angle infantile exotropia can be associated with an X pattern as a result of all four oblique

muscles overacting. In these cases the exotropia is larger in up and down gaze than is found in primary gaze.

Refractive Errors That Are Not Causative

In one study involving 13 patients, all cycloplegic refractions were within 3.50 D of emmetropia, with astigmatism not exceeding 2 D.[42] Significant myopia was not detected for any patient. In another study on 6 patients, all refractive errors were hyperopic and considered normal for age (maximum 2.50 D and no anisometropia exceeding 1 D).[45] Prescribing the glasses did not alter the size of the exotropia for any of these patients.

Limited Potential for Normal Binocular Vision

The prognosis for obtaining normal single binocular vision after treatment is poor. To our knowledge, the best that has been achieved is peripheral fusion, as measured for example with the near Worth four dot test, with rarely any stereopsis.[46] This contrasts with infantile esotropia, in which fusion and some stereopsis is frequently achieved if the residual angle of deviation after treatment is 10 PD or smaller.[47-49] The fact that treatment for infantile exotropia relative to infantile esotropia is usually later may account for the poorer fusion. On the other hand, lack of better fusion may be a part of the infantile exotropia syndrome, that is, the cause of infantile exotropia may be more extensive or serious in nature.

Treatment

Treatment for infantile exotropia is primarily surgical. Prisms are usually not helpful because of the large angle of constant exotropia and the poor fusion. As with other types of strabismus, surgery should only come after (1) the refractive error and fundus have been assessed, (2) amblyopia has been shown not to exist, and (3) the angle of exotropia is relatively stable on repeated examinations.

Careful follow-up is necessary, as indicated by the following case.

CASE 3

A 9-month-old boy was examined in March, 1991. The child was full-term and developing normally. The mother reported that his eyes began turning out 5 months earlier. There was no history of illness or trauma nor of closing of one eye by the child.

Our examination revealed a constant 50-PD right exotropia at distance and near. The child would occasionally fixate with the right eye. Versions were unrestricted, and there were no oblique muscle disorders. Visual acuity as determined with the Teller acuity cards was 20/100 for each eye. Cycloplegic refraction was emmetropia. Dilated ophthalmoscopy revealed normal findings. The diagnosis was infantile exotropia. The mother was instructed to alternately patch the child's eyes 4 to 5 hours each day to maintain equal visual acuity.

The patient returned 2 months later. The mother reported good compliance with the occlusion. Our findings showed a 50-PD constant alternating exotropia. Visual acuity for each eye remained similar. Occlusion therapy was terminated.

In January, 1992 the alternating exotropia measured 60 PD at distance and near, and a dissociated vertical deviation was noted. Visual acuities with the Teller acuity cards were 20/40 for each eye. Cycloplegic refraction was +0.50 D OU. At this time, surgical referral was made. The patient underwent a 9-mm recession of the lateral rectus combined with a 6-mm resection of the medial rectus of the left eye.

Two months following surgery, the patient manifested a 10-PD constant left exotropia at distance and near. A disso-

ciated vertical deviation, more for the right eye, was present. Visual acuities with the Broken Wheel test were 20/25 in the right eye and 20/40 in the left eye. Sensory testing with the Worth four dot test showed suppression of the left eye at distance and near. Cycloplegic refraction was OD +1.00 −1.00 × 180 and OS +1.00 −1.50 × 180. The parent was instructed to patch the child's right eye for 4 hours per day. Active therapy included accommodation, fixation, and eye-hand coordination exercises performed in conjunction with occlusion.

Two months later, visual acuity was 20/20 for each eye. A 10-PD constant alternating exotropia with a dissociated vertical deviation was measured at distance and near for the now 3-year-old child. The patient fused the Worth four dot test at near and showed suppression at distance. With the Randot stereotest no stereopsis was present. Base-in prisms equal to the angle of deviation did not improve fusion.

The patient did not return until 1½ years later. Visual acuity was now 20/20 for the right eye and 20/80 for the left eye. Cover testing showed a constant left exotropia of 12 PD, with a dissociated vertical deviation at distance and near. The patient suppressed the Worth four dot test at distance and near. Normal correspondence without second-degree sensory and motor fusion was found with the synoptophore. Amblyopia treatment was undertaken once again.

Comment

Surgery converted a large-angle alternating strabismus without amblyopia into a small-angle unilateral strabismus with amblyopia. Orthoptics/vision therapy may be attempted later. Achieving normal single binocular vision with high-grade stereopsis is probably not a realistic goal for this patient.

Compared with patients with esotropia, patients with large-angle exotropia are usually more willing to endure the strabismus and not seek treatment or seek it later. Adults with untreated infantile exotropia who alternately fixate and retain equal vision in each eye (see Fig. 9-2) have an enlarged field of peripheral binocular vision or panoramic vision. These patients should be warned that they will have a subjective loss in their binocular field of vision after their eyes are straightened.[50] This can be disturbing to patients, who may describe the sensation of "tunnel vision."

SECONDARY EXOTROPIA

An exotropia that results from a primary sensory deficit in a formerly nonstrabismic patient or from surgical or other intervention in a formerly esotropic patient is referred to as a *secondary exotropia*. Secondary exotropia can be sensory or consecutive.

SENSORY EXOTROPIA

Sensory exotropia is a constant unilateral exotropia following loss or severe reduction of vision in one eye. The loss of vision leads to disruption of fusion. Visually depriving factors causing sensory exotropia include uncorrected anisometropia, amblyopia, congenital cataracts, acquired cataracts, uncorrected aphakia, corneal opacities, optic nerve lesions, and retinal lesions. Sensory exotropia occurs in both adults and children, occurring in almost equal frequency with sensory esotropia when the onset of visual impairment occurs at birth or between birth and age 5.[51] It predominates over sensory esotropia in older children and adults because of the relative decrease in tonic convergence with age.

 CLINICAL PEARL

> Sensory exotropia is a constant unilateral exotropia following loss or severe reduction of vision in one eye.

Except for the direction of the deviation, the clinical features for sensory exotropia are similar to those for sensory esotropia. The deviation is often large, generally in the range of 30 to 60 PD at distance and near. Because of the poor vision in one eye, the Krimsky test rather than the alternating cover test with prisms is preferred to measure the deviation. The exotropia is frequently accompanied by overacting inferior and/or superior oblique muscles, which causes vertical deviations and A or V patterns. The overacting muscle is more likely in the poorer-seeing eye but can also be bilateral and also affect only the better-seeing eye.[51] Dissociated vertical deviations occur less frequently than with sensory esotropia.[52]

Reduced potential for normal binocular vision usually exists for cases with early childhood onset. Reestablishment of normal single binocular vision may not be possible, even when the sensory exotropia begins in adulthood. Fusion may be lost as a result of prolonged sensory deprivation. This is particularly true with patients who have unilateral acquired cataracts that remain in situ for many years.[53-55] Pratt-Johnson and Tillson[53] describe 24 patients who sustained traumatic unilateral cataract at an average age of 18. All patients become exotropic, hypotropic, and excyclotropic approximately 1 year or longer after the injury. The interval of time between the development of the cataract and the restoration of best possible visual acuity averaged 14 years. Although cataract surgery provided good visual acuity, all patients developed diplopia that could not be eliminated with either prisms or surgery. Sensory testing revealed that all patients had central fusion disruption (see Chapter 5) and were unable to superimpose any type of target on the synoptophore or with prisms, except momentarily. The prolonged monocular sensory deprivation caused by the cataracts apparently resulted in disruption of fusion and intractable diplopia for these patients. Regaining fusion with adult-onset sensory exotropia is more likely when the time interval between the onset

of the sensory deprivation and the restoration of visual acuity is less than 2 years.[53]

Intractable diplopia has also been reported in adults with childhood-onset strabismus who later developed unilateral cataracts and sensory exotropia and underwent cataract surgery.[54,55] The occlusion caused by the long-standing cataracts supposedly eliminated the suppression mechanism that developed in childhood for these patients.

CONSECUTIVE EXOTROPIA

Consecutive exotropia is usually a constant exotropia that has been preceded by an esotropia. It may occur spontaneously over time or more commonly can result following surgical correction of an esotropia. Consecutive exotropia is the most frequent type of constant exotropia seen in our clinic.

The following are predisposing factors that have been reported in spontaneous consecutive exotropia:

- Refractive error[56-59]
- Amblyopia[57,59-61]
- Reduced near point of convergence[59]
- Superficial anomalous correspondence[56]
- Low AC/A ratio[58]
- Reduced accommodative function[62]

Of these factors, high refractive error appears to be the most common. The prevalence of consecutive exotropia has been reported to occur in as many as 10% to 20% of esotropic patients treated with hyperopic glasses.[56] The exotropia can develop during childhood, within 1 year after the first pair of glasses, or later in adult life, as the patient's amplitude of accommodation decreases. It is sometimes precipitated by late correction of hyperopia.

Groves[57] first reported the relationship between hyperopia and consecutive exotropia. The patients with esotropia and wearing hyperopic glasses greater than 7 D eventually developed exotropia. Aichmar[63] followed 61 patients with esotropia, ages 4 to 11 years. Nine of the patients (14.7%) became exotropic after wearing hyperopic glasses. Of the nine, three had hyperopia ranging from 6 to 9 D, four had hyperopia ranging from 3 to 5 D, and two had smaller amounts of hyperopia. Moore[64] reviewed the records of 125 children with esotropia who wore hyperopic glasses. Of the group, 14 (11%) became exotropic by age 9. Nine had hyperopia greater than 4.50 D. Beneish and associates[59] report on 22 patients with esotropia, in whom exotropia developed after correction of hyperopia. The mean hyperopia was 5.50 D. The mean time interval between giving the hyperopic glasses and the appearance of the exotropia was 20½ months. The exotropia first become manifest at distance in most patients, with the average size being 10.8 PD at distance and 8.3 PD at near. Swan[60] reported six of 39 (15.3%) patients with esotropia who wore hyperopic glasses who became exotropic. Their median hyperopic refractive error was over 6 D, and all had amblyopia in one eye. Parker,[65] however, followed 23 patients with esotropia over the years and reported none developing consecutive exotropia. Parker's patients presumably had high AC/A ratios and none had high hyperopia.

Based on these studies and our clinical experience, moderately sized esotropia with 4.50 D or more hyperopia presents a risk factor for the development of consecutive exotropia. It is probably more likely with amblyopia, but this appears not to be essential.

❊ CLINICAL PEARL

Moderately sized esotropia with 4.50 D or more hyperopia presents a risk factor for the development of consecutive exotropia.

We do not see consecutive exotropia developing in individuals with totally accommodative esotropia with normal binocular vision potential. The high-grade stereopsis these patients achieve with glasses likely prevents the eyes from diverging over the years. The exception is the older patient with a history of refractive accommodative esotropia, who, for some unexplainable reason, was treated in childhood with surgery rather than hyperopic glasses. Substituting surgery for glasses in refractive accommodative esotropia goes against the pathophysiology of the condition. Many of these patients develop asthenopic symptoms in their mid-to-late teenage years because of the uncorrected hyperopia. Correction of the hyperopic refractive error relieves the accommodative strain, but exotropia and diplopia frequently occur.

Whether other factors, such as anomalous correspondence, the AC/A ratio, and poor accommodation, play a significant role in spontaneous consecutive exotropia is unclear. With the development of consecutive exotropia, the status of retinal correspondence may change from anomalous to normal for some patients.[66]

We treat consecutive exotropia that is optically induced by reducing the power of the hyperopic glasses, in some cases by as much as 50%. This is more appropriate in young children and when the deviation exceeds 20 PD. In the short term these patients tend to do well but must be followed for a long time before the clinician can be certain that their deviation is controlled. With older patients, reduction in the hyperopic correction usually results in accommodative asthenopia, and alternative treatment may be needed. Prisms are rarely helpful, because fusion ability is generally not present. When treating children with esotropia, high hyperopia, and poor potential for normal binocular vision, the possibility of consecutive exotropia should be considered, as indicated by the following case.

CASE 4

In April, 1983 a 3-year-old girl was examined. The parents had noticed the left eye turning in for about 3 months. The child was in good health and there had been no trauma.

Our examination showed visual acuities of 20/80 for each eye with the Broken Wheel test. The child manifested a constant alternating esotropia of 20 PD at distance and near. Versions were normal. Stereopsis with the Random-dot E stereotest was not present. Cycloplegic refraction was 6 D hyperopia OU. Biomicroscopy revealed diffuse, deep, bilateral corneal opacities consistent with posterior polymorphous dystrophy. Intraocular pressures were 12 mm in each eye. Ophthalmoscopic findings were normal.

It was presumed that the child had refractive accommodative esotropia, and glasses were prescribed.

Progress evaluation indicated visual acuity of 20/60 for each eye and a 7-PD residual esotropia at distance and near. Stereopsis testing with the Titmus test showed 200 seconds of arc. The child was monitored every 3 months.

In August, 1985, visual acuity was 20/40 in each eye. The patient was orthophoric at distance and 20-PD esotropic at near. Cycloplegic refraction was OD +7.00 D and OS +8.50 D. Treatment consisted of the refractive findings and a +2.00 D bifocal.

Three months later, visual acuity was 20/25 for each eye. However, with the glasses the child now manifested a 25-PD constant, alternating exotropia at distance and a 20-PD constant exotropia at near (Fig. 9-3, *A*). She denied any diplopia. When the glasses were removed, a 5-PD constant esotropia was present (Fig. 9-3, *B*). The hyperopic correction was reduced by 2 D, and the bifocal was eliminated. Subsequent evaluations revealed 15-PD exotropia at distance and 6-PD exotropia at near. There was no evidence of fusion with the Worth four dot test, the synoptophore, or stereopsis testing. The magnitude of the exotropia and the visual acuity have remained stable over the years.

Consecutive exotropia also occurs in 4% to 20% of all cases of esotropia treated surgically.[67-71] Immediate consecutive exotropia may occasionally be planned as a deliberate surgical overcorrection of esotropia, with good prognosis for a functional result. A surgically-induced exotropia supposedly causes a convergence impulse to regain fusion and avoid diplopia, provided the patient has the ability to fuse. It may also follow overliberal surgery (excessive weakening of the medial rectus muscles), especially when restriction of ocular motility is present.

Consecutive exotropia can occur a considerable time after surgery, many years in some instances. As mentioned in Chapter 8, as many as 25% of individuals with infantile esotropia may develop consecutive exotropia 5 or more years following surgery.[72] The mechanism of surgically-induced consecutive exotropia may be similar to that of the spontaneous type, and it may be difficult to say after surgery whether surgery was a predisposing factor or whether a spontaneous exotropia occurred independently of the surgery.

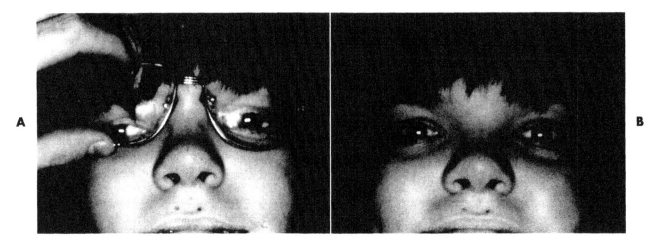

FIG. 9-3 Consecutive exotropia that is optically induced (Case 4). **A,** Exotropia exists with hyperopic glasses. **B,** Small-angle esotropia exists without glasses.

Folk, Miller, and Chapman[69] report on 250 patients with surgically-treated esotropia who subsequently developed exotropia. Sixty percent had an onset of esotropia at 1 year of age or younger. The majority of patients developed a consecutive exotropia after a single surgical procedure. Only 28 patients (11%) showed hyperopia in excess of 2.5 D. Sixteen percent had consecutive exotropia at the first postoperative visit, 44% within 4 years of the surgery, and 15% as long as 8 years following surgery. The presence of amblyopia and medial rectus restriction were the most common features associated with the development of surgically-induced consecutive exotropia. Bradbury and Doran[73] report consecutive exotropia occurring for patients with surgically treated esotropia as early as 2 weeks and as late as 4 years postoperatively. The presence of A or V patterns, medial rectus restriction, and absence of binocular function were more frequently associated with patients who developed consecutive exotropia than for patients who did not develop consecutive exotropia.

Persistent diplopia may accompany consecutive exotropia. This is more likely when the exotropia begins in adults and there is no suppression zone on the temporal hemiretina. We have used overcorrecting Fresnel press-on prisms base-in before the spectacle lens of the exotropic eye to move the diplopia image back into the already existing suppression zone on the nasal hemiretina (see Chapter 5, Case 1). If this proves successful, prisms can be ground into the patient's spectacles. If prisms are not feasible, a second operation using adjustable sutures to more exactly place the image in the nasal suppression zone can be attempted.[74]

INTERMITTENT EXOTROPIA

Intermittent exotropia is an occasional divergent misalignment of the eyes that is part of the time latent and part of the time manifest. Exophoria supposedly precedes the development of intermittent exotropia, but this is probably not always the case. The deviation becomes manifest when the fusional convergence amplitudes are exceeded. The period of manifest exotropia is variable for each patient. It is precipitated by factors such as anxiety, inattention, poor health, exposure to bright light, and excessive fatigue. At the beginning, it may be present only when the patient is tired, sleepy, or daydreaming. Illness and fatigue lessen the patient's control.

> **❊ CLINICAL PEARL**
>
> Intermittent exotropia is an occasional divergent misalignment of the eyes that is part of the time latent and part of the time manifest.

Intermittent exotropia is a common though enigmatic form of strabismus constituting about 25% of all the cases of strabismus and 1% of the general population.[75] As mentioned earlier, it can go unreported because of the infrequency of the strabismic phase. Patients with this type of strabismus demonstrate a duality of visual behavior in that they seem to be completely normal during ocular alignment and totally "turned off" during periods of exotropia.

In intermittent exotropia, the cover test reveals that when the cover is placed before the eye, the eye turns out under cover, just as the phoric eye does. However, when the cover is removed, the eye may act differently than the phoric eye. It may remain turned

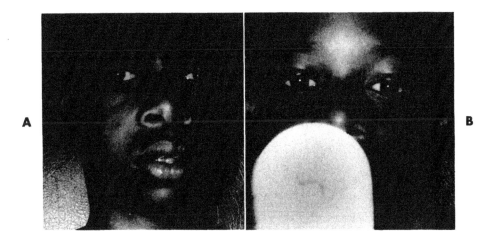

FIG. 9-4 Divergence excess intermittent exotropia. **A,** Exotropia when viewing at distance. **B,** Alignment when viewing at near.

out for a variable period, after which it will refixate and the eyes become realigned. At times the patient will only straighten the eye when it is suggested by the examiner. Quite often the patient will blink just before the realignment is attained, as if the blink aids in regaining fusion.

The exotropia may occur only or mostly for distance, only or mostly for near, or approximately equal at distance and near fixation distances. If the exotropia begins in early childhood, when sensory adaptations are easily developed, the patient may remain symptom free. An older patient may be quite symptomatic, because the onset of the deviation began at an age when sensory adaptations are less readily developed. Symptoms associated with intermittent exotropia include diplopia, headaches, photophobia, eye strain, pulling sensation, and reading problems.

CLASSIFICATION

Similar to exophoria, intermittent exotropia is classified in three categories, based on the distance at which the deviation is greater.[75-84]

Divergence Excess (Distance Exotropia)

Divergence excess exotropia is manifest for distance viewing either exclusively or much more frequently than near viewing and is larger by at least 10 PD at distance than at near (Fig. 9-4). Approximately 7% of the strabismic population consists of divergence excess.[75] It represents 5% to 17% of all cases of intermittent exotropia.[75]

Basic (Distance and Near Exotropia)

In basic type exotropia, the exotropia is approximately the same in frequency and magnitude at distance and near. It represents about 50% of all intermittent exotropias.[76,83]

Convergence Insufficiency (Near Exotropia, Convergence Weakness Exotropia, Innervational Exotropia)

Convergence insufficiency exotropia is manifest for near viewing either exclusively or much more frequently than for distance viewing and is larger by at least 10 PD at near (Fig. 9-5). The near point of convergence in these patients is usually receded. Convergence insufficiency represents approximately 33% of all intermittent exotropias.[76]

CLINICAL FEATURES
Age Distribution

The type of intermittent exotropia diagnosed is related to the age of the patient at the time of evaluation. Divergence excess is a strabismus that is diagnosed mostly in young children.[22,76-80] It is rare to find it in adults. On the other hand, basic and convergence insufficiency intermittent exotropias are vastly more frequent in the older population and are rarely diagnosed in very young patients.[76,81,82] The strong tonic convergence and accommodation in young children lessens, and with it the exodeviation at near likely increases, resulting in more convergence insufficiency and basic intermittent exotropia in the adult population.

Size of Deviation

For divergence excess intermittent exotropia, the average deviation while viewing at distance is 29 PD and while viewing at near is 9 PD.[84] Larger deviations in as many as one third of patients may be uncovered when viewing at 30 m rather than at 6 m.[85] Some clini-

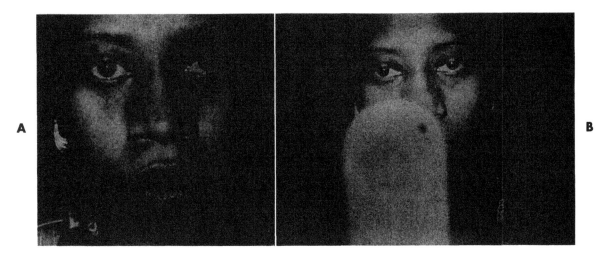

FIG. 9-5 Convergence insufficiency intermittent exotropia. **A,** Alignment when viewing at distance. **B,** Exotropia when viewing at near.

cians have the patient look out a window at a distant object while cover testing is carried out to detect the maximum exodeviation. With basic intermittent exotropia, an average angle of deviation of 16.6 PD at distance and 17 PD at near has been reported.[83] With convergence insufficiency the angle of deviation at distance varies usually from orthophoria to 10 PD of exophoria or intermittent exotropia, and the near deviation ranges from 10- to 25-PD intermittent exotropia.[82]

Laterality

Regardless of the category of intermittent exotropia, alternating fixation is frequent and amblyopia is uncommon. Corrected visual acuity is equal or within one line difference between the two eyes in 88% of the patients.[22] The difference in visual acuity between the eyes in the remaining patients can usually be directed to the presence of anisometropic amblyopia. The amblyopia in a few cases may also be the result of the exotropic phase becoming very frequent with one eye and therefore favored for fixation.[86]

Photophobia

Photophobia is particularly common in intermittent exotropia. Exposure to bright light frequently causes reflex closure of one eye for these patients.[87] Whereas normal individuals exposed to bright light will partially close either both eyes or the eye nearer the sun, those with intermittent exotropia close only the nonpreferred eye when exposed to bright sunlight. This is most likely to be reported by the parents of children with intermittent exotropia.[88] Closure of the deviating eye in bright light is strongly suggestive of di-

vergence excess intermittent exotropia and can be the presenting sign even when the exotropia has not been noticed. Some clinicians believe this to be pathognomonic, so as to allow a tentative diagnosis of childhood intermittent exotropia until proven otherwise.[8] Absence of this sign, however, does not speak against intermittent exotropia.

The reason for the eye closure in intermittent exotropia is unclear. It has been suggested that when the patient is outdoors and looking at a distant object, there are no near visual clues to stimulate convergence. The bright sunlight dazzles the retina, so that fusion is interrupted and the patient goes from exophoria to exotropia. Diplopia and visual confusion are avoided by monocular eye closure. This agrees with Wang and Chryssanthou,[89] who found monocular eye closure to be much greater for individuals with intermittent exotropia who have normal correspondence (90%) when strabismic than for those with intermittent exotropia who have anomalous correspondence (35%) when strabismic.

It is by no means certain that these patients close one eye to avoid diplopia. In fact, individuals with intermittent exotropia rarely complain of diplopia. It may be that the person shuts one eye in bright sunlight to avoid the many perceptual visual field changes that take place in bright light diffusion. Eye closure is more likely a mechanism to avoid visual discomfort in bright light in those with a low binocular photophobia threshold.[8]

It may be that bright light adversely affects the amplitude of fusional convergence and contrast sensitivity.[90,91] Under laboratory conditions, increasing illumination causes fusional amplitudes to decrease in the majority of patients, both exotropic and normal.[88] The deviating eye in intermittent exotropia has also been shown to have reduced contrast sensitivity when compared with the fellow eye and the contrast sensitivity in normals.[91] Some clinicians recommend using photochromatic lenses to reduce the photophobia in the treatment of intermittent exotropia.[6]

Suppression, Retinal Correspondence, and Panoramic Vision

When intermittent exotropia begins, the patient experiences diplopia. Suppression and/or anomalous correspondence usually develop to protect the child from diplopia. When exotropia begins later, these sensory adaptations are more infrequent than with the child in whom there is almost constant suppression when the eyes are exotropic. Suppression is switched off when the eyes are straight. The switching on and off of suppression is rapid. With alternating exotropia, the switch in suppression begins as soon as the eyes start to move and is completed in approximately 80 ms before the end of the saccade used to make the switch.[92]

The traditional belief is that the suppression zone in intermittent exotropia extends over the entire temporal retina.[93] As discussed in Chapter 5, the nature of the test stimuli greatly influences the degree and patterns of suppression. Patients with intermittent exotropia may also demonstrate suppression of the images falling on the nasal, as well as the temporal, hemiretina or have only two dense suppression regions, one corresponding to the fovea of the good eye and the other at the zero measure point, with nonsuppression of all points between the fovea and the zero measure point.[94-96] Melek and others,[97] evaluated suppression in 21 patients with intermittent exotropia using a Goldmann type of perimeter while the patients viewed the fixation target with the Bagolini striated lenses. Fixation and ocular position were monitored, with frequent occlusion of the fixating eye. They reported that 53% of the patients had an entire temporal retina suppression, whereas the remaining 47% showed regional suppression zones. During alignment, none of the patients demonstrated suppression.

According to some investigators, however, as many as 75% of individuals with intermittent exotropia suppress physiologic diplopia when phoric, suggesting the persistence of subtle hemiretinal suppression under fused conditions.[96-98] This suppression may also occur during dichoptic viewing of first-degree targets in the synoptophore and with cheiroscopic tracings. That the sensory status of some patients with intermittent exotropia when phoric is not perfectly normal is supported further by the reduced stereopsis reported in some studies.[99-103] In addition, as the frequency and du-

ration of the exotropic phase progress, some patients experience a further decline in stereopsis during the phoric phase.[101,103] The decline in stereopsis is frequently used as the basis for more aggressive treatment.

In intermittent exotropia, normal correspondence exists when the eyes are straight, and anomalous correspondence frequently exists when the exotropia is manifest. When the deviating eye turns out, there apparently is a simultaneous displacement of the egocentric localization of the eye so that no diplopia occurs. The angle of anomaly covaries with the objective angle.[104] With the Hering-Bielschowsky afterimage test, patients when phoric see a perfect cross and when exotropic see a displaced cross. This duality of correspondence is more likely in divergence excess intermittent exotropia. Interestingly, the testing conditions that elicit the greater number of anomalous responses in intermittent exotropia are opposite to those of esotropia. In intermittent exotropia, the more natural, or less dissociative, the testing conditions, (the Bagolini striated lenses), the greater the chance for normal correspondence, whereas the more artificial, or more dissociative, the testing conditions (the Hering-Bielschowsky afterimage test), the greater the chance for anomalous correspondence.[105]

 CLINICAL PEARL

In intermittent exotropia, normal correspondence exists when the eyes are straight, and anomalous correspondence frequently exists when the exotropia is manifest.

Despite having suppression and/or anomalous correspondence, the patient may be aware of when the exotropia occurs by either "feeling" the eyes diverge or by noticing an extension of the binocular peripheral visual field. The latter is known as *panoramic vision* and is characteristic of animals with wide eye separation. When exotropic, each eye surveys independently the full extent of its own visual field. Because these patients can alternately fixate and quickly turn one eye on or off, they have a much larger field to each side of the head than a person with normal binocular vision.[106] We find that this panoramic viewing is much more readily appreciated in adults with large-angle alternating exotropia. Panoramic viewing can be demonstrated by first measuring and plotting a binocular confrontation field with the eyes aligned and then repeating the procedure with the eyes exotropic. The panoramic vision allows the patient to increase peripheral vision and motion detection. The enlargement of spatial shift of the visual field exactly matches the angular measurement of the deviation.[105] The peripheral vision is reduced following treatment of the intermittent exotropia. The patient's awareness of the reduction of the peripheral field eventually disappears.

Accommodation

Several investigators have described adolescents and young adults with intermittent exotropia and abnormal accommodation.[62,81,107-111] This condition is more likely with convergence insufficiency intermittent exotropia. The condition of intermittent exotropia with abnormal accommodation can occur following diphtheria, mononucleosis, upper respiratory infection, encephalitis, head trauma, and endocrine dysfunction. It can be idiopathic and occur in patients without any obvious cause. For these patients the accommodative disorder appears to be the primary defect and the exotropia secondary, resulting from the reduced accommodative-convergence.

Rutstein and Daum[62] report on 13 patients, ages 8 to 31, with intermittent exotropia and abnormal accommodation. Most patients had a long history of visual symptoms, including diplopia and blurred vision that had not responded to therapy in the past. Clinical testing indicated orthophoria or minimal exophoria at distance and intermittent exotropia at near. The size of the exotropia ranged from 5 to 20 PD. The mean amplitude of accommodation was 3 D. Evaluating accommodation with dynamic retinoscopy indicated that these patients could not sustain accommodation. This involuntary fluctuation of accommodation was related to the appearance of the exotropia. With appropriate accommodation, the exotropia was not present, whereas with an extended lag of accommodation, the exotropia was manifest. Unlike other patients with convergence insufficiency intermittent exotropia, orthoptics/vision therapy was not beneficial, and most patients required bifocal lenses and base-in prisms. This type of intermittent exotropia requires careful assessment of the patients' accommodation. (See Case 5.)

CASE 5

A 14-year-old girl was referred for treatment of an exotropia. Five years previously, she had a severe case of chicken pox. Since then, she had experienced intermittent diplopia and blurred vision. Prisms were prescribed by the referring clinician but did not relieve her symptoms. She was in good health and not taking any medications. There was no history of trauma.

On examination the patient had 20/20 vision with each eye. A 4-PD exophoria at distance and a 15-PD intermittent exotropia at near were found. Version testing was normal. Stereopsis was 50 seconds of arc with the Randot stereotest. The patient fused the Worth four dot test at distance and had crossed diplopia at near. Fusional vergences could not be measured at near.

It was suspected that the patient had a typical convergence insufficiency intermittent exotropia. However, the amplitude of accommodation by the push-up method was 1 D for each eye. Dynamic retinoscopy fluctuated but mostly revealed a 2.50-D lag of accommodation. Cycloplegic refraction was emmetropia. Treatment with +2.00 D lenses and 6-PD base-in prisms for near relieved all symptoms.

An accommodative spasm can mask an exotropia. Some individuals with exotropia may employ excessive accommodative convergence at the cost of blurred vision to align the eyes. Intermittent exotropia can be missed, and constant exotropia can appear to be intermittent, as indicated by the following case.

CASE 6

A 24-year-old accountant with exotropia presented in the clinic. He had two surgical procedures supposedly for esotropia at 6 years and 14 years. He had also been treated with orthoptics/vision therapy. He denied any diplopia but reported intermittent blurred vision.

The examination revealed emmetropia and visual acuity of 20/20 for each eye. A constant left exotropia of 25 PD at distance and 30 PD at near was measured with the cover test. Version testing revealed bilateral superior oblique overactions that resulted in an **A** pattern; the exotropia was 20 PD in upgaze and 50 PD in downgaze. With the Worth four dot test the patient alternately suppressed at distance and near. Stereopsis was not present with the Randot stereotest. The synoptophore and the Hering-Bielschowsky afterimage test both showed anomalous correspondence.

The diagnosis was consecutive exotropia. The patient indicated that he could voluntarily "align" his eyes, which he did during job interviews. He had learned to do this when undergoing orthoptics/vision therapy as a child. During "alignment" there was no evidence of sensory fusion, and dynamic retinoscopy indicated an accommodative spasm of 4 D.

Accommodative Convergence/Accommodation (AC/A) Ratio

Because the AC/A ratio is used to explain differences in distance-near esotropia measurements, it has also been used to explain differences in distance-near exotropia measurements. Greater exodeviations at distance or at near supposedly result from an abnormal AC/A ratio. Patients with divergence excess intermittent exotropia have high AC/A ratios.[112-115] This idea is based on the fact that the average deviation is 29 PD at distance and only 9 PD at near, resulting in an average calculated distance-near AC/A ratio of approximately 12/1 (assuming an interpupillary distance of 60 mm). It has been suggested that the AC/A in young children is pliable to the extent that it can be adjusted to assist offsetting the exodeviation for the benefit of maintaining single binocular vision.[115,116] Because young children seem to have a more pliable overall sensory-motor innervation system than older patients, this could account for the fact that a high AC/A ratio occurs more frequently among children with intermittent exotropia. By this reasoning, divergence excess intermittent exotropia results from an attempt on the part of the child to compensate for the excessive divergence innervation rather than from excessive divergence innervation itself.

With convergence insufficiency intermittent exotropia, the average calculated AC/A ratio based on the distance-near measurements is 2.7/1, whereas with basic intermittent exotropia the average ratio is 6.1/1.[82,83]

All differences between the distance and near deviation in patients with intermittent exotropia are not manifestations of the AC/A ratio. Clinical measurement of the distance-near AC/A ratio is confounded by various factors. It is often assumed, for example, that the accommodative response is the same as the stimulus to accommodation. However, the accommodative response is usually less than the accommodative stimulus at near and more at distance.[117] Alteration in pupillary size from distance to near and proximal convergence factors also cause variation in the distance-near AC/A ratio for these patients. These factors tend to overestimate the AC/A ratio, particularly in young children with divergence excess intermittent exotropia. When using the gradient method to measure the AC/A ratio with spheric lenses over a range of +3.00 D to −3.00 D, the ratio ranges from as low as 3/1 to as high as 14/1.[*] Also with the gradient method, not all patients with convergence insufficiency intermittent exotropia have a low AC/A ratio.

Cooper, Cuiffreda, and Kruger[119] used an objective infrared optometer and infrared eye movement monitor to measure simultaneously and continuously both accommodation and accommodative vergence to near stimuli in four patients with divergence excess intermittent exotropia. Standard clinically determined stimulus AC/A ratios were also measured. The mean group response AC/A ratio was 5.9/1. They concluded that the reduced ocular deviation at near compared with distance in divergence excess intermittent exotropia is the result of fusional convergence and/or proximal convergence aftereffects and not an abnormally high AC/A ratio.

Kushner[121] quantified the AC/A ratio in patients with divergence excess by (1) comparing the distance-near deviations with the cover test, (2) using the gradient method with −2.00 D at 6 m, and (3) using the gradient method with +3.00 D at 33 cm. Measurements were done both before and after 1 hour of occlusion. Only 11% of the patients had a high AC/A ratio with both distance-near and gradient methods. For these patients, it was presumed that the risk of consecutive esotropia was high if surgical treatment was given. Another 9% had a high AC/A ratio using the distance-near relationship, a normal gradient AC/A with −2.00 D at 6 m, and a low gradient AC/A with +3.00 D at 33 cm. Another 59% had normal gradient AC/A, with −2.00 D at 6 m and normal or high AC/A with +3.00 D at 33 cm. The remaining patients had basic exotropia, with normal AC/A ratios with all three

methods. Thus it appears that the AC/A ratios in most patients with divergence excess intermittent exotropia are not abnormally high but are only slightly above the normal range.

True Versus Simulated, or Pseudo, Divergence Excess Intermittent Exotropia

Exuberant functioning of vergence aftereffects, the tonic near reflex, accommodative convergence and/or tenacious proximal convergence tonus in young children can make the near exodeviation look smaller. As a result the prevalence of divergence excess intermittent exotropia tends to be overestimated. Accordingly, the differentiation between true divergence excess and simulated, or pseudo, divergence excess exotropia has been used mostly by ophthalmic surgeons to help determine the muscles to be operated on for correction of the exotropia.[122,123] With simulated, or pseudo, divergence excess, the near exodeviation increases significantly after either disrupting fusion or eliminating accommodative convergence. Simulated divergence excess intermittent exotropia represents a basic exodeviation with a powerful convergence mechanism that conceals the entire exodeviation at near. It occurs more frequently than true divergence excess.[76,124]

The occlusion test and the +3.00-D lens tests have been used clinically to differentiate simulated from true divergence excess intermittent exotropia. With the occlusion test, an occluder is placed over one eye from 30 minutes to 3 hours to thoroughly dissociate the eyes.[122] Patching of one eye disrupts the excessive fusional and tonic convergence. Before removal of the occluder the opposite eye is covered to prevent binocular exposure, which may be sufficient to again obscure the near deviation by fusional convergence. The alternate prism cover test is repeated at near. With simulated divergence excess, the near deviation may reach or even exceed the distance deviation. With true divergence excess, the near deviation will essentially measure the same magnitude as measured before occlusion. Basic and convergence insufficiency intermittent exotropias usually demonstrate minimal effects with the occlusion test.

The +3.00-D lens test is based on the premise that patients with divergence excess use exuberant accommodative convergence to conceal some of their exodeviation at near.[123] If the exodeviation at near approaches the exodeviation at distance when repeating the alternate prism cover test at near while wearing the +3.00-D lenses that suspend accommodation and accommodative convergence, simulated divergence excess exists. If the near exodeviation remains the same, the diagnosis is true divergence excess.

Because different mechanisms are involved in the occlusion test and +3.00-D lens test, patients may respond differently to each test. In two studies with a combined total of 74 patients that used the occlusion

---

[*]References 77, 79, 85, 115, 116, 118-120.

test, only 24 (32%) were found to have true divergence excess.[76,124] In another study the near exodeviation increased with the occlusion test in 70% of the patients with divergence excess.[122] Simulated divergence excess, as determined with the +3.00-D lens test, is much less frequent.[124] This agrees with previously mentioned studies that indicate that the AC/A ratio for most patients with divergence excess is not excessive.[119,121] Of the two tests, we prefer the occlusion test.

TREATMENT

The ideal management for intermittent exotropia is a continuous discussion. The goal of treatment is to reduce the frequency of the eye turn by enhancing the fusional processes. The forms of treatment beyond correcting the refractive error include (1) minus lenses, (2) occlusion, (3) prisms, (4) orthoptics/vision therapy, and/or (5) surgery.[125] Factors determining the type of treatment include (1) the patient's age, (2) the size of the deviation, (3) the role of accommodation and the presence of refractive errors, (4) the frequency and duration of the exotropia, (5) the degree of deterioration, (6) the cosmetic appearance, and (7) the motivation and compliance of the patient and/or parents.

Correction of Refractive Error

Lenses that neutralize the refractive condition and balance accommodative effort should be prescribed when indicated. Full correction is advisable in myopic patients to achieve clear retinal imagery and maintain active accommodative convergence. Some authors report a higher incidence of myopic astigmatism and anisometropia in patients with intermittent exotropia who are poorly controlled; therefore the full amount of correction should be given to create sharp retinal images that in turn will increase the stimulus to fuse.[126,127]

With hyperopia, use of corrective glasses can aggravate the exotropia by relaxing accommodation. Whether hyperopia should be fully corrected, partially corrected, or not corrected at all depends on its degree, the age of the patient, the status of accommodation, and the AC/A ratio. Generally, we do not correct hyperopic refractive errors less than 2 D in young children with intermittent exotropia. The rationale is based on the assumption that young children can easily accommodate to compensate for moderate degrees of hyperopia, and that the associated accommodative convergence may be beneficial in helping to control their exodeviation. Larger amounts of hyperopia in children with intermittent exotropia frequently are corrected, at least partially.

Spectacle correction of hyperopia can cause paradoxic resolution of intermittent exotropia in some cases. Iacobucci, Archer, and Giles[127] report on seven children with exotropia who had uncorrected hyper-

opic refractive errors ranging from 2 to 7 D. All but one had intermittent exotropia that was converted with full hyperopic correction to a small esophoria. Apparently, if the hyperopia is large, some individuals with exotropia may not make the effort to overcome the hyperopia because they are unable to sustain the amount of accommodation necessary for a clear image. Full hyperopic correction may be warranted in selected children with intermittent exotropia, particularly if there is a low accommodative amplitude or other evidence of abnormal accommodation.

Minus Lenses

Overcorrecting, or added minus, lenses (glasses or contact lenses with more minus or less plus power than necessary for best refractive correction) are used temporarily to stimulate convergence by inducing accommodation, thus reducing and adding control of the intermittent exotropia. The idea is to use the accommodative-convergence response to start the vergence system in motion. It is hoped that the fusional vergence system will take over and maintain fusion.[128] A little accommodative effort can often trigger a large vergence response, which can be enough to keep the exodeviation latent. Ideally, after fusion has been improved, the minus lens power is gradually reduced to zero. The positive aspect of minus lenses is control of the exotropia without need for additional treatment in many cases. An obvious limitation of minus lens therapy is that its use is restricted to younger patients with sufficient accommodative amplitude; also, it has not been shown to be of value in the older patient. In addition, for some patients, it may require the wearing of glasses not otherwise required.

Minus lens therapy is frequently our treatment of choice for young children with intermittent exotropia (Fig. 9-6). It provides a more continuous form of therapy, especially when patient compliance with orthoptics/vision therapy is poor. The amount of minus lens power that is prescribed varies among patients and clinicians. Generally, the minimum amount that provides constant fusion is given. Clip-on minus lenses can be used in the office while the child views an accommodative target at distance. A good clinical guideline for the appropriateness of the minus prescription is a more rapid recovery of fusion after removal of the occluder following the alternate cover test. The power usually ranges from 0.75 to 3.00 D. A common starting point is 2.00 D added to the distance prescription. Because it may take some time for patients to adjust to new accommodative demands, immediate improvement may not be seen in some cases. We prescribe the appropriate minus lenses and bring the child back in 2 to 4 weeks to determine the results. Fresnel press-on lenses can be used if the patient already wears glasses.

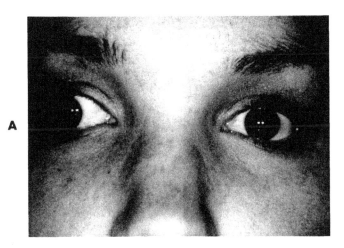

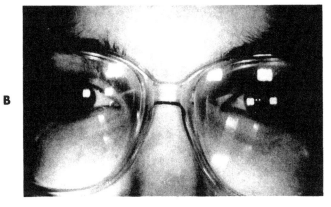

FIG. 9-6 Minus lens therapy for a patient with intermittent exotropia. **A,** Exotropia without minus lenses. **B,** Fusion with minus lenses.

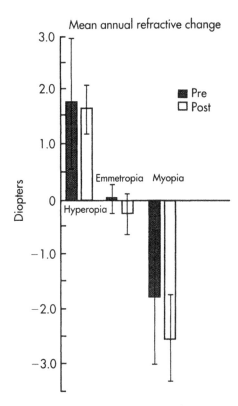

Mean annual refractive change

FIG. 9-7 Mean annual refractive changes for 40 patients with exotropia treated with minus lenses. (From Rutstein RP, Marsh-Tootle W, London R: Changes in refractive error for exotropes treated with overminus lenses, *Optom Vis Sci* 66:490, 1989.)

Discontinuation of this treatment should occur when the frequency and duration of the intermittent exotropia remain unchanged despite wearing minus lenses. Minus lenses are contraindicated in patients whose exotropia is associated with abnormal accommodation.

> ### CLINICAL PEARL
> Minus lens therapy is frequently our treatment of choice for young children with intermittent exotropia.

During this treatment, the patient's accommodation and near deviation must be carefully monitored. A large increase in the lag of accommodation, as determined with dynamic retinoscopy, indicates that the child is having difficulty at near with the minus lenses. A bifocal lens or accommodative training can be given in these cases. A large esophoria or intermittent esotropia at near also warrants a bifocal lens. Such induced near esodeviations are rare because of the fact that most children with intermittent exotropia have normal rather than high AC/A ratios.

A concern of some clinicians is that the added accommodative effort required with minus lenses may alter the natural refractive progression by either inducing myopia or enhancing myopia progression. Rutstein, Marsh-Tootle, and London[129] monitored the refractive error in 10 children treated with minus lenses and found the mean annual refractive error changes to be similar to those found in children without exotropia (Fig. 9-7).

The efficacy of minus lenses has been reported.[130-135] On the average, approximately 65% of patients will show improved fusion at least temporarily. Caltrider and Jampolsky[132] categorized the response to minus lenses for 35 patients into 3 groups. The duration of therapy was from 2 to 15 months, with the median being 18 months. Group 1 (Fig. 9-8, *A*), which consisted of 46% of the patients, involved a qualitative change in which a poorly controlled intermittent exotropia changed to a well-controlled exophoria. Group 2 (Fig. 9-8, *B*), which consisted of 26% of the patients, involved a quantitative change, as well. In these cases, there was also a decrease of at least 15 PD in the exodeviation, and the deviation

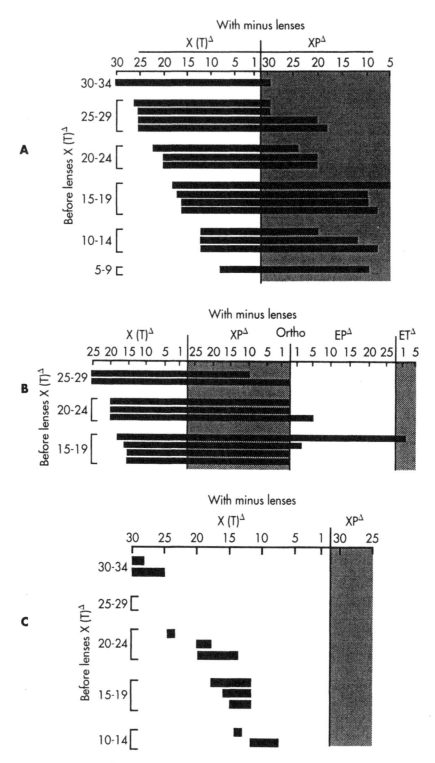

FIG. 9-8 Responses of 35 patients with exotropia treated with minus lenses. **A,** Group 1, qualitative improvement only. **B,** Group 2, qualitative and quantitative improvement. **C,** Group 3, no improvement. X(T) indicates intermittent exotropia in prism diopters and XP indicates exophoria in prism diopters. (From Caltrider N, Jampolsky A: Overcorrecting minus lens therapy for treatment of intermittent exotropia, *Ophthalmology* 90:1162, 1983.)

remained latent while wearing the minus lenses. Group 3 (Fig. 9-8, *C*), which consisted of 28% of the patients, involved neither qualitative nor quantitative changes with the minus lenses, and the therapy was ineffective. Caltrider and Jampolsky[132] slowly weaned the minus lenses in 10 patients and found that seven patients maintained a phoric posture for at least a year.

Reynolds, Wackerhagen, and Olitsky[136] correlated the efficacy of minus lenses with the size of the intermittent exotropia. Of 74 patients, 92% were successful with deviations less than 20 PD, 62.5% were successful with deviations of 20 to 25 PD, and only 23.5% were successful with deviations exceeding 25 PD.

Occlusion

A somewhat more controversial form of treatment is occlusion.[137-142] Although optometrists rarely use occlusion with intermittent exotropia, it is the most commonly used nonsurgical therapy among medical eye care practitioners in the United States and Canada.[143] It is used in intermittent exotropia to eliminate or prevent suppression. It serves as a form of passive antisuppression therapy applicable to very young patients, as opposed to active techniques involving diplopia awareness. Its proponents claim that by reducing or eliminating suppression, sensory fusion and fusional ranges are enhanced, with increased control of the deviation.[143,144] Occlusion for days or weeks has been reported to result in significant reduction in the size of the exodeviation. Treatment regimens vary from constant occlusion to only 1 to 2 hours per day. Alternating or dominant eye occlusion can be used.

CLINICAL PEARL

Although optometrists rarely use occlusion with intermittent exotropia, it is the most commonly used nonsurgical therapy among medical eye care practitioners in the United States and Canada.

It would be expected that occlusion therapy might increase the risk of the intermittent exotropia deteriorating even further. Prolonged occlusion can disrupt the fusional mechanism in a child who is intermittently fusing at distance and/or near. Occlusion may also increase the size of the exodeviation. Studies that have used constant occlusion in intermittent exotropia have reported such cases.[138] Part-time occlusion is less risky.[137] Freeman and Isenberg[139] treated 11 patients with intermittent exotropia, ages 9 months to 5 years, with patching of the dominant eye from 4 to 6 hours a day. Of the patients, 10 had divergence excess intermittent exotropia. After 6 months of treatment, all patients converted to heterophoria or orthophoria, at least temporarily. Three patients remained orthophoric without further treatment. Three other patients later developed

"constant" exotropia and underwent surgery. Similar findings were reported in older children.[137]

The success rate for occlusion therapy varies from 30% to 40%.[125] Patching for shorter periods (1 to 2 hours) likely achieves the same goals as longer periods, without the possibility of precipitating more strabismus by disrupting an already fragile binocular vision system. We feel that occlusion by itself is not an effective therapy for intermittent exotropia and use it only in patients with amblyopia.

Prisms

Prism therapy for intermittent exotropia involves prescribing base-in prisms to compensate for a portion of the deviation or prescribing base-in prisms to neutralize the entire deviation in an attempt to achieve more continuous binocular sensory fusion.[145-147] Giving a partial prism correction is preferred, because with prisms equal to the deviation, the patient may continue to suppress, resulting in no stimulus for fusional vergence. The amount of prisms will vary but generally can be prescribed to place the patients' deviation in balance with his or her fusional vergence amplitudes, so that the patient is able to maintain alignment without excessive effort. The criteria used in prescribing prisms for exophoria, as discussed in Chapter 6, can be applied with intermittent exotropia. An appropriate amount can also be determined by performing the unilateral cover test with base-in prisms. The minimum prism permitting a rapid fusional movement can be prescribed. The prisms should be worn constantly, with the aim of tapering them over time as fusional status improves.

Prisms can be used in all age groups because they require no active participation by the patient. They are more frequently used for basic and convergence insufficiency intermittent exotropias than for divergence excess esotropia, in which minus lenses are preferable. Prisms can be combined with minus lenses in patients with divergence excess and combined with plus lenses in patients with intermittent exotropia and abnormal accommodation. Prisms are frequently combined with orthoptics/vision therapy. Once convergence is more easily sustained, the prisms can be reduced and in some cases eliminated entirely while orthoptics/vision therapy is continued. The success rate for prisms has been estimated as 28%.[125] Deviations less than 20 PD respond better to prisms than do larger deviations.[146]

Potential adverse effects associated with prolonged wearing of prisms for intermittent exotropia remain largely unexplored in the clinical literature.[148,149] A few patients may experience an increase in the angle of exodeviation following the wearing of prisms.[147] The consensus is that prism adaptation does not alter significantly the magnitude of the deviation in exotropia as it does with esotropia.[149]

Orthoptics/Vision Therapy

Orthoptics/vision therapy for intermittent exotropia includes expanding fusional vergence amplitudes and facility, eliminating suppression, and improving accommodation.[110,150-164] The goals of these procedures are to facilitate increased vergence control of the exotropia and enhance sensory fusion by involving the patient actively.

Various approaches have been used with intermittent exotropia. One approach is to develop pathologic diplopia awareness, so that the patient will perceive crossed diplopia when the eyes deviate. Diplopia awareness is taught by placing a red filter over the nondeviating eye while the patient views a fixation light in a darkened room. The patient is required to maintain diplopia while the room illumination is slowly increased. Then the red filter is replaced by progressively less dense red filters. This can be done with the Bagolini filter bar. The last step is awareness of diplopia of the fixation light without any filter. Once the patient achieves diplopia awareness, therapy consists of conditioning the vergence system to eliminate the diplopia using the fusional vergence system. Many patients have deep suppression when the exotropia is manifest; therefore training may not be successful when the patient's eyes are in the exotropic position and may be more successful when the eyes are aligned.

We prefer the development of eye position awareness on the part of the patient rather than pathologic diplopia awareness. The way to address the suppression in intermittent exotropia is to enforce binocular vision which can be done by improving motor vergence skills. Training involves procedures that make the patient's eyes converge to the orthoposition and not be exotropic. This treatment is based on the fact that individuals with intermittent exotropia will be binocular when there is an advantage, (i.e., in the presence of stereopsis) and exotropic when disparity cues are lacking. Therapy employs operant conditioning techniques in which the patient can more readily maintain normal ocular alignment, (i.e., detailed near stereotargets). Instead of awareness of pathologic diplopia, awareness of physiologic diplopia is encouraged while the patient is trained to bifixate more readily. Training starts either with stereoscopes and/or filtered procedures (vectograms and tranaglyphs) and continues with procedures such as the aperture rule trainer and, eventually, chiastopic fusion techniques with eccentric circles or lifesaver cards.[160] Orthoptics/vision therapy for intermittent exotropia is essentially the same as that for exophoria, as discussed in Chapter 6, except that the former may require some additional support, such as using minus lenses and/or prisms to get started.

Auditory biofeedback has been used for treating intermittent exotropia.[153,164,165] Using an infrared eye movement monitor with a variable pitched tone, auditory biofeedback can be provided for the positional sense of the eyes. The goal is to have the patient use biofeedback to maintain normal alignment of the eyes, usually in an environment such as a darkened room, while performing a nonvisual task. Additional studies are needed to determine the efficacy of this innovative technique.

The advantages of orthoptics/vision therapy over other forms of treatment is that it provides a more complete treatment in that successful treatment not only eliminates the manifest strabismus, but frequently results in overall improvement in the quality of binocular vision. Orthoptics/vision therapy is noninvasive and relatively risk free. With intermittent exotropia, this therapy has an overall calculated success rate of 59%.[125]

The disadvantages of orthoptics/vision therapy are that it is time consuming, often requiring numerous repeat visits, and requires considerable commitment and motivation on the part of the patient and, with young children, on the part of the family.[151,156,160,164] In addition, it must be realized that this form of therapy does not actually "cure" the intermittent exotropia, if "cure" is meant to indicate that the exodeviation is abolished. The exodeviation becomes less obvious. Orthoptics/vision therapy can assist patients, particularly those having intermittent exotropia of 20 to 25 PD or less, in developing improved control of the deviation. It converts a sometimes manifest exodeviation into an always latent deviation.

Surgery

Extraocular muscle surgery is another therapy option for intermittent exotropia. Some physicians regard it as the treatment of choice for intermittent exotropia.[3,26] In a deviation in which vision is usually normal in each eye and fusion with stereopsis and motor fusion amplitudes are present, the muscles are recessed or resected to alter an alignment that is likely exophoric a large portion of the time. There is no evidence that this form of treatment has any effect on improving vergences or fusional ability. Simply reducing the angle of intermittent exotropia may not be helpful, because the same intermittent exotropia sensory pattern with suppression persists and the size can increase postoperatively. Based on a review of 2530 cases, surgery has a 46% rate of success.[125] The surgical techniques used in intermittent exotropia are discussed in Chapter 11.

The need for this form of treatment is determined by the state of fusional control, the size of the deviation, the age of the patient, and whether less invasive treatment modalities have been used. Nonsurgical management of the patient with intermittent exotropia should be considered before recommending surgical treatment. Surgical treatment is considered when (1) nonsurgical therapy is unsuccessful, (2) there is deterioration in binocularity manifested by increasing exotropia, and/or (3) there is parental or personal unhappiness with alternative therapies. The appropriateness of surgery for convergence insufficiency intermittent exotropia and other intermittent exotropias when there is less than 20 PD of deviation is not without controversy.[167]

✣ CLINICAL PEARL

Nonsurgical management of the patient with intermittent exotropia should be considered before recommending surgical treatment.

The question arises regarding the optimum age for surgery in children with intermittent exotropia.[168,169] Proponents of early surgery claim its advantages as being the prevention of sensory and motor changes (i.e., deepening suppression and lessening of fusional amplitudes) that may become untreatable later. Early surgery also minimizes the reinforcement of the habit of becoming exotropic. Proponents of later surgery claim (1) that the progress of the exotropia can be monitored (occasionally spontaneous improvement occurs); (2) that a more accurate diagnosis can be made, including assessment of fusion, as well as more exact measurements in upgaze and downgaze; (3) the patient can cooperate more with orthoptics/vision therapy; and (4) the risk of consecutive esotropia is less. Reoperation rates for patients age 3 or younger have been estimated as being more than 4 times greater than if the surgery is performed at age 7 or older.[169]

An increased success rate has been reported with moderate surgical overcorrection in the immediate postoperative period.[170-172] The ideal postoperative position is 10- to 15-PD esotropia.[173] This purposeful production of a small overcorrection may only occur by chance in some instances.[174] Immediate postoperative diplopia has been thought to be therapeutic in eliminating suppression and stimulating fusional vergence to allow for long-term stability. Spontaneous reduction in the esotropic angle of deviation should occur within 6 to 8 weeks after surgery. In some cases there is still a significant tendency toward divergence between the sixth and twelfth postoperative month.[173] Reduced preoperative stereopsis does not preclude long-term alignment stability, suggesting possibly that the peripheral rather than central fusion keeps the eyes aligned after surgery.[175]

Postoperative esotropia does not disappear in all cases, however. Persistent consecutive esotropia of 3 PD or more occurs in nearly 12% of patients operated on for intermittent exotropia.[176] Some patients may become constantly esotropic and diplopic (see Chapter 8, Case 19), whereas other patients develop suppression, amblyopia, and loss of stereopsis. That this result is age-dependent has been demonstrated.[176-179] Of 79 patients with surgically-induced consecutive esotropia, 7 of 24 patients (30%) under age 4 lost stereopsis, and 5 of the 24 (22%) became amblyopic.[178] Of 35 patients, 7 (20%) ages 4 to 6 lost stereopsis, and 2 of 35 (6%) became amblyopic. No patient over age 6 developed amblyopia or lost stereopsis, although 10% had diminished stereopsis. In addition, after surgery for intermittent exotropia, patients with consecutive esotropia are more likely to develop A or V patterns than patients who become orthophoric.[180] Because the consecutive esotropia can be small and go unnoticed by the parents, the child's visual problem may become difficult to treat, as illustrated by the following case.

CASE 7

A 9-year-old boy was referred to an optometrist because he failed the school vision screening. The parents indicated that at age 2 his eyes began to turn out occasionally. Six months later he underwent surgery to correct the problem. His last eye exam was at age 3, and everything was fine.

Our evaluation revealed visual acuities of 20/20 and 20/200 for the right and left eyes, respectively. A 5-PD constant left esotropia was present at distance and near. The deviation was comitant. The patient suppressed the left eye with the Worth four dot test and the Bagolini striated lens test at all distances. Stereopsis was not present. Refraction was +0.50 D OU.

Dilated ophthalmoscopy showed normal findings. Visuoscopic evaluation of the left eye revealed 3 degrees nasal eccentric fixation. Attempts to treat the amblyopia with occlusion and orthoptics/vision therapy were not successful.

Comment

For this patient, an occasional exotropia with supposedly good visual acuity and high-grade stereopsis was converted to a cosmetically acceptable microtropia with deep amblyopia and no stereopsis. Because the child's eyes no longer turned outward, the parents assumed good vision. Care must be exercised in balancing the desire for a "real cure" apparently more readily achieved with early surgery versus the potential complications of microtropia, amblyopia, and loss of stereopsis in the young visually developing child.

Because of the kind of situation described in Case 7, we rarely recommend surgery for children younger than age 6, unless the intermittent exotropia is large and very poorly controlled (manifest more than 50% of the time). We prefer the use of minus lenses. For older children, we add orthoptics/vision therapy. With adolescents and adults in whom the exotropia is more likely to be basic or convergence insufficiency, prisms and/or orthoptics/vision therapy can be given. In all age groups, when the exotropia persists after other forms of therapy have been unsuccessful or is larger than 20 PD, surgical therapy can be considered.

 CLINICAL PEARL

Because of the kind of situation described in Case 7, we rarely recommend surgery for children younger than age 6, unless the intermittent exotropia is large and very poorly controlled.

CLINICAL COURSE

The natural history of intermittent exotropia is unclear. Untreated cases can become progressive throughout life, both in degree and frequency, and eventually become constant.[181] The lessened role with age of dynamic factors such as accommodative convergence and powerful fusional convergence likely account for this.

Others have reported that the exotropia remains intermittent and of similar magnitude if untreated.[3,182] It may even improve. There are patients who manifest intermittent exotropia in early childhood and as adults became exophoric without any treatment. Hiles, Davies, and Costenbader[40] followed 48 patients with intermittent exotropia for an average of 11.7 years who for various reasons were never treated. Although there was a general trend toward a small reduction in the exotropia (5 PD), most patients maintained deviations of approximately the same magnitude. Moreover, 31 of 48 patients (64%) ceased to show an exotropic deviation and became exophoric. In a review by von Noorden[3] on 51 untreated patients who were followed for an average of 3.5 years, 75% showed increased frequency and duration of the exotropic phase, whereas 25% either stayed the same or became entirely exophoric.

Our clinical experience agrees with these observations. Intermittent exotropia is a "safe" strabismus. Delay in treatment is unlikely to result in permanently worsened visual status for very young children. When left untreated over the years, its frequency and duration may increase, but fusion will likely not be lost, regardless of the type of intermittent exotropia.[182] The size of the exodeviation remains relatively stable, with the exception of simulated divergence excess intermittent exotropia. Here, the exodeviation at near becomes larger coincident with the general reduction of the patient's convergence function. (See the following cases.)

 CLINICAL PEARL

Intermittent exotropia is a "safe" strabismus. Delay in treatment is unlikely to result in permanently worsened visual status for very young children.

CASE 8

A 5-year-old girl was first examined in April, 1981. The parents reported that the right eye turned out at times. Two years earlier, the child was diagnosed with a muscle imbalance and told to return in a year. The condition has worsened since then, according to her parents. The parents also reported that the child had a tendency to close her right eye when outside and in the sun.

Visual acuities were 20/20 for each eye. A 22-PD right intermittent exotropia was measured at distance, and a 6-PD exophoria was measured at near. Near point of convergence was to the nose. The near exodeviation increased to 14 PD after 2 hours of occlusion. Versions were normal. The youngster suppressed the Worth four dot test at distance and fused at near. With the Titmus stereotest, 60 seconds of arc was perceived. The amplitude of accommodation was adequate for the patient's age, and dynamic retinoscopy revealed a 0.75-D lag OU. Refraction was +0.50 D OU.

The diagnosis was divergence excess intermittent exotropia. Treatment consisted of minus lenses (−2.00 D) and orthoptics/vision therapy. The latter consisted of the TV trainer and vergence training using vectograms and tranaglyphs.

Progress evaluations revealed better control of the exotropia while wearing the minus lenses. Over a period of 2 years the minus lenses were weaned completely, and the patient has remained exophoric. During the last evaluation, the cover test showed 20-PD exophoria at distance and 8-PD exophoria at near. The refractive error had not changed. The parents never noticed an exotropia.

Comment

This is an example of a divergence excess intermittent exotropia treated successfully with minus lenses and orthoptics/vision therapy. The angle of deviation changed little after therapy, as expected. The child's control of the deviation improved, and the exodeviation is now entirely latent.

CASE 9

A 9-year-old girl was referred to our clinic because of an exotropia. The strabismus supposedly began at age 4. Previous treatment consisted of glasses and surgery 1 year earlier. The parents noticed the eye turning out again.

Our examination revealed 20/25 vision for each eye with her habitual glasses (OD −1.00 −1.50 × 50 and OS −1.00 −1.25 × 155). The patient manifested a constant 20-PD alternating exotropia at distance and near. Bilateral inferior oblique overactions and a V pattern with more exodeviation (28 PD) in upgaze were present.

The patient suppressed the right eye with the Worth four dot test at distance and near. No stereopsis was appreciated with the Randot stereotest. Normal correspondence and some fusion were present with the synoptophore. Refraction was identical to her present glasses. Accommodation was normal for the patient's age.

The diagnosis was recurring exotropia. Because of the possibility of fusion, minus lenses over her glasses (−1.50 D) and prisms (total 6 base-in) were provided, as well as orthoptics/vision therapy. The latter consisted mainly of vergence procedures using the minivectogram and the aperture rule. Bar reading and the TV trainer were also included.

Three months later the patient manifested a 15-PD intermittent exotropia at distance and near and had 55 seconds of arc with the TNO stereotest. Orthoptics/vision therapy was changed to include procedures that trained vergence ranges and vergence facility without filters or instruments such as the eccentric circles and lifesaver cards.

We followed the patient for 10 years. Presently, she is 10-PD exophoric at distance and near. She no longer uses added minus lenses, and the prisms have been reduced (total 3 base-in). With the Randot stereotest, 20 seconds of arc exists, and the patient fuses the Worth four dot test at all distances. More importantly, the eyes never drift out, according to the parents.

Comment

This case represents a deteriorated intermittent exotropia that appeared "constant." The exotropia was not helped greatly by surgery. The finding of fusion potential with the synoptophore justified the use of minus lenses and prisms. Excellent compliance with orthoptics/vision therapy was also a factor with the success of this case.

CASE 10

A 20-month-old boy presented to the clinic in October, 1986. The mother reported the child's eyes crossing over the previous 8 months. The child was in good health and had not suffered any trauma.

The child was orthophoric at distance and intermittently esotropic of 15 PD at near. Versions were normal and there was no A or V pattern. Visual acuities could not be measured. Cycloplegic refraction was +1.50 D in both eyes. Ocular health examination was normal. The diagnosis was nonrefractive accommodative esotropia. Treatment consisted of prescribing the refractive findings. The patient was to return in 4 weeks.

Six months later the child, while wearing the glasses, was noted to be exotropic. A 25-PD intermittent exotropia was measured at distance and orthophoria at near. Refraction and versions were similar to the earlier examination. We instructed the parent to not have the child wear the glasses any more and return in 1 month.

Two months later, the child continued to manifest intermittent exotropia at distance and alignment at near. A slight A pattern was now detected, with exodeviation increasing in downgaze. The diagnosis was divergence excess intermittent exotropia. Minus lenses (−1.50 D) were prescribed for constant wear.

In April, 1987, following 1 month of treatment with minus lenses, the patient was orthophoric at distance and near. The mother had not noticed the eye turn out with the glasses.

In October, 1987, alignment was still present with the glasses. When the glasses were removed, a 20-PD exotropia was measured. Refraction was +0.50 D OU.

In April, 1988 the 3-year-old child had 20/20 visual acuity for each eye with the Broken Wheel test. Cover testing with the minus lenses showed 14-PD exophoria at distance and 6-PD exophoria at near. The patient was monitored on a yearly basis.

In April, 1989 the patient had lost the glasses and had not worn them for 2 months. A 25-PD intermittent exotropia at distance and a 15-PD intermittent exotropia were measured at near. The patient was not diplopic. Visual acuity was 20/20 for each eye. No stereopsis was present with the Random-dot E stereotest. Minus lenses were again given.

Over the next 6 years the patient's exodeviation remained well controlled with the minus lenses. However, during that time, he lost his glasses four times and the exotropia became more apparent. Orthoptics/vision therapy was given on a limited basis because of poor compliance. During the last examination the now 9-year-old child again had lost his glasses. A "constant" 25-PD alternating exotropia at distance and a 4-PD exophoria were measured at near. With minus lenses (−1.50), much better control of the exotropia was apparent. Refraction was emmetropia. The child showed 70 seconds of arc with the Randot stereotest. Minus lenses were again prescribed.

Comment

Despite the favorable response with minus lenses, the poor compliance (losing glasses, no orthoptics/vision therapy, missed follow-up visits) should prompt consideration of alternative therapy, such as surgery. Interestingly, this patient at first had a nonrefractive accommodative esotropia and then a divergence excess exotropia. A high AC/A ratio is consistent with the nonrefractive accommodative esotropia and the favorable response with minus lenses.

CASE 11

A 50-year-old man presented with asthenopic symptoms. Specifically, he felt a pulling sensation when reading. He denied any diplopia. Previous treatment had consisted only of glasses. There was no other significant ocular history. The patient was in excellent health.

The patient had 20/20 vision when wearing his glasses (+1.25 −0.75 × 180 OU with +2.00 add). Cover testing revealed an 8-PD intermittent left exotropia at distance and a 20-PD intermittent exotropia at near. Versions were normal, and there was no A or V pattern. The patient fused the Worth four dot test at distance and had crossed diplopia at near. Stereopsis with the Randot stereotest was 60 seconds of arc. Compensensatory vergences (break/recovery) at near were 4/0 for base-out and 20/16 for base-in. The near point of convergence was 15 cm.

The diagnosis was convergence insufficiency intermittent exotropia. Treatment consisted of orthoptics/vision therapy by building up vergence ranges and vergence facility. The patient started with vectographic procedures and was seen on a biweekly basis. Computer orthoptics were done in the clinic. Over a period of 3 months the patient had developed better control of the exotropia and was now using lifesaver cards to exercise chiastopic fusion. Prisms were subsequently prescribed (total 5 base-in) to maintain the results of the therapy.

On his last examination 4 years after undergoing therapy, the patient reported no asthenopia and showed orthophoria at distance and 10-PD exophoria at near. Stereopsis was 30 seconds of arc with the Randot stereotest. Compensatory vergences at near were 18/14 for base-out and 20/16 for base-in. The patient is seen on an annual basis.

Comment

We treat convergence insufficiency intermittent exotropia with orthoptics/vision therapy. Base-in prisms can be helpful, especially in adults, in preventing regression. Not only did the quality of fusion improve, but the magnitude of the deviation became smaller, which was unexpected.

CASE 12

A 12-year-old boy complained of increasing blurred vision and diplopia when reading. These symptoms began about 2 years previously and have become progressively worse. The child is in good health and there had not been any trauma. The patient presently wears glasses for myopia (−0.75D).

Our examination showed corrected vision of 20/20 for each eye. A 2-PD exophoria existed at distance, and a 12-PD intermittent exotropia existed at near. Versions were normal. The patient fused the Worth four dot test at distance and had crossed diplopia at near. Stereopsis of 30 seconds of arc was present with the Randot stereotest. Compensatory vergences (break/recovery) at near were 4/2 base-out and 12/10 base-in. The near point of convergence was 20 cm. Amplitude at accommodation was 13 D for each eye, and dynamic retinoscopy showed a lag of 0.5 D.

The diagnosis was convergence insufficiency intermittent exotropia. The treatment consisted of orthoptics/vision therapy. Over a period of 6 weeks, the patient used physiologic diplopia, minivectograms, tranaglyphs, and eccentric circles to enhance vergence ranges and vergence facility.

At the last visit the patient was asymptomatic. Cover testing showed 2-PD exophoria at distance and 10-PD exophoria at near. Compensatory near vergences were 40/35 (base-out) and 16/12 (base-in). The near point of convergence was to the nose. Maintenance therapy (lifesaver cards) was given, and the patient is presently seen annually and remains exophoric without symptoms.

Comment

The patient had convergence insufficiency intermittent exotropia, which was treated successfully with orthoptics/vision therapy. Usually, this type of deviation is seen in somewhat older patients.

REFERENCES

1. Hugonnier R, Hugonnier S: *Strabismus, heterophoria, and ocular motor paralysis,* St Louis, 1969, Mosby.
2. Nordlow W: Squint: The frequency of onset and different ages and the incidence of some defects in a Swedish population, *Acta Ophthalmol* 42:1015, 1964.
3. von Noorden GK: *Binocular vision and ocular motility: therapy and management of strabismus,* ed 5, St Louis, 1996, Mosby.
4. Krzystkowz K, Pajakowa J: The sensorial state in divergent strabismus. In Mein J, Bierlaagh JJM, Brummel Kamp-Dons TEA, editors: *Proceedings of the Second International Orthoptic Congress,* Amsterdam, 1972, Excerpta Medica.
5. Jenkins R: Demographics, geographic variations in the prevalence and management of exotropia, *Am Orthopt J* 42:82, 1992.
6. Eustace P, Wesson ME, Drury DJ: The effect of illumination on intermittent divergent squint of the divergence excess type, *Trans Ophthalmol Soc U K* 93:559, 1973.
7. Romano PE: The relationship between light and exotropia, *Binoc Vis Eye Muscle Surg* 5:11, 1990.
8. Costenbader FD: The physiology and management of divergent strabismus. In Allen JH, editor: *Strabismic ophthalmic symposium I,* St Louis, 1950, Mosby.
9. Holland G: On the time of onset and the cause of strabismus in early childhood, *Klin Monatsbl Augenheilkd* 147:498, 1965.
10. Lang J: *Strabismus,* Thorofare, NJ, 1984, Slack.
11. Nixon RB and others: Incidence of strabismus in neonates, *Am J Ophthalmol* 100:798, 1985.
12. Sondhi N, Archer SM, Helveston EM: The development of ocular alignment, *J Pediatr Ophthalmol Strab* 25:210, 1988.
13. Archer SM, Sondhi N, Helveston EM: Strabismus in infancy, *Ophthalmology* 96:133, 1989.
14. Cooper J: Intermittent exotropia of the divergence excess type, *J Am Optom Assoc* 48:1261, 1977.
15. Schlossman A, Boruchoff SA: Correlation between physiological aspects of exotropia, *Am J Ophthalmol* 40:53, 1955.
16. Donders FC: *An essay on the nature and the consequences of anomalies of refraction,* Philadelphia, 1899, Blakiston & Son.
17. Burian HM: Pathophysiology of exodeviations. In Manley DR, editor: *Symposium on horizontal ocular deviations,* St Louis, 1971, Mosby.
18. Gregersen E: The polymorphous exo patient: analysis of 231 consecutive cases, *Acta Ophthalmologica* 47:579, 1969.
19. Melek N, Zabulo S, Domingue Z: Intermittent exotropia with bilateral axial high hyperopia: case reports of large but harmless surgical overcorrection, *Binoc Vis Eye Muscle Surg* 8:37, 1993.
20. Abrahamsson M, Fabian G, Sjostrand J: Refraction changes in children developing convergent or divergent strabismus, *Br J Ophthalmol* 76:723, 1992.
21. Davies GT: Vertical deviations associated with exodeviations. In Manley DR, editor: *Symposium on horizontal ocular deviations,* St Louis, 1971, Mosby.
22. Moore S, Stockbridge L, Knapp P: A panoramic view of exotropias, *Am Orthopt J* 27:70, 1977.
23. Wilson ME, Parks MM: Primary inferior oblique overaction in congenital esotropia, accommodative esotropia, and intermittent exotropia, *Ophthalmology* 98:950, 1989.
24. Capo H, Mallette RA, Guyton D: Overacting oblique muscles in exotropia: a mechanical explanation, *J Pediatr Ophthalmol Strab* 25:281, 1988.
25. Moore S: The prognostic value of lateral gaze measurements in intermittent exotropia, *Am Orthopt J* 19:69, 1969.
26. Knapp P: Management of exotropia. In Burian HM and others, editors: *Symposium on strabismus,* St Louis, 1971, Mosby.
27. Martin LP: The effect of lateral incomitance in intermittent exotropia, *Br Orthopt J* 46:49, 1989.

28. Repka MX, Arnold KA: Lateral incomitance in exotropia: fact or artifact? *J Pediatr Ophthalmol Strab* 28:125, 1991.
29. Vargas ME, Warren FA, Kupersmith MJ: Exotropia as a sign of myasthenia gravis in dysthyroid ophthalmopathy, *Br J Ophthalmol* 77:822, 1993.
30. Burke JP, Shipman TC, Watts MT: Convergence insufficiency in thyroid eye disease, *J Pediatr Ophthalmol Strab* 30:127, 1993.
31. Knapp P: Intermittent exotropia: evaluation and therapy, *Am Orthopt J* 3:27, 1953.
32. Carruthers JDA: Strabismus in craniofacial dysostosis, *Graefes Arch Clin Exp Ophthalmol* 226:230, 1988.
33. Blatt AN, Tychsen L: Frequency of infantile esotropia vs exotropia and associated neurologic abnormalities, *Invest Ophthalmol Vis Sci* 36S:593, 1995.
34. Roper-Hall G: Exotropia in neurological disease, *Am Orthopt J* 42:74, 1992.
35. Miller M, Folk E: Strabismus associated with craniofacial anomalies, *Am Orthopt J* 25:27, 1975.
36. Izquierdo NJ, Traboulsi EJ: Strabismus in Marfan syndrome, *Am J Ophthalmol* 117:632, 1994.
37. Tamler E, Jampolsky A: Is divergence active? An electromyographic study, *Am J Ophthalmol* 63:452, 1967.
38. Brenin GM, Moldaver J: Electromyograph of the human extraocular muscles, *Arch Ophthalmol* 54:200, 1955.
39. Ogle KW, Dyer JA: Some observations on intermittent exotropia, *Arch Ophthalmol* 73:58, 1965.
40. Hiles DA, Davies GT, Costenbader FD: Long-term observations on unoperated intermittent exotropia, *Arch Ophthalmol* 80:436, 1968.
41. Hiles DA, Biglan AW: Early surgery of infantile exotropia, *Trans Pa Acad Ophthalmol Otolaryngol* 30:161, 1983.
42. Moore S, Cohen RL: Congenital exotropia, *Am Orthopt J* 35:68, 1985.
43. Rubin SE and others: Infantile exotropia in healthy children, *Ophthalmic Surg* 19:792, 1988.
44. Brodsky MC, Fritz KJ: Hereditary congenital exotropia: a report of three cases, *Binoc Vis Eye Muscle Surg* 8:133, 1993.
45. Biedner B and others: Congenital constant exotropia: surgical results in six patients, *Binoc Vis Eye Muscle Surg* 8:137, 1993.
46. Williams F and others: Congenital exotropia, *Am Orthopt J* 34:92, 1984.
47. Ing MR: Early surgical alignment for congenital esotropia, *Ophthalmology* 90:132, 1983.
48. von Noorden GK: Infantile esotropia: a continuing riddle, *Am Orthopt J* 34:52, 1984.
49. Scheiman M, Ciner E. Gallaway M: Surgical success rates in infantile esotropia, *J Am Optom Assoc* 60:22, 1989.
50. Herzau V, Bleher I, Joos-Kratch E: Infantile exotropia with homonymous hemianopia: a rare contraindication for strabismus surgery, *Graefes Arch Clin Exp Ophthalmol* 226:148, 1988.
51. Sidikaro Y, von Noorden GK: Observations in sensory heterotropia, *J Pediatr Ophthalmol Strab* 19:12, 1982.
52. Kutluk S, Avilla CW, von Noorden GK: The prevalence of dissociated vertical deviation in patients with sensory heterotropia, *Am J Ophthalmol* 119:744, 1995.
53. Pratt-Johnson JA, Tillson G: Intractable diplopia after vision restoration in unilateral cataract, *Am J Ophthalmol* 107:23, 1989.
54. Sharkey JA, Sellar PW: Acquired central disruption following cataract extraction, *J Pediatr Ophthalmol Strab* 31:391, 1994.
55. Kushner BJ: Abnormal sensory findings secondary to monocular cataracts in children and strabismic adults, *Am J Ophthalmol* 102:349, 1986.
56. Ciner EB, Herzberg C: Optometric management of optically induced consecutive exotropia, *J Am Optom Assoc* 63:266, 1992.

57. Groves JS: Spontaneous divergence in cases of convergence strabismus, *Br Orthopt J* 12:79, 1955.
58. Burian HM: Hypermetropia and esotropia, *J Pediatr Ophthalmol Strab* 9:135, 1972.
59. Beneish R and others: Consecutive exotropia after correction of hyperopia, *Can J Ophthalmol* 16:16, 1981.
60. Swan KC: Accommodative esotropia: long-range follow-up, *Ophthalmology* 90:1141, 1983.
61. Fitton MH, Jampolsky A: A case report of spontaneous consecutive esotropia, *Am Orthopt J* 14:144, 1964.
62. Rutstein RP, Daum KM: Exotropia associated with detective accommodation, *J Am Optom Assoc* 58:548, 1987.
63. Aichmar H: *Der Einfluss der Refraktion auf die Operation des Einwartsschielens,* Wissensch Zschur, Mathem Naturwiss Reihe, Leipzig, Karl Marx University, 18:303, 1969.
64. Moore S: The natural course of esotropia, *Am Orthopt J* 21:80, 1971.
65. Parker AR: Effect of passage of time on accommodative strabismus of the convergence excess type, *Br Orthopt J* 17:93, 1960.
66. Rutstein RP and others: Changes in retinal correspondence following changes in ocular alignment, *Optom Vis Sci* 68:325, 1991.
67. Yazawa K: Postoperative exotropia, *J Pediatr Ophthalmol Strab* 18:58, 1981.
68. Cooper EL: The surgical management of secondary exotropia, *Trans Am Acad Ophthalmol Otolaryngol* 65:595, 1961.
69. Folk RF, Miller MR, Chapman L: Consecutive exotropia following surgery, *Br J Ophthalmol* 67:546, 1983.
70. Bietti GB, Bagolini B: Problems related to surgical overcorrections in strabismus surgery, *J Pediatr Ophthalmol Strab* 2:11, 1965.
71. Dunnington JH, Regan EF: Factors influencing the postoperative result in concomitant convergent strabismus, *Arch Ophthalmol* 44:813, 1950.
72. Caputo AR and others: Preferred postoperative alignment after congenital esotropic surgery, *Ann Ophthalmol* 22:269, 1990.
73. Bradbury JA, Doran RML: Secondary exotropia: a retrospective analysis of matched cases, *J Pediatr Ophthalmol Strab* 30:163, 1993.
74. Eskridge JB: Persistent diplopia associated with strabismus surgery, *Optom Vis Sci* 70:849, 1993.
75. Cooper J, Medow N: Intermittent exotropia: basic and divergence excess type, *Binoc Vis Eye Muscle Surg* 8:185, 1993.
76. Burian HM, Franceschetti AT: Evaluation of diagnostic methods for the classification of exodeviations, *Trans Am Ophthalmol Soc* 68:56, 1970.
77. Kran BS, Duckman R: Divergence excess exotropia, *J Am Optom Assoc* 58:921, 1987.
78. Pickwell LD: Prevalence and management of divergence excess, *Am J Optom Physiol Opt* 56:78, 1979.
79. Noorden GK von: Divergence excess and simulated divergence excess, *Doc Ophthalmol* 26:719, 1969.
80. Daum KM: Divergence excess: characteristics and results of treatment with orthoptics, *Ophthalmic Physiol Opt* 4:15, 1984.
81. Matsuo T, Ohtsuki H: Follow-up results of a combination of accommodation and convergence insufficiency in school-age children and adolescents, *Graefes Arch Clin Exp Ophthalmol* 230:166, 1992.
82. Daum KM: Convergence insufficiency, *Am J Optom Physiol Opt* 61:16, 1984.
83. Daum KM: Equal exodeviations: characteristics and results of treatment with orthoptics, *Aust J Optom* 67:53, 1984.
84. Bair DR: Symposium: intermittent exotropia—diagnosis and incidence, *Am Orthopt J* 2:12, 1952.
85. Burian HM, Smith DR: Comparative measurement of exodeviations at twenty and one hundred feet, *Trans Am Ophthalmol Soc* 69:188, 1971.

86. Smith K, Kaban TJ, Orton R: Incidence of amblyopia in intermittent exotropia, *Am Orthopt J* 45:90, 1995.

87. Backman HA: Monocular photophobia, *Am J Optom Physiol Opt* 64:299, 1987.

88. Wiggins RE, Noorden GK von: Monocular eye closure in sunlight, *J Pediatr Ophthalmol Strab* 27:16, 1990.

89. Wang FM, Chryssanthou G: Monocular eye closure in intermittent exotropia, *Arch Ophthalmol* 106:941, 1988.

90. Wirtschafler JR, von Noorden GK: The effect of increasing luminance on exodeviatioin, *Invest Ophthalmol* 3:549, 1964.

91. Williams F, Lachapelle P, Beneish R: Evaluation of the contrast sensitivity function in patients with intermittent exotropia, *Am Orthopt J* 41:77, 1991.

92. Steinbach MJ: Alternating exotropia: temporal course of the switch in suppression, *Invest Ophthalmol Vis Sci* 20:129, 1981.

93. Jampolsky A: Physiology of intermittent exotropia: symposium—intermittent exotropia, *Am Orthopt J* 2:5, 1952.

94. Cooper J, Record CD: Suppresion and retinal correspondence in intermittent exotropia, *Br J Ophthalmol* 70:673, 1986.

95. Pratt-Johnson JA, Pop A, Tillson G: The complexities of suppression in intermittent exotropia. In Mein J, Moore S, editors: *Orthoptics, research, and practice*, London, 1981, Kimpton.

96. Awaya S and others: Studies of suppression in alternating, constant, exotropia and intermittent exotropia with reference to the effects of fusional background. In Moore S, Mein J, Stockbridge L, editors: *Orthoptics, past, present, and future*, New York 1976, Stratton Intercontinental.

97. Melek N and others: Intermittent exotropia: a study of suppression in binocular visual field in 21 cases, *Binoc Vis Eye Muscle Surg* 7:25, 1992.

98. Pritchard C, Flynn JT: Suppression of physiologic diplopia in intermittent exotropia, *Am Orthopt J* 31:72, 1981.

99. Baker JD, Davies GT: Monofixational intermittent exotropia, *Arch Ophthalmol* 97:93, 1979.

100. Galloway-Smith K and others: Monofixation exotropia, *Am Orthopt J* 42:125, 1992.

101. Stathacopoulos RA and others: Distance stereoacuity: assessing control in intermittent exotropia, *Ophthalmology* 100:495, 1993.

102. Rutstein RP, Fuhr P, Schaafsma D: Distance stereopsis in orthophores, heterophores, and intermittent strabismus, *Optom Vis Sci* 71:415, 1994.

103. Rosenbaum AL, Stathacopoulos RA: Subjective and objective criteria for recommending surgery in intermittent exotropia, *Am Orthopt J* 42:46, 1992.

104. Daum KM: Covariation in anomalous correspondence with accommodative vergence, *Am J Optom Physiol Opt* 59:146, 1982.

105. Cooper J, Feldman J: Panoramic viewing, visual acuity of the deviating eye, and anomalous retinal correspondence in intermittent exotropia of the divergence excess type, *Am J Optom Physiol Opt* 56:422, 1979.

106. Gote H, Gregerson E, Rindzunski E: Exotropia and panoramic vision compensating for an occult congenital homonymous hemianopsia: a case report, *Binoc Vis Eye Muscle Surg* 8:129, 1983.

107. von Noorden GK, Brown DJ, Parks M: Associated convergence and accommodation insufficiency, *Doc Ophthalmol* 34:393, 1973.

108. Bugola J: Hypoaccommodative and convergence insufficiency, *Am Orthopt J* 27:85, 1977.

109. Lieppman ME: Accommodative and convergence insufficiency after decompression sickenss, *Arch Ophthalmol* 99:453, 1981.

110. Stark L and others: Accommodative disfacility presenting as intermittent exotropia, *Ophthalmic Physiol Opt* 4:233, 1984.

111. Mazow ML and others: Acute accommodative and convergence insufficiency, *Trans Am Ophthalmol Soc* 87:158, 1989.

112. Plenty JV: The AC/A ratio in intermittent exotropia, *Br Orthopt J* 44:59, 1987.

113. Jampolsky A: Ocular divergence mechanisms, *Trans Am Ophthalmol Soc* 68:703, 1970.

114. Brown W: Accomodative convergence in exodeviation, *Int Ophthalmol Clin* 11:39, 1971.

115. Parks M: Concomitant exodeviation. In Tasman W, Jeager EA, editors: *Duane's clinical ophthalmology,* vol 1, Philadelphia, 1990, JB Lippincott.

116. Manley DR: Classification of the exodeviations. In Manley DR, editor: *Symposium on horizontal ocular deviations,* St Louis, 1971, Mosby.

117. Cooper J: Accommodative dysfunction. In Amos J, editor: *Diagnosis and managment in vision care,* Boston, 1987, Butterworth-Heinemann.

118. Ogle KN, Dyer JA: Some observations on intermittent exotropia, *Am Orthopt J* 13:20, 1963.

119. Cooper J, Ciuffreda KJ, Kruger PB: Stimulus and response AC/A ratios in intermittent exotropia of the divergence excess type, *Br J Ophthalmol* 66:398, 1982.

120. Jampolsky A: Physiology of intermittent exotropia, *Br Orthopt J* 44:59, 1987.

121. Kushner BJ: Exotropic deviations: a functional classification and approach to treatment, *Am Orthopt J* 38:81, 1988.

122. Niederecker O, Scott W: The value of diagnostic occlusion for intermittent exotropia, *Am Orthopt J* 25:90, 1975.

123. Burian HM, Spivey BE: The surgical management of exodeviations, *Trans Am Ophthalmol Soc* 62:276, 1964.

124. Noorden GK von: Divergence excess and simulated divervence excess: diagnosis and surgical management, *Doc Ophthalmol* 26:719, 1969.

125. Coffey B and others: Treatment options in intermittent exotropia: a critical appraisal, *Optom Vis Sci* 69:386, 1992.

126. Kushner BJ: Surgical pearls for the management of intermittent exotropia, *Am Orthopt J* 42:65, 1992.

127. Iacobucci IL, Archer SM, Giles GL: Children with exotropia responsive to spectacle correction of hyperopia, *Am J Ophthalmol* 116:79, 1993.

128. London R: Passive treatments for early onset strabismus. In Scheiman MM, editor: *Problems in optometry*, Philadelphia, 1990, JB Lippincott.

129. Rutstein RP, Marsh-Tootle W, London R: Changes in refractive error for exotropes treated with overminus lenses, *Optom Vis Sci* 66:487, 1989.

130. Kennedy JR: The correction of divergent strabismus with concave lenses, *Am J Optom* 31:605, 1954.

131. Merrick F: Use of concave lenses in the management of intermittent divergent squint, *Aust Orthopt J* 12:13, 1975.

132. Caltrider N, Jampolsky A: Overcorrecting minus lens therapy for treatment of intermittent exotropia, *Ophthalmology* 90:1160, 1983.

133. Goodacre H: Minus overcorrection: conservative treatment of intermittent exotropia in the young child—a comparative study, *Aust Orthopt J* 22:9, 1985.

134. Iacobucci SL, Mertanyi EJ, Giles CL: Results of overminus lens therapy on post-operative exodeviations, *J Pediatr Ophthalmol Strab* 23:287, 1986.

135. Donaldson PJ, Kemp EG: An initial study of the treatment of intermittent exotropia by minus overcorrection, *Br Orthopt J* 48:41, 1991.

136. Reynolds JD, Wackerhagen M, Olitsky SE: Overminus lens therapy for intermittent exotropia, *Am Orthopt J* 44:86, 1994.

137. Berg PH, Isenberg SJ: Treatment of unilateral exotropia by part-time occlusion, *Am Orthopt J* 41:72, 1991.

138. Iacobucci I, Henderson JW: Occlusion in the preoperative treatment of exodeviaions, *Am Orthopt J* 15:42, 1965.

139. Freeman BS, Isenberg SJ: The use of part-time occlusion for early onset unilateral exotropia, *J Pediatr Ophthalmol Strab* 26:94, 1989.

140. Mims JL, Wood RC: The effect of preoperative alternate day patching on surgical results in intermittent exotropia: a retrospective study of 66 cases, *Binoc Vis Eye Muscle Surg* 5:189, 1990.

141. Chutter CP: Occlusion treatment of intermittent divergent strabismus, *Am Orthopt J* 27:80, 1977.

142. Spoor DK, Hiles DA: Occlusion therapy for exodeviations occurring in infants and young children, *Ophthalmology* 86:2152, 1979.

143. Romano PE, Wilson MF: Survey of current management of intermittent exotropia in the USA and Canada. In Campos EC, editor: *Strabismus and ocular motility disorders,* Indianapolis, Ind, 1990, Macmillan.

144. Flynn JT, McKenney S, Rosenhouse M: Management of intermittent exotropia. In Moore S, Mein J, Stockbridge L, editors: *Orthoptics, past, present, and future,* New York, 1976, Stratton Intercontinental.

145. Hardesty HH: Management of intermittent exotropia, *Binoc Vis Eye Muscle Surg* 5:145, 1990.

146. Pratt-Johnson, JA, Tillson G: Prismotherapy in intermittent exotropia: a preliminary report, *Can J Ophthalmol* 14:243, 1979.

147. Veronneau-Troutman S, Shippman S, Clahane AC: Prisms as an orthoptic tool in the management of primary exotropia. In Moore S, Mein J, Stockbridge L, editors: *Orthoptics, past, present, and future,* New York: 1976, Stratton Intercontinental.

148. Shippman S and others: Prisms in the pre-operative diagnosis of intermittent exotropia, *Am Orthopt J* 38:101, 1988.

149. Baker JD: Future research directions in intermittent exotropia, *Am Orthopt J* 42:98, 1992.

150. Singh V, Roy S, Sinha S: Role of orthoptic treatment in the management of intermittent exotropia, *Indian J Ophthalmol* 40:83, 1992.

151. Frantz KA: The importance of multiple treatment modalities in a case of divergence excess, *J Am Optom Assoc* 61:457, 1990.

152. Gallaway M, Vaxmonsky T, Scheiman M: Management of intermittent exotropia using a combination of vision therapy and surgery, *J Am Optom Assoc* 60:428, 1989.

153. Letourneau JE, Giroux R: Using biofeedback in an exotropic aphake, *J Am Optom Assoc* 55:909, 1984.

154. Daum KM: Modelling the results of the orthoptic treatment of divergence excess, *Ophthalmic Physiol Opt* 4:25, 1984.

155. Sanflippo S, Clahane A: Effectiveness of orthoptics alone in selected cases of exodeviation: the immediate results and several years later, *Am Orthopt J* 20:104, 1970.

156. Flax N, Duckman RH: Orthoptic treatment of strabismus, *J Am Optom Assoc* 49:1353, 1978.

157. Duckman RH: Management of binocular anomalies: efficacy of vision therapy—exotropia, *Am J Optom Physiol Opt* 64:421, 1987.

158. Goldrich SG: Optometric therapy of divergence excess strabismus, *Am J Optom Physiol Opt* 57:7, 1980.

159. Griffin JR: *Binocular anomalies: procedures for vision therapy,* ed 2, Chicago, 1982, Professional.

160. Rosner J, Rosner J: *Vision therapy in primary care practice,* New York, 1988, Professional.

161. Daum KM: Characteristics of exodeviations. II. Changes with treatment with orthoptics, *Am J Optom Physiol Opt* 63:244, 1986.

162. Goldrich SG: Oculomotor biofeedback therapy for exotropia, *Am J Optom Physiol Opt* 59:306, 1982.

163. Chryssanthou G: Orthoptic management of intermittent exotropia, *Am Orthopt J* 24:69, 1974.

164. Etting GL: Strabismus therapy in private practice: cure rates after three months of therapy, *J Am Optom Assoc* 49:1367, 1978.

165. Alfanador AJ: Auditory biofeedback and intermittent exotropia, *J Am Optom Assoc* 53:481, 1982.

166. Deleted in galleys.

167. Newman J, Mazow ML: Intermittent exotropia: is surgery necessary? *Ophthalmol Surg* 12:199, 1981.

168. Veronneau-Troutman S: Intermittent exotropia, *Ophthalmol Clin* 11:114, 1971.

169. Reynolds JD, Wackerhagen M: Early onset exodeviations, *Am Orthopt J* 38:34, 1988.

170. Seaber JH: Orthoptic treatment of divergence excess type deviation, *Am Orthopt J* 28:119, 1968.

171. Jampolsky A: Treatment of exodeviations: pediatric ophthalmology and strabismus. In *Transactions of the New Orleans Academy of Ophthalmology,* New York, 1986, Raven.

172. Raab EL, Parks MM: Recession of the lateral recti, *Arch Ophthalmol* 82:203, 1969.

173. Souza-Dias C, Uesuguci CF: Postoperative evolution of the planned initial overcorrection in exotropia: 61 cases, *Binoc Vis Eye Muscle Surg* 8:141, 1993.

174. Scott WE, Keach RV, Mash AJ: The postoperative results and stability of exodeviations, *Arch Ophthalmol* 99:8114, 1981.

175. Beneish R, Flanders M: The role of stereopsis and early postoperative alignment in long-term surgical results of intermittent exotropia, *Can J Ophthalmol* 29:119, 1994.

176. Keech RV, Stewart SA: The surgical overcorrection of intermittent exotropia, *J Pediatr Ophthalmol Strab* 27:218, 1990.

177. Cooper EL: Purposeful overcorrection in exotropia. In Arruga A, editor: *International strabismus symposium,* (University of Giessen, 1966), New York, 1968, S Karger.

178. Edelman PM and others: Consecutive esotropia....then what? *Am Orthopt J* 38:111, 1988.

179. Pratt-Johnson JA, Barlow JM, Tillson G: Early surgery in intermittent exotropia, *Am J Ophthalmol* 84:689, 1977.

180. Miller MM, Guyton DL: Loss of fusion and the development of A or V patterns, *J Pediatr Ophthalmol Strab* 31:220, 1994.

181. Jampolsky A: Differential diagnostic characteristics of intermittent exotropia and true exophoria, *Am Orthopt J* 4:48, 1954.

182. Goldstein JH, Schneekloth BB: The potential for binocular vision in constant exotropia, *Am Orthopt J* 43:67, 1993.

An incomitant (noncomitant, nonconcomitant) deviation is a heterophoric or strabismic deviation that changes by more than 5 PD for a given fixation distance in the different directions of gaze and/or with each eye fixating in turn. There is consistency in the way the deviation changes, so that it is always greater in one particular direction for any particular patient each time the eyes are turned in that direction. The angle of deviation increases as the eyes make a version movement in one direction and decreases when the eyes make a version movement in another direction. The misalignment of the visual axes is markedly asymmetric between one position of gaze and the other. In incomitant strabismus, the magnitude of the angle changes in different gaze positions, and, on occasion, the direction of the strabismus may also reverse. A patient manifesting an incomitant deviation may be strabismic in one position of gaze and heterophoric or orthophoric in another. A deviation may be either horizontally or vertically incomitant. Most vertical deviations greater than a few prism diopters are incomitant.

For a deviation to be classified as incomitant, it must vary in amount by more than 5 PD, depending on the direction of gaze and not according to changes in fusional status. A patient with a 15-PD exophoria in downgaze and 15-PD exotropia in upgaze therefore does not have an incomitant deviation, because the magnitude does not vary; only the frequency varies.

Incomitant deviations are either paretic or the result of mechanical restriction. They are caused by lesions in the final motor pathway, such as may occur in the nuclear region, the peripheral nerve, the extraocular muscle, or adjacent structures. Paretic deviations account for the majority of incomitant deviations.

The doll's-head maneuver (the oculocephalic reflex) is useful in differentiating supranuclear and infranuclear ocular motility restrictions. Forced gentle rotation of the head from side to side or vertically will normally produce eye movement in the opposite direction. If the site of the lesion is supranuclear, the eyes will deviate fully in the direction of the ocular motility restriction. If the site is nuclear or infranuclear, which is the case with incomitant deviations, the ocular motility restriction is still present.

Incomitant deviations are accompanied by extraocular muscle underactions and/or extraocular muscle overactions in particular directions of gaze. Underactions result from (1) involvement or weakness of the muscle itself, (2) mechanical or structural disorders adjacent to the muscle, or (3) innervational disturbances to either the oculomotor (third), trochlear (fourth), or abducens (sixth) cranial nerves that innervate the extraocular muscles. Mechanical disorders may include abnormal muscle insertion, abnormal adhesion between the muscles or surrounding tissues, variation in orbital shape such as occurs in Apert's and Crouzon's syndromes, contracture or tightening of the conjunctiva, scar tissue formation following muscle surgery, cheek ligament abnormalities, and abnormal insertion of the muscle tendons into the globe. These physical factors interfere with muscle contraction or relaxation and prevent free movement of the globe.

Muscle overactions also result from mechanical disorders. More commonly, they are attributed to Hering's law of equal innervation. Hering's law states that corresponding, or yoke, muscles of each eye, such as

TABLE 10-1   CLINICAL FEATURES OF CONGENITAL VERSUS RECENTLY ACQUIRED INCOMITANT DEVIATIONS

Features	Congenital	Acquired
Diplopia	Infrequent (may occur with decompensation)	Frequent (always greatest in at least one position of gaze)
Abnormal head posture	Usually present (patient is not aware of it)	Usually absent
Difference between primary and secondary angles of deviation	Absent for paretic deviations; present with mechanically restrictive deviations	Present
Amblyopia/suppression	May be present	Absent
Limitation in ocular motility	Not severe with paretic deviations; marked with mechanically restrictive deviations	Severe
Course	Static	Dynamic
Onset	Uncertain	Sudden and distressing
Associated neurologic findings or systemic disease	Rare	Frequent

Modified from Rutstein RP: Incomitant deviations in children. In Scheiman MM, editor: *Problems in optometry,* vol 2, Philadelphia, 1990, JB Lippincott.

the left lateral rectus and right medial rectus, receive equal innervation so that the eyes move together. When a muscle in one eye is paretic or mechanically restricted and the patient fixates with that eye, overaction of the yoke muscle will occur because of the excessive innervation required of the paretic eye.

Certain extraocular muscle overactions, cannot always be attributed to mechanical causes or Hering's law. These overactions usually involve the oblique muscles and are frequently seen accompanying other types of strabismic deviations. Overaction of the inferior oblique, which causes elevation of the eye in adduction, is considered to be a primary overaction and is not secondary to a mechanical or paretic etiology. It is a frequent incomitant deviation seen in clinical practice.

The prognosis for maintaining or achieving normal binocular vision is likely greater for incomitant deviations than for comitant deviations. Amblyopia, suppression, and anomalous correspondence are less frequent with incomitant deviations and even when present may not be as detrimental to the establishment of normal binocular vision. Three explanations account for this. First, because many incomitant deviations are paretic, their onset may occur later in life than the onset of comitant strabismus. The later onset prevents sensory adaptations from developing, because such adaptations are limited to the period of early childhood. Second, sensory adaptations may be prevented in all positions of gaze and fusion maintained in the other positions by the acquisition of a compensatory head posture. Third, sensory adaptations, when present, may only be superficially established. Because of the changing size of the deviation in the different positions of gaze, the intensity of suppression, for example, may be lessened. The suppression zone is not fixed, as with comitant strabismus.

 CLINICAL PEARL

The prognosis for maintaining or achieving normal binocular vision is likely greater for incomitant deviations than for comitant deviations.

Incomitant deviations may be congenital or acquired. These deviations frequently present with different clinical features and case histories (Table 10-1).[1] Congenital deviations include deviations for which the onset is either before, during, or shortly after birth and all deviations whose onset is before 6 months of age. Some clinicians also include as congenital any incomitant deviation whose onset dated back to early life, with the absence of a specific cause located at a later point in time. Supporting evidence of a congenital incomitant deviation is a history of abnormal eye position, photographs of abnormal childhood head posture, and no history of head trauma.

Congenital incomitant deviations frequently occur as isolated defects in otherwise normal patients. They may also occur in children with developmental neurologic disorders, such as hydrocephalus and cerebral palsy, or may be associated with antenatal infections and birth trauma.[2,3]

Acquired incomitant deviations refer generally to deviations that commence after 6 months of age. Such deviations are frequently the presenting feature of an underlying disease. Common causes of acquired incomitant deviations in children include trauma, tumor, and neoplasm; vascular etiologies, such as diabetes and hypertension, are more common causes for adults.[4,5] In some cases, there may be no definite cause. In a report on 4176 patients with incomitant deviations that were paretic in origin, the cause remained undetermined for 1037 patients (24.8%), despite extensive neurologic and medical tests.[6]

Generally, patients who complain of little or no visual disturbance despite having an obvious incomitant deviation usually have had the deviation from early life. Childhood-onset deviations may as a result of some transient illness, increasing stress, or an unknown cause decompensate when the patient is older and present all the symptoms of a recently acquired deviation. Previous photographs may be needed to confirm the diagnosis of a decompensated congenital deviation. Decompensation can occur with patients who have early-onset superior oblique paresis, as indicated by the following case.

CASE 1

A 22-year-old woman presented with intermittent vertical diplopia of 1 month's duration.[7] There was no preceding illness or recent trauma. Corrected vision in each eye with a mild myopic correction was 20/20. The cover test showed an intermittent right hypertropia in primary position. Versions and the three-step test were consistent with a right superior oblique paresis. The patient showed no torsion with the double Maddox rod test and was unaware of any image tilting. The patient's mother recalled that when the patient was 2 years old, she fell from her crib and suffered a head injury. An "eye muscle problem" was diagnosed at that time. It was concluded that the patient had a long-standing superior oblique paresis that had recently decompensated from hyperphoria to hypertropia. Treatment with prisms eliminated the diplopia.

EXAMINATION AND DIAGNOSIS

The methods used in evaluating incomitant deviations should include (1) detection of an abnormal head posture, (2) the alternating cover test with prisms in the different positions of gaze, (3) evaluation of ductions and versions, (4) diplopia fields, (5) the Hess-Lancaster test, (6) the three-step test, (7) tests for torsion, and (8) sensory fusion testing in the different positions of gaze.

ABNORMAL HEAD POSTURE

An abnormal, or compensatory, head posture becomes readily apparent during the initial part of the examination. Although there are several causes of abnormal head posture, such as unilateral deafness, enlarged or tender cervical lymph nodes, a tight sternomastoid muscle on one side, or even uncorrected refractive error, ocular movement abnormalities associated with incomitant deviations are the most common. Assessment of head posture can frequently assist in determining the extraocular muscle at fault. Patients with incomitant deviations frequently adjust their heads in positions that compensate for the deviation and permits binocular vision, eliminates diplopia, or places the fixating eye in the most comfortable position. This is

known as *ocular torticollis*. Patients usually position their heads to reduce the need for the affected muscle to contract. In the case of a paretic deviation, the head is placed in the field of action of the involved muscle, and the doll's-head maneuver causes the eyes to move out of the field of action of the involved extraocular muscle.

CLINICAL PEARL

Patients with incomitant deviations frequently adjust their heads in positions that compensate for the deviation and permits binocular vision, eliminates diplopia, or places the fixating eye in the most comfortable position.

Abnormal head posture may be one of three types. The first type is a head turn to either the right or left. This can be a sign of weakness of either the medial or lateral rectus muscle. For example, diplopia may be avoided and fusion maintained with left lateral rectus weakness by turning the face to the left so that contraction of the left lateral rectus is not required (Fig. 10-1). The second type of abnormal head posture is a head or chin elevation or a head or chin depression. This may occur with weakness to either of the vertically acting muscles or in A or V patterns with which the size of the horizontal deviation changes significantly between up and down gaze. With an A-pattern esodeviation the patient may use a chin elevation to place the eyes in downgaze, in which fusion is more likely to be achieved (Fig. 10-2). The third type is a head tilt to counteract torsional and vertical diplopia. A head tilt is more likely for patients with inferior or superior oblique paresis (Fig. 10-3).

Frequently, abnormal head posture consists of multiple components. Because the cyclovertical muscles (superior rectus, inferior rectus, superior oblique, inferior oblique) have three actions, the head posture becomes more complex and may include all three types. The position of the head will mimic the action of the affected cyclovertical muscle. A patient with a hypertropia caused by a paretic superior oblique, for example, may not only tilt the head to the opposite side but also depress the chin and occasionally turn the head to the opposite side. With this posture, the patient is more likely to maintain binocular vision and/or avoid diplopia.

Table 10-2 lists the possible compensatory head postures according to the extraocular muscle involved. It is apparent that the head posture the patient uses is fairly consistent for the horizontal rectus and oblique muscles but not the vertical rectus muscles. For the latter the descriptions of head position are likely based more on theoretic considerations than actual observation of the patient.

Abnormal head postures are not always present with incomitant deviations. Patients with expanded fu-

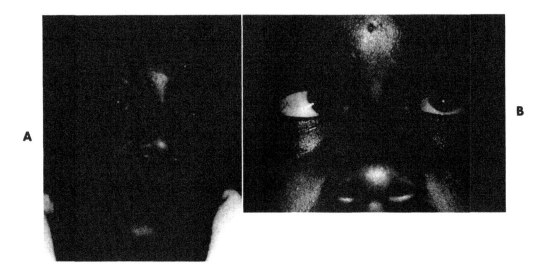

FIG. 10-1 Compensatory head posture for patient with left lateral rectus weakness. **A,** Head turn to left. **B,** No abduction for left eye. (From Rutstein RP: Incomitant deviations in children. In MM Scheiman, editor: *Problems in optometry,* vol 2, Philadelphia, 1990, JB Lippincott.)

TABLE 10-2 PROBABLE HEAD POSITION FOR PATIENTS WITH INCOMITANT DEVIATIONS

Muscle Involved	Face Turn	Chin	Head Tilt
Right medial rectus	Left	—	—
Right lateral rectus	Right	—	—
Right superior rectus	Right	Up	Right
	Left	Up	Left
Right inferior rectus	Right	Down	Left
	Left	Down	Right
Right superior oblique	Left	Down	Left
Right inferior oblique	Left	Up	Right
Left medial rectus	Right	—	—
Left lateral rectus	Left	—	—
Left superior rectus	Left	Up	Right
	Right	Up	Left
Left inferior rectus	Left	Down	Right
	Right	Down	Left
Left superior oblique	Right	Down	Right
Left inferior oblique	Right	Up	Left

sional vergence amplitudes or amblyopia and no fusion ability may not need to adjust their heads.[8] Also, not all patients adjust their heads to permit fusion. Some patients may place their heads in the opposite field so that the eyes are moved into the field of the involved muscle. This head posture supposedly increases the separation between diplopic images, and the patient is less troubled with diplopia.

Furthermore, the head posture in congenital and long-standing deviations may not follow the expected pattern, particularly if the patient fixates with the involved eye or if marked contracture or tightening of the antagonist muscle develops. For example, with paresis of the left superior rectus, the head is usually expected to be tilted to the right (see Table 10-2). If the patient fixates with the paretic eye, according to Hering's law, overaction of the right inferior oblique occurs, with subsequent inhibitional palsy and underaction of the right superior oblique. Because the right superior oblique is a greater intorter than the left superior rectus, the patient may tilt the head to the left to confuse the picture.

Any abnormal head posture should always raise concern because it may cause neck strain; if left untreated, secondary scoliosis, contracture of the neck muscles, and, possibly, facial asymmetry may result.

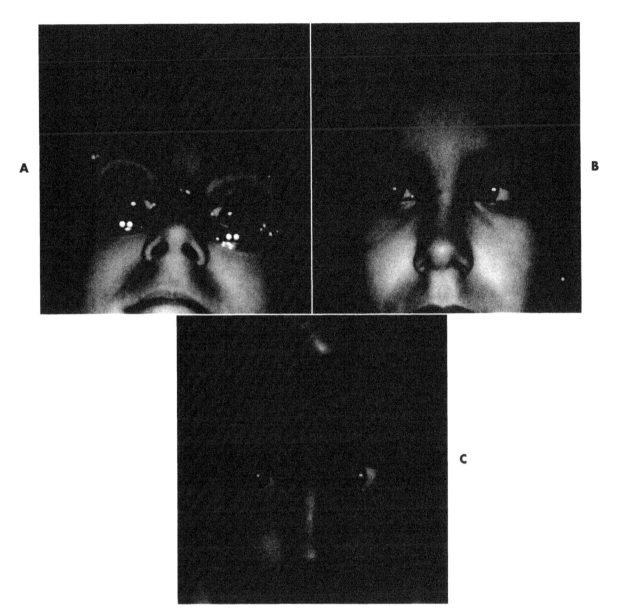

FIG. 10-2 Compensatory head posture for patient with A-pattern esotropia. **A,** Chin elevation allows fusion in downgaze. **B,** Esotropia exists in primary position and **(C)** in upgaze.

COVER TEST

With incomitant deviations, the alternate cover test with prisms is done initially with the sound eye fixating (the prisms are placed before the eye with the involved muscle), and the deviation is measured in the primary position, right and left gaze, and in 30 degrees of elevation and depression. If there is also a vertical deviation, oblique and head tilt measurements are added. Loose hand-held prisms are preferred when measuring combined horizontal and vertical deviations.

The cover test is repeated with the involved eye fixating (the prisms are placed over the sound eye). The detection of a larger movement of redress in one eye than the other helps identify the weak member of a yoke muscle pair. In accordance with Hering's law of equal innervation, with one eye covered, the fixating eye will determine the amount of innervation transmitted to both eyes. Excessive innervation is required to move and maintain the eye in primary position. The same amount of innervation flows simultaneously to the yoke muscle in the sound eye, and the angle of deviation is larger when the patient uses the eye with the weak muscle for fixation than when the patient fixates with the sound eye. The deviation with the sound eye fixating is known as the *primary angle* and the devia-

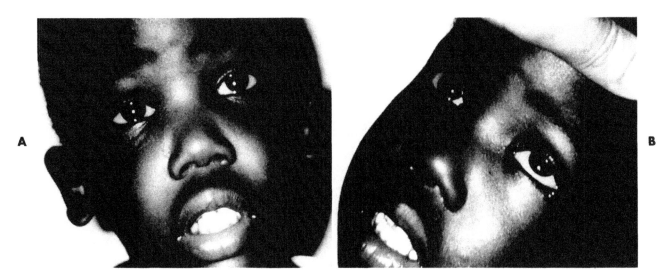

Fig. 10-3 Compensatory head posture for a patient with left superior oblique paresis. **A,** Head tilt to right allows fusion. **B,** Left hypertropia is manifest with head tilt left. (From Rutstein RP: Incomitant deviations in children. In MM Scheiman, editor: *Problems in optometry,* vol 2, Philadelphia, 1990, JB Lippincott.)

tion with the involved eye fixating is the *secondary angle.* In recently acquired paretic deviations, the secondary angle exceeds the primary angle. In congenital and chronic paretic deviations, these measures tend to become similar. In deviations caused by mechanical restriction, the secondary deviation exceeds the primary deviation, regardless of time of onset. Although usually measured for primary position, primary and secondary deviations can exist for any direction of gaze.

 CLINICAL PEARL

In recently acquired paretic deviations, the secondary angle exceeds the primary angle. In congenital and chronic paretic deviations, these measures tend to become similar.

When there is marked mechanical restriction to ocular motility, the Hirschberg or Krimsky tests, rather than the alternating cover test with prisms, can be used to quantify the incomitancy.

TESTS FOR OCULAR MOTILITY

Ocular motility testing evaluates extraocular muscle for overactions and underactions. It may also be used to differentiate incomitant deviations that are paretic from those that are mechanically restricted. Ocular motility is investigated by evaluating duction and version eye movements. Both tests are best performed with the patient's glasses removed.

Ductions are monocular eye movements. The movements are described as adduction, abduction, supraduction, and infraduction for the secondary posi-

tions of nasal, temporal, up, and down. While one eye is occluded and the head is erect, the patient is asked to follow a fixation target, preferably a penlight, with the uncovered eye, from the primary position to each of the secondary and tertiary positions. In the case of a young child, a toy can be used. The clinician notes any limitations in eye movement that persist despite vigorous encouragement. Abduction, adduction, and infraduction should have at least 10 mm of rotation. Supraduction is normal at 5 to 7 mm.

Versions are binocular conjugate movements of the eyes, allowing the lines of sight to move in a parallel direction. In the secondary positions, these are termed *dextroversion, levoversion, supraversion,* and *infraversion* for right, left, up, and down version movements. As with ductions, the head is erect and motionless while the patient binocularly follows the fixation target in all positions. The clinician notes whether both eyes move fully and simultaneously or there is limitation or excessive movement of the nonfixating eye in a particular gaze position. By using a penlight and noting differences in the corneal reflections in the various positions, the test becomes more sensitive. If there is a change in the position of the corneal reflection of the two eyes, there is either an overaction or underaction in the movement of one of the eyes in that direction. It is important for the clinician to keep aligned with the penlight. This is achieved most easily if the patient's head is rotated during fixation of a stationary penlight. This method is especially valuable when facial asymmetries, such as hypertelorism, ptosis, or epicanthal folds give a false impression of incomitance.

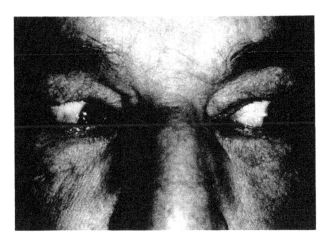

FIG. 10-4 Slight (−1) underaction of left eye in abduction.

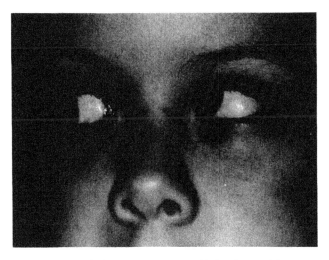

FIG. 10-5 Slight (+1) overaction of left inferior oblique.

At the extreme of the version movement, an end-point nystagmus may be noted. Although end-position nystagmus is usually considered normal, accentuated end-point nystagmus may indicate an internuclear ophthalmoplegia or muscle paresis.

Results of ductions and versions can be recorded on a 4-point scale. Overactions are considered positive and rate +1 to +4, whereas underactions are considered negative and are rated −1 to −4. A normal movement is rated 0. Supposedly, each number represents a difference of 25% compared with normal movement. With a lateral rectus weakness, for example, −1 represents slight (25%) underaction (Fig. 10-4), and −4 means the eye does not extend beyond the midline (Fig. 10-1, *B*). Similarly, with inferior oblique overaction, +1 represents slight overaction (Fig. 10-5), and +4 means a good portion of the cornea disappears during adduction (Fig. 10-6).

Duction testing may not be as sensitive as version testing. Normal ductions rule out mechanical restriction of ocular motility but do not exclude the possibility of paresis of an extraocular muscle. When a patient performs a duction movement with an eye that has a paretic muscle, excessive innervation will flow to that eye in accordance with Hering's law, so that the needed movement may actually be made. This can conceal any ocular motility restriction. Version testing, however, will show the overacting and underacting muscles. Comparing ductions and versions is used as a method for differentiating incomitant deviations that are paretic from those that are caused by mechanical restriction. Ductions will equal versions in mechanically restrictive deviations and will exceed versions in recently acquired paretic deviations.[9] We have used duction versus versions to help distinguish the deficient elevation in adduction caused by an inferior oblique paresis from that caused by Brown's syndrome.

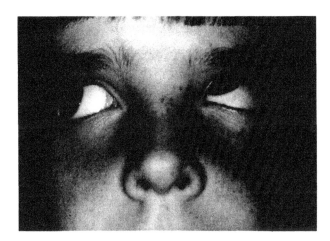

FIG. 10-6 Marked (+4) overaction of left inferior oblique.

A form of duction test used to further differentiate paretic from mechanically restrictive incomitant deviations is the forced duction test, or traction test. This test requires use of topical anesthetic such as tetracaine or cocaine. The patient is asked to fixate an object toward the side of limited gaze. It is important to instruct the patient to look up when there is restriction to elevation. The patient's eye is then grasped at the conjunctiva and moved by the clinician using forceps or a cotton-tipped applicator at the limbus to determine if any obstruction to motility exists (Fig. 10-7). The patient looks at his or her hand, which is extended in the direction of limitation of movement. Care is taken not to press the eye into the orbit during the test, because this may simulate a negative finding when, in fact, restrictions are present. If the clinician can rotate the eye with forceps past the point of the patient's voluntary

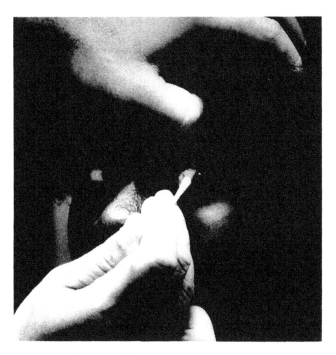

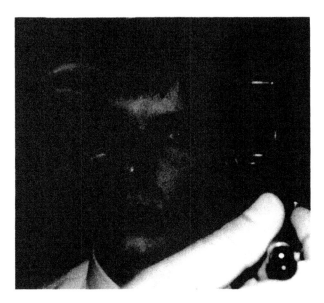

FIG. 10-8 Diplopia fields testing with red lens.

FIG. 10-7 The forced duction test. (From Rutstein RP: Paretic muscle determination. In Eskridge JB, Amos JF, Bartlett JD, editors: *Clinical procedures in optometry,* Philadelphia, 1991, JB Lippincott.)

rotational limit during extreme gaze attempts, a paresis exists. This is indicated because a restriction has been ruled out. If the clinician cannot augment the eyes by the forced duction test, a mechanical restriction exists. In some case, restrictions cannot be determined until the extraocular muscle is exposed at surgery.[10] In addition, a long-standing paresis may result in the muscle's antagonist developing contracture or tightening and producing a positive forced duction test. For example, in recently acquired superior oblique paresis, the forced duction test would be negative. In superior oblique paresis of long standing, the forced duction test may become positive because of contracture or tightening of the ipsilateral inferior oblique.

A form of testing known as *saccadic velocity* has also been used to distinguish between paretic and mechanically restrictive incomitant deviations.[11-15] Saccadic velocity corroborates generation of muscle force. The patient's eye movements are charted by the electro-oculogram, a method not usually available in an office environment. The speed of saccadic movements produced by a paretic muscle is reduced in velocity in its field of action, whereas in a mechanically restrictive deviation, the speed of saccadic velocity in the affected position of gaze is normal.

Saccadic velocities can be estimated by direct observation.[16] The patient fixates first on the clinician's

nose in the midline, and then the clinician's index finger is held to either side. The clinician observes the relative speed of the two eyes as conjugate movements are made. If a muscle is paretic, the eye that is moving into the field of action of the paretic muscle will move more slowly than the other eye as the eyes conjugately fixate.

An increase in intraocular pressure of 5 mm or more when the eye is moved toward the position of limited motility compared with the opposite direction is diagnostic of a mechanically restrictive type of incomitant deviation. The best example is thyroid myopathy. A hand-held applanation type of tonometry is ideal for this measurement.

DIPLOPIA FIELDS (RED LENS TEST)

This subjective test differentiates comitant from incomitant deviations by determining the separation between diplopic images in the primary, secondary, and tertiary positions of gaze. If retinal correspondence is normal and suppression is not deep, this represents a measure of the deviation. This test lets the clinician monitor the improvement or deterioration of the incomitancy.

Two principles are important in this type of diplopia testing. The first is that the two images will be maximally separated when the patient looks in the direction of action of the weak muscle. The second is that the target seen by the involved eye is always projected more peripherally.

A red lens is placed before the sound eye while the patient views a penlight in the different directions of gaze (Fig. 10-8). The use of the red lens lets each eye see an object of different color, and the patient will

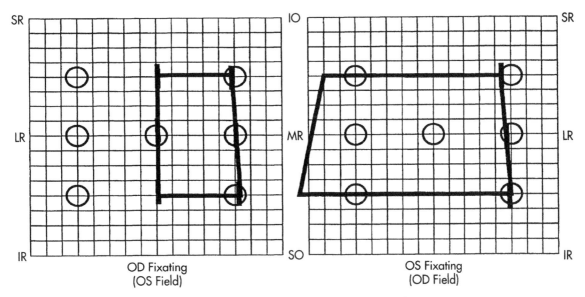

FIG. 10-9 Hess-Lancaster charts for patient with left lateral rectus paresis.

have less trouble distinguishing one image from the other. The test is performed at 1 m, and the patient describes the respective positions of the two images. With incomitance, the red and white images will be separated to a greater degree in the position in which the deviation is greatest. The furthest image belongs to the affected eye, which is identified by the color of the light. The affected muscle can be diagnosed when the field producing the greatest deviation is known. The separation can be quantified with prism until superimposition of the images occurs. Measurements should also be made with the red lens before the involved eye to determine the presence of primary and secondary angles of deviation. In recently acquired paretic deviations, when the paretic eye fixates (secondary deviation), the separation of the diplopic images will be greater than when the nonparetic eye fixates (primary deviation).

HESS-LANCASTER TEST

The Hess-Lancaster test provides another way of recording the degree of incomitance and other information that will help the assessment and progress of the condition. This subjective test measures the deviation in the primary, secondary, and tertiary positions but has additional value in giving a graphic representation of the deviation.[17] The apparatus consists of a screen marked in red lines on a white cloth, along with a red target projector and a green target projector. The screen is ruled into squares of 7 cm, so that at a 1-m test distance each square subtends approximately 7 PD. The patient is seated 1 m from the screen, with the head erect, stationary, and opposite the center of the screen. The patient wears red-green glasses while being tested and holds the green target vertically while the clinician holds the red target horizontally. The eye with the red filter becomes the fixating eye. The patient is asked to superimpose the green streak projected by the flashlight he or she holds on the red one projected on the screen by the clinician. When the subjective superimposition is complete, the positions of the streaks on the screen indicate the relative positions of the lines of sight. If the two streaks are separated, the distance between them is a measure of the deviation, assuming retinal correspondence is normal. An advantage of this method is that because it uses streaks as targets, it can give some indication of torsion. A tilting of the green streak indicates torsion. The test is performed in the various positions of gaze, and the positions of the patient's target are recorded on the chart. The demarcation of the physical position of the lights projected by the patient are joined with a solid line, forming four enclosures of various size. To measure the deviation with the other eye fixating, the patient switches the red-green glasses or the target projectors.

With an incomitant deviation, the graphs of the two eyes are unequal in size and distorted (Fig. 10-9). The smaller of the graphs is the primary deviation and indicates the eye with the affected muscle or restriction. Compression of space indicates muscle underaction, whereas expansion of space indicates muscle overaction. The most underacting muscle will be plotted farthest in restriction from the normal position. The larger graph is the secondary deviation and demonstrates the overaction of the yoke muscle in the noninvolved eye when the involved eye is fixating. The

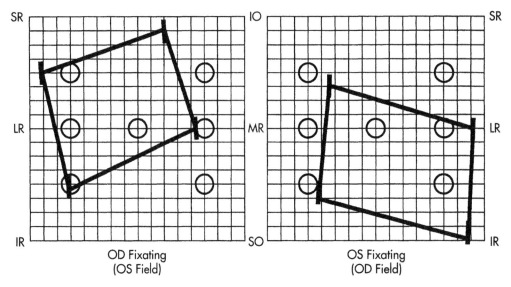

FIG. 10-10   Hess-Lancaster charts for patient with cyclovertical muscle paresis. Underactions for both left superior oblique and right superior rectus are indicated, as are overactions for left inferior oblique and right inferior rectus muscles.

greater the dissimilarity between the graphs, the more incomitant and more recent the deviation.

For long-standing paretic deviations in which near perfect comitance has evolved, the Hess-Lancaster test may not indicate the site of the primary defect, and more sensitive testing is needed. Also, in paresis of a cyclovertical muscle, secondary inhibitional palsy of the contralateral antagonist will show an underaction in the field of this muscle and may mislead the diagnosis (Fig. 10-10). Other tests, such as the three-step test, will confirm the correct diagnosis.

THREE-STEP TEST

The three-step test, or Bielschowsky head tilt test, is an objective clinical procedure used to determine whether or not a paretic cyclovertical muscle exists in a patient with a vertical deviation.[18] All patients with a vertical deviation in primary position should undergo the three-step test. Its most useful application is to confirm the diagnosis of superior oblique paresis. The three-step test is diagnostic in nearly 90% of all cases of superior oblique paresis, even when there has been a spread of comitance.[19] Its objective nature makes it very useful for noncommunicative or younger patients.

The three-step test is based on the torsional imbalance that results when a single cyclovertical muscle is paretic. It is also based on the premises that (1) cyclovertical muscles that are synergistic in one action are antagonistic in another, and (2) the vertical recti muscles have their greatest vertical action with the eye in abduction, whereas the oblique muscles have their greatest vertical action with the eye in adduction.[20] The

head tilt is explained on the basis of vestibular stimulation. When the head is tilted to one side, the vestibular system causes a compensatory cyclorotation in both eyes. For example, if the head is tilted to the left shoulder, the left superior rectus and the left superior oblique, which have opposing vertical actions, will produce an incycloduction of the left eye. Simultaneously, the right inferior rectus and the right inferior oblique, which also have opposite vertical actions, will produce an excyclodeviation of the right eye. When the cyclovertical muscles are intact, their opposing vertical actions cancel one another, so there is no vertical deviation of the eyes. If one of the cyclovertical muscles is paretic, tilting the head in the appropriate direction will produce not only a cyclodeviation but an elevation or depression, resulting in a greater vertical deviation of the eyes.

The procedure to determine the paretic cyclovertical muscle using the three-step test includes the following.

1. Step 1 determines the type of hyperdeviation that exists in the primary position. With the patient fixating a distant target and holding the head erect, the type of hyperdeviation, right or left, is determined by the cover test. If the patient's presenting sign is a hypodeviation, consider it a hyperdeviation of the opposite eye. This reduces the number of possible cyclovertical muscles involved from eight to four. For example, a left hyperdeviation indicates that there is either a weak left depressor muscle (i.e., left superior oblique or left inferior rectus) or a weak right elevator muscle (i.e., right superior rectus or right inferior oblique).

2. Step 2 determines whether the hyperdeviation in-

TABLE 10-3 PARETIC MUSCLE DETERMINATION

	Right Hyperdeviation in Primary Position		Left Hyperdeviation in Primary Position	
	Increases with Dextroversion	Increases with Levoversion	Increases with Dextroversion	Increases with Levoversion
Increases with head tilt right	Left inferior oblique	Right superior oblique	Right superior rectus	Left inferior rectus
Increases with head tilt left	Right inferior rectus	Left superior rectus	Left superior oblique	Right inferior oblique

From Rutstein RP, Eskridge JB: Clinical comparison of congenital or early onset paretic vertical strabismus vs. acquired paretic vertical strabismus, *Am J Optom Physiol Opt* 62:726, 1984.

creases in dextroversion or in levoversion. When the patient fixates the target in dextroversion and levoversion positions, the magnitude of the hyperdeviation is measured with the alternate cover test and prisms. This step reduces the number of muscles involved from four to two—one muscle in each eye. One is an oblique muscle and the other is a rectus muscle, but both are either superior muscles (intortors) or inferior muscles (extortors). For example, if a left hyperdeviation increases in dextroversion and decreases in levoversion, this indicates there is a weak depressor in the left eye (left superior oblique) or a weak elevator in the right eye (right superior rectus).

3. Step 3 determines whether the hyperdeviation increases when the head is tilted toward the right shoulder or toward the left shoulder. While the patient is fixating the target, the patient's head is tilted toward each shoulder and the amount of the vertical deviation is measured with the alternate cover test and prisms. For example, if a left hyperdeviation decreases with right head tilt and increases with left head tilt, the paretic muscle is the left superior oblique.

While measuring the deviation with the head tilted, prisms should also be tilted and positioned so that their bases are parallel to the floor of the orbit, not parallel to the floor of the room. For any simultaneous exodeviation or esodeviation, the bases of the horizontal prisms are placed parallel to the lateral wall of the orbit.

Various tables and flowcharts to assist the clinician with the three-step test have been used. A useful one is given in Table 10-3.[21]

The three-step test tends to bias the diagnosis more toward paretic oblique muscles than toward paretic vertical recti muscles. Studies that have used the alternate cover test and prism in the nine positions of gaze, rather than the three-step test, to diagnose a paretic cyclovertical muscle have shown a higher incidence of paretic vertical recti muscles.[22] When doing the three-step test with the head tilted to the right and left shoul-

ders, there is less difference in the vertical deviation between the two positions with paretic vertical rectus muscles than with paretic oblique muscles. This is because the vertical action of the oblique muscles is less than the vertical action of the vertical recti muscles. Thus an isolated vertical rectus paresis, although uncommon, may be even more difficult to diagnose with the three-step test. Furthermore, because the three-step test also assumes that the patient has a single cyclovertical muscle paresis and that there are no mechanical restrictions to eye movements, it may incorrectly diagnose an oblique muscle paresis in conditions such as dissociated vertical deviation, skew deviation, ocular myasthenia, orbital floor fracture, inferior rectus fibrosis, and mechanical restrictions associated with prior extraocular muscle surgery.[23-25] In these cases, tests such as the forced duction test, electromyography, and saccadic velocity testing will establish the true diagnosis.

TESTS FOR TORSION

The double Maddox rod test is a subjective test used to measure the torsion or cyclodeviation that may be associated with vertical deviations. Testing for torsion is done whenever a patient reports tilting of one or both double images in the differential diagnosis of a cyclovertical muscle paresis or for a patient with a head tilt. The most common cause of torsion is superior oblique paresis. The test is performed in the primary position at 40 cm and also in downgaze, or the reading position, as the patient is fixating on a light and wearing the proper refractive correction. Testing is done in dim illumination.

 CLINICAL PEARL

Testing for torsion is done whenever a patient reports tilting of one or both double images in the differential diagnosis of a cyclovertical muscle paresis or for a patient with a head tilt.

Red and white Maddox rods are placed in a trial frame or a phoropter so that the Maddox rods can be

The double Maddox rod test

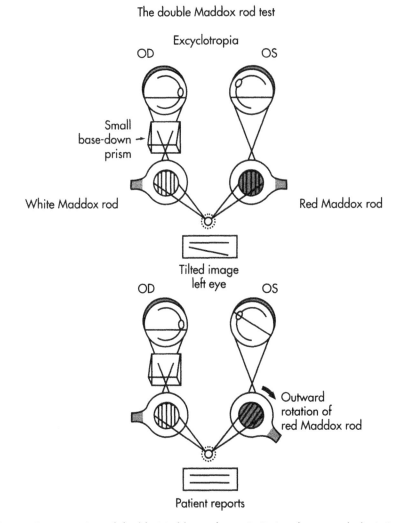

Fig. 10-11 Interpretation of double Maddox rod test. **A,** Patient has excyclodeviation of left eye associated with superior oblique paresis. Red line is seen as tilted by patient. **B,** Red Maddox rod is rotated outward for alignment, indicating excyclodeviation. (Modified from Nelson LB, Catalano RA: *Atlas of ocular motility,* Philadelphia, 1989, WB Saunders.)

rotated. The red Maddox rod is placed before the right or left eye. The patient's head should be erect and not tilted during testing. The axes of the Maddox rods are placed to 90 degrees. Vertical prism (6 PD) is placed before one eye to separate the two lines. When the patient views the fixation light, he or she will see two horizontal lines that are vertically displaced, one red and one white. If the patient reports seeing both of the horizontal lines appearing parallel to the floor, no torsion exists. If one line is tilted with respect to the floor, torsion exists (Fig. 10-11). The Maddox rod in front of the eye seeing the tilted line is rotated until the lines appear parallel to each other and the floor.

The number of degrees that the Maddox rod must be rotated for parallelism to occur from 90 degrees indicates the amount of torsion. If the axis of the Mad-

dox rod before the right eye was rotated clockwise, an intorsion is present, and if the axis was rotated counterclockwise, an extorsion is present. If the Maddox rod before the left eye is used to measure the torsion, a clockwise rotation indicates extorsion and a counterclockwise rotation indicates intorsion. Because consecutive measurements in the same patient can vary, recording the average of three readings is the preferred method.[26]

Torsion, as measured with the double Maddox rod test, may occur paradoxically. Paradoxic indicates that the nonparetic, or noninvolved, eye manifests the torsion, rather than the paretic, or involved eye.[27] This is more likely when the visual acuity of the paretic eye is better than the nonparetic eye, and the patient prefers to fixate with the paretic eye under dissociative conditions.[28] On the other hand, the standard two-color format (red and white Maddox rods) can give rise to an artifactual localization of the cyclodeviation to the eye with the red Maddox rod.[29] The laterality of the cyclodeviation has been found to be more reliable if Maddox rods of the same color (red) are used before both eyes.[29]

Torsion can also be determined objectively using the techniques of binocular indirect ophthalmoscopy or fundus photography.[30,31] These methods detect rotation of the posterior pole of the globe, as revealed by an alternation of the normal anatomic relationship between the fovea and the optic disc. Supraplacement or infraplacement of the macula relative to the optic disc with indirect ophthalmoscopy indicates the presence of torsion.

The double Maddox rod test will reveal torsion for cyclovertical deviations whose onset is after the period of visual immaturity.[7,21] The objective techniques should reveal torsion, regardless of the age of onset of the deviation. Apparently, the early onset of the deviation permits patients to develop a sensory adaption to torsion.[31,32] It is as though the patient had developed "torsional anomalous correspondence." This adaptation prevents the deviation from entering the patient's conscious awareness.

CLINICAL PEARL

The double Maddox rod test will reveal torsion for cyclovertical deviations whose onset is after the period of visual immaturity.

The clinical implication of this is significant. Some patients with childhood-onset superior oblique paresis may remain entirely asymptomatic until adulthood and then suddenly report visual symptoms and diplopia. The absence of a cyclodeviation, as determined by the double Maddox rod test, in these cases allows the clinician to better differentiate an acquired paresis from a childhood-onset paresis that has likely decompensated (see Case 1).

Torsion can also be measured with the synoptophore. Using first-degree superimposition targets, a tilt of one target relative to the other target perceived by the patient indicates torsion. The amount of torsion is determined by adjusting the tubes of the synoptophore until there is no tilt of the targets.

SENSORY FUSION TESTING

Sensory fusion testing for patients with incomitant deviations should be performed not only in the primary position but also in the secondary and tertiary positions to determine the chance for fusion. The Worth four dot test, the Bagolini striated lens test, the synoptophore, and stereopsis tests may be used to assess sensory status in the different positions. The presence of normal binocular vision in any position of gaze improves the prognosis considerably. (See Case 2.)

CASE 2

A 7-year-old girl was evaluated for an esotropia.[34] The parents were told that the child had no binocular vision ability, and treatment would not be of functional benefit. The child had experienced head trauma to the right side at 9 months of age. The parents first noticed the strabismus when the child was 2 years old. At this time, the child also began occasionally turning her head. All previous medical and neurologic evaluations were normal. The child was wearing glasses for hyperopia. She did not experience diplopia in everyday life.

Our examination revealed that the patient had a pronounced head turn to the right that permitted ocular alignment (Fig. 10-12). Without the head turn, she manifested a 20-PD constant right esotropia at distance and near. Corrected visual acuity with a +2.00-D refraction was 20/20 for each eye.

Versions were full for the left eye but showed marked underaction in abduction for the right eye. The motility for the right eye improved slightly with duction testing. Testing with the Worth four dot test showed suppression in primary position and dextroversion and fusion in levoversion. The Randot stereotest indicated that the patient exhibited 20 seconds of arc with the head turn and absence of stereopsis without the head turn.

The diagnosis was right lateral rectus paresis, likely caused by the earlier head trauma. Because fusion existed with the head turn, base-out prisms were prescribed to reduce the head turn.

Two weeks later the patient returned with a minimal head turn and fused with the prisms in primary position. Subsequent extraocular muscle surgery eliminated the need for any prisms.

PARETIC DEVIATIONS

Incomitant deviations that are paretic consist of oculomotor, or third cranial nerve, paresis; trochlear, or fourth cranial nerve, paresis; and abducens, or sixth cranial nerve, paresis. Paretic deviations demonstrate limited versions in the field of action of the affected extraocular muscle, accompanied by negative forced duction testing. The type of paretic deviation (oculomotor, trochlear, abducens) that is most frequent varies according to the kind of practice. In neurology practice, abducens nerve, or lateral rectus, paresis is the most common, representing nearly 45% of paretic deviations.[6] This is likely attributed to the abducens nerves' susceptibility to raised intracranial pressure as they pass over the petrous portion of the temporal bones. In our practice, trochlear nerve, or superior oblique, paresis is the most frequently seen variety of paretic deviation.

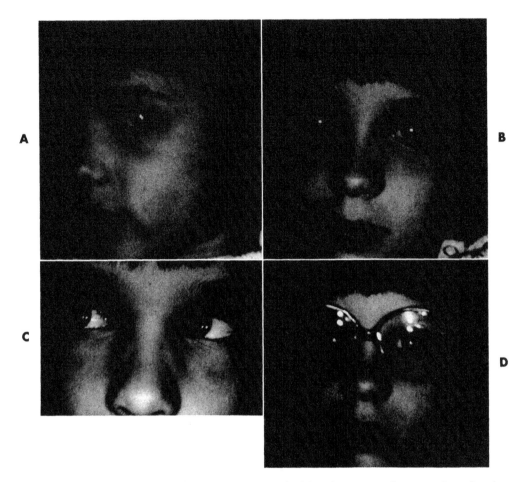

FIG. 10-12 Patient examined in Case 2. **A,** Marked head turn to right. **B,** Without head turn, right esotropia exists in primary position. **C,** Underaction of right lateral rectus. **D,** Prisms alleviate head posture and thereby permit fusion in primary position. (From Rutstein RP: Therapy for early acquired noncomitant esotropia, *J Am Optom Assoc* 54:161, 1983.)

OCULOMOTOR NERVE PARESIS

The oculomotor, or third cranial, nerve supplies the superior rectus, inferior rectus, inferior oblique, medial rectus, and levator muscle and the autonomically innervated sphincter muscle of the pupil and ciliary muscle. Complete paresis of the oculomotor nerve causes restricted motility and an exotropia, hypotropia, ptosis, fixed dilated pupil, and diminished accommodation (Fig. 10-13). The eye is in a down-and-out position because of continued action of the uneffected superior oblique and lateral rectus. Abduction and intorsion are the only remaining oculomotor functions. With oculomotor nerve paresis the vertical deviation switches from hypotropia in primary position and upgaze to hypertropia in downgaze. Depending on the degree of ptosis, the patient may or may not be diplopic.

 CLINICAL PEARL

Complete paresis of the oculomotor nerve causes restricted motility and an exotropia, hypotropia, ptosis, fixed dilated pupil, and diminished accommodation.

Congenital and bilateral cases are relatively rare. The former usually has a benign nature with respect to neurologic disease. It may occur as an isolated defect in an otherwise normal child or be associated with other neurologic abnormalities.[2] Congenital deviations without a history of infection or trauma can also be indicative of a developmental anomaly or birth trauma. Injury to the nerve itself is more likely than hypoplasia of the nucleus.[35]

The causes of acquired oculomotor nerve paresis from a series of 1130 patients are illustrated in Fig. 10-14.[6] The leading cause in adults is ischemic or vascular,

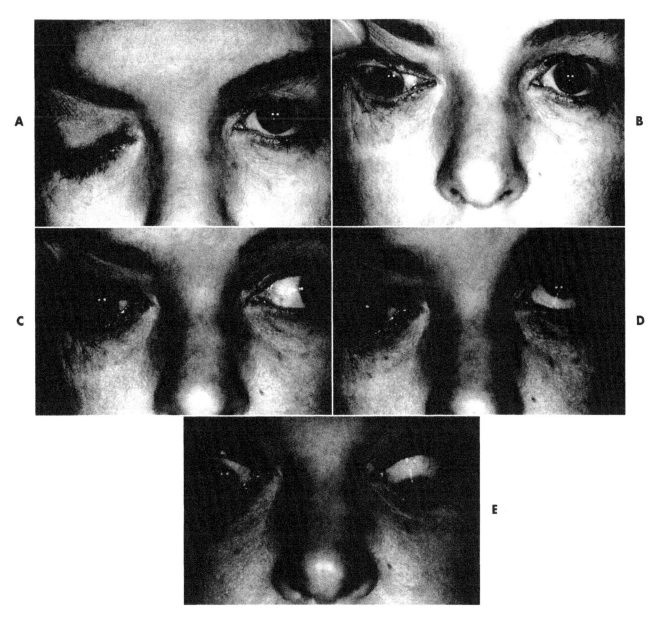

FIG. 10-13 Oculomotor nerve paresis of right eye. **A,** Complete ptosis. **B,** Eye is down and out in primary position and pupil is dilated. Impaired **(C)** adduction, **(D)** elevation, and **(E)** depression.

such as diabetes, hypertension, and atherosclerosis, in which the pupil is usually spared. Generally, with pupillary involvement, the cause is more ominous. Undetermined causes, despite extensive neurologic and medical work-up, comprise 24% of the cases.[6] Acquired cases in children are most commonly the result of blunt trauma or infectious processes, either local or systemic.

Oculomotor nerve paresis may be partial or incomplete. Anatomically, the oculomotor nerve bifurcates into superior and inferior branches at the anterior

cavernous sinus. The superior division innervates the superior rectus and levator muscles, whereas the inferior division innervates the remaining muscles. This explains the relative infrequency of isolated paresis of the superior rectus, inferior rectus, inferior oblique, and medial rectus. Paresis of a single muscle innervated by the oculomotor nerve should be differentiated from ocular motility disorders associated with mechanically restrictive causes, such as thyroid myopathy, and trauma, as well as ocular myasthenia, and congenital absence of a muscle. Rather than medial rectus paresis, for ex-

N = 1,130

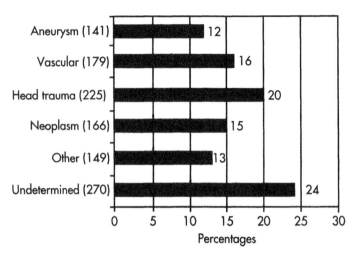

FIG. 10-14 Causes of acquired oculomotor nerve paresis. (Modified from Richards BW, Jones FR, Younge BR: Causes and prognosis in 4728 cases of paralysis of the oculomotor, trochlear, and abducens cranial nerves, *Am J Ophthalmol* 113:489, 1992.)

ample, limited adduction is more likely the result of injury, prior eye muscle surgery, contracture of the lateral rectus, Duane's syndrome type II, thyroid myopathy, or internuclear ophthalmoplegia. Rather than inferior oblique paresis, limited elevation in adduction is more likely caused by Brown's syndrome. When it does occur, paresis of isolated muscles innervated by the oculomotor nerve is more likely to be congenital than acquired. However, permanent vertical rectus muscle paresis following cataract surgery, presumably the result of anesthetic myotoxicity, and inferior oblique paresis following trauma have been reported.[36,37] The clinical features associated with paresis of single muscles innervated by the oculomotor nerve are listed in Table 10-4. Some of these features may only be theoretic, as indicated by the following cases from our clinic.

CASE 3

In January, 1988 a 68-year-old man was referred to the clinic complaining of almost constant diplopia that increased when looking up and to the left. Three months earlier the patient underwent retinal detachment surgery in the left eye. The diplopia was noted immediately after surgery. The patient has bilateral aphakia.

On observation, there was no compensatory head posture or ptosis. Pupillary reflexes were normal. Corrected vision was 20/20 and 20/30, with a refraction of +11.00 −1.50 × 74 and +8.25 −4.00 × 95 for the right and left eye. The patient manifested a 6-PD left hypotropia and 8-PD esotropia in the primary position. With the three-step test the vertical deviation increased in levoversion and slightly with left head tilt. Version testing revealed restriction of the left

eye when looking up and to the left. The patient could elevate the left eye more during duction testing. Overaction of the right inferior oblique occurred when the patient looked up and to the left and fixated with the paretic eye. The Hess-Lancaster test indicated left superior rectus underaction (Fig. 10-15). No torsion was measured with the double Maddox rod test. It was presumed that the retinal detachment surgery caused the subtle left superior rectus paresis.

With prism correction (4PD vertical and 6PD horizontal, divided equally between the eyes) the diplopia was eliminated in the primary and reading positions, and the patient achieved 50 seconds of arc with the Randot stereotest.

CASE 4

A 50-year-old woman was first seen in the clinic because of an increasing strabismus. The patient had diabetes. At age 12 she supposedly developed a strabismus after having a high fever. There was no history of head trauma. She was only occasionally bothered by diplopia, mostly when she was upset or tired.

The patient had corrected vision of 20/20 for each eye with a refraction of −0.50 −0.75 ×150 for the right eye and +0.75 −0.50 × 165 for the left eye. A slight head tilt to the left existed. Pupillary reflexes were normal. By cover test a constant 20-PD exotropia with a 12-PD hypotropia for the left eye was measured at distance (Fig. 10-16). At near the exotropia and hypotropia increased to 25 PD. An A-pattern exotropia, 45 PD in downgaze and 20 PD in upgaze, existed. With the three-step test the hypotropia increased in dextroversion and right head tilt. Version testing showed limited motility of the left eye when looking up and to the right that improved on duction testing.

TABLE 10-4 **FEATURES OF DEVIATIONS CAUSED BY PARESIS OF ISOLATED MUSCLES INNERVATED BY THE OCULOMOTOR NERVE**

Muscle	Major Deviation in Primary Position	Head Posture	Versions	Three-Step Test	Cyclodeviation*	Other	Differential Diagnosis
Medical rectus	Exotropia of involved eye	Turn toward opposite side	Limited adduction	Not applicable	Not applicable	Adults with untreated childhood-onset exotropia may develop limited adduction as a result of lateral rectus contracture	Internuclear ophthalmoplegia; Duane's syndrome type II, thyroid myopathy; ocular myasthenia
Superior rectus	Hypotropia and ptosis of involved eye	Inconsistent (see Table 10-2); some patients elevate the chin and tilt the head to the opposite side	Limited elevation in abduction	Hypotropia increases in abduction and with head tilted to involved side (less consistent than in oblique muscle paresis)	Excyclodeviation (if acquired after visual immaturity)	Ptosis may be pseudo and disappear when patient fixates with paretic eye	Thyroid myopathy; trauma; ocular myasthenia; inhibitional palsy of contralateral antagonist in cases of superior oblique paresis
Inferior oblique	Hypotropia of involved eye	Head tilt toward involved side, chin is elevated and face is turned to noninvolved side	Limited elevation in adduction	Hypotropia increases in adduction and on head tilt to unaffected side	Incyclodeviation (if acquired after visual immaturity)	A-pattern; least likely cyclovertical muscle to be paretic	Brown's syndrome; ocular myasthenia
Inferior rectus	Hypertropia of involved eye	Inconsistent (see Table 10-2); slight chin depression with face turned to involved side	Limited depression in abduction	Hypertropia increases in abduction and with head tilt to opposite side (less consistent than in oblique muscle paresis)	Incyclodeviation (if acquired after visual immaturity)	Most frequent muscle to become fibrotic; when involved eye fixates, pseudoptosis can occur in the nonparetic eye	Trauma, thyroid myopathy, ocular myasthenia

*As measured with the double Maddox rod test.

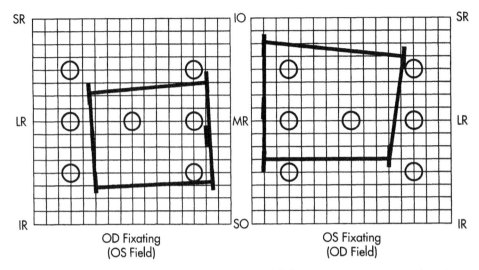

FIG. 10-15 Hess-Lancaster charts for patient with left superior rectus paresis (Case 3).

A 9-degree incyclodeviation of the left eye was measured with the double Maddox rod test. The patient suppressed the left eye with the Worth four dot test at distance and near. With the synoptophore, normal correspondence without second-degree sensory and motor fusion was elicited.

The diagnosis was a long-standing left inferior oblique paresis. Surgical treatment was recommended, but the patient declined. Subsequent neurologic evaluations were normal.

CASE 5

A 38-year-old functionally illiterate woman was first seen in February, 1985. She was under a physician's care for a thyroid disorder and diabetes. She had suffered head trauma 2 years previously as a result of a beating by her husband. She denies any diplopia.

On examination, the patient was noted to have a head tilt to the right and a slight chin depression (Fig. 10-17). Her vision was 20/20 for each eye, with no significant refractive error. Pupillary reflexes were normal. A 20-PD left hypertropia and 6-PD exotropia were measured with the cover test at distance and near. With the three-step test the hypertropia increased to 30 PD in levoversion and decreased to 4 PD in dextroversion. The vertical deviation measured 20 PD on both right and left head tilt. Version testing indicated underaction of the left inferior rectus, which did not improve with duction testing. Testing with the double Maddox rod test was not reliable. The patient suppressed the left eye with the Worth four dot test and showed no stereopsis when tested in all positions of gaze.

The diagnosis was acquired left inferior rectus paresis. Secondary mechanical restrictive changes in the muscles were suggested by the finding of equal ductions and versions. Surgical treatment was recommended. Subsequent neurologic evaluations were normal.

Oculomotor nerve paresis may involve only the nerve's superior division.[38] Weakness of the superior

rectus and levator is associated with ptosis and hypotropia of the involved eye in primary position (Fig. 10-18). The intraocular musculature is spared. The greatest motility defect occurs when the patient attempts to elevate the eye while it is abducted. It may be associated with overaction of the contralateral inferior oblique and/or ipsilateral inferior rectus. The ptosis in some cases may be solely the result of the hypotropic position of the paretic eye and may disappear when the paretic eye fixates. Any lid lag that remains with the paretic eye fixating is a true ptosis.

An inferior division paresis of the oculomotor nerve is extremely rare.[39,40] Affected are the medial rectus, inferior rectus, and inferior oblique muscles, as well as the intraocular musculature. An exotropia is present in primary position, with any vertical deviation depending on the involvement of the two vertically acting muscles. Some have associated a residual tonic pupil with inferior division paresis.[41]

The clinician should suspect an early-onset oculomotor nerve paresis in patients who have a long history of constant exotropia, hypotropia, and ptosis of the involved eye, with various degrees of limitation in elevation, depression, and adduction. Amblyopia exists in approximately three-fourths of patients with childhood-onset oculomotor paresis.[42] The amblyopia is usually deep, because with the accompanying ptosis, deprivation amblyopia and strabismic amblyopia occur. In rare cases, amblyopia may occur in the contralateral eye if the patient fixates with the paretic eye. Suppression and anomalous correspondence prevent normal binocular vision in the majority of cases. Exceptions may occur for patients who adopt a compensatory head posture. In these cases, binocular vision accompanied by normal visual acuity can exist in certain positions of gaze, despite the paresis. However, a com-

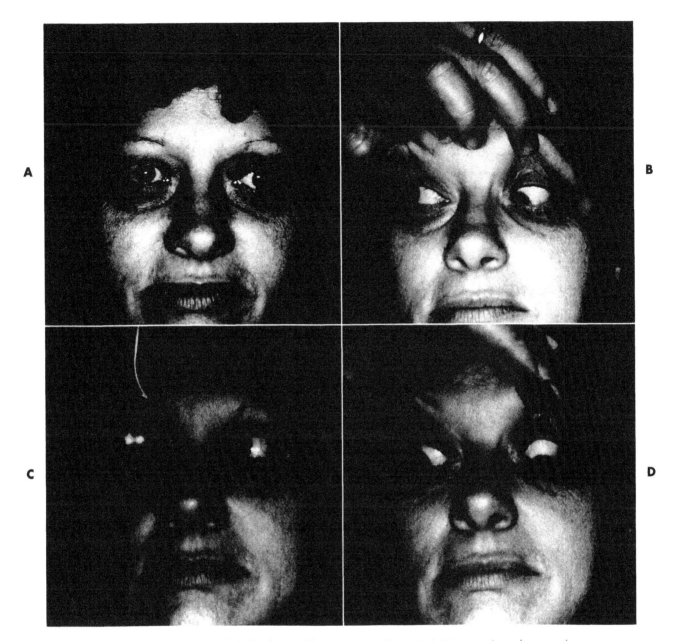

FIG. 10-16 Patient with left inferior oblique paresis (Case 4). **A,** Hypotropia and exotropia exist in primary position. **B,** Underaction of left inferior oblique. **C,** Improved motility with duction testing. **D,** Overaction of ipsilateral superior oblique resulting in A-pattern exodeviation.

pensatory head posture usually is not adopted because of the ptosis and large amounts of incomitance.

Approximately two thirds of patients with oculomotor paresis develop aberrant regeneration. Aberrant regeneration occurs mostly during the recovery of acquired paresis, although it may also occur with congenital deviations. It does not occur in cases that are caused by diabetes. It manifests mostly as a failure of the upper lid to follow the involved eye as it moves downward or retraction of the upper lid in downgaze

(Fig. 10-19). The lid retraction may be accompanied by constriction of the pupil. Aberrant regeneration may also include widening of the palpebral fissure on adduction and narrowing of the fissure on abduction; a dilated fixed pupil that does not react to direct or consensual light stimulation but reacts slightly on convergence and adduction; and retraction and adduction of the globe on attempted upgaze.[43,44] The exact cause of aberrant regeneration remains unclear. Most authorities believe that it is caused by the nerve fibers origi-

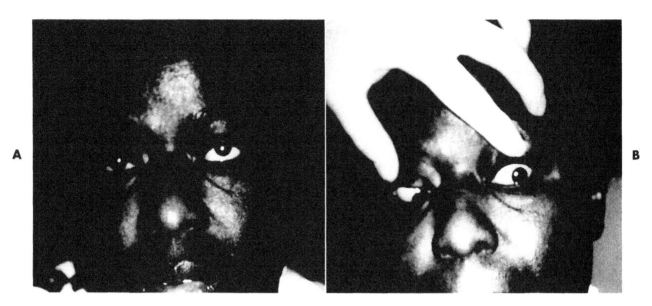

FIG. 10-17 Patient with left inferior rectus paresis (Case 5). **A,** Head tilt to right and chin depression with left hypertropia in primary position. **B,** Underaction of left inferior rectus.

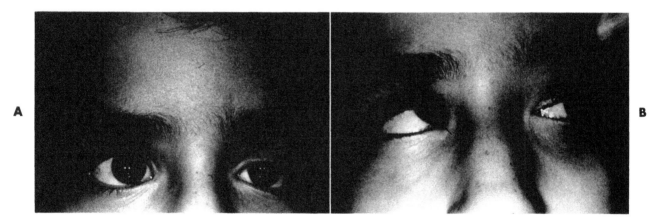

FIG. 10-18 Superior division oculomotor nerve paresis of left eye. **A,** Ptosis and hypotropia in primary position. **B,** Hypotropia increases when looking up and to left. (From Amos JF, editor: *Diagnosis and management in vision care,* Boston, 1987, Butterworth-Heinemann.)

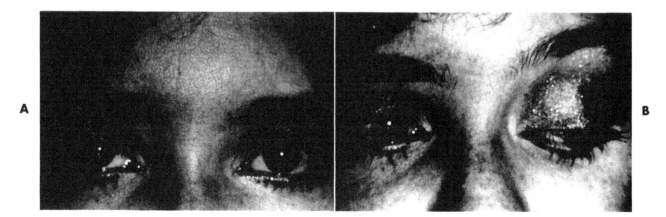

FIG. 10-19 Aberrant regeneration for patient with oculomotor nerve paresis. **A,** Ptosis and hypotropia exist in primary position. **B,** Lid retraction when looking down and to left.

nally connected with the inferior rectus growing into the sheath of the levator, so that the impulses to look down increase the innervation to the levator.[43,44] The presence of aberrant regeneration assists in the diagnosis of a congenital oculomotor nerve paresis in cases that present in adulthood as being "relatively" comitant with unilateral visual loss. (See Case 6.)

CASE 6

A 24-year-old woman was referred to the clinic in May, 1990. The patient indicated that she had been diagnosed during childhood as having "poor vision." Treatment consisted only of glasses. Because of the extent of the visual acuity reduction, an organic rather than a functional cause was suspected by the referring clinician.

Our examination revealed corrected vision of 20/20 for the right eye with +2.00 D and 20/120 for the left eye with +2.50 D. The patient had a slight left ptosis. There was no pupillary defect. With the cover test a 20-PD constant left exotropia and 4-PD hypotropia were measured at distance and near. Versions showed slight restriction of the left eye in elevation, depression, and adduction. On downgaze, left lid retraction occurred, indicating aberrant regeneration. Ophthalmoscopic findings were normal.

It was concluded that the reduced vision in the left eye was associated with amblyopia secondary to childhood-onset oculomotor nerve paresis.

Unlike congenital cases, acquired cases occur precipitously with maximal involvement. Within weeks, there may be indications of partial recovery. Recovery may be complete in many cases by 3 to 6 months after the onset. The latter is more likely to occur with cases associated with ischemic causes. During the initial stages when the deviation is severely incomitant, occlusion can be used to eliminate the diplopia. When the deviation becomes less incomitant and starts to recover, prisms can be given to maintain fusion in primary position and downgaze, which are the positions most frequently used by most patients. (See Case 7.)

CASE 7

In December, 1991 a 67-year-old man complained of diplopia that began 1 week previously. The patient had diabetes. Ten years previously, he had a lateral rectus paresis that resolved in 3 months.[45]

Our examination revealed corrected vision of 20/40 for each eye with a mild myopic correction. A 2- to 3-mm ptosis existed for the right side. The pupils were symmetric and responded to light. With the cover test, a 20-PD constant right exotropia and 8-PD right hypotropia were measured at distance and a 14-PD exotropia and 8-PD right hypotropia at near. The right hypotropia switched to a right hypertropia in downgaze. Version testing revealed limited motility of all extraocular muscles innervated by the right oculomotor nerve (see Fig. 10-20, *A*). Ophthalmoscopy showed mild background diabetic retinopathy.

Because of the extreme incomitance, an occluder lens was placed before the right eye to alleviate the diplopia. A neurologic evaluation concluded that the deviation was diabetically induced.

The patient returned to the clinic in February, 1992. The magnitude of the deviation and the ptosis were similar to that measured previously. Prisms could not give fusion. Occlusion for the right eye was continued. Two months later, the patient showed complete resolution of the paresis (see Fig. 10-20, *B*).

TROCHLEAR NERVE (SUPERIOR OBLIQUE) PARESIS

The most common cause of a vertical deviation is a trochlear nerve, or superior oblique, paresis. As many as 90% of all vertical deviations can be attributed to a paresis of the superior oblique.[46] Exclusive innervation of the superior oblique by the trochlear nerve and the nerve's long exposed course account for the high prevalence of this condition. Adults who suddenly develop superior oblique paresis complain of vertical and torsional diplopia that is worse when reading. As mentioned earlier, superior oblique paresis is the most common paretic extraocular muscle seen in our clinic.

 CLINICAL PEARL

The most common cause of a vertical deviation is a trochlear nerve, or superior oblique, paresis.

Congenital superior oblique paresis accounts for 29% to 66% of all cases.[47] The diagnosis of congenital cases is usually presumptive, based on a history of early-onset of findings and exclusion of findings that could produce an acquired paresis. Congenital cases may be the result of hypoplasia or hemorrhage, which can affect the trochlear nuclei, or may be associated with an anomalous loose tendon or misdirection of the superior oblique muscle. Facial asymmetry has been reported in association with congenital superior oblique paresis. The facial asymmetry typically is manifested by midfacial hypoplasia on the side opposite the paretic muscle, with deviation of the nose and mouth toward the hypoplastic side.[48]

Of all the paretic deviations, superior oblique paresis tends to be least indicative of serious underlying disease. Acquired cases are most often caused by head trauma, especially blunt frontal injury. Intracranial aneurysm and neoplasm are rarely associated with superior oblique paresis (Fig. 10-21). Undetermined etiologies account for about one-third of all cases.[6] In cases of superior oblique paresis presenting suddenly in adulthood without any apparent cause, the presumption is frequently made that the deviation was controlled for many years, but with time the same fusional effort could no longer be maintained and the deviation

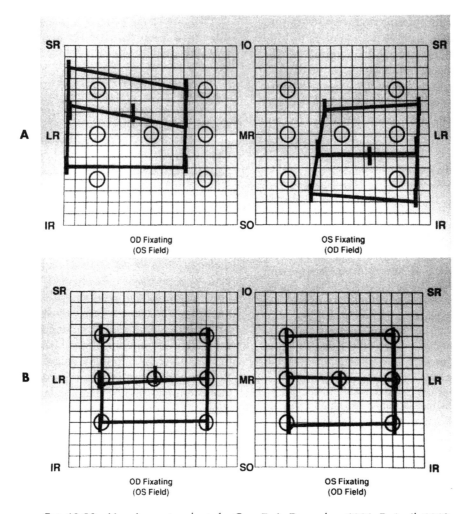

FIG. 10-20   Hess-Lancaster charts for Case 7. **A,** December, 1991. **B,** April, 1992.

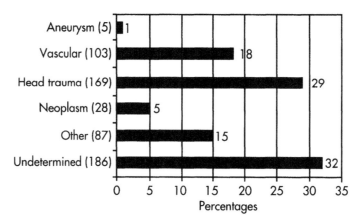

FIG. 10-21   Causes of acquired superior oblique paresis. (Modified from Richards BW, Jones FR, Younge BR: Causes and prognosis in 4728 cases of paralysis of the oculomotor, trochlear, and abducens cranial nerves, *Am J Ophthalmol* 113:489, 1992.)

presented. This is referred to as *decompensated superior oblique paresis* (see Case 1).

The diagnosis of superior oblique paresis (Fig. 10-22) includes the presence of (1) a vertical deviation in primary position, either a hyperphoria or a hypertropia that increases in the nasal field of the involved eye and also when tilting the head toward the paretic side; (2) underaction of the paretic superior oblique and/or overaction of the ipsilateral inferior oblique muscle; (3) a compensatory head posture consisting mostly of a head tilt to the nonparetic side and occasionally a chin depression; and (4) an excyclodeviation. Superior oblique paresis frequently produces a V-pattern deviation.

The paretic eye is always the hyperdeviated eye in cases of superior oblique paresis. This is true whether the paretic or nonparetic eye is fixating. When the paretic eye fixates, there is a hypotropia of the nonfixating eye. The magnitude of the vertical deviation in the primary position averages 11 PD.[32] The vertical deviation is usually greater for near than for distance viewing.[7]

Version testing reveals underaction of the paretic superior oblique and/or overaction of the antagonist inferior oblique. Underaction of the involved superior oblique may be subtle and escape detection on examining ductions and versions. In congenital and long-standing cases, the inferior oblique overaction may be more apparent than the underaction of the superior oblique. The Hess-Lancaster test assists in the diagnosis, but, as mentioned earlier, frequently it is necessary to differentiate an ipsilateral superior oblique paresis from a contralateral superior rectus paresis because of secondary inhibitional palsy (see Fig. 10-10). The latter is likely when the patient fixates with the paretic eye. For example, a patient with a right superior oblique paresis who fixates with the right eye may appear to have left superior rectus paresis because of the overaction of the yoke left inferior rectus. The three-step test will distinguish between these two muscles.

A "comitant" vertical deviation can be the sequelae of a superior oblique paresis. The direction of maximal deviation need not remain in the field of action of the paretic superior oblique. A spread of the deviation to all positions of gaze can occur as early as 3 weeks after the onset, and the superior oblique paresis may become less incomitant. Secondary inhibitional palsy may involve not only the contralateral superior rectus but also the contralateral inferior oblique. If the patient habitually fixates with the paretic eye, the inferior rectus in the hypotropic eye can undergo contracture and limit elevation. In such instances, mechanical restrictions develop on both versions and ductions and the forced duction test will be positive. In the majority of cases, the maximal vertical deviation remains either in the field of action of the antagonist inferior oblique or the paretic superior oblique.

The three-step test is diagnostic in nearly all cases, even when there has been a spread of comitance. The vertical deviation becomes larger while forcibly tilting the head to the paretic side. In long-standing cases in which there has been a spread of comitance, there may be little variation in the deviation to the right and left gaze.

Superior oblique paresis is the most common cause of a head tilt encountered in optometric practice. Approximately 70% of these patients develop compensatory head postures to maintain single binocular vision and avoid diplopia.[32] The head is placed in the direction of action of the weak superior oblique muscle. A patient with a paretic left superior oblique (see Fig. 10-3) will usually tilt the head to the right, depress the chin, and occasionally turn the face to the right. As indicated earlier, patients with a head tilt from infancy often develop facial asymmetry, with the fuller facial features on the side of the abnormal superior oblique. This is a valuable sign to date the onset of the strabismus.

A compensatory head posture does not ensure bifoveal fusion. In some cases of superior oblique paresis the head posture may permit fusion on the basis of anomalous correspondence.[49,50] Furthermore, for approximately 3% of patients, the head position may be paradoxic and tilted toward the paretic side.[32] The latter supposedly widens the diplopic image separation but more likely eliminates discomfort that may have been associated with a fusional effort.

Most patients with superior oblique paresis have a high level of binocular vision with good stereopsis and, rarely, significant amblyopia. Amblyopia of less than 20/25 and at least a line difference between the two eyes occurs in only 12% of these patients.[51]

Adults who develop superior oblique paresis manifest an excyclodeviation of the affected eye and frequently complain of images being tilted. The magnitude of the excyclodeviation in primary position averages 3.5 degrees.[32] Approximately 15% will have a paradoxic excyclodeviation when measured with the double Maddox rod test.[32] In cases of childhood-onset superior oblique paresis, torsional diplopia is not present, and little or no torsion is measured with the double Maddox rod test. Expanded vertical fusional amplitudes are also characteristic of childhood-onset cases and not adult-onset cases.[52]

With torsion, the eyes will rotate around the line of sight to the physiologic position of rest under monocular viewing conditions, but under fused binocular viewing conditions a cyclofusional movement will occur. Thus torsion associated with superior oblique paresis can alter the patient's refractive correction. The change in the axis of astigmatism when determined monocularly versus binocularly has been found to be

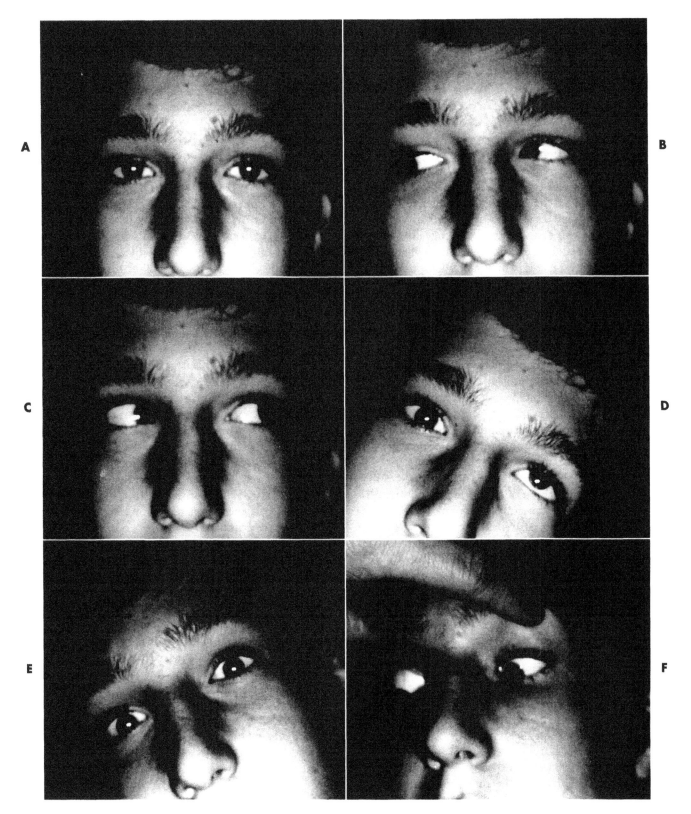

FIG. 10-22 Left superior oblique paresis. **A,** Intermittent left hypertropia in primary position. **B,** Hypertropia increases in dextroversion. **C,** No hypertropia in levoversion. **D,** Hypertropia is greatest on left head tilt. **E,** Hypertropia absent on right head tilt. **F,** Underaction of the left superior oblique.

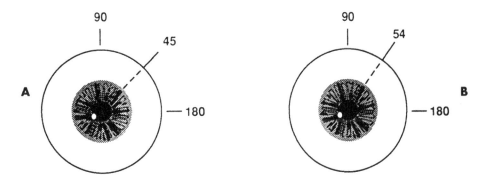

FIG. 10-23 Change in the axis of astigmatism associated with excyclodeviation of left eye. A, Left eye axis under monocular viewing conditions and (B) binocular viewing conditions. (Modified from Rutstein RP, Eskridge JB: Effect of cyclodeviations on the axis of astigmatism (for patients with superior oblique paresis), *Optom Vis Sci* 67:80, 1990.)

similar to the amount and direction of the cyclodeviation as measured with the double Maddox rod test (Fig. 10-23).[28] Patients with acquired superior oblique paresis and having astigmatism of 1 D or more, fusion ability, and an excyclodeviation exceeding 5 degrees are best refracted under binocular viewing conditions rather than refracted under monocular viewing conditions.[28]

Patients with superior oblique paresis and a vertical deviation of 10 PD or smaller in the primary position usually benefit from prisms. The minimum amount of prismatic correction needed to provide comfortable fusion in the primary position and downgaze is given. Confounding the usefulness of prisms is the simultaneous excyclodeviation. Many patients, however, will cyclofuse successfully if the vertical deviation is treated with prisms.

❖ CLINICAL PEARL

Patients with superior oblique paresis and a vertical deviation of 10 PD or smaller in the primary position usually benefit from prisms.

It has been estimated that as many as 25% of all cases of superior oblique paresis involve both eyes.[53] The clinical features usually include (1) a small vertical deviation in the primary position, (2) a V-pattern deviation with esotropia in downgaze and exotropia in upgaze, (3) a hyperdeviation that switches from right hyperdeviation in left gaze to left hyperdeviation in right gaze, and (4) an excyclodeviation usually exceeding 10 degrees as measured with the double Maddox rod test. In addition, with the three-step test, a right hyperdeviation exists on right head tilt and a left hyperdeviation exists on left head tilt. Version testing can reveal underaction of both superior obliques and overaction of both inferior obliques.

Bilateral superior oblique paresis is almost always caused by head trauma. The vertical deviation in primary position rarely exceeds 5 PD.[32] These patients experience both image tilting and diplopia. Amounts of excyclodeviation exceeding 10 degrees should raise suspicion of a bilateral paresis. (See Case 8.)

CASE 8

A 59-year-old man suffered head trauma as a result of a car accident 14 years before presenting for examination. He experiences occasional diplopia, especially when looking to the right and left but closes one eye when this occurs. For a long time, he has also seen images turned at an angle. He has a slight head tilt to the left. He is in excellent health and is presently not taking any medications.

The examination revealed corrected vision of 20/20 for the right eye with +3.25 −0.50 × 10 and 20/25 for the left eye with +3.00 −1.50 × 180. The deviation as measured with the cover test in primary position was 6-PD exophoria combined with a 2-PD right hyperphoria at distance and 10-PD exophoria combined with 2-PD right hyperphoria at near. In levoversion the right hyperdeviation increased to 6 PD and in dextroversion the vertical deviation changed to 12-PD left hypertropia. With head tilt to the right, 10-PD right hypertropia existed, and with the head tilted to the left, 10-PD left hypertropia existed. Version testing revealed bilateral superior oblique underaction. The patient manifested a V pattern, being exotropic in upgaze and esotropic in downgaze. Only gross stereopsis was appreciated with the Titmus stereotest. A 17-degree excyclodeviation was measured with the double Maddox rod test. Despite the large amount of torsion, prism therapy was attempted and the patient reported that it reduced the incidence of diplopia.

In some cases of superior oblique paresis the bilaterality may be "masked" and diagnosed as a unilateral superior oblique paresis. Only after treatment, do the bilateral features become apparent. (See Case 9.)

CASE 9

A 61-year-old man complained of occasional diplopia of approximately 3-years duration. He denied any trauma. He was treated for tuberculosis 7 years previously. There was a history of childhood exotropia for which he received no treatment. He is presently in good health.

The patient manifested a 20-PD exotropia, with 12-PD left hypertropia in primary position. The hypertropia increased in right gaze and left head tilt. Versions revealed overaction of the left inferior oblique and underaction of the left superior oblique. Motility of the right eye was normal. There was no V-pattern. Normal retinal correspondence with poor fusion ability existed with the synoptophore. The double Maddox rod test revealed 21 degrees of excyclodeviation. The diagnosis was acquired left superior oblique paresis with long-standing exotropia. Neurologic and medical evaluations were normal.

Because of the amount of torsion, a bilateral SOP was suspected. Subsequent extraocular muscle surgery was performed to reduce the deviation.

Follow-up examination revealed increased diplopia; the diplopia was absent only in upgaze. The patient now manifested a 6-PD right hypertropia and 6-PD esotropia in primary position. There was a right hypertropia with left gaze and right head tilt and a left hypertropia with right gaze and left head tilt. Version testing revealed bilateral inferior oblique overaction and bilateral superior oblique underaction. A V-pattern deviation, with exotropia in upgaze and esotropia in downgaze now existed. The double Maddox rod test showed 12 degrees of excyclodeviation. Applying base-out prisms and placing the extrafoveal image in the suppression zone on the temporal hemiretina reduced the patient's diplopia significantly.

ABDUCENS NERVE (LATERAL RECTUS) PARESIS

Abducens nerve, or lateral rectus, paresis causes an incomitant esotropia that increases on gaze toward the involved side (Fig. 10-24). The esotropia may disappear entirely in the direction of gaze in which the lateral rectus works least, in adduction. This is where patients will most likely want to position their eyes. This frequently results in a compensatory face turn toward the paretic side (see Fig. 10-12). In acquired cases, lateral rectus paresis results in uncrossed diplopia that is greatest when viewing at distance. The paretic eye demonstrates limited abduction with overaction of the ipsilateral medial rectus when fixating with the nonparetic eye. Overaction of the contralateral medial rectus occurs when fixating with the paretic eye. The amount of movement of the paretic eye in abduction increases with duction testing.

Acquired cases are frequent, whereas congenital cases are rare. Limitation of abduction in a young child with significant esotropia in primary position is usually caused either by cross-fixation in infantile esotropia or by nystagmus with a null point in adduction, which

can be a part of infantile esotropia. Lateral rectus paresis in infants is often transient and without further sequelea. Acquired cases in older children are ominous and frequently the result of tumor, hydrocephalus, or head trauma.[54] Upper respiratory infection of viral origin has been associated with acquired lateral rectus paresis in some children. Its course is benign, and full restoration of function usually occurs. Intracranial neoplasm is the cause in approximately 22% of all acquired lateral rectus paresis in adults, whereas 26% of the cases are idiopathic (Fig. 10-25).[6]

Lateral rectus paresis may be bilateral. In these cases the esodeviation is smallest in the primary position and greatest in right and left gaze. These patients may cross-fixate as in infantile esotropia, using their right eye in left gaze and their left eye in right gaze. Compensatory head postures are unlikely in bilateral cases but may occur if the paresis is asymmetric.

Patients with recently acquired lateral rectus paresis manifest greater primary-position esotropia when fixating with the paretic eye and lesser primary-position esotropia when fixating with the nonparetic eye. Over time, a spread of comitance may occur, and the amount of esotropia with each eye fixating in turn becomes similar. With chronic lateral rectus paresis, secondary contracture, or tightening of the antagonist medial rectus, may cause restriction of abduction with the forced duction test.

If the paresis occurs when the patient is visually immature, suppression, anomalous correspondence, and amblyopia may develop. Amblyopia is usually prevented and normal binocular vision maintained in patients who adapt a compensatory head posture (see Case 2). Amblyopia occurs only in cases in which a head position is not used or a nonalternating constant esotropia remains even with the head turn.

Lateral rectus paresis should always be suspected in older children, adolescents, and adults with acute-onset esotropia (see Chapter 8). The classic features of lateral rectus paresis may not be obvious, and in some cases the esotropia may appear as being almost comitant. Limitation of abduction may be very subtle. Side gaze measurements of the deviation should be performed at distance fixation. Any esotropia that is greater at distance than at near should always alert the clinician to search for neurologic causes. The potentially serious nature of a recent-onset lateral rectus paresis is illustrated by the following case.

❋ CLINICAL PEARL

Lateral rectus paresis should always be suspected in older children, adolescents, and adults with acute-onset esotropia.

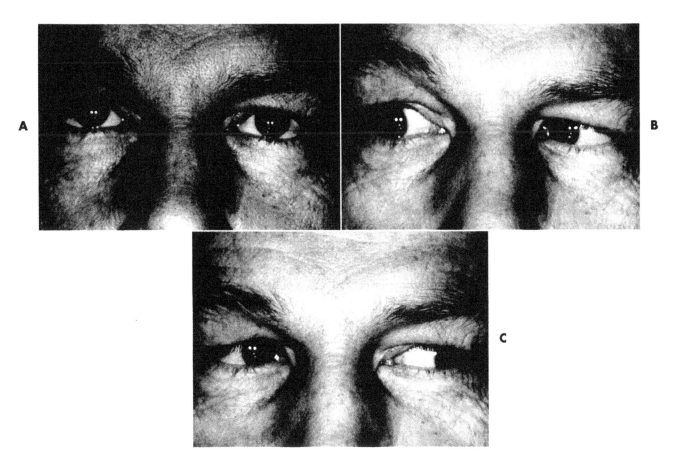

FIG. 10-24   Right lateral rectus paresis. **A,** Right intermittent esotropia exists in primary position. **B,** Increased esotropia with limited abduction exists in dextroversion. **C,** Full motility and orthophoria exist in levoversion.

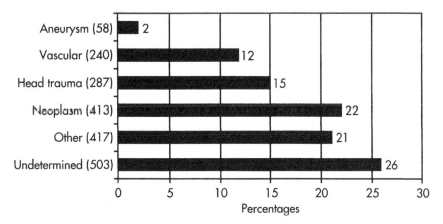

FIG. 10-25   Causes of acquired lateral rectus paresis. (Modified from Richards BW, Jones FR, Younge BR: Causes and prognosis in 4728 cases of paralysis of the oculomotor, trochlear, and abducens cranial nerves, *Am J Ophthalmol* 113:489, 1992.)

CASE 10

An apparently healthy 19-year-old female exchange student from France was referred to the clinic because of recent onset of diplopia and strabismus.[55] According to the patient the diplopia had begun approximately 1 month previously. There had not been any recent illness or physical or emotional trauma. The patient's medical history was unremarkable, except for a history of mitral valve prolapse that was being treated with nadolol (Corgard). This was the patient's first eye examination.

The examination revealed visual acuity of 20/20 for each eye. A 35-PD constant esotropia at distance and a 25-PD constant esotropia at near was present. The size of the deviation was similar in right and left gaze and with each eye fixating in turn. Versions and ductions were full, with slight overaction of the medial recti. With the Worth four dot test, the patient reported homonymous diplopia at distance and near. The separation of the diplopic images decreased during right gaze. Fusion could be achieved with prisms, 35-PD base-out.

Refraction revealed 6-D hyperopia for both eyes. It was suspected that the patient possibly had a late-onset refractive accommodative esotropia. Ophthalmoscopy, however, revealed bilateral papilledema. Lateral rectus paresis secondary to increased intracranial pressure was now suspected. The patient was referred for neurologic examination.

The neurologist's findings indicated a large neoplasm in the left frontal lobe. Surgery was attempted to remove the tumor. Postsurgically, the patient's condition worsened. She developed lower back pain, extremity pain, and general weakness. Further neurologic testing revealed metastases of the neoplasm to the spinal cord. Despite radiation and chemotherapy, the patient's condition deteriorated. Three months after developing the strabismus, the patient died.

The differential diagnosis of lateral rectus paresis includes other causes of impaired abduction, such as Duane's syndrome, cross-fixation in infantile esotropia, spasm of the near reflex, and mechanically restrictive causes, such as thyroid myopathy. The features of these clinical entities are summarized in Table 10-5.

Similar to the other paretic deviations, congenital lateral rectus paresis generally remains stable. Some patients with a head turn can benefit from base-out prisms. This may obviate the need for the head turn to view in forward position (see Fig. 10-2 and Case 2). Acquired deviations follow a dynamic course. They remiss completely or tend to become less incomitant with time. Complete resolution tends to occur within 6 months after the onset of the deviation and is more likely if the cause is vascular and less likely if the cause is related to trauma.[56] In the meantime, Fresnel prisms can be used to maintain fusion. Because the esodeviation is usually greater at distance, use of two base-out prisms may be necessary, one for the upper portion of the lens and another for the reading portion. We prefer

if possible to put all the Fresnel prism before the paretic eye, because this encourages fixation with the nonparetic eye, avoiding a larger secondary deviation. As the paresis recovers, the prism can be reduced. Deviations that persist and exceed 15 PD in the primary position can be considered for either extraocular muscle surgery or chemodenervation.

Patients with divergence insufficiency esotropia may at times actually represent the sequelae of a lateral rectus paresis. As described in Chapter 8, the esotropia occurs only for distance viewing and its magnitude remains the same in right and left gaze.[57,58] The patient is frequently either heterophoric or orthophoric for near viewing. Versions are normal, as are the amplitude and speed of horizontal saccades. The amount of fusional divergence amplitude is diminished or absent. (See Case 11.)

CASE 11

In March, 1982 a 59-year-old man with diabetes was first seen in the clinic. He complained of diplopia beginning 1week previously. He had continuously rubbed his right eye to eliminate the diplopia. Past ocular history was unremarkable, except for a mild myopic refractive error for which spectacles were prescribed. His medical history was significant only for diabetes.

The examination showed corrected vision of 20/20 for each eye. The patient manifested a constant right esotropia of 30 PD at distance and 20 PD at near. When fixating with his right eye, the esotropia increased to 45 PD. Versions showed marked underaction of the right lateral rectus, which improved with ductions. Homonymous diplopia was elicited with the Worth four dot test at distance and near.

A 30-PD base-out Fresnel prism before the right spectacle lens eliminated the diplopia and was prescribed. The patient was referred for a neurologic evaluation. It was concluded that the lateral rectus paresis was the result of diabetic neuropathy.

One month later, the deviation was essentially the same, and the patient continued with the prism.

In July the patient manifested signs of a divergence insufficiency esotropia. The deviation measured 20 PD esotropia at distance with each eye fixating and 12 PD esophoria at near. Version testing revealed full motility of the right lateral rectus. With the Worth four dot test, homonymous diplopia was noted at distance and fusion existed at near. The prism was reduced to 14 PD, which allowed the patient to fuse all the time.

In September a 14-PD intermittent esotropia was measured at distance and a 6-PD esophoria was measured at near. Versions were full. Fusional divergence amplitudes were deficient for distance fixation. Diplopia was still present at distance with the Worth four dot test. Because the deviation had persisted for 7 months, prism (8 PD base-out, 4 PD each lens) was ground into the patient's glasses. Subsequent evaluations over the years continued to show a divergence insufficiency esotropia.

TABLE 10-5 DIFFERENTIAL DIAGNOSIS OF LATERAL RECTUS PARESIS

	Lateral Rectus Paresis	Infantile Esotropia	Duane's Syndrome	Spasm of Near Reflex	Thyroid Myopathy
Onset	Childhood or adulthood	Before 6 months of age	Infancy	Childhood and adolescence mostly	40-60 yr
Diplopia	Present in acquired cases	Absent	Usually absent	Present with blurred vision	Present
Head Posture	Turn to involved side in unilateral cases	Absent except in cases with nystagmus	Turn to involved side in unilateral cases	Absent	Rare
Deviation in primary position	Esophoria or esotropia; greater at distance	Esotropia of 40-60 PD; Same at distance and near	Frequently orthophoria	Variable esotropia; may exist only at near	Esophoria or esotropia (more commonly seen with a vertical deviation)
Forced duction test	Negative	Negative	Positive	Negative	Positive
Abduction limitation	Usually unilateral; remains the same with doll's-head maneuver	Usually bilateral, eliminated with doll's-head maneuver	Usually unilateral; left eye more than right eye	Bilateral and intermittent	Usually bilateral and asymmetric
Size of deviation on lateral gaze	Increases toward affected side	Similar to primary position	Increases toward affected side	Variable; during spasm it increases	Increases toward affected side
Lid signs	Absent	Absent	Present; narrowing of palpebral tissue in adduction	Absent	Lid retraction on versions; more on down gaze
Pupils	Normal	Normal	Normal	Miotic	Normal
Normal binocular vision	Usually present	Absent	Usually present	Usually present	Present
Associated with neurologic or system disease	Frequent	Rare	Rare	Mostly psychogenic	Yes

We have also seen cases in which a divergence insufficiency esotropia has evolved into a frank lateral rectus paresis.[59,60] (See Case 12.)

CASE 12

In November, 1983 a 55-year-old man presented with symptoms of occasional diplopia that began 3 weeks earlier. Temporal arteritis had been recently diagnosed. Twelve years previously the patient had a slight stroke with full recovery.

The examination revealed 20/20 vision for each eye. A 10-PD intermittent esotropia was measured at distance and a 2-PD esophoria was measured at near. Version testing revealed normal findings, and the magnitude of the deviation did not change in dextroversion and levoversion. With the Worth four dot test, homonymous diplopia occurred at distance and fusion at near. Fusional divergence amplitudes as measured with the prism bar(break/recovery) were 2/1 for distance and 6/2 for near.

The diagnosis was divergence insufficiency esotropia. A

letter summarizing the findings was sent to the patient's internist. Because the diplopia was occasional and not too bothersome, no treatment was given.

Two months later the patient returned, complaining of increased diplopia. The patient now manifested a constant 12-PD right esotropia at distance and 10-PD intermittent esotropia at near. The esotropia increased to 30 PD in dextroversion, as did the separation between the diplopic images with the red lens test. Version testing revealed abduction deficiency for the right eye. The diagnosis was right lateral rectus paresis. A 6-PD base-out Fresnel press-on prism was placed before the patient's right spectacle lens to give fusion. The patient then underwent neurologic evaluation. An intracranial neoplasm was found and radiation therapy followed.

In August, 1984 the patient had not experienced any diplopia for 2 months. He now showed a 2-PD esophoria at distance and orthophoria at near with normal versions. The lateral rectus paresis had resolved.

TABLE 10-6 CLINICAL FEATURES FOR PATIENT'S WITH DUANE'S SYNDROME

Patient Number	Gender	Laterality	Type	Anisometropia (1 D or more)	Amblyopia (2 lines or more difference)	A or V Pattern	Stereopsis	Compensatory Head Posture
30	37% M 63% F	60% OS 20% OD 20% OU	60% I 3% II 37% III	27%	10%	13%	93%	57%

Modified from Rutstein RP: Duane's retraction syndrome, *J Am Optom Assoc* 63:426, 1992.

MECHANICALLY RESTRICTIVE DEVIATIONS

Incomitant deviations that are nonparetic and mechanically restricted in origin can occur where an extraocular muscle is tethered or a systemic disease reduces the elasticity of one or more muscles. These deviations have the following in common (1) gross limitation of ocular movement in one or more directions of gaze of the same amount, as shown clinically on ductions and versions; (2) frequently, a small angle of deviation or orthophoria in primary position; (3) positive forced duction testing; (4) diverse causative factors; and (5) frequent preservation of normal binocular vision aided by a compensatory head posture. As mentioned earlier, the measurement of the deviation in many of these cases cannot be accurately made by the alternate cover test and prisms, because the affected eye is restricted to a greater or lesser extent from taking up fixation when the nonaffected eye is covered. A Maddox rod and prism bar may be placed before the affected eye to measure the deviation. If both eyes are restricted, the Hirschberg test or the Krimsky test can be used to measure the deviation.

Congenital mechanically restrictive deviations include Duane's syndrome, Brown's syndrome, and the fibrosis syndrome. Acquired deviations include thyroid myopathy and deviations caused by trauma.

DUANE'S SYNDROME (DUANE'S RETRACTION SYNDROME)

Duane's syndrome, or Duane's retraction syndrome, consists of limitation of abduction, adduction, or both, as well as globe retraction, enophthalmos, and palpebral fissure narrowing on adduction. Rarely is there a large strabismus in primary position. The incidence is generally reported to be about 1% of the strabismic population.[61] The limited abduction in Duane's syndrome must be differentiated from the abduction deficiencies associated with other causes (see Table 10-5). A patient with limited abduction in the absence of a significant strabismic deviation in primary position should be considered to have Duane's syndrome until proven otherwise.

CLINICAL PEARL

A patient with limited abduction in the absence of a significant strabismic deviation in primary position should be considered to have Duane's syndrome until proven otherwise.

Duane's syndrome usually occurs as an isolated disorder, and most patients are otherwise normal. However, additional ocular and nonocular defects, such as deafness, brain stem abnormalities, and skeletal deformities have been associated with Duane's syndrome.[62-66] Sporadic onset is far more common than hereditary origin, and we rarely see Duane's syndrome among family members.

Etiologically, Duane's syndrome has been attributed to a fibrotic lateral rectus or a medial rectus that is inserted too far posteriorly.[67] Electromyographic studies have revealed anomalous innervation.[68,69] With restricted abduction, the lateral rectus does not fire during abduction but fires with the medial rectus in adduction. Clinicopathologic reports have shown absence of the abducens nucleus and peripheral nerves of the affected side and innervation of the lateral rectus with branches of the inferior division of the oculomotor nerve.[70-72]

The features for 30 patients with Duane's syndrome evaluated in our clinic are summarized in Table 10-6. Duane's syndrome consists of three types, I, II, III. In type I, the most common, abduction is markedly restricted and adduction is normal or only slightly restricted (Fig. 10-26). These patients may manifest orthophoria or a small esodeviation in primary position, with an increasingly larger esodeviation in abduction. In type II, the least common, adduction is markedly defective and abduction is normal or minimally restricted (Fig. 10-27). These patients may manifest orthophoria or a small exodeviation in primary position, with increasing exodeviation in adduction. In type III, both abduction and adduction are defective (Fig. 10-28). These patients manifest an esodeviation during abduction and an exodeviation during adduction. An esodeviation, or orthophoria, is more likely in primary position. In all

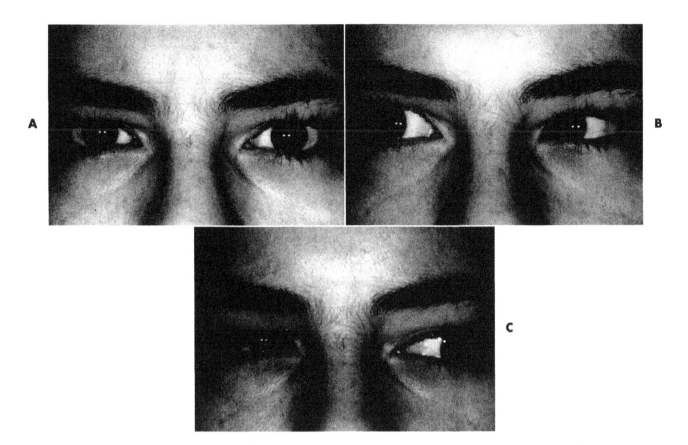

FIG. 10-26 Duane's syndrome type I. **A,** Orthophoria in primary position. **B,** Minimal abduction for right eye. **C,** Retraction of right eye and occurrence of palpebral fissure narrowing.

three types, retraction of the globe and narrowing of the palpebral fissure occurs during adduction. Some patients also show an upshoot and/or a downshoot of the affected eye during adduction, which mimics overaction of the inferior oblique and/or superior oblique muscles. It is believed that a taut, or tethering, effect occurs secondary to the tight and fibrotic lateral rectus muscle. Surgically weakening the oblique muscles thus has been ineffective in eliminating the occurrence of the patient's upshoot or downshoot.[73] Patients with Duane's syndrome can also have A and V patterns.

Duane's syndrome is mostly unilateral, occurs more commonly in the left eye than the right eye, and is more frequent in females than males. Bilateral cases occur in 15% to 20% of all patients.[61]

A high level of binocular vision usually exists with Duane's syndrome. Many patients develop a head turn toward the field of limited motility to permit fusion. Without the head turn, most patients manifest a strabismus in the primary position. In some cases, the head turn may be used to improve visual acuity rather than permit fusion. Amblyopia is rare in Duane's syndrome

and is limited to patients who do not have a compensatory head posture and who manifest a nonalternating strabismus in primary position. Deep suppression and anomalous correspondence are also uncommon. The lack of diplopia for many of these patients may result more from ignoring the extrafoveal image than from suppression.[74,75]

Treatment for Duane's syndrome is usually surgical and is reserved for those patients manifesting a significant strabismic deviation in primary position, a marked head posture, or a marked upshoot or downshoot and/or retraction of the globe in adduction. The surgical procedures for treatment of Duane's syndrome are discussed in Chapter 11. Surgery rarely improves the deficient abduction and/or adduction for these patients but does improve the field of binocular vison.[76,77]

As with lateral rectus paresis, prisms can be used in selected cases to alleviate compensatory head postures.[78] For example, a patient with unilateral Duane's syndrome type I of the left eye frequently will have a head turn to the left. Base-out prisms can reduce the head turn and allow fusion in the primary position. In

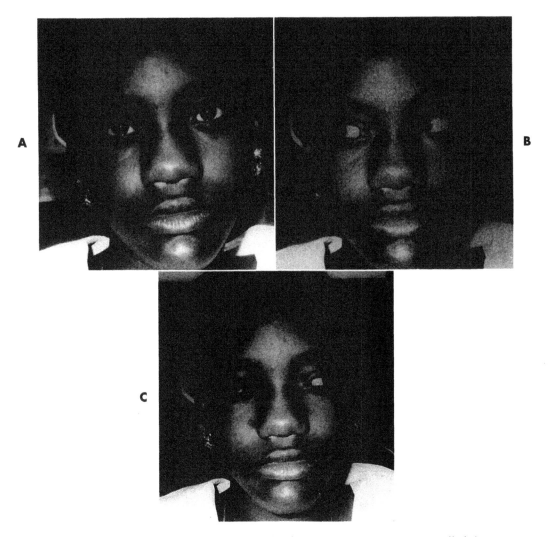

Fɪɢ. 10-27 Duane's syndrome type II. **A,** Orthophoria in primary position. **B,** Full abduction for right eye. **C,** Limited adduction of right eye, with retraction and palpebral fissure narrowing.

addition, because of the minimal sensory adaptations, prisms are also appropriate for use in patients who, despite having strabismus in the primary position, still possess normal fusion ability when the angle is compensated for either with prisms or with the synoptophore.

BROWN'S SYNDROME (SUPERIOR OBLIQUE TENDON SHEATH SYNDROME)

Patients with Brown's syndrome or the superior oblique tendon sheath syndrome show restricted elevation of an adducted eye around the midhorizontal plane (Fig. 10-29). Most cases are unilateral, with the right eye being more frequently involved.[16] Approximately 10% are bilateral.[16] Brown's syndrome is sup-

posedly more common in females than males and more common in children than adults. The motility deficiency is usually constant. However, intermittent episodes sometimes do occur. These episodes are usually associated with injury and inflammation in the region of the trochlea and may improve with time. Brown's syndrome is differentiated from the rarely occurring condition of inferior oblique paresis (Table 10-7).

✤ CLINICAL PEARL

Patients with Brown's syndrome or the superior oblique tendon sheath syndrome show restricted elevation of an adducted eye around the midhorizontal plane.

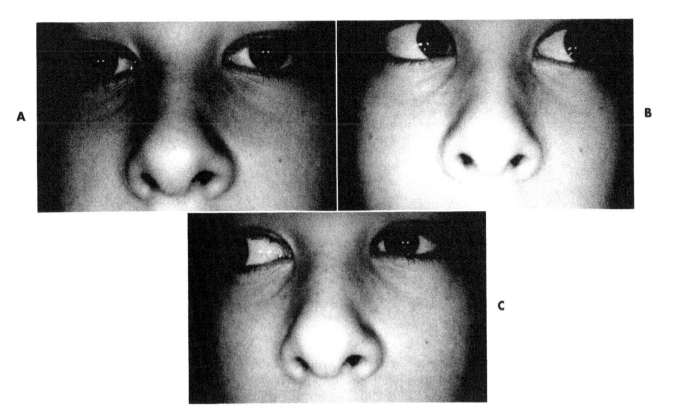

FIG. 10-28 Duane's syndrome type III. **A,** Orthophoria in primary position. **B,** Marked abduction restriction for left eye. **C,** Limited adduction of left eye, with retraction and palpebral fissure narrowing.

TABLE 10-7 CLINICAL DIFFERENTIATION OF BROWN'S SYNDROME VERSUS INFERIOR OBLIQUE PARESIS

	Brown's Syndrome	Inferior Oblique Paresis
Vertical deviation in primary position	Minimal or absent	Hypotropia of affected eye
Major motility disorder	Limited elevation in adduction	Limited elevation in adduction
Head posture	Frequently chin elevation	Usually a head tilt to affected side; a face turn toward the uninvolved side and chin elevation may also occur
Three-step test criteria	Not fulfilled	Fulfilled
A or V pattern	V pattern exo in upgaze	A pattern exo in downgaze
Duction versus version	Duction equals version	Duction exceeds version
Amblyopia	Rare	Rare
Binocular vision	Present	Usually present; may be absent in children without a head tilt
Overaction of antagonist superior oblique	Absent	Present
Forced duction test	Criteria fulfilled	Criteria not fulfilled
Symptoms	Rare; may have diplopia and/or pain and discomfort on elevation in adduction	Diplopia and asthenopia in adult-onset cases
Cyclodeviation*	None	Intorsion if onset after period of visual immaturity

Modified from Rutstein RP: Incomitant deviation in children. In Scheiman MM, editor: *Problems in optometry,* vol 2, Philadelphia, 1990, J Lippincott.
*As measured with the double Maddox rod test.

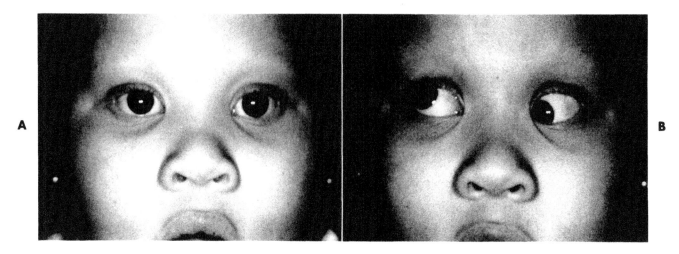

FIG. 10-29 Brown's syndrome. **A,** Patient is orthophoric in primary position. **B,** Inability to elevate left eye in adduction. Note downshoot of left eye.

Etiologically, it is presumed that the trochlea to the superior oblique tendon insertion distance cannot be increased because of mechanical causes. Commonly, thickening of the superior oblique tendon impairs its movement through the trochlea. Although mostly congenital, acquired cases associated with trauma, inflammatory disease processes, and iatrogenic causes may occur.[79-82] Trauma to the orbit may cause the muscle itself to become entrapped in the roof of the orbit. Iatrogenic cases occur following a tight surgical tuck of the superior oblique if the tendon sheath is not adequately stripped away or if surgery is performed too close to the trochlea.[83,84] In addition, Brown's syndrome may occur following blephoplasty and sinus surgery. Inflammation of the superior oblique tendon has occurred with rheumatoid arthritis. The inflammation causes pain on local palpation and when elevation of the involved eye is attempted.

A patient with Brown's syndrome will manifest (1) restricted elevation or absence of elevation in adduction that is the same on version and duction testing; (2) normal elevation in abduction for the affected eye; (3) a positive forced duction test with marked resistance to forcible elevation of the eye only in adduction; (4) usually, widening of the palpebral fissure with adduction; (5) absence of overaction of the ipsilateral superior oblique; (6) a V-pattern exodeviation; (7) a compensatory head posture frequently consisting of a chin elevation and pointing toward the opposite shoulder; (8) a mild downshoot of the affected eye in adduction; and (9) minimal or no vertical deviation in the primary position. Not all patients with Brown's syndrome manifest all of these findings.

The restricted elevation is present only in adduc-

tion. As the eye gradually rotates from the adducted position toward the abducted position, there is a corresponding increase in elevation. This change from left to right gaze differentiates Brown's syndrome from other causes of monocular elevation deficiency that are mechanically restrictive. Most patients with Brown's syndrome also have a V exo pattern in upgaze. The greater exotropia in upgaze helps differentiate Brown's syndrome from inferior oblique paresis, which usually causes an A pattern that is greater exotropia in downgaze. For some patients, the ocular movements may improve with repeated testing. In cases that are intermittent, an audible click frequently is heard when the patient eventually is able to elevate the adducted eye.[79] This may cause some discomfort to the patient.

Most patients with Brown's syndrome have a high level of binocular vision when the eyes are in primary position and downgaze. Many are orthophoric in primary position. Amblyopia is uncommon. In one study, 38% of patients with congenital Brown's syndrome exhibited perfect stereopsis in the primary position.[84] Another 23% had some stereopsis. The remaining patients were unable to appreciate any stereopsis. Amblyopia was present in 14%. As with Duane's syndrome, ignoring rather than suppressing of the diplopic image most likely occurs in the affected position of gaze.

The majority of patients with Brown's syndrome do not require treatment. Treatment is reserved for those patients with either a significant hypotropia in primary position or a compensatory head posture that is cosmetically displeasing. Orthoptics/vision therapy procedures to improve the elevation of the affected eye in adduction are usually unsuccessful. Prism therapy has limited application. Because a chin elevation pos-

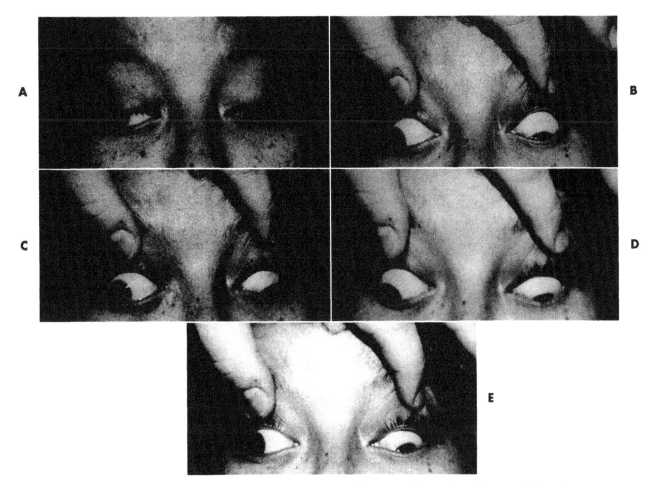

FIG. 10-30 Generalized fibrosis syndrome. Bilateral ptosis and limited motility are exhibited in all positions of gaze. **A,** Primary gaze. **B,** Right gaze. **C,** Left gaze. **D,** Downgaze. **E,** Upgaze.

ture may be present, conjugate base-up or yoked prisms can be given in an attempt to reduce the head posture. The amount of prisms used can rarely exceed 10 PD.

Treatment of Brown's syndrome is primarily surgical. The results can be unpredictable. Cases of iatrogenically induced superior oblique paresis accompanied with a head tilt toward the opposite side have been reported in patients treated surgically for Brown's syndrome.[85] Surgery solely to improve elevation in adduction in a patient without a compensatory head posture and who is orthophoric in primary position and downgaze is unjustified.

FIBROSIS SYNDROME

In the fibrosis syndrome, the tissue of the extraocular muscles is abnormal, and replacement of the normal contractile tissue with fibrous tissue takes place. Extreme restrictions in ocular motility exist.[86] Fibrosis

of the extraocular muscles is usually a bilateral condition and present at birth. It is transmitted as an autosomal dominant trait and typically affects multiple family members.[87,88] In many cases, however, it occurs sporadically. Fibrosis may be generalized and affect all of the muscles of both eyes or affect only one muscle. With generalized fibrosis, there is ptosis, all extraocular muscles are involved, and the eyes can barely move (Fig. 10-30). Patients with generalized fibrosis of the extraocular muscles are generally healthy.

When only the medial rectus is involved, strabismus fixus exists. In this rare condition, the eye (or both eyes) is fixed in extreme adduction. The eye cannot be moved either actively or passively from the habitually adducted position. The esotropia is very large and may exceed 100 PD (Fig. 10-31). Rarely, patients may adapt a compensatory head turn toward the side of the fixating eye. Unlike most strabismic patients who use an abnormal head posture, those with strabismus fixus do

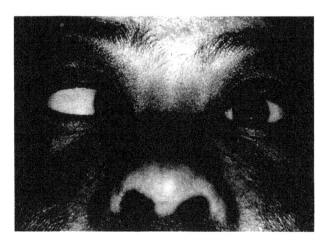

FIG. 10-31 Strabismus fixus. Right eye is fixed in extreme adduction.

not have fusion. Although strabismus fixus is mostly congenital, it may result from infection, trauma, or surgery. Strabismus fixus can also occur secondary to fibrosis of muscles contracted as the ipsilateral antagonists of a previous paresis; the esotropia would be secondary to a lateral rectus paresis. Strabismus fixus is differentiated from Duane's syndrome by having no globe retraction, palpebral fissure aperture changes on attempted horizontal rotations of the eye, and a very large strabismic deviation in primary position.

Of the individual extraocular muscles, the inferior rectus is most likely to become fibrotic.[89] This condition has also been referred to as *double elevator palsy.* However, it is caused by a mechanical restriction, not a paretic muscle. With fibrosis of the inferior rectus, one or both eyes are drawn downward. If bilateral, the involvement is usually asymmetric. Ptosis and hypotropia exist in primary position. The eyes are fixed 20 to 30 degrees below the horizontal. Versions and ductions are equally restricted, and the forced duction test is positive to passive elevation. The eyes frequently become spastically esotropic on attempted upgaze. On downgaze, the eyes may become exodeviated. Occasionally, patients may use an elevated chin position to centrally fixate straight ahead. A high degree of hyperopia and astigmatism has been reported in patients with fibrotic inferior rectus muscles.[90] Amblyopia is common.

For the rare patient with a fibrotic inferior rectus muscle who is capable of fixating with the involved eye or who uses a compensatory head posture, amblyopia may be prevented and normal binocular vision preserved. (See Case 13.)

CASE 13

A 5-year-old boy was first examined in our clinic in July 1986. The parents had noted a variable left ptosis since in-

fancy. There was no history of trauma, illness, or abnormal birth. A year earlier, the patient was examined by another clinician and no treatment was recommended. According to the parents, the patient occasionally elevated his chin.

Our examination confirmed the presence of a left ptosis. The ptosis was much less apparent when the patient fixated with the left eye. Visual acuity was 20/20 for each eye. A 15-PD left hypotropia existed in the primary position. The hypotropia increased in upgaze, and in extreme downgaze the patient was orthophoric. With the Randot stereotest, 70 seconds of arc was measured in this position. Version testing showed restriction of elevation of the left eye, greater in abduction than in adduction. The motility defect was similar when ductions were tested. The diagnosis was probable fibrosis of the left inferior rectus.

The parents desired surgical treatment. At the time of surgery, the surgeon documented the left inferior rectus as being quite tight and fibrotic. Its insertion was also noted to be quite anomalous, bending anteriorly as close as 3½ mm from the limbus nasally and arching away from the limbus temporally. The muscle's insertion also extended further posteriorly along the sclera than normal. A 5-mm left inferior rectus recession was performed.

The patient returned to the clinic in October, 1986. According to the parents, the ptosis was now less frequent, as was the chin elevation. Our examination now showed a 10-PD left hypotropia in primary position. The patient continued to fuse in downgaze and maintained the stereopsis. The ability to elevate the left eye had not improved. The patient was subsequently lost to follow-up.

Patients with fibrosis of the extraocular muscles usually have a visual and cosmetic handicap. Amblyopia should be treated for younger patients, and any refractive correction given when needed. Because normal binocular vision is the exception, prisms and orthoptics/vision therapy are rarely used. Surgical treatment is the therapy of choice.[91] Multiple procedures are frequently necessary. Ptosis surgery is often required as a secondary procedure. Ocular motility is rarely improved by surgery for fibrotic muscles; however, moving the eyes closer to primary position is a cosmetic advantage, and the head position may improve as a result. Generally, if there is no significant head posture or strabismus in primary position, patients can be followed without surgical intervention.

THYROID MYOPATHY (GRAVES' OPHTHALMOPATHY)

Thyroid myopathy, or Graves' ophthalmopathy, is an autoimmune inflammatory condition that involves mostly the orbital tissues, primarily the muscles and fat. Abnormalities encountered in patients with thyroid disorders include chemosis, periorbital congestion, lid retraction and lid lag, exophthalmos, optic neuropathy, and impaired ocular motility. Enlargement of the extraocular muscles, as determined by orbital ultrasonography and computed tomography, results from an in-

TABLE 10-8 **CLINICAL FINDINGS OF FOUR PATIENTS WITH THYROID MYOPATHY**

Patient	1	2	3	4
Gender	Female	Female	Male	Female
Age	69	59	64	65
Symptoms	Diplopia, words run together	Diplopia; left eye is not working well	Diplopia	Occasional diplopia
Deviation in primary position (distance and near)	8 PD right hypotropia and 5 PD exotropia; 10 PD right hypotropia and 5 PD exotropia	12 PD right hypotropia and 15 PD exotropia; 6 PD right hypotropia and 20 PD exotropia	12 PD right hypotropia and 12 PD exotropia at distance and near	12 PD left hypotropia and 10 PD exotropia at distance and near
Versions	Restriction of upgaze for both eyes in abduction and adduction	Restriction of upgaze in field of right superior rectus	Restriction of upgaze in field of right superior rectus	Restriction of upgaze for both eyes in field of superior rectus
Other ocular signs	Lid retraction; dry eye	Lid retraction	Right ptosis	Lid retraction
Cyclodeviation	Not tested	None	None	7° left excyclo
Head posture	Normal	Normal	Chin elevation	Normal
Medical history	Hypothyroidism	Hypothyroidism	Euthyroid	Euthyroid
Treatment	Prisms (5 PD vertical)	Prisms (5 PD vertical and 8 PD horizontal)	Prisms (8 PD vertical)	None

crease in intraorbital tissue occurs.[92-94] These histologic changes consist of lymphocytic infiltration and fibrosis of the muscles, which impair their elasticity. This reduces the motility of the affected extraocular muscle and results in an incomitant deviation. Usually, both eyes are affected, although one eye is usually affected more than the other. Thyroid myopathy is probably the most common cause of spontaneous diplopia in middle age. Diplopia may be worse in the morning. Compensating head postures, such as chin elevation, may be used to maintain fusion and avoid diplopia.

 CLINICAL PEARL

Thyroid myopathy is probably the most common cause of spontaneous diplopia in middle age.

The inferior rectus is involved the most with thyroid myopathy, followed by the medial rectus, the superior rectus, and least the lateral rectus.[95] A fibrous union between the inferior rectus and inferior oblique leads to a restriction in upgaze and a hypotropia of the affected eye (Fig. 10-32). In severe cases the eye may be tethered down. Adhesions between other muscles and adjacent orbital structures cause restrictions in the other gaze positions, thereby resulting in A and V patterns.

Thyroid myopathy is more common with females, peaking in the third and fourth decades of life; however, it may occur at any age. In a recent study the average age at the time of diagnosis was 44.7 plus or minus 17.4 years of age.[96] Thyroid myopathy is rarely the cause of an incomitant deviation in children. In children, the condition tends to be more benign, with no

sight-threatening complications and fewer restrictions in ocular motility.

Clinically, the presence of other ocular signs, such as lid retraction, exophthalmos, and lid lag caused by sympathetic stimulation of Mueller's muscle, assist with the diagnosis. The lid retraction may be a primary effect of the disease or may be secondary to inferior rectus fibrosis. Advanced cases may present with periorbital edema and exposure keratitis secondary to exophthalmos. In some patients with thyroid myopathy, symptoms and signs are minimal and diagnosis may be difficult. The motility dysfunction may occur before, at the same time as, or after systemic signs of Graves' disease. In euthyroid patients without a history of thyroid disease but with typical thyroid myopathy, the association between thyroid gland dysfunction is difficult to establish. In other patients it appears with hypothyroidism secondary to treatment of hyperthyroidism.

For most patients, a restriction of the affected eye in elevation occurs (Table 10-8). This causes a hypotropia in primary position. Esotropia and exotropia may coexist. Because the deviation usually commences in adulthood, torsion with the double Maddox rod test may also be present.[97] Thyroid myopathy involving the inferior rectus is frequently misdiagnosed as superior rectus paresis. In thyroid myopathy, limited elevation may occur in adduction and abduction and is similar with ductions and versions. The forced duction test indicates marked restriction in upgaze, and intraocular pressure will be elevated in upgaze by 5 mm or more, relative to downgaze. Measuring the intraocular pressure in upgaze, primary position, and downgaze can help with the diagnosis.

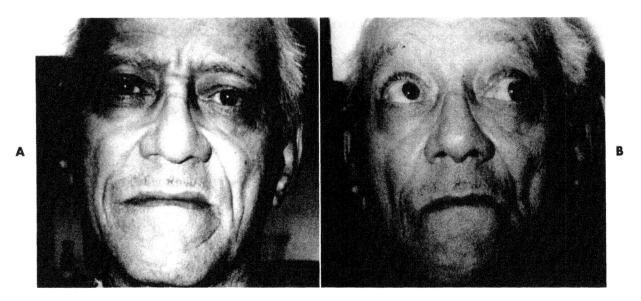

FIG. 10-32   Thyroid myopathy. **A,** Small left hypotropia exists in primary position. **B,** Limited elevation of left eye when looking up and to left. Note left eyelid retraction.

Although some patients may spontaneously improve or show reversal with time, more commonly there is persistence of the deviation, even following normalization of the endocrine imbalance by medical control.[98,99] Improvement in ocular motility may occur as a result of resolution of orbital edema, but regression of the portion of restricted motility because of muscle fibrosis is unlikely.

In mild cases, prism therapy is quite successful. The least amount of prism to allow fusion in primary position and downgaze is the appropriate prismatic correction. Because the deviation may change over time, Fresnel press-on prisms can be given initially. We prefer to place the entire prism before the more involved eye. Prisms should be avoided in patients with diplopia only in extreme positions of gaze.

With marked ocular deviations and restrictions, corrective surgery is needed. This can be delayed for 2 to 3 years and performed during the quiescent phase of the disease. Stability in the measurements for at least 6 months is generally required before surgery. Perfect results are rarely achieved in one operation because of the great variability that occurs secondary to swollen muscles. Surgery can be successful in restoring binocular vision in primary and reading positions, but a normal conjugate type of eye movement is seldom achieved. The adjustable suture technique increases the chance of better results for these patients and is described in Chapter 11.[100,101]

DEVIATIONS ASSOCIATED WITH TRAUMA

Trauma to the globe produced by blunt objects, such as a ball, fist, knee, elbow, or automobile dash-

board may cause a blow-out fracture to the thin orbital floor and, less commonly, to the medial orbital wall. Often there are other severe injuries to the eye. The most likely site of orbital fracture is the posterior medial aspect of the floor, which is the thinnest part of the maxillary bone. Ocular motility is impaired because of proptosis and edema from original trauma, intraorbital hemorrhage, herniation of the orbital fascia, and muscle entrapment. An orbital fracture may also damage the trochlea or the origin of the inferior oblique muscle.

When the orbital floor is involved, the inferior rectus and inferior oblique, along with other orbital structures, such as nerves, blood vessels, and Tenon's connective tissue, can become incarcerated in a linear crack in the maxillary bone. In some cases, hemorrhage and edema involving orbital fat rather than entrapment of muscles may occur.

The clinical findings for patients with recently acquired fracture of the orbital floor include enophthalmos, ecchymosis, lid edema, and painful and limited motility of the affected eye in upgaze.[102,103] A vertical strabismus with diplopia is noted, and a restriction in motility is seen in a direction opposite to the defect. There may be orthophoria in the primary position (Fig. 10-33). The entrapment of the orbital tissue by bone fragments in the affected site is the cause of the vertical deviation. With limited upgaze, this condition simulates a combined superior rectus and inferior oblique paresis. The degree of restriction is similar for ductions and versions, and the forced duction test is positive. As with thyroid myopathy, measuring the intraocular pressure in primary position and then once again in elevation shows an increase in pressure. When limitation

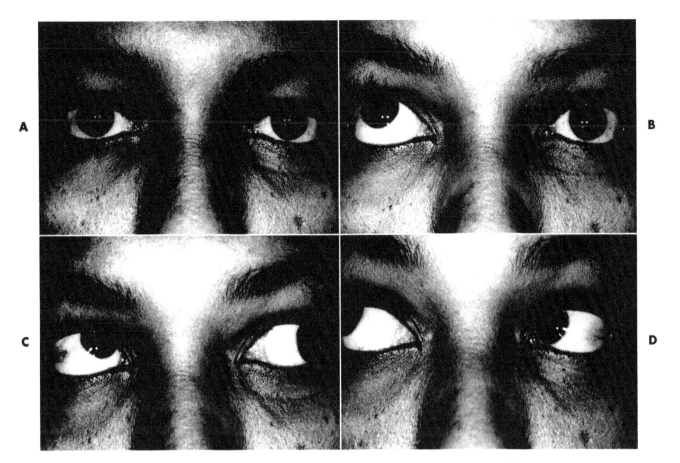

FIG. 10-33 Deviation associated with history of blow-out fracture of left orbital floor. **A,** Orthophoria in primary position. **B,** Marked restriction of elevation of left eye when looking up, **C,** looking up and to left, and **D,** looking up and to right.

in downgaze is also found, damage to the inferior rectus nerve or to the muscle itself secondary to direct trauma must be ruled out. If the nerve to the inferior rectus is primarily damaged, the eye will be elevated in primary position. Patients with traumatically induced deviations may adapt a head posture to avoid diplopia and permit fusion.

The thin ethmoid bone of the medial wall of the orbit may be involved. In these cases, limited abduction as a result of medial rectus entrapment occurs and esotropia is present. This simulates lateral rectus paresis. The degree of restriction on ductions and versions is similar, and the forced duction test is positive.

Most traumatically induced deviations follow a variable course. Although surgery is the treatment of choice, it is rarely done on an emergency basis.[104] Time should elapse, with frequent evaluation of the diplopia, before surgery is considered. Indications for surgery are enophthalmos and diplopia secondary to entrapment. Enophthalmos is evaluated after the swelling resolves, and entrapment is diagnosed with the forced duction test and can be seen radiographically. Entrap-

ment generally requires surgical treatment within weeks of the trauma.

Patients with orbital floor fracture who have no diplopia or in whom diplopia disappears within 14 days may be spared surgery unless there is an extensive defect of the orbit that may cause enophthalmos.[104]

Other patients may not require surgery and will have a satisfactory recovery in a few months. This group is usually associated with limitation of eye movement secondary to hemorrhage and edema in the orbit without entrapment, as well as paresis of the inferior rectus muscle.[83] In the interim, occlusion or prisms can be used to alleviate the diplopia.[105] Because surgical therapy is rarely totally curative, prisms may still be useful for patients years after the trauma. (See Case 14.)

CASE 14

A 20-year-old man was examined in November, 1983. In 1972 he had a bicycle accident that resulted in an orbital floor fracture on the left side. Surgery was performed to repair the fracture. The patient presently experiences diplopia in upgaze and when he reads. The latter is the most troublesome. He states that when he looks down, he has to raise his chin slightly to maintain single binocular vision.

The examination revealed 20/20 vision for each eye, with a slight hyperopic correction. The patient was orthophoric at distance and 3-PD exophoric at near in the primary position. When viewing straight up a 15-PD left hypotropia and 4-PD exotropia were measured. In downgaze a 2-PD left hypertropia and 4-PD exotropia existed.

Version testing revealed marked restriction of the left eye on upgaze and slight restriction of the left eye when looking down. The forced duction test was positive, and ductions were similar to versions.

The patient had 40 seconds of arc in the primary position with the Titmus stereotest and fused the Worth four dot test except when viewing up and down. Compensatory fusional vergence ranges at near were reduced.

Because the patient was bothered by the diplopia mostly when reading, prisms (4 PD base-in and 1 PD base-up OD) were given for near vision only, along with orthoptics/vision therapy to expand his horizontal fusional ranges. Subsequent evaluations revealed resolution of the diplopia.

OTHER INCOMITANT DEVIATIONS

Incomitant deviations that are neither paretic nor mechanically restrictive in origin include ocular myasthenia, dissociated vertical deviation, and oblique muscle dysfunction.

OCULAR MYASTHENIA

Myasthenia gravis is a neuromuscular disorder manifested by weakness and fatigability of voluntary striated muscle, especially muscles involved in mastication and breathing. It is caused by a failure to release or produce acetylcholine, so that the muscle does not contract sufficiently and its action is weakened. Circulating antibodies against acetylcholine probably occur at the neuromuscular endplate.

Clinicians should always consider myasthenia gravis as a possible cause of any acquired deviation. Half of all patients with myasthenia gravis initially present with ocular symptoms, and almost all eventually develop the eye movement and lid abnormalities of ocular myasthenia.[106,107] Ocular myasthenia may mimic almost any type of strabismus and ocular muscle paresis. Diplopia and abnormal ocular motility may be the sole symptoms of the disease. Although it has an onset mostly between ages 20 and 40 and occurs slightly more frequently in females, ocular myasthenis can occur at any age. Cases in early childhood and infancy have been reported. A familial, usually benign form of the disease occurs in children, typically involving the extraocular muscle.[108]

 CLINICAL PEARL

Clinicians should always consider myasthenia gravis as a possible cause of any acquired deviation.

Ptosis is almost always present in ocular myasthenia (Fig. 10-34). The ptosis is unilateral or bilateral but always variable. If unilateral, it is usually asymmetric and may alternate from one eye to the other. The ptosis is also progressive, that is, it is brought out more, for example, by attempted sustained upgaze. In addition, extraocular muscle restrictions occur in approximately 90% of all these patients.[106-108] Such motility disorders may be preceded by an emotional upset or upper respiratory infection. Any of the extraocular muscles may be involved, with upgaze restriction being more common. The ocular muscle disorder can resemble any type of incomitant deviation, paretic or mechanically restrictive. The motility disorders are fleeting. They may affect one, some, or all of the extraocular muscles, and the restriction can range from subtle to severe. Unusual combinations, such as ipsilateral superior oblique and inferior rectus weaknesses, have been associated with myasthenia. The disease may have predilection for the inferior rectus. As mentioned earlier, isolated weakness of the inferior rectus is rare and should lead to consideration of ocular myasthenia rather than inferior branch oculomotor nerve palsy.[109] Isolated medial rectus involvement may also occur, simulating the supranuclear disorder of internuclear ophthalmoplegia. Usually, the levator is the first muscle involved, resulting in the ptosis. Additional eyelid signs, such as lid flutter and lid twitch may occur. If the patient is asked to look downward for 15 seconds and then quickly back to the primary position, an upward twitch of the upper lid (retraction) is frequently seen before it resumes the ptotic position.[110] Also, when myasthenia is suspected, the patient, when asked to blink rapidly 20 times, will usually demonstrate an increase in the ptosis.

The presence therefore of a fleeting and inconsistent deviation, ptosis, and restricted ocular motility should make the clinician suspect ocular myasthenia. Accommodative and convergence insufficiency of sudden onset may also be a manifestation of the disease.[111,112] However, perhaps the earliest and most sensitive signs of extraocular involvement are abnormalities of saccades and quick phase of nystagmus. In large saccades the eye may start off rapidly, but slow in midflight and creep up to the desired eye position. During prolonged optokinetic nystagmus, quick phases may become slow.

On examination there is generally fatigability of the extraocular muscles and the levator. The signs are usually more apparent later in the day. Rapid forced repetitive version movements fatigue the extraocular muscle. Ocular movement can also be fatigued by sustaining fixation on a target well above eye level or by repeated saccadic eye movements. Measurement of the deviation by alternate cover test and prisms is difficult and frequently inaccurate because of the extreme variability of the deviation.

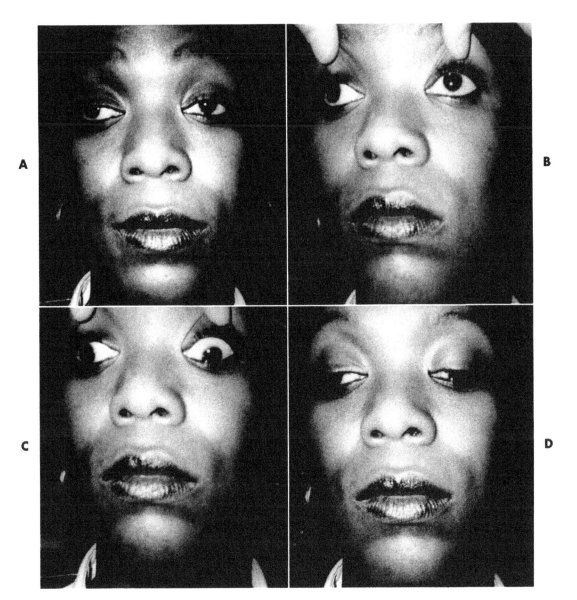

FIG. 10-34 Ocular myasthenia. **A,** Bilateral ptosis and exotropia exist in primary position. Versions show **B,** limited elevation, and **C,** limited depression. **D,** Increased ptosis occurs following prolonged testing.

Electromyography is a useful diagnostic test and shows reduced potentials as the extraocular muscles fatigue.[113] Administering systemic anticholinesterase agents, such as edrophonium chloride (Tensilon) and neostigmine intravenously improves the ptosis and eliminates the ocular motility restriction. The ocular deviation is measured before and after administration of edrophonium chloride. Changes in motility are much less reliable predictors of a diagnosis of ocular myasthenia than are improvement in ptosis. Occasionally, the ocular deviation worsens after administration of edrophonium if one muscle is more susceptible to the effects of the drug than others. Thus only the direct observation of a weak muscle becoming stronger after administration of edrophonium is reliable evidence of myasthenia. Side effects, such as gastrointestinal and respiratory problems, may occur following the test.

Ocular myasthenia is the great mimicker. The strabismus can measure comitant or appear to be an oculomotor, trochlear, or abducens nerve palsy. We have examined patients with the classic features of superior oblique paresis who, during medical evaluation, were diagnosed as having ocular myasthenia. Acute-onset esotropia in adolescents, which is more likely to be associated with lateral rectus paresis, can also be the first sign of ocular myasthenia (see Cases 10 and 15.)

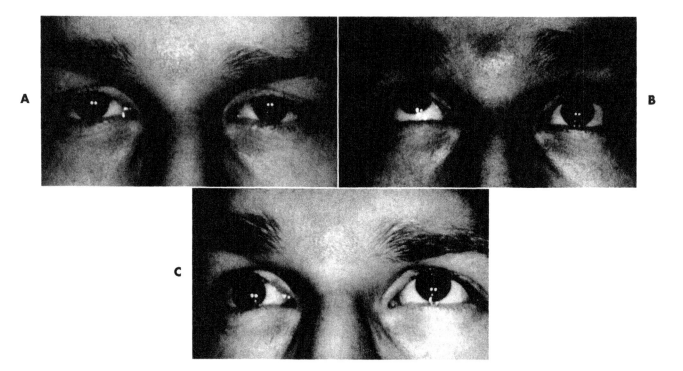

FIG. 10-35 Dissociated vertical deviation. **A,** Orthophoria. **B,** Right hypertropia after right eye occlusion. **C,** Left hypertropia after left eye occlusion. (From Amos JF, Rutstein RP: Vertical deviations. In Amos JF, editor: *Diagnosis and management in vision care,* Boston, 1987, Butterworth-Heinemann.)

CASE 15

A 14-year-old girl presented with the complaint of diplopia that began about 6 months earlier. The diplopia existed mostly for distance viewing. Two months earlier another clinician concluded that the diplopia was psychogenic in origin and recommended psychiatric counseling. The patient was in good health and taking no medication. There was no history of trauma or recent illness.

Our examination indicated corrected vision of 20/20 for each eye with a mild myopic correction. There was no ptosis. The patient manifested a constant alternating esotropia of 20 PD at distance and 12 PD at near. The deviation was the same with each eye fixating in turn. Version testing revealed slight abduction deficiency in each eye.

Sensory testing with the Worth four dot test showed homonymous diplopia at distance and near. With the synoptophore, normal correspondence and second-degree fusion existed. The patient perceived 20 seconds of arc with the Randot stereotest with compensatory prisms. Funduscopic examination indicated normal findings.

It was presumed that the patient had developed a lateral rectus paresis, and, over time, the deviation had become less incomitant. Fresnel prisms (20 PD, base-out) were placed on the left spectacle lens. The patient was referred to a pediatric neurologist to determine the etiology of the deviation.

During the neurologic evaluation the patient responded positively to the Tensilon test and the electromyogram showed reduced action potentials. The diagnosis was ocular myasthenia. The patient is presently being treated with steroids and anticholinesterase agents.

The lack of a stable deviation generally prevents deep suppression, anomalous correspondence, and amblyopia from developing in very young children. Despite this, ocular myasthenia has been the cause of amblyopia in some children.[114] Because of the variability of the deviation, prism therapy usually is not helpful, and strabismus and ptosis surgery generally are not indicated at first. Diplopia can be eliminated with occlusion. Spontaneous remission may occur in as many as 30% of patients with ocular myasthenia.[114]

The use of steroids, immunotherapy, thymectomy, and plasmapheresis has been attempted by some physicians, mostly in younger patients who do not improve with anticholinesterase agents. Extraocular muscle surgery may be considered when there is no improvement from medical therapy and weakness of a particular muscle becomes chronic and does not undergo further changes.[115]

DISSOCIATED VERTICAL DEVIATION

Dissociated vertical deviation (DVD), also referred to as *alternating hyperphoria, double dissociated hypertropia, dissociated vertical divergence,* and *alternating sursumduction,* is characterized by the spontaneous turning of one or both eyes upward when the patient is fatigued or inattentive or when fusion is interrupted by covering one eye (Fig. 10-35). On alternating cover test, the clinician notes a slow introduction of the eye being uncovered.[116] The deviation occurs either in a manifest form with both eyes open or as a latent deviation in which each eye will drift up when covered. The upward movement is typically asymmetric and sometimes absent in one eye. Unlike other vertical deviations, in DVD there is absence of a hypodeviation of the nonfixating eye when the hyperdeviated eye fixates. Neither eye drops below midline during cover testing. The eyes violate Hering's law of equal innervation. With DVD, equal innervation is not going to the yoke muscles, and the eyes appear to move independently of one another. The hyperdeviation shows appreciable variation and usually increases with prolonged occlusion. Because each eye drifts upward under cover and moves downward on removal of the cover, the deviation is difficult to accurately measure. The alternate cover test with prisms, with first one eye fixating and then the other eye fixating, can be used to measure the deviation. A base-down prism is placed over the more involved eye, and the strength of the prism is adjusted until no movement occurs as the cover is shifted to the fixating eye. This is repeated with the prism placed before the lesser involved eye. Most clinicians prefer to grade it as being slight (+1), moderate (+2, +3), or marked (+4) rather than actually quantifying it.

With DVD, if a photometric neutral filter is placed before one eye while the other is occluded, the eye behind the cover makes a gradual downward movement as the density of the filter is increased in front of the fixating eye. This is known as the *Bielschowsky phenomenon*. In addition, when placing a red lens before one eye and having the patient view a muscle light at distance, the red light will always be below the white light, regardless of which eye fixates.

DVD generally begins when the patient is young and visually immature, usually before age 3. It has been reported as early as 8 months.[117] DVD is unrelated to trauma or any systemic or neurologic disorder. It is seen mostly in patients with underlying fusion anomalies, such as esotropia, exotropia, or other vertical deviations. Approximately 50% to 90% of all individuals with infantile esotropia will eventually develop DVD.[118] This is frequently seen following reduction of the large-angle esotropia. As many as 12% of patients with sensory strabismus also have DVD.[119] DVD occurs much less commonly in patients who are heterophoric and have no other apparent binocular vision disorder.

Because either eye may be hypertropic, DVD is frequently confused with bilateral inferior oblique overaction, which also causes a hyperdeviation of the eyes. Unlike inferior oblique overaction, in which the hyperdeviation occurs only in adduction, the hyperdeviation in DVD occurs in adduction, primary position, and abduction. Also, unlike inferior oblique overaction, the nonfixating eye is always the hyper eye in DVD. There is no hypotropia in DVD when either eye is fixating or

in right or left gaze. Oblique muscle dysfunctions and other types of vertical deviations may coexist with DVD, making the diagnosis of DVD difficult.

As many as 50% of patients with DVD have latent nystagmus. This consists of a conjugate lateral jerk or a conjugate cyclorotary nystagmus accentuated by covering one eye; both eyes drift to the side of the covered eye with oppositely directed quick phases. Using a high plus lens (6 D) or double polarizing lenses instead of an opaque occluder held before the eye not being tested will prevent a falsely worse visual acuity threshold.[120,121]

In most cases of DVD, a cyclodeviation coexists with the vertical deviation. By alternate cover test, the covered eye elevates and extorts and the just uncovered eye depresses and intorts. In some cases, the excyclodeviation may be more prominent than the hyperdeviation. By observing the iritic, or conjunctival, vessels the cyclodeviation becomes more apparent. The cyclodeviation cannot be measured with the double Maddox rod test, because the deviation begins during visual immaturity. Patients with DVD also do not demonstrate objective cyclodeviation with the eye in primary position, as determined with binocular indirect ophthalmoscopy, unless there is also inferior oblique overaction.[29,122]

Oblique muscle dysfunction frequently occurs with DVD. DVD has been described as part of a syndrome consisting of an A-pattern exotropia with overaction of the superior oblique muscles and underaction of the inferior oblique muscles.[123] Incomitance is also demonstrated by the unequal amounts of hyperdeviation, depending on which eye is fixating and the variability of the deviation.

Patients with DVD have poor potential for normal binocular vision and are rarely symptomatic. Suppression is well developed and prevents diplopia from occurring when the deviation becomes manifest.[124] The poor fusion ability is probably the result of the frequent association of DVD with infantile esotropia. However, even patients with heterophoria and no history of any other binocular vision disorder who have DVD apparently do not bifixate, as indicated by the reduced stereopsis.[116,117,121]

 CLINICAL PEARL

Patients with DVD have poor potential for normal binocular vision and are rarely symptomatic.

With regard to treatment, some investigators have reported that DVD improves with time.[125,126] It is less frequent in adults than in children. It has been suggested that when the manifest hypertropia is less established than the latent hyperphoria, the hypertropic phase will eventually diminish and even disappear.[117] However, we have seen dissociated vertical deviation in adults. Longitudinal studies are needed to clarify the clinical course of DVD.

Unfavorable cosmesis is the major indication of

treatment. If the DVD remains latent, no treatment is needed, because these patients are generally asymptomatic. Attempts at prism therapy usually fail because of poor fusion ability and the extreme variability of the deviation. We aggressively treat any amblyopia. Caution should be exercised with occlusion therapy for patients who also have latent nystagmus, because this may intensify the nystagmus. In our experience, any form of orthoptics/vision therapy to establish sensory fusion and expand fusion ranges is rarely successful.

Surgery is the most accepted form of treatment.[126,127] Because DVD may improve with time, we generally wait before referring the patient for surgery. Interestingly, although 50% to 90% of all patients with infantile esotropia have or will develop DVD, only 5% have a vertical deviation significant enough to require surgery.[128] Surgery is recommended for those patients with an unsightly, predominantly unilateral DVD who do not wish to wait for the effect, if any, of age. The surgical techniques for DVD are discussed in Chapter 11.

In patients beyond the amblyopiagenic age with nearly equal vision but predominantly unilateral DVD, optical blur before the dominant eye (+3.00 D) may cause a change in fixation preference and result in improved cosmetic appearance, thus avoiding surgery.

OBLIQUE MUSCLE DYSFUNCTIONS

Oblique muscle dysfunctions include overactions of the inferior or superior oblique muscles.

Inferior Oblique Overaction

Probably the most frequently occurring incomitant deviation involves an upshoot, or overelevation, of the adducted eye caused by overactivity of the inferior oblique.[1] On horizontal version testing, one eye may move first toward the nose, as expected, but may then make a jerky upshoot (see Figs. 10-5 and 10-6). In these cases, there is minimal or no vertical deviation in the primary position. Only when the patient adducts the affected eye does the hypertropia become manifest. The hyperdeviation can present a few degrees in adduction, in full adduction only, or only in the field of action of the inferior oblique. If the patient is forced to fixate with the involved eye on versions, the other eye will become hypotropic during abduction. This condition is referred to as *strabismus sursoadductorius, spasm of the inferior oblique,* or *primary overaction of the inferior oblique.* The latter is preferred, because the overaction is not associated with underaction of the antagonist superior oblique or any muscle paresis. Its cause is speculative, ranging from a structural anomaly in the fascia surrounding the insertion of the inferior oblique and medial rectus to reduced tonus in the ipsilateral superior oblique, where esotropia is present. It

commences mostly during early childhood, usually before age 4.[129] Upshoot of the adducted eye related to a tethering effect and not to inferior oblique overaction can occur in Duane's syndrome.

CLINICAL PEARL

Probably the most frequently occurring incomitant deviation involves an upshoot, or overelevation, of the adducted eye caused by overactivity of the inferior oblique.

Inferior oblique overaction can also occur secondary to a superior oblique paresis in the ipsilateral eye or, rarely, to a superior rectus paresis in the contralateral eye. Patients with inferior oblique overaction secondary to superior oblique paresis manifest a significant vertical deviation in primary position, usually underaction of the superior oblique, a compensatory head tilt to the contralateral side, a positive finding with the three-step test, and, frequently, an excyclodeviation with the double Maddox rod test. Patients with the more common primary inferior oblique overaction have minimal or no vertical deviation in primary position, usually normal motility of the antagonist superior oblique, no head tilt, a negative finding with the three-step test, and absence of torsion, as measured with the double Maddox rod test. Also, the vertical deviation with primary inferior oblique overaction is always greatest in upgaze rather than downgaze.

Primary inferior oblique overaction occurs mostly with other forms of strabismus.[129] A high incidence exists with infantile esotropia and sensory strabismus.[130,131] It may also occur with intermittent exotropia and the accommodative esotropias. Inferior oblique overaction may exist by itself and be the only sign of a binocular vision disorder.

Primary inferior oblique overaction can be unilateral or bilateral, the latter being more frequent. It may be unilateral at onset and then become bilateral. In bilateral cases, a right hypertropia occurs for left gaze and a left hypertropia occurs for right gaze. The degree of overaction in each eye is usually asymmetric and can be graded on a scale of +1 to +4. In +4 overaction, the amount of hyperdeviation may be as much as 45 PD, and the affected eye's cornea nearly disappears during adduction (see Fig. 10-6).

Because of its tertiary action of abduction, the overacting inferior oblique muscle causes not only excessive elevation but also excessive abduction in upgaze. Inferior oblique overaction causes the horizontal deviation of the eyes to become divergent in upgaze, resulting in a V-pattern deviation (Figs. 10-36 and 10-37). A horizontal deviation whose angle changes more than 15 PD in the divergent direction between 30 degrees upward and 30 degrees downward has a V pattern (exotropia with a V pattern has greater exodevia-

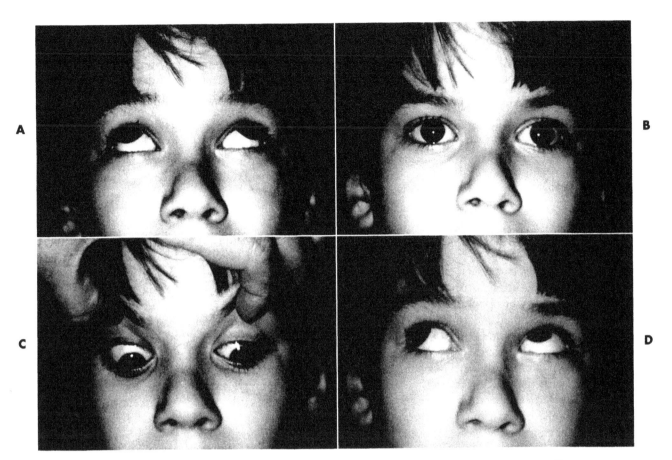

FIG. 10-36 V-pattern exodeviation. **A,** Upgaze. **B,** Primary position. **C,** Downgaze. **D,** Marked overacting left inferior oblique.

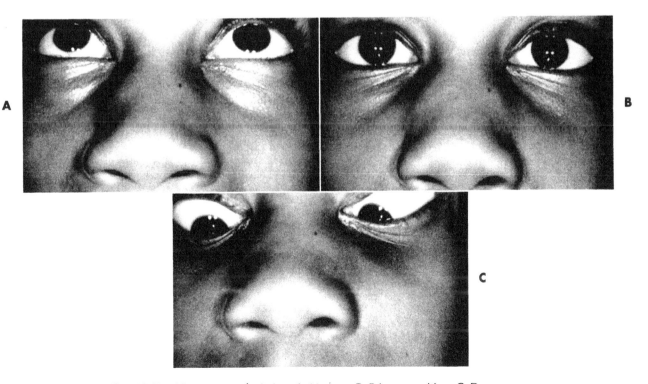

FIG. 10-37 V-pattern esodeviation. **A,** Upgaze. **B,** Primary position. **C,** Downgaze.

tion in upgaze; esotropia with a V pattern has greater esodeviation in downgaze). These measurements are best taken with distance fixation. Patients with a V exo pattern may use a chin-up head posture to maintain fusion. A chin-down posture may be used by patients with a V eso pattern.

It is unclear why all patients with inferior oblique overaction do not develop a V-pattern deviation. Also, some V patterns occur in patients with normally functioning inferior oblique muscles. Anatomic variations in the horizontal rectus muscles that permit greater effect of the lateral rectus in upgaze and the medial rectus in downgaze have been reported in some of these cases.[132] Vertical rectus overactions and underactions may also cause V patterns.

The level of binocular vision is dependent on the type of deviation existing in primary position and whether a compensatory head posture is present. With constant strabismus acquired in early childhood, a high degree of fusion is unlikely and amblyopia is probable if nonalternating fixation occurs. Amblyopia is more likely to be present in bilateral inferior oblique overactions in the eye with the greatest overaction.[133] When inferior oblique overaction occurs with fully accommodative esotropia, intermittent exotropia, or heterophoria, normal fusion with stereopsis is expected in the primary position and amblyopia is unlikely. If marked bilateral overaction is present, however, the patient has only a narrow range of comfortable binocular vision to either side of primary position.

Patients with primary inferior oblique overaction rarely exhibit symptoms of diplopia. Because the deviation begins early in life, adequate suppression or ignoring usually exists. When diplopia occurs, the area may be avoided by the patient elevating or depressing the chin or limiting horizontal movement of the eyes.

Superior Oblique Overaction

The opposite condition, overdepression, or downshoot, of the adducted eye caused by overaction of the superior oblique is referred to as *strabismus deorsoadductorius*. It is considerably less frequent than inferior oblique overaction. Antagonist inferior oblique function is usually normal but occasional underactions can be demonstrated. Because a paresis of either the inferior oblique or the inferior rectus is rare, the cause of superior oblique overaction remains elusive. Similar to inferior oblique overaction, the onset of superior oblique overation generally is before age 4. Downshoot of the adducted eye that is unrelated to superior oblique overaction can also occur in Duane's syndrome, Brown's syndrome, and alternating skew deviation on lateral gaze. The latter can be associated with posterior fossa tumors.[134]

Superior oblique overaction usually coexists with esotropia or exotropia. It is more common in ex-

otropia, especially of large degree. Some patients have a smaller vertical strabismus in primary position. A lack of any associated strabismus may also occur.

Similar to inferior oblique overaction, superior oblique overaction is more likely bilateral than unilateral. On levoversion, a right hypotropia is manifest, and on dextroversion, a left hypotropia is manifest (Fig. 10-38). The amount of hypotropia is usually asymmetric. The extent of superior oblique overaction is graded on a scale of +1 to +4, with +1 indicating mild and +4 indicating severe.

Because of its tertiary action of abduction, the overaction of the superior oblique produces not only more depression but also more abduction when the eyes view in downgaze. Superior oblique overaction usually causes an A-pattern deviation. A horizontal deviation whose angle changes more than 10 PD between 30 degrees upgaze and 30 degrees downgaze gaze (greater in upgaze in esotropia and greater in downgaze in exotropia) has an A pattern. Patients with A exodeviations (Fig. 10-39) may use a chin-down posture, and patients with an A esodeviation may use a chin-up posture to maintain fusion (see Fig. 10-2). Not all patients with superior oblique overaction have an A pattern nor are all A-pattern deviations caused by superior oblique overaction.

Superior oblique overaction may represent a clinical marker for an associated neurologic dysfunction and require further medical evaluation. A high incidence of A-pattern strabismus and superior oblique overaction are found in children with certain neurologic diseases, such as hydrocephalus, meningomyelocele, and cerebral palsy.[135] In a study of 168 children with strabismus who had superior oblique overaction, 40.2% had concurrent neurologic abnormalities compared with only 17.3% of control patients with strabismus who did not have superior oblique overaction.[135]

Inferior and Superior Oblique Overaction

In rare cases, all four oblique muscles may overact. This is more likely in large, long-standing exotropia that is constant. This causes an X-pattern deviation, with the exotropia being smaller in primary position than it is in upgaze and downgaze.

Treatment

Treatment of inferior and superior oblique muscle disorders consists of surgery, prisms, or orthoptics/vision therapy. As with other incomitant deviations, the most important positions functionally are primary position and downgaze. Rarely does a patient view more than 15 degrees from the primary position. Diplopia, or loss of binocular vision, in only extreme positions may not be a hindrance to a patient. A patient who is exophoric in primary position and orthophoric in downgaze, who also manifests a slight right hyperdevi-

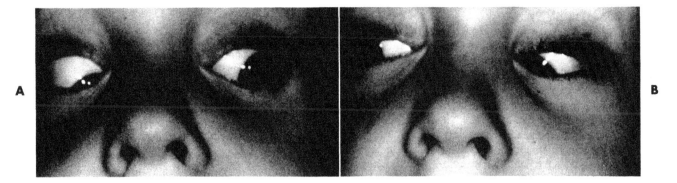

FIG. 10-38   Bilateral superior oblique overaction. **A,** Right hypotropia on left gaze. **B,** Left hypotropia on right gaze.

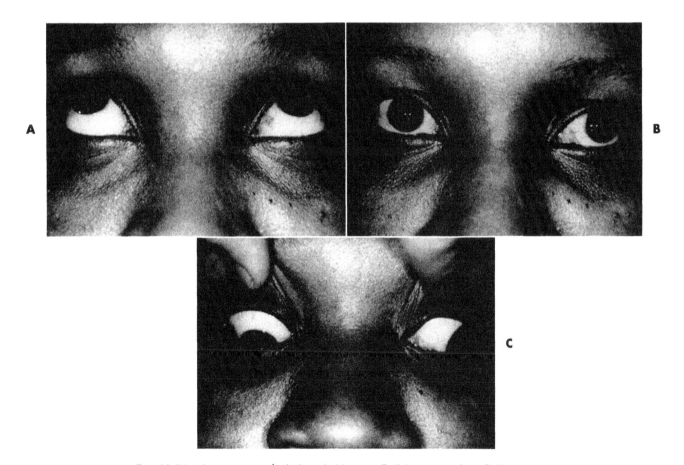

FIG. 10-39   A-pattern exodeviation. **A,** Upgaze. **B,** Primary position. **C,** Downgaze.

ation in levoversion and a slight left hyperdeviation on dextroversion, with a minimal V exodeviation, may not need treatment.

We have used conjugate, or yoked, prisms in some patients with oblique muscle dysfunction associated with V or A patterns. Bilateral base-down prisms may be used for patients with mild V-pattern esodeviations, as well as A-pattern exodeviations. Similarly, bilateral base-up prism can be used for mild A-pattern esodeviations and V-pattern exodeviations. Such treatment is limited to smaller deviations and for patients in whom fusion in at least one position of gaze occurs. (See Case 16.)

CASE 16

A 25-year-old woman was referred to the clinic. She experienced headaches in the frontal area, associated mostly with near tasks. She also noticed occasional diplopia when reading. She always remembered having an eye turn. No treatment was ever given.

Our examination revealed visual acuities of 20/20 for each eye, with a refraction of +1.25 for the right and left eyes. No compensatory head posture was noted. With the cover test, the patient manifested a 15-PD constant alternating esotropia at distance, which increased to 25 PD at near. Versions showed bilateral superior oblique overaction and bilateral inferior oblique underaction. There was an A pattern, with the esodeviation increasing to 25 PD in upgaze and decreasing to 6-PD intermittent esotropia in downgaze. The patient, with extreme effort, fused occasionally in downgaze

and had 70 seconds of arc with the Randot stereotest. Ophthalmoscopic findings were normal.

The patient was treated by giving the hyperopic correction and 5 PD base-up in each lens to move the eyes more in downgaze. Follow-up examination revealed alleviation of the patient's symptoms.

Orthoptics/vision therapy has not proven effective in resolving oblique muscle dysfunction. Surgery is generally recommended for patients with grade +3 and +4 overactions. When surgery is performed on the horizontal recti for any associated primary position esotropia or exotropia, the oblique muscles, if overacting, can also be altered.

REFERENCES

1. Rutstein RP: Incomitant deviations in children. In Scheiman MM, editor: *Problems in optometry,* vol 2, Philadelphia, 1990, JB Lippincott.
2. Hiles DA, Wallar PH, MacFarlane F: Current concepts in the management of strabismus in children with cerebral palsy, *Ann Ophthalmol* 7:789, 1975.
3. Murphee AL, Edelman PM: Strabismus associated with congenital anomalies, *Am Orthopt J* 32:22, 1982.
4. Sanflippo S: Acquired ocular palsy in children, *Am J Orthopt* 27:134, 1977.
5. Harley RD: Paralytic strabismus in children: etiologic incidence and management of the third, fourth, and sixth nerve palsies, *Ophthalmology* 87:24, 1980.
6. Richards BW, Jones FR, Younge BR: Causes and prognosis in 4278 cases of paralysis of the oculomotor, trochlear, and abducens cranial nerves, *Am J Opthalmol* 113:489, 1992.
7. Rutstein RP: Superior oblique palsy. In London R, editor: *Problems in optometry* vol 4, Philadelphia, 1992, JB Lippincott.
8. Burian H, Rowan P, Sullivan M: Absence of spontaneous head tilt in superior oblique muscle palsy, *Am J Ophthalmol* 79:972, 1975.
9. Scott W: Differential diagnosis of vertical muscle palsies: symposium on strabismus. In Helveston Em and others, editors: *Transactions of the New Orleans Academy of Ophthalmologists,* St Louis, 1978, Mosby.
10. Goldstein JH: The intraoperative forced duction test, *Arch Ophthalmol* 72:647, 1964.
11. Metz H, Scott A, O'Meara D: Saccadic velocity in infants and children, *Am J Ophthalmol* 72:1130, 1971.
12. Scott W: Clinical study of saccadic eye movements: symposium on strabismus. In Helveston Em and others, editors: *Transactions of the New Orleans Academy of Ophthalmologists,* St Louis, 1978, Mosby.
13. Rosenbaum A, Carlson M, Gaffney R: Vertical saccadic velocity determination in superior oblique palsy, *Arch Ophthalmol* 95:821, 1977.
14. Metz H: III nerve palsy saccadic velocity studies, *Ann Ophthalmol* 5:526, 1973.
15. Metz H: Saccades with limited downgaze, *Arch Ophthalmol* 98:2204, 1980.
16. Dale R: *Fundamentals of ocular motility and strabismus,* New York, 1982, Grune and Stratton.
17. Lancaster W: Detecting, measuring, plotting, and interpreting ocular deviations, *Arch Ophthalmol* 22:867, 1939.
18. Parks MM: Isolated cyclovertical muscle palsy, *Arch Ophthalmol* 60:1027, 1958.
19. Khawam E, Scott AB, Jampolsky A: Acquired superior oblique palsy: diagnosis and management, *Arch Ophthalmol* 77:761, 1967.
20. Rutstein RP: Paretic muscle determination. In Eskridge JB, Amos JF, Bartlett JD, editors: *Clinical procedures in optometry,* New York, 1991, JB Lippincott.
21. Rutstein RP, Eskridge JB: Clinical comparison of congenital or early onset paretic vertical strabismus vs. acquired paretic vertical strabismus, *Am J Optom Physiol Opt* 62:725, 1985.
22. Getman I, Goldstein JH: Diagnosis of an isolated vertical muscle palsy, *Acta Ophthalmol (Copenh)* 61:85, 1983.
23. Kushner BJ: Simulated superior oblique palsy, *Ann Ophthalmol* 2:337, 1981.
24. Kushner BJ: Errors in the three-step test in the diagnosis of vertical strabismus, *Ophthalmology* 96:127, 1989.
25. Wonjo TH: The incidence of extraocular muscle and cranial nerve palsy in orbital blow-out fractures, *Ophthalmology* 94:682, 1987.
26. Kraft SP and others: Cyclotorsion in unilateral and bilateral superior oblique palsies, *J Pediatr Ophthalmol Strab* 30:361, 1993.
27. Oliver P, von Noorden GK: Excyclotropia of the nonparetic eye in unilateral superior oblique paralysis, *Am J Ophthalmol* 93:30, 1982.
28. Rutstein RP, Eskridge JB: Effect of cyclodeviations on the axis of astigmatism (for patients with superior oblique paresis), *Optom Vis Sci* 67:80, 1990.
29. Simons K, Arnoldi K, Brown MH: Colored association artifacts in double Maddox rod cyclodeviation testing, *Ophthalmology* 101:1897, 1994.
30. Morton G, Lucchese N, Kushner B: The role of funduscopy and fundus photography in strabismus diagnosis, *Ophthalmology* 90:1186, 1983.
31. Levine M, Zahoruk R: Disc-macula relationship in diagnosis of vertical muscle paresis, *Am J Ophthalmol* 73:262, 1982.
32. von Noorden GK, Murray E, Wong SY: Superior oblique paralysis: a review of 270 cases, *Arch Ophthalmol* 104:1771, 1986.

33. Guyton DL, von Noorden GK: Sensory adaptations to cyclodeviations. In Reinecke RD, editor: *Strabismus: Proceedings of the Third Meeting of the International Strabismological Association,* Kyoto 1978, New York, 1978, Grune and Stratton.
34. Rutstein RP: Therapy for early acquired noncomitant esotropia, *J Am Optom Assoc* 54:161, 1983.
35. Norman MG: Unilateral encephalmalacia in cranial nerve nuclei in neonates: report of two cases, *Neurology* 24:424, 1974.
36. Esswein MB, von Noorden GK: Paresis of vertical rectus muscle after cataract extraction, *Am J Ophthalmol* 116:424, 1993.
37. Pollard ZF: Diagnosis and treatment of inferior oblique palsy, *J Pediatr Ophthalmol Strab* 30:15, 1993.
38. Stefanis L, Przedborski S: Isolated palsy of the superior branch of the oculomotor nerve due to chronic erosive sphenoid sinusitis, *J Clin Neuro Ophthalmol* 13:229, 1993.
39. Susac JD, Hoyt WF: Inferior branch palsy of the oculomotor nerve, *Ann Neurol* 2:336, 1977.
40. Cunningham ET, Good WV: Inferior branch nerve palsy: a case report, *J Clin Neuro Ophthalmol* 14:21, 1994.
41. Musarella MA, Bunic JR: Isolated palsy of the inferior division of the oculomotor nerve: a case report and review of the literature. In Reinecke RD, editor: *Strabismus II: Proceedings of the Fourth Meeting of the International Strabismological Association, Asilomar,* 1982, New York, 1984, Grune and Stratton.
42. Victor DI: The diagnosis of congenital unilateral third-nerve palsy, *Brain* 99:711, 1976.
43. Glaser JS: *Neuro-ophthalmology,* Hagerstown, Md, 1987, Harper and Row.
44. Walsh TJ: *Neuro-ophthalmology: clinical signs and symptoms,* Philadelphia, 1978, Lea and Febiger.
45. Rutstein RP: Acute esotropia in the adult, *J Am Optom Assoc* 53:917, 1982.
46. Bielschowsky A: *Lectures on motor: anomalies,* Hanover, NH, 1940, Dartmouth College.
47. Harris DJ and others: Familial congenital superior oblique palsy, *Ophthalmology* 93:88, 1986.
48. Paysee EA, Coats DK, Plager DA: Facial asymmetry and tendon laxity in superior oblique palsy, *J Pediatr Ophthalmol Strab* 32:158, 1995.
49. Bagolini B, Campos EC, Chiesi C: Plagiocephaly causing superior oblique deficiency and ocular torticollis: a new clinical entity: *Arch Ophthalmol* 100:1093, 1982.
50. Bellizzu M, Lamorgese C, Gross T: Ocular torticollis: diagnosis and prognosis, *J Fr Ophthalmol* 6:589, 1983.
51. Ellis FD, Helveston EM: Superior oblique palsy: diagnosis and classification, *Int Ophthalmol Clin* 16:127, 1976.
52. Rutstein RP, Corliss DA: The relationship between duration of superior oblique palsy and vertical fusional vergence, cyclodeviation, and diplopia, *J Am Optom Assoc* 66:442, 1995.
53. Scott WE, Kraft SP: Classification and treatment of superior oblique palsies. II, Bilateral superior oblique palsies: pediatric ophthalmology and strabismus. In *Transactions of the New Orleans Academy of Ophthalmology,* New York, 1986, Raven.
54. Aroichane M, Repka MX: Outcome of sixth nerve palsy or paresis in young children, *J Pediatr Ophthalmol Strab* 32:152, 1995.
55. Rutstein RP: Acute acquired comitant esotropia simulating late onset accommodative esotropia, *J Am Optom Assoc* 59:446, 1988.
56. Rush JA, Younge BR: Paralysis of cranial nerves III, IV, and VI, *Arch Ophthalmol* 99:76, 1981.
57. Scheiman M, Gallaway M, Ciner E: Divergence insufficiency: characteristics, diagnosis, and treatment, *Am J Optom Physiol Opt* 63:425, 1986.
58. Moore S, Harbinson JR, Stockbridge L: Divergence insufficiency, *Am Orthopt J* 21:59, 1971.
59. Bedrossian EH: Bilateral sixth nerve paresis simulating divergence paralysis, *Am J Ophthalmol* 45:417, 1985.
60. Curran RE: True and simulated divergence palsy as a precursor of benign sixth nerve palsy, *Binoc Vis Eye Muscle Surg* 4:125, 1989.
61. Rutstein RP: Duane's retraction syndrome, *J Am Optom Assoc* 63:419, 1992.
62. Terashima M, Hayasaka A: Multiple congenital anomalies associated with Duane's syndrome, *Ophthalmic Pediatr and Genet* 11:113, 1990.
63. Sachdev JS, Harrington JL: Duane's retraction syndrome associated with cerebral arteriovenous malformation, *South Med J* 79:623, 1986.
64. Miller MT: Association of Duane's retraction syndrome with craniofacial malformations, *J Craniofac Genet Dev Biol (suppl)* 1:273, 1985.
65. Hayes A, Costa T, Polomeno RC: The Okihiro syndrome of Duane's anomaly, radial ray abnormalities, and deafness, *Am J Med Genet* 34:139, 1985.
66. Taylor MJ, Rolomeno RC: Further observations on the auditory brainstem responses in Duane's syndrome, *Can J Ophthalmol* 18:238, 1983.
67. Duane A: Congenital deficiency of abduction, associated with impairment of adduction, retraction movement, contraction of the palpebral fissure and oblique movements of the eye, *Arch Ophthalmol* 34:133, 1905.
68. Huber A: Electrophysiology of the retraction syndromes, *Br J Ophthalmol* 58:293, 1974.
69. Scott AB, Wong GY: Duane's syndrome: an electromyographic study, *Arch Ophthalmol* 87:140, 1972.
70. Miller NR and others: Unilateral Duane's retraction syndrome (type I), *Arch Ophthalmol* 100:1468, 1982.
71. Hotchkiss MG and others: Bilateral Duane's retraction syndrome: a clinical-pathologic case report, *Arch Ophthalmol* 98:870, 1980.
72. Mulhern M, Keohane C, O'Conner G: Bilateral abducens nerve lesions in unilateral type 3 Duane's retraction syndrome, *Br J Ophthalmol* 78:588, 1994.
73. von Noorden GK, Murray E: Up- and downshoot in Duane's retraction syndrome, *J Pediatr Ophthalmol Strab* 23:212, 1986.
74. Hoogesteger MF, Everhard-Halm YS: Suppression behavior in Duane's patients older than 17 years of age, *Br Orthopt J* 43:34, 1986.
75. MacDonald AL, Crawford S, Smith DR: Duane's retraction syndrome: an evaluation of the sensory status, *Can J Ophthalmol* 9:458, 1974.
76. Kraft SP: Surgical approach for Duane's syndrome, *J Pediatr Ophthalmol Strab* 25:119, 1988.
77. Pressman SH, Scott WE: Surgical treatment of Duane's syndrome, *Ophthalmology* 93:29, 1986.
78. Mende A: Duane's retraction syndrome and the relief of secondary torticollis and near point asthenopia with prism, *J Am Optom Assoc* 61:556, 1990.
79. Wang FM, Wertenbacker C, Beharens MM: Acquired Brown's syndrome in children with juvenile rheumatoid arthritis, *Ophthalmology* 91:23, 1984.
80. Beisner DM: Acquired Brown's syndrome of inflammatory origin, *Arch Ophthalmol* 97:173, 1979.
81. Jackson OB, Nankin SJ, Scott WE: Traumatic stimulated Brown's syndrome: a case report, *J Pediatr Ophthalmol Strab* 16:160, 1979.
82. Herman JS: Acquired Brown's syndrome of inflammatory origin, *Arch Ophthalmol* 96:1228, 1978.
83. von Noorden GK: *Binocular vision and ocular motility: theory and management of strabismus,* ed 5, St Louis, 1996, Mosby.
84. Sato S and others: Superior oblique overaction in patients with true Brown's syndrome, *J Pediatr Ophthalmol Strab* 24:282, 1987.

85. Parks MM: Surgery for Brown's syndrome. In *Symposium on strabismus*, St Louis, 1978, Mosby.

86. Hiatt RL, Halle AA: General fibrosis syndrome, *Ann Ophthalmol* 15:1103, 1983.

87. Apt L, Axelrod RN: Generalized fibrosis of the extraocular muscles, *Ophthalmology* 85:822, 1978.

88. Traboulsi EI and others: Congenital fibrosis of the extraocular muscles: report of 24 cases illustrating the clinical spectrum and surgical management, *Am Orthopt J* 43:45, 1993.

89. von Noorden GK: Congenital hereditary ptosis with inferior rectus fibrosis, *Arch Ophthalmol* 83:378, 1970.

90. Harley RD, Rodrigues MM, Crawford JS: Congenital fibrosis of the extraocular muscles, *Trans Am Ophthalmol Soc* 76:197, 1978.

91. Stavis MI, Niemann SJ: Medical and surgical treatment of vertical deviations. In London R, editor: *Problems in optometry*, vol 4, Philadephia, 1992, JB Lippincott.

92. Knapp P: Special types of muscle abnormalities associated with Graves' disease, *Ophthalmology* 86:2081, 1979.

93. Uretsky S, Kennerdell J, Gutai J: Graves' ophthalmopathy in childhood and adolescence, *Arch Ophthalmol* 98:1963, 1980.

94. Chen YI and others: Relationship of eye movement to computed tomographic findings in patients with Graves' ophthalmopathy, *Acta Ophthalmol* 72:472, 1994.

95. Smith JL: Recent advances in therapy of thyroid eye disease. In Smith JL, editor: *Neuro-ophthalmology*, St Louis, 1972, Mosby.

96. Bartley GE and others: The treatment of Graves' ophthalmopathy in an incidence cohort, *Am J Ophthalmol* 121:200, 1996.

97. Trobe J: Cyclodeviation in acquired vertical strabismus, *Arch Ophthalmol* 102:717, 1984.

98. Hales I, Rundle E: Ocular changes in Graves' disease: a long-term follow-up study, *Q J Med* 29:113, 1960.

99. Greaves B, Mein J, Gibb J: A long-term follow-up of patients presenting with dysthyroid eye disease. In Moore S, Mein J, Stockbridge L, editors: *Orthoptics: past, present, and future*, New York, 1976, Grune and Stratton.

100. Keech RV, Scott WE, Christensen LE: Adustable suture strabismus surgery, *J Pediatr Ophthalmol Strab* 24:97, 1987.

101. McNeer K: Adjustable sutures of the vertical recti, *J Pediatr Ophthalmol Strab* 19:259, 1982.

102. Converse J: The blow-out fracture of the orbit: some common sense. In Brockhurst R, Boruchoff S, Hutchinson B, editors: *Controversy in ophthalmology*, Philadelphia, 1977, WB Saunders.

103. Putterman A: Nonsurgical management of blow-out fractures of the orbital floor. In Brockhurst R, Boruchoff A, Hutchinson B, editors: *Controversy in ophthalmology*, Philadelphia, 1977, WB Saunders.

104. Emery J, von Noorden GK, Schlernitzauer D: Orbital floor fractures: long-term follow-up of cases with and without surgical repair, *Trans Am Acad Ophthalmol Otolaryngol* 75:802, 1971.

105. Reinecke R and others: An improved method of fitting resultant prism in treatment of two-axis strabismus, *Arch Ophthalmol* 95:1255, 1977.

106. Osher RH: Myasthenic oculomotor palsy, *Ann Ophthalmol* 11:31, 1979.

107. Osserman KE: Ocular myasthenia gravis, *Invest Ophthalmol* 6:277, 1967.

108. Berkovitz S, Belkin M, Tenenbaum A: Childhood myasthenia gravis, *J Pediatr Ophthalmol Strab* 14:269, 1977.

109. Cleary PE: Ocular manifestations of myasthenia gravis, *Br Orthopt J* 30:38, 1973.

110. Cogan DG: Myasthenia gravis: a review of the disease and a description of lid twitch as a characteristic sign, *Arch Ophthalmol* 74:217, 1965.

111. Morris JE: Ocular presentation of juvenile myasthenia gravis, *Am Orthopt J* 32:51, 1982.

112. Cooper J, Kruger P, Panariello GF: The pathognominic pattern of accommodative fatigue in myasthenia gravis, *Binoc Vis Eye Muscle Surg* 3:141, 1987.

113. Teasdall RD, Sears M: Myasthenia gravis: electromyographyic evidence for myopathy, *Am J Ophthalmol* 54:541, 1962.

114. Ellenhorn N, Lucchese N, Greenwald M: Juvenile myasthenia gravis and amblyopia, *Am J Ophthalmol* 101:214, 1986.

115. Hamed LM and others: Strabismus surgery in selected patients with stable myasthenia gravis, *Binoc Vis Eye Muscle Surg* 9:283, 1994.

116. Amos JF, Rutstein RP: Vertical deviations. In Amos JF, editor: *Diagnosis and management in vision care*, Boston, 1987, Butterworth-Heinemann.

117. Parks MM: *Ocular motility and strabismus*, New York, 1975, Harper & Row.

118. Helveston E, Ellis F: *Pediatric ophthalmology practice*, St Louis, 1980, Mosby.

119. Kutluk S, Avilla CW, von Noorden GK: The prevalence of dissociated vertical deviationin patients with sensory heterotropia, *Am J Ophthalmol* 119:744, 1995.

120. Raab E: Dissociated vertical deviation, *J Pediatr Ophthalmol Strab* 7:146, 1970.

121. Helveston E: Dissociated vertical deviation: a clinical and laboratory study, *Trans Am Ophthalmol Soc* 78:734, 1980.

122. Guyton D: Clinical assessment of ocular torsion, *Am Orthopt J* 33:7, 1983.

123. Helveston E: A pattern exotropia, alternating sursumduction and superior oblique overaction, *Am J Ophthalmol* 67:377, 1969.

124. MacDonald A, Pratt-Johnson J: The suppression pattern and sensory adaptation in dissociated vertical divergent strabismus, *Can J Ophthalmol* 9:113, 1974.

125. Fleming A: Dissociated vertical deviation, *Arch Ophthalmol* 98:2083, 1980 (letter).

126. Pratt-Johnson J: Surgery of dissociated vertical deviation, *Int Ophthalmol Clin* 16:171, 1976.

127. Noel L, Park S: Dissociated vertical deviation: associated findings and results of surgical treatment, *Can J Ophthalmol* 17:10, 1982.

128. Knapp P: Dissociated vertical deviations. In Fells P, editor: *The second congress of the International Strabismological Association, Marseilles: Diffusion*, Marseilles, 1976, Generale de Librairie.

129. Wilson ME, Parks MM: Primary inferior oblique overaction in congenital esotropia, accommodative esotropia, and intermittent exotropia, *Ophthalmology* 96:950, 1989.

130. von Noorden, GK: A reassessment of infantile esotropia: XLIV Edward Jackson Memorial Lecture, *Am J Ophthalmol* 105:1, 1988.

131. Sidikaro Y, von Noorden GK: Observations in sensory heterotropia, *J Pediatr Ophthalmol Strab* 19:12, 1982.

132. Knapp P: Vertically incomitant horizontal strabismus: the so-called "A" and "V" syndromes, *Trans Am Opthalmol Soc* 67:304, 1969.

133. Weakley DR Jr, Urso RG, Dias CL: Asymmetric inferior oblique overaction and its association with amblyopia in esotropia, *Ophthalmology* 99:590, 1992.

134. Hamed LM and others: Intact binocular function and absent ocular torsion in children with alternating skew on lateral gaze, *J Pediatr Ophthalmol Strab* 33:164, 1996.

135. Hamed LM and others: The prevalence of neurologic dysfunction in children with strabismus who have superior oblique dysfunction, *Ophthalmology* 100:1483, 1993.

CHAPTER 11

Medical and Surgical Management of Strabismus

Martin S. Cogen
Andrew Mays

Correction of strabismus generally should be considered functional or reconstructive (i.e., to restore the normal order and balance between the eyes designed by "Mother Nature"). If a more pleasant appearance is gained, this is simply a beneficial side-effect. Medical and surgical intervention will, for certain types of strabismus, remain secondary to established optical and orthoptic/vision therapy regimens. For other cases, medical management and surgical intervention will represent the cornerstones of initial therapy. Refinement of current drugs and available surgical techniques, along with the inevitable expansion of knowledge and introduction of better pharmaceutics and surgical procedures for strabismus will eventually affect the doctor-patient decision in selecting a particular treatment plan. Additionally, an "outcome-based" approach will increasingly be adopted by government and third-party payers attempting to control spiraling health care costs, and clinicians will have to "prove" that an intervention is not only beneficial but cost effective.

PHARMACOLOGIC TREATMENT

The use of pharmacologic agents to treat strabismus is limited to accommodative esotropia, refractive or nonrefractive. Pharmacologic management of accommodative esotropia can be considered when compliance with glasses has proven unsuccessful, especially in patients with a greater esodeviation at near (high AC/A ratio). Occasionally, clinicians prescribe this therapy before glasses to determine the effectivness of antiaccommodative treatment in patients with esotropia who have relatively low amounts of hyperopia to help determine whether glasses will be beneficial. Approximately 5% of the patients we see with accommodative esotropia are given pharmacologic treatment.

 CLINICAL PEARL

The use of pharmacologic agents to treat strabismus is limited to refractive and nonrefractive accommodative esotropia.

The principle behind such management is related to the mechanism of action of two agents: echothiophate iodine (Phospholine Iodide) and isoflurophate (Floropryl). Both are long-acting cholinesterase inhibitors that indirectly enhance the action of endogenously released acetylcholine. By altering the sensitivity of the acetylcholine receptors in the ciliary body, these drugs cause the eye to react appropriately to much smaller amounts of acetylcholine. Less input from the brain along the parasympathetic pathway is required to cause accommodation, hence less convergence occurs, because accommodation and convergence are both part of the synkinetic near reflex.

Isoflurophate ointment is used as follows: 1/4 inch of ointment is applied topically to each eye daily for 1 to 2 weeks. The dose is then tapered from every day to every other day to once or twice each week for 2 months. Close observation during this period is recommended. The drug is discontinued if an effective dosing interval of 48 hours or greater cannot be achieved. The dosing interval should be tapered to the greatest length compatible with acceptable benefit. Echothiophate iodide 0.125% solution is administered one drop to each eye daily for 2 to 3 weeks. Thereafter the dose is tapered to every other day and the strength reduced to 0.06% or, in some cases, 0.03%. Again, the goal is to reach the maximum dosing interval with the minimum concentration of drug to achieve satisfactory results. Recent studies[1] show fewer systemic side effects with isoflurophate than with echothiophate iodide. The most important side effects are some patients' extreme sensitivity to depolarizing muscle relaxants such as succinylcholine, frequently used during induction of general anesthesia, and the tendency to develop iris cysts. Iris cysts are seen mostly in brown-eyed people, will usually resolve when the drug is discontinued, and can be controlled with concomitant use of topical phenylephrine HCl 2.5%. However, these pigment epithelial cysts usually form at the pupillary border and, in a miotic patient, may become large enough to obstruct the visual axis and cause amblyopia.

TABLE 11-1   COMMON TYPES OF EXTRAOCULAR MUSCLE SURGERY

Type	Description
Recession	Involves weakening of a muscle by first securely fastening an absorbable suture through the tendon near the insertion and then detaching the muscle from the globe and reattaching it to superficial sclera a measured distance posterior to the original insertion.
Resection	Involves tightening a muscle by removing a distal segment of tendon and muscle and then suturing the cut muscle back to the globe at the original insertion.
Myectomy	Involves weakening a muscle by excising a section of the muscle belly.
Tenotomy	A weakening procedure in which part or all of the superior oblique tendon is divided between the trochlea and the tendon insertion on the globe.
Faden procedure	Involves fixation of the rectus muscle belly posterior to the equator of the globe with a nonabsorbable suture to reduce the effect of muscle contracture without altering the resting position of the eye.
Y-Splitting procedure	Involves dividing the lateral rectus tendon lengthwise and reinserting the tendon halves 10-15 mm apart in the shape of the letter Y to stabilize the muscle during cocontraction and prevent the vertical forces of a "slipping leash."
Adjustable suture	Involves placing a suture through the edge of a muscle and securing it with locked knots on both sides. The muscle is detached from the globe and then the ends of the sutures are placed through the original insertion. The surgeon then may leave the ends of the suture in a temporary knot that can be loosened or tightened when the patient has recovered from anesthesia and is fully awake.
Jensen procedure	Involves tying the lateral halves of the superior and inferior recti to the lateral rectus without disinserting the tendons.
Hummelscheim procedure	Involves disinserting the lateral halves of the superior and inferior recti and suturing these to the lateral rectus.
Full-muscle transposition	Involves disinserting the complete rectus muscle and suturing it to the paretic muscle.
Harado-Ito procedure	Involves dividing the superior oblique tendon lengthwise and suturing the anterior one-third of the tendon to the globe near the superior edge of the lateral rectus to strengthen intorsion without affecting the vertical position of the globe.
Superior oblique tuck	Involves strengthening the superior oblique by doubling-over the loose tendon and securing it with a nonabsorbable suture woven in a double figure-of-eight fashion through its base.
Knapp procedure	Involves full muscle transposition of the medial and lateral recti to the superior rectus insertion.
Vertical offset-setting the horizontal recti muscle	Involves re-attaching the muscles to superficial sclera ½-1 tendon width higher or lower than the original muscle insertion, usually combined with simultaneous recession or resection of the muscle to alter the horizontal pull of the muscle in upgaze and downgaze (i.e., moving the medial recti downward will decrease adduction in downgaze and moving the lateral recti upward will decrease abduction in upgaze and vice-versa).

SURGICAL TREATMENT

When nonsurgical methods of correcting ocular misalignment are unsuccessful, surgical intervention is warranted. Generally, nonaccommodative esotropia greater than 12 to 15 PD, exotropia greater than 15 to 20 PD, and vertical strabismus greater than 8 to 10 PD in the primary position can be treated surgically. Also, patients with significant horizontal or vertical incomitance may benefit from surgical correction. The major types of surgery are described in Table 11-1.

 CLINICAL PEARL

> Nonaccommodative esotropia greater than 12 to 15 PD, exotropia greater than 15 to 20 PD, and vertical strabismus greater than 8 to 10 PD in the primary position can be treated surgically.

ESOTROPIA
Infantile Esotropia

Surgery is the major form of treatment in infantile esotropia. Infantile esotropia is noted before 6 months of age. The refraction may show a mild hyperopic error, considered normal in young infants. A large angle of esotropia with cross-fixation is frequently observed, and nystagmus and vertical deviations are frequently present in these cases. We prefer to do surgery before 18 months of age for best results, but only after amblyopia and clinically significant refractive errors have been corrected. A bilateral medial rectus muscle recession procedure is successful in realigning the eyes in approximately 70% to 80% of the cases. Additional surgery is required in the remaining patients and is often secondary to vertical deviations, which may only become apparent after the esotropia has been corrected and frequently do not appear until ages 2 to 4. During surgery, A and V patterns can be addressed by vertically off-setting the reinsertion of the horizontal muscles.[2] Overaction of the inferior oblique muscles can be treated intraoperatively with inferior oblique myectomies or inferior oblique recessions. The goal of surgery is to align the eyes to within 10 prism diopters of the ortho position. This often results in a stable microtropia with peripheral fusion. Overcorrection of the esotropia can lead to a consecutive exotropia, requiring additional muscle balancing.

Nystagmus blockage syndrome is a rare type of infantile esotropia in which a purposeful esotropia is used to dampen horizontal nystagmus. A bilateral medial rectus muscle recession with or without a Faden (retroequatorial myopexy, posterior fixation suture) may be helpful to facilitate dampening of the nystagmus in primary gaze.

Adults with a history of untreated infantile esotropia can benefit from surgical intervention. A bilateral medial rectus recession, a unilateral medial rectus recession combined with lateral rectus resection, or a supramaximal unilateral medial rectus muscle recession with or without a posterior fixation suture (Faden procedure) can result in ocular realignment. An adjustable suture technique can also be used in these cases to refine the muscle balance when the patient is fully awake. As mentioned in Chapter 8, studies have shown that even adult patients can regain some "binocularity" after this procedure.[3] Visual rehabilitation through an expanded peripheral field of vision is also a goal of surgery in this group.[4]

Duane's Syndrome Type I

Duane's syndrome type I can be seen as esotropia in primary gaze. Disturbances of innervation of the lateral rectus muscle cause esotropia, limited abduction, and globe retraction, with palpebral narrowing on adduction. Vertical deviations and upshooting or downshooting on adduction can also be seen.[5] A head turn toward the affected side to achieve bifoveal fusion is often present. We generally limit surgery to patients manifesting either significant esotropia in primary position, a marked head turn, or extreme upshoot or downshoot of the adducted eye. Surgically, lateral rectus resections should be avoided because they will aggravate the retraction component of the syndrome. Medial rectus muscle recession in the abnormal eye is the procedure of choice for correction of primary-position esotropia and/or significant head turn, although abduction limitation usually persists. If severe upshooting or downshooting is present, we will perform a Y-splitting and recession of the lateral rectus muscle or use a posterior fixation suture to alleviate the "slipping

leash" phenomenon thought to be responsible for these abnormal eye movements.

 CLINICAL PEARL

Surgery is generally limited to patients manifesting either significant esotropia in primary position, a marked head turn, or extreme upshoot or downshoot of the adducted eye.

Lateral Rectus Paresis

The lateral rectus muscle is innervated solely by the abducens cranial nerve. Paresis of this nerve or muscle will result in an incomitant esotropia. Some causes of lateral rectus weakness may resolve spontaneously, but others may indicate the presence of more serious diseases. If spontaneous resolution has not occurred after 6 months and the presence of ocular myasthenia and an intracranial tumor has been excluded, surgery can realign the eyes. A large medial rectus muscle recession with lateral rectus muscle resection is often successful when residual lateral rectus function exists. An adjustable suture technique is useful in cooperative patients to refine ocular alignment. In the case of total sixth cranial nerve paralysis, a Jensen, Hummelscheim, or full-muscle transposition procedure using the healthy superior and inferior recti may be required to realign the eyes.[6] Risks associated with these procedures include anterior segment ischemia and iatrogenic vertical muscle imbalance. We have had good success with botulinum-A toxin (Botox) injection in patients with acute lateral rectus paresis (see Chemodenervation).

Partly Accommodative Esotropia

In partly accommodative esotropia a residual angle of esotropia will remain after full spectacle correction is given or pharmacologic therapy is started. Furthermore, some patients with high AC/A ratios initially corrected with glasses can deteriorate and develop a superimposed nonaccommodative esotropia at a later time. When the nonaccommodative esotropia exceeds 15 PD, surgery can be considered. In cases of amblyopia and esotropia, we recess the medial rectus muscle and resect the lateral rectus muscle of the same eye to correct the nonaccommodative esotropia. With equal vision and esotropia, we recess both medial rectus muscles equally, and in selected cases of small- or moderate-angle residual esodeviation, a large unilateral medial rectus recession is useful. Large medial rectus recessions and/or placement of posterior fixation sutures (Faden) on the medial recti can effectively dampen or eliminate the excess esodeviation at near fixation in patients with high AC/A ratios.

CLINICAL PEARL

When the nonaccommodative esotropia exceeds 15 PD, surgery can be considered.

Decompensated Esophoria

Some patients harbor an esophoria that progresses to esotropia for various reasons, including trauma, stress, illness, and aging. These patients with decompensated nonaccommodative esotropia respond well to surgical correction. The angle of esotropia should generally be 15 PD or greater before surgery is considered. A bilateral medial rectus muscle recession procedure will often re-align the eyes to within 10 prism diopters of orthophoria. In selected cases involving cooperative older patients, an adjustable suture technique can be used to refine the correction after general anesthesia has worn off. Binocular vision and fusion are often restored.[3] There is an ever-present risk of overcorrection, which leads to a consecutive exotropia. This may resolve spontaneously or may require further surgery to align the eyes. Because of the length of time and effort required, we do not routinely use the prism adaptation test in determining the amount of surgery to be done in either partly accommodative esotropia or decompensated esophoria.

EXOTROPIA

Exodeviations are seen less frequently than esodeviations. Nonetheless, surgical management is often successful in realigning the eyes and restoring normal binocular vision.

Infantile Exotropia

Congenital, or infantile, exotropia noted before 6 months of age is rare. Correction of pre-existing refractive errors and amblyopia is necessary, just as in cases of infantile esotropia. Early surgical treatment (before 18 months of age) is preferred and usually consists either of bilateral lateral rectus muscle recession or a recession of the lateral rectus combined with a resection of the ipsilateral medial rectus. Success is defined as realignment to within 10 PD of the ortho position and may be achieved in approximately 80% of cases after one surgery.[7]

Intermittent Exotropia

Intermittent exotropia is the most common exodeviation. We rarely do surgery initially on these patients. We prefer to observe over time, prescribe glasses with added minus lens power, give prisms, or recommend orthoptics/vision therapy or alternate part-time patching. Surgical measures are necessary when the intermittent exotropia progresses in spite of other therapy and usually relates more to the fre-

quency rather than the magnitude of the exodeviation. We rarely intervene surgically when the exotropia is less than 15 to 20 PD.

 CLINICAL PEARL

Surgical measures are necessary when the intermittent exotropia progresses in spite of other therapy and usually relates more to the frequency rather than the magnitude of the exodeviation.

The different forms of intermittent exotropia warrant different surgical approaches.[8] A true divergence excess exotropia often requires a bilateral lateral rectus muscle recession. Patients with pseudo divergence excess intermittent exotropia or basic intermittent exotropia usually benefit from a resection of the medial rectus muscle combined with recession of the ipsilateral lateral rectus muscle. Convergence insufficiency intermittent exotropia is treated surgically only when orthoptics/vision therapy fails to treat this deviation. A minimal unilateral or bilateral medial rectus muscle resection can be done. Postoperative diplopia can be a side effect of surgery for these exodeviations, especially those involving resection of a medial rectus muscle.

In most cases of intermittent exotropia, our goal is mild-to-moderate overcorrection (approximately 15 PD of esotropia) in the early postoperative period. This will eventually settle into heterophoria as healing progresses over the next 6 to 8 weeks. Persistent surgical overcorrection of exotropia results in a consecutive esotropia (see Chapter 8, Case 19 and Chapter 9, Case 7). Frequently, these resolve spontaneously, and part-time patching may help prevent amblyopia in younger patients. Reoperation may be necessary if satisfactory realignment does not occur after 6 months. Undercorrection leads to persistent and recurrent exotropia. However, some patients will demonstrate only mild exophoria and can use fusional amplitudes to maintain binocularity. Success with surgical treatment is age-dependent. Children under age 4 show an increased risk of amblyopia with overcorrection. Therefore we prefer to perform surgery between ages 4 and 8. Children older than age 8 show a decreased success rate and a greater tendency to drift back into intermittent exotropia.[9]

Sensory Exotropia

Sensory deprivation can cause exotropia, more commonly in older patients. Corneal scars, dense cataracts, vitreous opacities, retinal lesions, and optic nerve atrophy can cause disparate retinal images and an exodeviation in the neglected eye. These are often large-angle exotropias. Surgical correction of the underlying problem, if possible, is attempted first. Subsequently, the misalignment is addressed. Usually, a medial rectus muscle resection combined with an ipsilateral lateral rectus muscle recession and possibly a posterior fixation suture is necessary to realign the eyes. Often, this is a reconstructive procedure, and vision remains poor in the affected eye. Exotropia associated with craniofacial anomalies, such as Apert's and Crouzon's syndromes, is best treated after the underlying structural bony abnormalities have been corrected.

Duane's Syndrome Type II

Duane's syndrome type II can present with an exotropia in the primary position and limited adduction. A and V patterns are common. Prisms may be helpful when the deviation is small; however, large exodeviations or extreme head turning is treated surgically. The lateral rectus muscle on the affected side is recessed to help realign the eyes and is often combined with a Y-splitting, because these patients frequently exhibit vertical upshoots and downshoots on adduction.

VERTICAL STRABISMUS

Vertical deviations are usually the result of problems with muscle innervation or muscle restriction. These deviations as a whole are more difficult to manage and treat than esotropia and exotropia.

Dissociated Vertical Deviation

Dissociated vertical deviation (DVD) is of unknown cause. Usually, the gaze in the observed eye floats upward with occlusion or inattention. As mentioned earlier, it is usually bilateral and asymmetric, making measurement of the angle of deviation variable. Surgical indications with DVD include a large angle of deviation, frequent drifting of the eye off axis, and obvious and disturbing misalignment of the eyes. If a bilateral approach is chosen, a large bilateral superior rectus muscle recession is performed. A unilateral approach involves a moderate superior rectus muscle recession with a posterior fixation (Faden) suture.[6] Surgery will often improve the DVD, but in our experience recurrence is not unusual. Care must be taken when a unilateral procedure is performed, because this may "unmask" a latent DVD in the opposite eye.

Inferior Oblique Overaction

Inferior oblique muscle overaction is a frequent cause of vertical deviation and V-pattern deviations. Primary overaction of the inferior oblique muscles is not well understood; secondary overaction is often the result of weakness of the antagonist superior oblique muscle or the yoke superior rectus muscle in the contralateral eye. This causes elevation of the eye in adduction and increasing exodeviation in upgaze (V pattern). It is important to differentiate inferior oblique muscle overaction from DVD. Significant elevation in adduction warrants surgical intervention.

We weaken the inferior oblique muscles, either through bilateral inferior oblique muscle recession or inferior oblique myectomies.[10] When inferior oblique overaction and DVD coexist, anterior transposition of the inferior oblique muscle, transforming the muscle to a depressor, is useful, but this procedure should not be performed unilaterally, or a hypotropia may result.[11]

 CLINICAL PEARL

Significant elevation in adduction warrants surgical intervention.

Superior Oblique Overaction

Superior oblique overaction may present with a hypotropia on the affected side, an associated exotropia in downgaze, (A-pattern deviation), and depression on adduction of the involved eye. Exotropia in downgaze (e.g., reading position) will invariably spread to the primary position over time, and if the deviation is clinically significant and fusion is impossible, superior oblique tenotomy is appropriate.[12] The major disadvantage with this procedure is the risk of disturbing vertical and/or torsional symptoms in patients with good fusion potential.

Superior Oblique Paresis

Superior oblique palsies present diagnostic and surgical challenges. They can be congenital or acquired. When acquired, the condition is frequently traumatic. Clinically, the patient may present with a hypertropia or hypotropia, depending on which eye is used for fixation. Extorsion may cause objects to appear tilted, and a compensatory head tilt toward the normal side is common. In our experience, bilateral "masked" cases of superior oblique palsy are seen in 15% to 18% of cases and must be differentiated from unilateral cases (see Chapter 10, Case 9). Bilateral superior oblique palsy usually presents with a V-pattern esotropia, less than 10 PD of hypertropia in primary gaze, and greater than 10 degrees of excyclodeviation in primary gaze. The three-step test is often positive to both sides.[13]

Surgical treatment is indicated if diplopia has not resolved spontaneously in 6 months in acquired cases, if prisms and patching have failed, if head position is abnormal, or if a large vertical deviation in primary position (10 PD or more) is present. The surgery is designed to treat the field of gaze in which the vertical deviation is the greatest.[14] Less than 15 PD of hypertropia in primary position can be treated by recessing the antagonist inferior oblique muscles. Greater than 15 PD of hypertropia can be treated with an ipsilateral inferior oblique recession combined with recession of the contralateral inferior rectus muscle. If the inferior oblique muscle is not overacting, then recession of the contralateral inferior rectus muscle is preferred. Congenital laxity of the superior oblique tendon is best managed by a superior oblique tuck, although a mild side effect of this procedure is the creation of Brown's syndrome. Symptomatic excyclotorsion can be treated with the Harada-Ito procedure, involving anterior and lateral displacement of the anterior one third of the superior oblique tendon. This corrects the excyclotorsion without affecting the vertical alignment in primary gaze.[15]

 CLINICAL PEARL

Surgical treatment is indicated if diplopia has not resolved spontaneously in 6 months in acquired cases, if prisms and patching have failed, if head position is abnormal, or if a large vertical deviation in primary position (10 PD or more) is present.

Brown's Syndrome

Brown's syndrome refers to restrictions of the superior oblique tendon sheath.[16] Limitation of elevation in adduction is noted on examination. Cases are most often congenital. However, acquired Brown's syndrome should raise the suspicion of direct trauma or inflammation involving the trochlea, and computerized tomography can be helpful.[17] Observation in acquired cases is indicated, because many cases resolve either spontaneously or with treatment of the underlying disease (e.g., contiguous sinusitis). Corticosteroids may be useful in decreasing swelling caused by inflammation.[18] Indications for surgery include a large manifest hypotropia in primary gaze or fusion, which is possible only with a large compensatory head posture. Most surgeons perform a procedure to weaken the superior oblique tendon. This may induce a manifest superior oblique muscle paresis, necessitating subsequent recession of the ipsilateral inferior oblique in approximately 30% of cases.

Double Elevator Palsy

Double elevator palsy (infantile monocular elevation deficiency) may represent a supranuclear disorder. Patients may exhibit a manifest hypotropia, pseudoptosis, or a chin-up head posture to fuse. Three types have been identified. The first and most common involves significant fibrosis of the inferior rectus muscle. This is managed surgically by recessing the involved inferior rectus muscle. The second type involves significant elevator weakness of both the superior rectus and inferior oblique. It is treated by a Knapp procedure involving transposition of the medial and lateral muscles toward the superior rectus muscle in the involved eye.[6] A third type combines elements of the first two, and appropriate surgery involves a combination of recession and transposition procedures.

Thyroid Myopathy

Thyroid eye disease can cause significant ocular muscle inflammation. Restrictions as a result of acute and chronic inflammation of the extraocular muscles can be extreme and frequently involve the inferior rectus muscles. This can be demonstrated during the patient examination with positive forced ductions. Treatment of the thyroid disorder and a short course of systemic corticosteriods should be followed by observation. Often, partial resolution of the restrictions can be observed as the ocular inflammation subsides. Persistent restrictions and diplopia can be managed surgically. The goal of surgery is to restore binocular vision in primary gaze and reading position. This is accomplished by appropriate recession of the restricted muscle, and adjustable suture techniques are sometimes useful. Residual horizontal and vertical restrictions may occur as a result of persistent or recurrent inflammation or muscle weakness.

CHEMODENERVATION

A recent development as an alternative to incisional strabismus surgery is chemodenervation of an extraocular muscle.[19] Botulinum-A toxin, a potent neurotoxin that is lethal in large doses, has been shown to affect specific nerve receptors in striated muscles when used in minute (0.1 to 0.5 ng) doses.[20] By interfering with the calcium-dependent release of acetylcholine from nerve terminals, botulinum toxin functionally denervates the muscle. The onset of action begins within 12 to 24 hours after injection, peak effect is observed in 2 to 7 days, and a recovery phase is observed within 3 months. Although the target muscle paralysis is transient, the resulting change in static eye muscle position can be permanent and is ideal in small-angle strabismus. Such deviations seen after primary muscle surgery (overcorrection and undercorrection) and after scleral buckling/encircling band procedures respond well to chemodenervation.[21,22] The toxin, when injected directly into the overacting muscle of the involved eye, purposefully weakens the target muscle to balance it with its counterpart. The advantages of such a procedure are that it involves local anesthesia and may be performed in an office setting. The disadvantages are that it requires a reasonable amount of patient cooperation, is not as powerful as surgery, and its effects may not be fully appreciated by the patient until 6 to 8 weeks after the injection. Repeat injections may be needed, and transient vertical strabismus and ptosis can occur. Rarely, serious complications, such as perforation of the globe and retrobulbar hemorrhage, can be observed. However, under the right conditions, botulinum toxin injection into the extraocular muscles offers a good option to surgery, especially for patients who present a high anesthetic risk, such as those in a compromised cardiovascular status or those with a previous episode or family history of malignant hyperthermia. Although it has been used in different types of strabismus, including infantile esotropia, we use botulinum-A toxin mostly in adults with small- or intermediate-angle esotropia, hypotropia, and recently acquired lateral rectus paresis. In the latter case the drug induces a muscle paresis when injected into the antagonist medial rectus muscle, which lasts 2 to 4 months. This allows the patient with lateral rectus paresis to obtain an area of single binocular vision in primary gaze while waiting for potential recovery and helps also prevent contracture or tightening of the medial rectus muscle.

CONCLUSION

Pharmacologic and surgical management of strabismus can be a great challenge. Sound medical practices and thorough examination techniques can help identify and treat most eye muscle misalignments. In selected cases, good surgical techniques can help correct or improve misalignments and restore binocular vision.

REFERENCES

1. Mims JL, Wood RC: Isoflurophate (Floropryl) ointment as the initial treatment of various esotropias: a survey and a review of 279 cases, *Binoc Vis Eye Muscle Surg* 8:11, 1993.
2. Knapp P: A and V patterns. In *Symposium on strabismus: transactions of the New Orleans Academy of Ophthalmology,* St Louis, 1971, Mosby.
3. Kushner BJ, Morton GV: Postoperative binocularity in adults with long-standing strabismus, *Ophthalmology* 99:316, 1992.
4. Kushner BJ: Binocular field expansion in adults after surgery for esotropia, *Arch Ophthalmol* 112:639, 1994.
5. Rogers GL, Bremer DL: Surgical treatment of the upshoot and downshoot in Duane's retraction syndrome, *Ann Ophthalmol* 16:841, 1984.
6. Helveston E: *Atlas of strabismus surgery,* ed 3, St Louis, 1985, Mosby.
7. Biedner B and others: Congenital constant exotropia: surgical results in six patients, *Binoc Vis Eye Muscle Surg* 8:137, 1993.
8. von Noorden GK: *Binocular vision and ocular motility,* ed 5, St Louis, 1996, Mosby.
9. Parks MM: *Ocular motility and strabismus,* Hagerstown, Md, 1975, Harper & Row.
10. Parks MM: The overacting inferior oblique muscle, *Am J Ophthalmol* 77:787, 1974.
11. Bremer DL, Rogers GL, Quick LD: Primary position hypotropia after anterior transposition of the inferior oblique, *Arch Ophthalmol* 104:229, 1986.
12. Harley RD, Manley DR: Bilateral superior oblique tenectomy in A-pattern exotropia, *Trans Am Ophthalmol Soc* 67:324, 1969.
13. Kushner BJ: The diagnosis and treatment of bilateral and masked superior oblique palsy, *Am J Ophthalmol* 105:186, 1988.
14. Knapp P: Classification and treatment of superior oblique palsy, *Am Orthopt J* 24:18, 1974.
15. Metz HS, Lerner H: The adjustable Harada-Ito procedure, *Arch Ophthalmol* 99:624, 1981.
16. Parks MM: Superior oblique tendon sheath syndrome of Brown, *Am J Ophthalmol* 79:82, 1975.
17. Meyer E and others: Computerized tomographic radiology of traumatic simulated Brown's syndrome, *Bin Vis Eye Muscle Surg* 3:135, 1988.
18. Saunders R and others: Acute onset of Brown's syndrome associated with pansinusitis, *Arch Ophthalmol* 108:58, 1990.
19. Scott AB: Botulinum toxin injection of eye muscles to correct strabismus, *Trans Am Ophthalmol Soc* 79:735, 1981.
20. Chen I: Toxins to the rescue, *Science News* 139:42, 1991.
21. Mindel J, Mishima S: Botulinum-A toxin in ophthalmology, *Surv Ophthalmol* 36:28, 1991.
22. Petitto VB, Buckley EG: Use of botulinum toxin in strabismus after retinal detachment surgery, *Ophthalmology* 98:509, 1991.

CHAPTER 12

Binocular Vision in Private Practice

Paul B. Freeman

The diagnosis of binocular visual anomalies is a significant part of every optometric practice.[1] Failure to diagnose can cause needless visual disability and/or poor visually related performance by the patient as well as engendering significant legal risks to the clinician.

EMPHASIS

The emphasis that a particular clinician places on dealing with binocular vision anomalies varies over a wide continuum (Table 12-1). The extremes include clinicians expert in dealing with all kinds of binocular vision anomalies to clinicians hesitant to diagnose and treat even the simplest binocular vision problem. Conveniently, the same anomaly can be handled to suit the emphasis of the clinician and still provide the patient with the best possible visual care. Managing various binocular vision anomalies can be a general diagnosis and referral or can be a specific diagnosis and treatment plan managed entirely by the initial clinician. Each of these approaches may be effective and appropriate and are neither better nor worse but simply different.

Clinicians placing marked emphasis on binocular vision usually are more experienced and have developed an interest in binocular visual problems. Their practices often include space dedicated to orthoptics/vision therapy and have allied personnel adept at teaching and monitoring the results of such therapy (Fig. 12-1).

Clinicians placing a limited emphasis on binocular vision anomalies often restrict both their diagnosis and

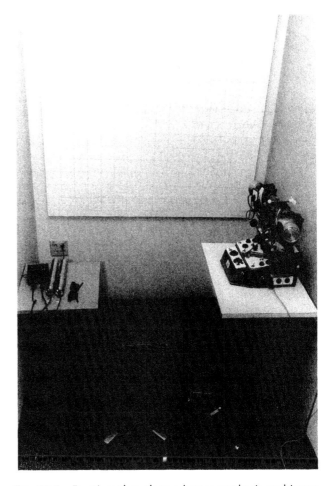

FIG. 12-1 Practices that place a heavy emphasis on binocular vision usually have special equipment and dedicated space.

treatment of binocular vision anomalies to procedures that can be concluded during their comprehensive examination. Usually, they do not prescribe extensive orthoptics/vision therapy, and their diagnosis of strabismic anomalies often is general in nature. They are frequently reluctant to undertake complicated cases, such as incomitant strabismus, aniseikonia, and amblyopia. On the other hand, they often prescribe adds for accommodative dysfunction or convergence excess esophoria. Most also include prescribing prisms, horizontal and vertical, when it appears helpful.

TABLE 12-1   DIFFERENCES IN EMPHASIS ON BINOCULAR VISION IN CLINICAL PRACTICE

Topic	Limited Emphasis	Marked Emphasis
Diagnosis	Limited and general	Extensive and specific
Treatment	• Generally within the context of comprehensive examination. • Largely limited to spectacles, prisms, and adds. • Little orthoptics/vision therapy.	• Treatment often extends beyond comprehensive examination. • Emphasizes orthoptics/vision therapy. • Largely in-office orthoptics/vision therapy.
Amblyopia	• Prescribing proper refractive correction within the normal examination process. • Prescribing occlusion therapy requires some additional equipment (occluder patches, etc.) and additional time spent instructing, counseling, and monitoring the patient.	• Limited emphasis, plus: • Some additional testing (additional assessment of binocular status, psychometric visual acuity testing, visuoscopy) and process may be involved. • Sometimes prescribes other forms of amblyopia treatment (i.e., entoptic phenomena, antisuppression therapy).
Suppression, Anomalous Correspondence, Aniseikonia	Limited.	Proper diagnosis and management usually extends beyond comprehensive examination. Additional testing (i.e., assessment of binocular status) and process may be involved. Prescribing therapy often requires additional equipment and additional time spent instructing, counseling, and monitoring the patient.
Accommodative Dysfunction	• Prescribing near plus adds within comprehensive examination process. • Prescribing accommodative training (amplitude and/or facility) requires some additional equipment (push-up paddles, flipper lenses, etc.) and additional time spent instructing, counseling, and monitoring the patient. • Often does not include complete diagnosis and management of spasm of accommodation or paresis of accommodation.	Limited emphasis, plus: Some additional testing (dynamic retinoscopy) and process may be involved. Diagnoses and manages spasm of accommodation and paresis of accommodation.
Convergence Excess Esophoria	• Prescribing near plus adds. • Some additional testing (accommodative amplitude and/or facility, dynamic retinoscopy) and process may be involved e.g., cycloplegic examination.	• Limited emphasis, plus: • Sometimes prescribes orthoptics/vision therapy for esophoria anomalies.
Vertical Phorias	• Prescribing vertical prisms requires additional equipment (fixation disparity device) and testing (vertical associated phoria, Maddox rod, vertical vergences).	• Limited emphasis, plus: • Includes full diagnosis and possible etiology of vertical deviation, including incomitancy and A and V deviations. • May include orthoptics/vision therapy for vertical deviations.
Horizontal Heterophoria, Vergence Anomalies	• Prescribing horizontal prisms may require additional equipment (fixation disparity device) and testing (associated phoria, Maddox rod, dynamic retinoscopy, vergences). • Prescribing vergence training (usually positive) requires some additional equipment (push-up paddles, vectograms, flipper bars, etc.) and additional time spent instructing, counseling, and monitoring the patient.	• Limited emphasis, plus: • May include vergence training for esophoria problems. • May include vergence training to maximize visual efficiency and performance, as in sports vision therapy.

TABLE 12-1   DIFFERENCES IN EMPHASIS ON BINOCULAR VISION IN CLINICAL PRACTICE—cont'd

Topic	Limited Emphasis	Marked Emphasis
Strabismus and Related Sensorimotor Anomalies	Limited.	• Prescribing refractive correction and vergence training in conjunction with antisuppression or anomalous correspondence therapy for intermittent or constant strabismus. • Management of various other types of strabismus by various means.
Staff	Limited or no assistance by technician.	• Technicians trained to assist. • Technicians may direct in-office training.
Equipment	Limited equipment may include occluders, push-up sticks, mini-vectograms, flip lenses.	• Substantial, includes limited, plus: • Flip prism, chiastopic cards, aperture rules, stereoscopes, synoptophore.

COMMUNICATION

Communication is the key to any successful practice and is crucial to the success of orthoptics/vision therapy. In dealing with establishing a successful orthoptics/vision therapy program, the following three individuals or groups must be addressed and their needs must be recognized and satisfied: (1) the patient who has a binocular vision problem that is interfering with some activity or the patient who has a binocular vision problem but does not appreciate the importance of the interference; (2) a school, work, or sports program in which the patient is involved; (3) the entities that may be sponsoring this individual financially to obtain the evaluation, services, or treatment that is being suggested.

 CLINICAL PEARL

Communication is the key to any successful practice and is crucial to orthoptics/vision therapy.

To be successful, each of the above must appreciate the importance of the problem, because this appreciation indirectly supports all of the other aspects of the treatment program. In short, "No problem, no leverage; no leverage, no compliance; no compliance, no program; no program, no problem." The most crucial aspect of the treatment program is that the patient recognizes the problem, why the problem is worthy of the treatment, and how the treatment will relieve the difficulties.

 CLINICAL PEARL

The most crucial aspect of the treatment program is that the patient recognizes the problem, why it is worthy of the treatment, and how the treatment will relieve the difficulties.

COMMUNICATION TO THE PATIENT

The clinician should initially define the visual problem to the patient and explain how the treatment will improve the situation. Appropriate caution should be used so that success is not always guaranteed. In a sense the patient about to undergo orthoptics/vision therapy is like an athlete, and the clinician and staff function as coach. If as a result of the orthoptics/vision therapy the skill level of the patient on various procedures increases and the problems encountered by the patient decreases, the training is successful. If the patient's performance on clinical tests improves but the problems remain, the clinician then should look elsewhere, because other variables may be preventing progress.

A hand-out may be useful to describe orthoptics/vision therapy (Table 12-2). This should be discussed with the patient and parents as treatment is initiated.

ARRANGEMENT OF THE PRACTICE

There are several aspects to efficiently dealing with binocular vision anomalies in private practice. Each clinician must include an integration of the treatment of these anomalies into the daily routine. When this is accomplished, dealing with binocular vision anomalies is handled smoothly and efficiently and the patient can recognize both the dedication of the practice to solving the patient's problem and the unique abilities of the clinician and staff.

FINANCIAL ASPECTS

The diagnosis of any binocular vision anomaly should be included in the examination codes routinely applied to clinical practice. These codes span the

TABLE 12-2   DESCRIPTION OF ORTHOPTICS/VISION THERAPY

Topic	Comments
Treatment sessions length	The treatment will consist of 1 or 2 45-minute in-office treatment sessions per week.
Treatment description	During the treatment the patient will work with lenses, prisms, or other devices that will help achieve more comfortable and efficient use of the eyes.
Home training activities	Home training may be used to supplement the in-office treatment.
Consultation with the doctor and staff	At the end of the treatment program, the progress will be discussed, along with what steps may be necessary to maintain success.
Letters to teachers, referral source, etc.	These letters will explain the problem and the treatment program, as well as what could be done otherwise to help the patient.
Questions	At the end of each treatment period, there will be a period available for answering questions regarding treatment progress or any other concerns.
Periodic examinations	At the completion of treatment, an appropriate schedule for a follow-up examination will be discussed.

gamut from technician only, brief, limited, intermediate examinations to comprehensive and extended comprehensive examinations.

The charge for the diagnosis and recommendation of treatment options should be reflected in the examination code (e.g., intermediate or comprehensive) and should be consistent with charges for these codes for other anomalies seen in the office. In a comprehensive examination, there should be no additional charge for providing the diagnosis and treatment recommendations to the patient. If the patient requires testing beyond the scope of the comprehensive examination, the patient should be informed of the binocular vision anomaly and that further testing will be required to verify the nature of the problem and the most appropriate recommendations for treatment. These patients should be charged an additional fee, based on the amount of time that is necessary and the complexity of the problem. A consultation fee is charged when the patient has been specifically referred by another clinician with the appropriate documentation.

If orthoptics/vision therapy is to be administered, a case-based fee schedule can be developed for each type of condition. A basic and a complex fee that are standard fees for typical patients in certain categories should be developed and should reflect professional time and effort. These fees typically represent estimates of the costs involved for the patient to complete a certain number of office visits for the complete remediation of the condition. For example, a patient with amblyopia may require more office visits than a patient with accommodative insufficiency. There also may be equipment rental fees, as described below, if any of the therapy is to be home-based.

An alternative to the case-based fee format is to charge the patient for each encounter with the clinician. Each encounter is charged at the clinician's current rate for an abbreviated, intermediate, extended, or comprehensive visit. Usually, the case-based technique is better, because with the fees paid before treatment is initiated the patient is motivated to take advantage of all of the treatment opportunities offered by the clinician. In the latter case, in which the pay-as-you-go approach is used, there is a not-so-subtle disincentive to see the doctor or technician, because a fee is administered at each encounter.

ONE ON ONE VERSUS GROUPS IN ORTHOPTICS/VISION THERAPY

Administering orthoptics/vision therapy to groups of patients at one time can be very helpful. This allows clinicians to keep the fees relatively low while also allowing maximum earnings for the practice, because many patients may be supervised by the technician at the same time. There are, however, some patients who are complex and require one-on-one care. Those patients should get individual care and, when possible, should be moved into one of the therapy groups. If group therapy sessions are used, the therapy times may be twice a week, immediately after school or some other time that is convenient for the majority of patients. Frequently, a training session of 30 to 45 minutes is effective.

EQUIPMENT REQUIREMENTS

The equipment necessary for diagnosing and treating binocular vision anomalies depends on the emphasis determined by the clinician. If the emphasis is to be limited, very little additional equipment that is not used during a comprehensive examination is necessary. Prism bars for vergences, tests of stereopsis, Maddox rods, push-up sticks for fixation, and accommodative amplitude and flipper lenses for accommodative facility are very useful equipment and are readily available.

If binocular vision anomalies are to be given marked emphasis, the above equipment should be augmented with several other devices and instruments. These include vectograms, tranaglyphs, stereoscopes, aperture rules, and computerized systems for vergence training, as well as cheiroscopes, TV trainers, or other devices for treating suppression. Clinicians diagnosing and managing amblyopia and strabismus should have a Macula Integrity Tester, Psychometric visual acuity cards, synoptophore, and Hess-Lancaster system available. Diagnosis and management of aniseikonia usually requires a set of afocal magnifiers.

Equipment can be sold, rented, lent, or given away to patients who do at-home training. Inexpensive devices such as eye patches and chiastopic cards can be given away and included in the examination fees. Other devices that are rarely used more than 1 to 2 months by the patient (i.e., flipper lenses, vectograms, stereoscopes) may be loaned to the patient. When receiving the equipment, the patient pays the full cost of the device. If the equipment is returned with normal wear and tear, this amount minus a small handling fee is returned to the patient. If the equipment has been damaged or not returned, no money is returned to the patient. Equipment should be conveniently located and assembled as needed.

Office space is also necessary to explain treatment alternatives to the patient and/or parent and to monitor the treatment being administered. Most offices have space outside of the examination room devoted to visual fields, fundus photography, or services such as teaching patients to manage their contact lenses. The orthoptics/vision therapy program can be conducted in the same area if patient flow allows. A dedicated area should be considered when several patients are undergoing orthoptics/vision therapy.

OFFICE VERSUS HOME TRAINING

Basing orthoptics/vision therapy as in-office versus at-home orthoptics/vision therapy is a very significant decision. In-office orthoptics/vision therapy has significant benefits for both the patient and the practice. The major advantage of in-office orthoptics/vision therapy is that it enhances compliance. We find that this is a significant advantage, because lack of compliance is a major reason for failure of orthoptics/vision therapy. Completing the therapy in the presence of the office assistant strongly reinforces the correct technique for the proper period. In-office orthoptics/vision therapy requires appropriate office space and the dedicated time of a staff member. In-office orthoptics/vision therapy also requires a greater commitment of time from the patient than does similar activity at home.

✿ CLINICAL PEARL

The major advantage of in-office orthoptics/vision therapy is that it enhances compliance.

At-home orthoptics/vision therapy is convenient for many patients, particularly for highly motivated and independent patients. At-home orthoptics/vision therapy can also be useful for patients who must complete periodic maintenance because of the chronic nature of their conditions. As discussed above, however, poor compliance is a very significant issue with at-home orthoptics/vision therapy. Patients often do not complete the required amount of therapy and often do not perform the therapy as instructed. A combination of in-office and at-home treatment is the best way to administer orthoptics/vision therapy.

STAFF REQUIREMENTS

Support from well-trained staff is a very important aspect of any practice and is particularly important if a heavy emphasis is to be placed on binocular vision or if orthoptics/vision therapy is to be administered. Without staff support, cost-effective management of treating binocular vision anomalies is hardly possible. In the same way that it is usually not feasible financially for doctors to explain insertion and removal of contact lenses and the use of various solutions when contact lenses are being fitted, it is usually not feasible for a doctor to explain all the therapy procedures to patients with binocular visual anomalies. Delegating this responsibility to an office assistant allows the clinician to see other patients, so that costs are contained and efficiency is maintained. The office assistant should be able to interpret directions and explain procedures correctly and communicate effectively. Because many orthoptics/vision therapy procedures require stereopsis, normal binocular vision is also very helpful. Because there are few if any formal educational programs, the clinician should train the office assistant to assist as necessary.

CASE PRESENTATION

The case presentation after the initial comprehensive vision examination should review the choices for treatment and associated costs, risks, and benefits, so that an informed choice can be made. This discussion should include the time and cost of each treatment, along with its benefits and any limitations or uncertainties.

If orthoptics/vision therapy is selected, the discussion should include a detailed description of the orthoptics/vision therapy to be done, duration of each session, number of times per day, number of days per week, and whether the orthoptics/vision therapy is to be in or out of the office (or, preferably, some combination). The patient should have specific goals to reach during orthoptics/vision therapy. These motivate the patient in achieving the endpoint results as soon as possible.

Whenever possible, some orthoptics/vision therapy should be completed in the office. Because one of the major problems in orthoptics/vision therapy is poor compliance, in-office treatment is an effective solution. Any orthoptics/vision therapy techniques should be demonstrated to the patient. If the treatment is to be completed entirely at-home, the patient should first demonstrate understanding of the prescribed orthoptics/vision therapy in the office. Using as much variety in orthoptics/vision therapy as possible is important. At a follow-up examination, the clinician should select several tests to evaluate progress, and the results should be shared with the patient. If treatment is performed at home, contact with the patient should be made at least once a week over the phone. Follow-up is critical to success of the treatment plan.

 CLINICAL PEARL

Because one of the major problems in orthoptics/vision therapy is poor compliance, in-office treatment is an effective solution.

Clear written instructions, frequent follow-up checks, attainable but challenging goals, and the use of a log to record progress all help with the important documentation of compliance.[1,2] Documentation of changes in vergence orthoptics/vision therapy with an operant conditioning paradigm and automated random-dot stereograms has been helpful.[3]

KEEPING PACE

Keeping pace with rapid developments in binocular vision is challenging. Continuing education seminars can help maintain an adequate knowledge of the area. Many such courses are available, particularly at state and national meetings of the profession. Another method of learning to deal with anomalies of binocular vision is to discuss cases that are encountered with a knowledgeable and interested colleague. Reading of other books and recent journal articles relating to binocular vision is essential. Extensive searches of the literature are now easily accessible over the Internet, as well as through more traditional library techniques. Finally, good residency opportunities in the area of binocular vision are available. Residency or fellowship training can be extremely beneficial for a person with a high degree of interest who intends to place a heavy emphasis on binocular visual anomalies.

REFERENCES

1. Rosner J, Rosner J: *Vision therapy in a primary-care practice,* New York, 1988, Professional.
2. Cooper J, Feldman J: Operant conditioning of fusional convergence ranges using random dot stereograms, *Am J Optom Physiol Opt* 57:205, 1980.
3. Grisham JD: Visual therapy results for convergence insufficiency: a literature review, *Am J Optom Physiol Opt* 65:448, 1988.

CHAPTER 13

Liability Issues in Binocular Vision Practice

John G. Classé

Reports of professional liability claims involving optometrists have established that the most important source of large claims is misdiagnosis of intraocular disease.[1-3] The conditions that most often lead to these claims are glaucoma, retinal detachment, and tumors affecting the visual system.[1-3] In the latter category, both intraocular and brain tumors may be the cause of claims. Anomalies of binocular vision—strabismus and reduced visual acuity (misdiagnosed as amblyopia)—are frequently the presenting conditions but are caused by the underlying tumor.[4] Children seem to be disproportionately affected, and damages resulting from the misdiagnosis and delay in treatment are substantial.[5] In addition, claims may result from failure to properly diagnose and manage true disorders of binocular vision, principally amblyopia and strabismus. In these cases, which inevitably involve children, the failure to institute treatment leads to impairment of visual development and loss of vision potential. Although damages are not as substantial as in the cases resulting from tumors, they can be significant, because the impairment extends over the lifetime of the affected individual.

This chapter describes both types of liability claims, to make optometrists aware of the circumstances under which these claims are most likely to be brought to assist in minimizing the risk of litigation. Although there is a greater risk of litigation from a case in which there is an underlying tumor, failure to properly manage a binocular vision disorder can also lead to a liability claim.[5] Because it is the diagnosis and treatment of strabismus or amblyopia that constitutes the usual reason for binocular vision evaluation, this discussion will begin with a review of representative liability claims in which failure to properly manage these anomalies resulted in liability for the eyecare practitioner.

BINOCULAR VISION DISORDERS

Binocular vision disorders may be encountered in any age population, from infants to the elderly. Although they may result in impairment at any age, children are particularly susceptible to these disorders because of detrimental effects on visual development. Optometrists often encounter children with complaints or clinical findings that indicate the child has a binocular vision disorder. The most significant disorders for legal purposes are constant strabismus and functional amblyopia. These conditions, if untreated, can lead to visual acuity decrement, loss of binocularity, and impairment of vision function. It is essential that clinicians recognize the importance of diagnosing these conditions at an early age and instituting timely treatment. Failure to detect these disorders and institute or refer for appropriate treatment may result in a successful action for damages being brought against the eye care clinician.

 CLINICAL PEARL

The most significant disorders for legal purposes are constant strabismus and functional amblyopia.

This discussion will describe representative legal claims arising out of an eye care clinician's failure to diagnose and manage constant strabismus or amblyopia in a child.

STRABISMUS

Constant strabismus in children can result in vision loss. The deviation creates diplopia, which is eliminated through the mechanism of suppression and/or anomalous correspondence. In addition, amblyopia usually develops if the child has a unilateral strabismus. Any age child may be affected with strabismus. Because of the detrimental effect that vision deprivation has when it occurs during the period of visual development, however, strabismus occurring in children under age 8 is the most important.[6] Constant esotropia is the most significant type of strabismus for purposes of litigation.

ESOTROPIA

As mentioned in Chapter 8, esotropia is estimated to affect 2% to 4% of the general population.[7] Deviations may be classified as infantile, accommodative, acute-onset, secondary to another condition (e.g., cataract, surgery), mechanically restrictive, or small-angle (microtropia). Although any of these deviations, if undiagnosed and untreated, can lead to amblyopia and the potential for litigation, infantile and acute-onset esotropias are most likely to produce a legal claim.

 CLINICAL PEARL

Infantile and acute-onset esotropias are most likely to produce a legal claim.

Infantile Esotropia

This disorder begins during the first 6 months of life and is usually a large, constant deviation that is frequently accompanied by amblyopia and other anomalies, such as dissociated vertical deviation, inferior oblique overaction, and nystagmus. Transient strabismus is common in neonates, but any newborn with an esotropia that persists past 3 months of age should receive a careful eye examination.[8] Treatment requires correction of clinically significant refractive errors, the use of occlusion therapy for amblyopia, possibly prisms, and extraocular muscle surgery to obtain ocular alignment. The following case illustrates that failure to comply with the standard of care may result in a liability claim.

CASE 1

A 2-year-old child with constant unilateral esotropia was taken by his parents to an optometrist for assessment of the strabismus.[9] The esotropia had begun in the first few months of the child's life but had not been previously treated. A hyperopic refractive error, deep amblyopia in the deviating eye, and normal ocular health were found. The optometrist prescribed glasses and instituted binasal occlusion without first attempting to use conventional occlusion therapy for the amblyopia.

After 18 months of this therapy the parents took the child to an ophthalmologist. The ophthalmologist told the parents that constant total direct occlusion was needed for the amblyopia, but that it was too late to attempt treatment to restore binocular vision. A lawsuit was filed against the optometrist, alleging that improper therapy had been attempted and that it had prevented more efficacious treatment from being timely employed.

Proper management of infantile esotropia requires that conventional occlusion therapy, not binasal occlusion, be instituted for any amblyopia, and that the refractive correction be provided when indicated. Although the ophthalmologist in this case erroneously asserted that the 3 1/2-year-old child was too old to achieve "fusion," accurate extraocular muscle surgery most likely would have resulted in some restoration of peripheral fusion. Although surgery should ideally be performed before age 2, even previously untreated adults with a history of infantile esotropia can sometimes achieve some degree of fusion with treatment (see Chapter 8, Table 8-2).[10-12]

Accommodative Esotropia

This type of deviation is caused by uncorrected hyperopia, a high AC/A ratio, or both. The age of onset in most cases is usually between ages 6 months and 7 to 8 years (2 1/2 years is the mean).[13] The deviation often begins gradually as an intermittent esotropia and may become constant. The deviation is usually moderate in size and, depending on the AC/A ratio, may be about the same magnitude at distance and near or larger at near.[14] In some cases the esotropia may occur only at near. There is an inferior oblique overaction in about one third of cases.[15] Usually, the hyperopic refractive error is between 2 and 6 D.[16] Correction of the hyperopia either significantly or completely reduces the strabismus in about two thirds of cases; if an esotropia remains at near, bifocal lenses may be prescribed.

Children who are suspected of having accommodative esotropia should be examined immediately. Failure to diagnose and treat the condition can result in the frequency changing from intermittent to constant and the development of a nonaccommodative deviation, amblyopia, or suppression and/or anomalous correspondence. Treatment usually requires full correction of the hyperopia, the institution of occlusion therapy for amblyopia if needed, and the use of orthoptics/vision therapy to enhance sensory and motor fusion. In some cases, additional esotropia may develop after glasses have been prescribed, thus necessitating further treatment to prevent the loss of binocular vision.[17]

Acute-Onset Esotropia

An acute-onset esotropia is one that develops suddenly in a patient with previously normal binocular vision. It is a much less frequent form of strabismus than either infantile or accommodative esotropia. As mentioned in Chapter 8, acute-onset esotropia has several types of presentations (see Table 8-3), and some of these conditions can be associated with underlying disease. Clinicians must be aware of the potential of a neurologic cause in these cases. It is the undiagnosed underlying disease that usually causes the injury and leads to a liability claim, especially in acute-onset esotropia that is paretic.

 CLINICAL PEARL

Acute-onset esotropia has several types of presentations, and some of these conditions can be associated with underlying disease.

The standard of care requires not only evaluation of the esotropia but also assessment of the child for ocular, systemic, and neurologic disease. This assessment often requires referral of the child for a neurologic examination. Failure to recognize that such an assessment is needed has been the cause of large liability claims involving optometrists.[18,19]

Mechanically Restrictive Esotropia

This type of esotropia is caused by a mechanical restriction or obstruction of motility (e.g., Duane's syndrome types I and III, fibrosis of the medial rectus muscles, and trauma to the orbit). Treatment sometimes includes prisms and/or extraocular muscle surgery, particularly if the patient manifests an abnormal or compensatory head posture. Litigation in these cases rarely occurs.

Secondary Esotropia

The two principal causes of secondary esotropias are sensory deficits and extraocular muscle surgery. Sensory deficits are often amblyopiagenic and require appropriate management. Typical causes of these deficits include cataract, uncorrected anisometropia, and also any eye disease or other condition that causes a reduction in visual acuity in one eye. Consecutive esotropias result from surgical overcorrection of an exotropia. When this occurs in young children, amblyopia may result, as well as suppression and/or anomalous correspondence.

Microtropia

A microtropia is a small-angle esotropia measuring less than 10 PD. It usually begins in young children and because of its small size it may go undetected by the parents. A constant unilateral deviation will be amblyopiagenic and most often is associated with anomalous correspondence and poor potential for normal binocular vision. Therefore early detection and treatment are essential.

In general, liability claims involving children with esotropia occur because a clinician has not recognized the need for treatment during the period of visual development or that a more serious, underlying condition was missed. The failure to institute appropriate treat-

ment (or to refer for treatment) results in permanent injury and becomes the basis for a liability claim.

 CLINICAL PEARL

In general, liability claims involving children with esotropia occur because a clinician has not recognized the need for treatment during the period of visual development or that a more serious, underlying condition was missed.

EXOTROPIA

In general, the clinical considerations described for esotropias also apply to exotropias. Most exotropias, however, are intermittent rather than constant. In fact, intermittent exotropia is common in neonates.[20,21] Also, acute onset exotropia and microexotropia are rare. The constant forms of exotropia are the most likely to produce a claim.

AMBLYOPIA

Amblyopia is estimated to affect a minimum of 2% of American children.[23] If the amblyopia is undiagnosed, the affected eye fails to develop its full visual potential, resulting in a loss of acuity. Amblyopia typically occurs before age 6.[24] The most common types of amblyopia are anisometropic, strabismic, and deprivation amblyopia.

DEPRIVATION AMBLYOPIA

This type of amblyopia occurs when there is an obstruction in the line of sight that prevents clear focus from being obtained. Because cataract and similar obstructions (i.e., ptosis, corneal opacification) are usually rather evident, there is less opportunity for misdiagnosis and thus a relatively small risk of litigation.

Anisometropic amblyopia and strabismic amblyopia are the most common causes of liability claims. Negligence may occur because the condition is undiagnosed and treatment is thereby delayed, or because the condition is detected but no treatment is undertaken. The latter cause is the more frequent source of claims.

 CLINICAL PEARL

Anisometropic amblyopia and strabismic amblyopia are the most common causes of liability claims.

ANISOMETROPIC AMBLYOPIA

Amblyopia may be caused by high but equal refractive errors (isoametropia) or by significantly unequal refractive errors (anisometropia). Of the two conditions, anisometropia is the more prevalent and more likely to produce a legal claim, usually from anisometropic hyperopia. A finding of anisometropic amblyopia requires treatment. Failure to undertake complete treatment prevents the eye from attaining its full vision potential, thus creating a cause of action against the clinician. The following case demonstrates the potential for liability.

CASE 2

A 6-year-old boy was examined by an optometrist and found to have anisometropic amblyopia that reduced acuity in the affected eye to 20/200.[25] The optometrist prescribed glasses but made no effort to treat the amblyopia that persisted following 1 month of wearing the glasses.

Another optometrist examined the child 2 years later and obtained similar results but likewise instituted no amblyopia therapy. A year and a half later (2 months short of the child's tenth birthday) an ophthalmologist performed an examination and commented to the child's parents that patching, if instituted 4 years earlier, could have improved vision to 20/40 in the amblyopic eye.

The parents subsequently sued both optometrists, alleging that they had been negligent in failing to institute or recommend occlusion therapy on a timely basis.

Reduced vision is a frequent reason for the examination of children. If the examination reveals decreased visual acuity, it is essential that the clinician determine the cause. A patient should not be dismissed from care without this determination, and the reason for the vision loss should always be documented in the record of care. In the above case example, however, documentation of anisometropic amblyopia was not the cause for the litigation. Failure to provide complete treatment was the cause.

STRABISMIC AMBLYOPIA

Amblyopia develops in children below age 6 with constant unilateral strabismus. Prompt diagnosis and aggressive treatment are required to provide proper visual stimulation to the amblyopic eye.

The standard of care for children with amblyopia is to correct any refractive error to obtain best visual acuity, use occlusion therapy to provide visual stimulus to the amblyopic eye, and—when appropriate—to institute orthoptics/vision therapy. Failure to adhere to this standard creates the potential for liability.[26] In amblyopia claims the most common deviation from the standard of care is failing to use appropriate occlusion therapy (see Case 1).

✦ **CLINICAL PEARL**

In amblyopia claims the most common deviation from the standard of care is failing to use appropriate occlusion therapy.

For children with irreversible amblyopia, protective eyewear should be provided, such as a sturdy frame with polycarbonate lenses. If the child is allowed to participate in sports that pose a risk of injury, athletic eyewear meeting the impact resistance standards of ASTM F803-94 should be prescribed.[27] Failure to provide protective eyewear, if the child sustains an injury to the non-amblyopic eye, can create a cause of action for damages. Studies have reported that monocular individuals have a greater risk of vision loss in the good eye than binocular individuals in either eye.[28] Therefore protective eyewear is both clinically and legally justifiable.

FAILURE TO DETECT BRAIN TUMORS

Brain tumors that affect the visual system may present as binocular vision disorders (i.e., reduced visual acuity mimicking amblyopia caused by the tumor's effect on the optic chiasm). Common symptoms include decreased visual acuity, acute-onset strabismus, and headache. Brain tumors with ocular manifestations are rare but are significant causes of liability claims involving children. These claims most often result from the failure to detect a craniopharyngioma.[29] Although optometrists are not responsible for the differential diagnosis of brain tumors, failure to perform a reasonable evaluation or to refer a patient for appropriate evaluation can create liability if the delay increases injury.

The symptoms produced by brain tumors may be vague, and the clinical signs of disease may be subtle (Box 13-1). Headaches are particularly difficult to evaluate because they are frequently a source of complaints but are rarely produced by tumors. Children in particular often complain of headache, and the clinician must resort to thorough history taking and appropriate testing to ascertain the headache's cause. In the rare case in which the cause is not apparent, referral may be necessary for neurologic testing. In such cases an appointment should be scheduled with the appropriate health care practitioner for a specific date and time, and a letter should be sent to the practitioner (by facsimile transmission if necessary), describing the reason for the referral. If disease is present, failure to make a timely referral may be a key part of a liability claim, as illustrated by the following case.

CASE 3

A 5-year-old child who had failed a vision screening and was suspected of having amplyopia was examined by an optometrist, who found that the child's fundus was "normal" and his visual field "full."[25] Despite the child's complaints of blurred vision in one eye, glasses were not prescribed. After the examination, the mother allegedly informed the optometrist that the child had often complained of headaches,

From: Classé JG: Liability for pediatric care, *Optom Clin* 5(2):161, 1996.

and the optometrist recommended that the boy be seen by the family physician.

About 3 months later the child began to exhibit clumsiness and to complain of poor acuity while watching television. Two months later the mother took the child to a physician, who found optic atrophy in one eye and papilledema in the other.

The child was referred to a hospital for further evaluation, and hydrocephalus secondary to an astrocytoma was diagnosed. Surgery was performed to remove the tumor, and the child received 25 radiation treatments thereafter.

A lawsuit was filed against the optometrist, alleging that he had been negligent for failing to recognize fundus changes indicative of increased intracranial pressure and for failing to refer the child for a medical evaluation.

Acute-onset strabismus, particularly esotropia in a child, is a significant finding. Generally speaking, the onset of strabismus in a child after age 5 is a more ominous indication of a possible underlying disease.[31,32]

CLINICAL PEARL

The onset of strabismus in a child after age 5 is a more ominous indication of a possible underlying disease.

CASE 4

An 8-year-old boy with a 1-week history of esotropia and diplopia was examined by an optometrist, who found unaided distance acuities of 20/25 in each eye and a 15- to 20-PD esotropia at both distance and near.[18,33] There was no lateral rectus paresis, and ophthalmoscopy through an undilated pupil was unremarkable.

The optometrist prescribed glasses and occlusion and scheduled the child for reevaluation in 2 weeks. The optometrist saw the child seven times over the next 8 months,

with no significant change noted in the child's status, although the use of occlusion was reduced. At the optometrist's last examination (approximately a year after the initial examination), corrected acuity was 20/20 in each eye, with constant esotropia of 15 PD at distance and 10 PD at near.

During a physical examination a month and a half later, however, a physician performed ophthalmoscopy and detected what he believed was papilledema. He sent the child to an ophthalmologist, who diagnosed optic atrophy and "amblyopia."

The child was referred to another ophthalmologist, who found chronic papilledema with pale swollen discs and arranged for a neurologist to perform radiographs and MRI. These tests revealed that ventricular dilatation had caused elevation of intracranial pressure; shunt surgery was performed to lower the pressure. A small midbrain tumor was ultimately found to be the cause of the ventricular changes. A lawsuit was filed against the optometrist, alleging that he had failed to refer the child for medical evaluation of an acute-onset esotropia and that the delay had adversely affected the child's prognosis.

For children with acute-onset strabismus, a finding that the deviation is incomitant is particularly important. However, the clinician should keep in mind that comitancy does not necessarily rule out underlying disease. Acute-onset strabismus must be carefully investigated to rule out the possibility of underlying disease. When assessing children, it is essential that clinicians adhere to generally accepted standards for examination. These standards have been compiled by the American Optometric Association and published as part of the *Optometric Clinical Practice Guidelines* series.[34] Clinicians should be familiar with these guidelines; of particular relevance are the guidelines for dilation of the pupil and assessment of the ocular fundus. The use of ophthalmoscopy through a dilated pupil will greatly assist in the effort to detect tumors affecting the visual system. Brain tumors in children are most likely to be detected by virtue of the compressive effect that they exert on the optic nerve, optic chiasm, or optic pathway, causing visual field loss or injury to the optic nerve. Worsening visual acuity unrelated to changes in refraction should raise suspicion. An example case reveals the potential for significant damages in such a case. (See Case 5.)

CASE 5

A 6-year-old boy who complained of headaches and vomiting was examined by a pediatrician, who diagnosed sinusitis and allergy and recommended a series of allergy shots.[19] Six weeks later, after the child's symptoms were aggravated by a bout of influenza, the physician allegedly recommended that the child be given an eye examination.

The child was examined by an optometrist 2 weeks later, who found that uncorrected distance visual acuity was 20/40 in each eye, corrected to 20/30 with +1.50-D glasses. The optometrist examined the interior of the eye through an undilated pupil and detected no evidence of disease. The mother was instructed to bring the child back for reassessment in 3 months, but 6 months passed before she returned with the child. At this examination the optometrist noted that binocular uncorrected distance visual acuities were 20/60 rather then 20/40. Because the mother reported that the child was not wearing the glasses, the optometrist asked the child to use the glasses regularly for 2 months and to return for reevaluation.

When the child was examined 2 months later, however, uncorrected distance acuities were 20/60 OD and undetermined OS (the child would not say that he could see the 20/400 line). The optometrist repeated retinoscopy, but mistakenly determined that the refractive error was plano; cycloplegia was not used. There was no examination of the interior of the eye. The mother was told to discontinue use of the glasses, and no further treatment was recommended.

About 2 weeks after the examination the mother called the optometrist, reporting that the child had severe headaches, vomiting, and was "shaking." The optometrist advised her to take the child to the pediatrician and called the mother a few days later to determine the child's status. The mother informed the optometrist that the pediatrician had treated the child for an infection and had recommended more allergy shots.

About 5 months later the mother brought the child to the optometrist because the child was wearing the glasses and she wanted the prescription to be checked again. At this examination the optometrist found the child's unaided distance acuities to be 20/200 OD and 20/400 OS. A week later the child was diagnosed as having bilateral optic atrophy secondary to craniopharyngioma. Following surgery, the child became completely blind.

A lawsuit was filed, with the optometrist and the pediatrician named as co-defendants, alleging that the child had suffered severe, recurring headaches and worsening visual acuity during their care, and that their failure to provide referral for neurologic testing constituted negligence.[19]

Visual field testing—if it can be performed—is essential to making the appropriate diagnosis. The most common field defects produced by craniopharyngiomas are central scotomas, bitemporal hemianopias, and homonymous hemianopias.[35] Even though children are not always the most cooperative of patients, at the very least, confrontation visual field testing should be attempted when an intracranial lesion is suspected.

FAILURE TO DETECT INTRAOCULAR TUMORS

Binocular vision disorders may also be produced by intraocular tumors. Depending on the location and size of the tumor, the patient may be symptomatic or asymptomatic. For infants the most common intraocular tumor is retinoblastoma; the most frequently af-

fected age group is 4 years and younger; and the most likely presenting signs are leukocoria and strabismus.[36,37] Failure to detect the tumor is most often caused by failure to perform a dilated fundus examination. Failing to adequately evaluate the retina can create a cause of action, as the following case demonstrates.

CASE 6

A 4 1/2-year-old girl who had been wearing glasses for refractive accommodative esotropia since age 2 was examined by an optometrist. He found that distance acuity was 20/30 in each eye, that both eyes were well aligned with the glasses, and that there was no ocular pathology observable by direct ophthalmoscopy through an undilated pupil. He suggested that the child's past eye care records be obtained, and that the child return for reassessment in 3 months.

At this second examination the optometrist found acuity to be reduced to 20/40 in one eye, which he attributed to amblyopia and prescribed occlusion. The mother was asked to bring the child back in another 3 months. At this examination, after finding that acuity was 20/30 in each eye, the optometrist performed cycloplegic retinoscopy and prescribed new glasses. Because of the improved acuity the optometrist discontinued the patching and asked the mother to bring the child back for reevaluation in 3 months, but because of complications related to her pregnancy the mother was not able to return with the child until more than 6 months had elapsed.

At this examination, which was approximately 13 months after the initial examination, the optometrist found that the child had developed unilateral leukocoria. A subsequent dilated fundus examination revealed the cause to be retinoblastoma; the tumor was located at the equator of the eye but was growing anteriorly and had seeded into the vitreous.

The child was referred to an eye hospital, where the parents were given a choice of therapies: enucleation—the usual outcome in such cases—or irradiation. They chose irradiation, and the course of treatment was successful in destroying the tumor. However, the irradiation caused a cataract and the tumor caused a retinal detachment. As a result, the child's best acuity in the eye was ultimately reduced to 20/300.

A lawsuit was filed, alleging that the optometrist had been negligent in failing to perform a dilated fundus evaluation with a binocular indirect ophthalmoscope at the initial examination, and that this omission had allowed the tumor to grow, worsening the likely outcome of therapy.[38]

Intraocular tumors present a significant diagnostic challenge to clinicians. For symptomatic children the standard of care requires a dilated fundus examination. For asymptomatic children at the initial examination the most likely means of detecting a "silent"" intraocular tumor is through a dilated fundus examination performed with a binocular indirect ophthalmoscope. For this reason all children, at initial examination and at reasonable periods thereafter, should receive an ophthalmoscopic assessment of the posterior pole and retinal periphery. The need for a thorough eye health assessment is particularly important when strabismus is present, as the following case demonstrates.

CASE 7

A mother took her infant daughter to a family medical center that conducted well-baby examinations and provided treatment for children with minor illnesses.[39] The mother had noticed that one of the child's eyes would frequently turn in, and although she described the intermittent esotropia to the pediatricians, they did not perform any assessment of the child's vision and did not refer her to an eye specialist for examination.

After several months elapsed, she consulted her optometrist about the problem, and he arranged an immediate referral to an ophthalmologist. The child was found to have bilateral retinoblastoma, and, despite irradiation therapy, both eyes eventually had to be enucleated.

A lawsuit was filed against the pediatricians, alleging that they had deviated from the standard of care by failing to appreciate the significance of the child's symptoms and to arrange a referral to an eye specialist.

Evaluation of the interior of the eye can be particularly difficult with small children. A clinician must use reasonable skill in performing the examination, but the degree of cooperation exhibited by the child will exert a substantial effect on the quality of the evaluation. It may be necessary to bring a noncooperative child back for another examination. If a suspicious finding is present, the parent or guardian must be informed of the finding and a reasonable effort made to determine its significance. If the child must be given further evaluation, an appointment should be scheduled for a specific date and time and documented in the child's record. Failure to provide necessary follow-up for a suspicious finding can form the basis for a liability claim, if it results in a delayed diagnosis that increases the child's injury.

Reduced visual acuity is always a suspicious finding; the cause of decreased acuity should always be determined and documented in the record of care. If the cause cannot be ascertained, the clinician must provide further testing or referral for such additional evaluation as would be deemed reasonable under the circumstances. The patient (or, if the patient is a child, the patient's parent or guardian) should be informed of the reduced acuity and of the clinician's plan to discover its cause.

In summary, for cases involving intraocular tumors the risk of liability is greatly diminished by periodic use of pupillary dilation and ophthalmoscopic assessment of the retinal pole and periphery. Clinicians should recommend to parents that children receive periodic eye health evaluations. The practice guidelines published by the American Optometric Association provide recommendations for periodic reexamination intervals.[40]

CONCLUSION

Anomalies of binocular vision, particularly in children, are an important cause of liability claims involving eye care providers. Ocular findings (such as decreased visual acuity and acute-onset strabismus) and presenting complaints (such as blurred vision and diplopia) may indicate the presence of underlying disease. Clinicians must perform an adequate assessment of eye health—even in infants and young children—to rule out the presence of pathology such as a tumor. The most certain means of performing an eye examination that satisfies the standard of care is to evaluate the interior of the eye through a dilated pupil and to employ binocular indirect ophthalmoscopy, to the extent that it is possible, so that the retinal periphery can be viewed.

Treatment of patients with binocular vision anomalies should follow recognized standards of care, using techniques of therapy and schedules of follow-up that are considered to be reasonable within the profession. Clinicians who are not familiar with prevailing standards for the diagnosis and treatment of binocular vision anomalies or who do not wish to manage binocular vision problems should refer patients to skilled practitioners, so that appropriate care can be timely scheduled and competently provided.

REFERENCES

1. Classé JG: Malpractice and optometry: a personal commentary, *South J Optom* 5:26, 1987.
2. Classé JG: A review of 50 malpractice claims, *J Am Optom Assoc* 60:694, 1989.
3. Classé JG: Liability and ophthalmic drug use, *Optom Clin* 2:121, 1992.
4. Classé JG, Rutstein RP: Binocular vision anomalies: an emerging cause of malpractice claims, *J Am Optom Assoc* 66:305, 1995.
5. Classé JG: Liability for pediatric care, *Optom Clin* 5(2):161, 1996 (in press).
6. Oliver M and others: Compliance and results of treatment for amblyopia in children more than 8 years old, *Am J Ophthalmol* 102:340, 1989.
7. Roberts J, Rowland M: Refractive status and motility defects of persons 4-74 years: United States 1971-1972, Vital and health statistics: series 11, DHEW Pub no (PHS) 78-1654, Hyattsville, Md, 1978, National Center for Health Statistics.

8. Nixon RB and others: Incidence of strabismus in neonates, *Am J Ophthalmol* 100:798, 1985.

9. *Brandt v Zettel,* A-8603897, District Court, Hamilton County, Ohio. In: *Medical Malpractice Verdicts: Settlements and Experts* 8(5):8. 1992.

10. Kushner BJ, Morton GV: Postoperative binocularity in adults with long-standing strabismus, *Ophthalmology* 99:316, 1992.

11. Kushner BJ: Postoperative binocularity in adults with long-standing strabismus: is surgery cosmetic only? *Am Orthopt J* 40:64, 1990.

12. Morris RJ, Scott WE, Dickey CF: Fusion after surgical alignment for long-standing strabismus in adults, *Ophthalmology* 100:135, 1993.

13. Parks MM: Management of acquired esotropia, *Br J Ophthalmol* 58:240, 1974.

14. Von Noorden GK: *Binocular vision and ocular motility: theory and management of strabismus,* ed 5, St Louis, 1996, Mosby.

15. Wilson ME, Parks MM: Primary inferior oblique overaction in congenital esotropia, accommodative esotropia, and intermittent esotropia, *Ophthalmology* 96:950, 1989.

16. Parks MM: Abnormal accommodative convergence squint, *Arch Ophthalmol* 59:364, 1958.

17. Wick B: Accommodative esotropia: efficacy of therapy, *J Am Optom Assoc* 58:562, 1987.

18. *Dickey v Long,* 575 NE 2d 339 (Ind App 1992).

19. *Medders v Woodruff,* CV-88-0885, Circuit Court, Jefferson County, Alabama, 1988.

20. Nixon RB, Helveston EM, Miller K: Incidence of strabismus in neonates, *Am J Ophthalmol* 100:798, 1985.

21. Archer SM, Sondhi N, Helveston EM: Strabismus in infancy, *Ophthalmology* 96:133, 1989.

22. Deleted in galleys.

23. Flom MC, Neumaier RW: Prevalence of amblyopia, *Public Health Rep* 81:329, 1988.

24. Harweth RS: Multiple sensitive periods in the development of the primate visual system, *Science* 232:235, 1986.

25. Classé JG: *Legal aspects of optometry,* Boston, 1989, Butterworth-Heinemann, 1989.

26. American Optometric Association: Care of the patient with amblyopia, St Louis, 1994, The Association.

27. American Society for Testing and Materials: Standard specification for eye protectors for use by players of racket sports, standard F-803-94, Philadelphia, 1994, The Society.

28. Vereecken EP, Brabant P: Prognosis for vision in amblyopia after the loss of the good eye, *Arch Ophthalmol* 102:220, 1984.

29. Leavesn ME and others: Nonadenomatous intrasellar and parasellar neoplasms. In Wilson JD and others, editors: *Harrison's principles of internal medicine,* ed 12, New York, 1991, McGraw-Hill.

30. *Castaneda v Pederson,* 89CV-4063, Circuit Court, Milwaukee County, Wisconsin. In: *Medical malpractice verdicts, settlements and experts,* 8(2):28, 1992.

31. Williams AS, Hoyt CS: Acute comitant esotropia in children with brain tumors, *Arch Ophthalmol* 107:376, 1989.

32. Astle WF, Miller SJ: Acute comitant esotropia: a sign of intracranial disease, *Can J Ophthalmol* 29:151, 1984.

33. Classé JG: Brain tumors, malpractice, and optometry, *Optom Clin* 3:127, 1993.

34. American Optometric Association: Care of the patient with strabismus: esotropia and exotropia, St Louis, 1995, The Association.

35. Trevino R: Chiasmal syndrome, *J Am Optom Assoc* 66:559, 1995.

36. Abramson DH, Servodidio RN: Retinoblastoma, *Optom Clin* 3:49, 1993.

37. Abramson DH: Retinoblastoma: diagnosis and management, *Cancer* 32:130, 1982.

38. *Keir v United States,* 853 F 2d 398, Sixth Cir, 1988.

39. *Shumaker v United States,* C-85-932-G, C-85-995-G, US District Court for the Middle District of North Carolina, 1989.

40. American Optometric Association: Pediatric eye and vision examination, St Louis, 1994, The Association.

A pattern Exotropia in which the deviation increases in straight downgaze or esotropia in which the deviation increases in straight upgaze.

aberrant regeneration Possible sequela of an oculomotor nerve palsy, resulting in abnormal lid and pupillary and horizontal or vertical movement of the eye.

abducens nerve Sixth cranial nerve, which innervates the lateral rectus muscle.

accommodation The dioptric adjustment of the eye to achieve maximal clarity of retinal imagery for an object of regard.

accommodative convergence/accommodation ratio (AC/A ratio) The convergence response of an individual to a unit stimulus of accommodation, usually expressed as the quotient of accommodative convergence in prism diopters divided by the accommodative stimulus in diopters.

accommodative esotropia Esotropia resulting from uncorrected hyperopia and/or a high AC/A ratio.

accommodative insufficiency The condition in which the amplitude of accommodation is below the minimal limits of the expected amplitude for the patient's age.

Adie's (tonic) pupil A pupil in which the reactions to light, direct or consensual, are almost absent. A reaction only occurs after prolonged exposure to light or dark.

afocal lens (size lens) A lens of zero focal power in which rays entering parallel emerge parallel.

afterimage test A test of retinal correspondence using afterimage projections of two flashing lights, one in the vertical direction and one in the horizontal direction.

alternate cover test The successively alternate placement of an opaque occluder in front of each eye without allowing interim fusion, to observe the magnitude of heterophoria or strabismus and to measure the deviation by repeating with varying amounts of prism until the deviation is neutralized, as indicated by no fixational movement.

alternating strabismus In strabismus, each eye not only takes up fixation but holds fixation while both eyes are open.

amblyopia Loss of vision in an eye without any overt pathologic changes in that eye.

    functional amblyopia Amblyopia resulting from disorders such as strabismus, anisometropia, or visual deprivation.

    occlusion amblyopia Amblyopia that develops in an eye that has been constantly occluded for a long time.

    organic amblyopia Amblyopia resulting from subophthalmoscopic anatomic or pathologic anomalies in the visual pathway.

    psychogenic amblyopia Psychic loss of vision caused by neurosis or psychosis, often characterized by constricted and tubular visual fields.

amblyopiagenic A condition such as anisometropia or strabismus that can cause amblyopia if it remains untreated in a young child.

angle kappa Angle between the pupillary axis and the visual axis subtended at the nodal point of the eye.

angle of anomaly The angular difference between the objective and the subjective angles of deviation in anomalous correspondence

angle of deviation Angle between the visual axis of the deviated eye and the visual axis of the fixating eye. It can be measured subjectively, that is, superimposing first-degree targets in the synoptophore, or objectively, that is, the alternate cover test with prisms.

aniseikonia A relative difference in size and/or shape of the ocular images of the eyes.

anisometropia A condition of unequal refractive state for the two eyes, one eye requiring a different lens correction from the other.

anomalous correspondence Correspondence occurs or has a tendency to occur between the fovea in the fixating eye and a peripheral point or area in the strabismic eye. Anomalous correspondence is usually either harmonious, in which the angle of anomaly equals the objective angle, or unharmonious, in which the angle of anomaly is less than the objective angle.

antagonist A muscle with opposite primary action to that of another muscle in the same eye, that is, the right lateral rectus is the antagonist of the right medial rectus.

associated phoria The amount of prism needed to neutralize a fixation disparity.

asthenopia Any symptoms or distress arising from use of the eyes; eyestrain.

attenuation A form of occlusion used in amblyopia therapy in which the transmission of light to the nonamblyopic eye is altered by means of certain filters.

Bagolini striated lenses Lenses with fine parallel striations that are used in the testing of retinal correspondence and suppression.

blind-spot esotropia Esotropia in which the magnitude of the deviation is such that the image of fixation falls on the optic disc of the deviating eye, making the development of a suppression zone unnecessary.

Brewster stereoscope A stereoscope with lenses and a septum to control what each eye sees when both eyes are open.

Brown's syndrome Limitation of elevation in adduction of the same degree on version and duction testing.

NOTE: Definitions of the common types of extraocular muscle surgery are defined in Chapter 11.

cheiroscope A haploscopic instrument to treat suppression that presents a line drawing to the view of one eye to be projected visually and traced with a pencil or crayon in the field of view of the other eye.

chiastopic fusion Fusion obtained by voluntarily converging to fixate directly two fusible targets, laterally separated in space, such that the right eye directly fixates the left target and the left eye fixates the right target.

comitant A condition in which the magnitude of deviation remains essentially the same in all positions of gaze and with either eye fixating.

congenital strabismus Strabismus present or existing on or before 6 months of age.

conjugate (yoked) prisms Prisms in which the bases are prescribed in the same direction before both eyes. Sometimes used in A- or V-pattern deviations to avoid the area where binocular vision is lost, that is, bilateral base-down prisms for V esotropia.

consecutive strabismus Strabismus in which the deviation differs in direction from that of a preexisting strabismus, as may occur following extraocular muscle surgery.

constant strabismus Strabismus present at all times.

contracture Inability of an extraocular muscle to relax, resulting in structural changes with the inelasticity becoming permanent.

convergence Turning inward of the eyes.

    accommodative convergence Convergence changes physiologically induced by, related to, or associated with changes in accommodation.

    fusional convergence Convergence induced by fusion stimuli without a change in accommodation.

    proximal convergence Convergence initiated by the awareness of a near object.

    tonic convergence Continuous convergence response maintained by the extraocular muscle tonus.

convergence excess A high esophoria at near associated with a relatively orthophoric condition at distance.

convergence insufficiency An inability to converge or maintain convergence usually associated with a high exophoria or intermittent exotropia at near and a relatively orthophoric condition at distance.

covariation A condition in strabismus in which the objective angle and the angle of anomaly change in concert with one another while the subjective angle remains zero.

cross fixation A condition in which a large, alternating esotropia is associated with the use of the adducted eye for fixation of objects in the contralateral temporal field. Frequently occurs with infantile esotropia.

crowding phenomenon A difficulty or inability of the amblyopic eye to discriminate small visual acuity targets when they are presented next to each other in a row, whereas the same size targets presented singly are resolved.

cycloplegia Paralysis of the ciliary muscle, resulting in a loss of accommodation.

cyclovertical muscle Any of the vertical recti or oblique extraocular muscles.

decompensated heterophoria The condition in which a heterophoria becomes a strabismus.

deviating eye The eye that is not straight in strabismus, as distinguished from the fixating eye.

diagnostic positions of gaze The primary, the four secondary, and the four tertiary positions of ocular fixation attempted to demonstrate normal or defective ocular motility.

diplopia A condition in which a single object is perceived as two rather than one. Homonymous, or uncrossed, diplopia is the condition in which the image seen by the right eye is to the right of the image seen by the left eye; heteronymous, or crossed, diplopia is the condition in which the image seen by the right eye is to the left of the image seen by the left eye.

Disparometer A device used to measure fixation disparity.

dissociated vertical deviation On dissociation (occlusion) of either eye, the eye behind the occluder deviates upward but reverts to its fixating position when dissociation ceases. When the right eye fixates, a left hyperdeviation exists, and when the left eye fixates, a right hyperdeviation exists.

divergence Movement of the eyes turning away from each other so that the lines of sight intersect behind the eyes.

divergence excess A high exophoria or intermittent exotropia at distance associated with a much lower exophoria at near.

divergence insufficiency A high esophoria or intermittent esotropia at distance associated with a much lower esophoria at near.

doll's-head maneuver (the oculocephalic reflex) Rotation of the eyes in a direction opposite to a sudden head movement, through an angle equal to the head movement, with a subsequent return toward the original position, in a case of a destructive lesion of the central mechanism for voluntary eye movements when the lesion is above the pontine centers.

Duane's syndrome Retraction of the eye into the orbit, associated with either limited abduction, limited adduction, or limited abduction and adduction.

Ductions Ability of the eyes to show a full range of motion under monocular viewing conditions.

    abduction The eye turns outward.

    adduction The eye turns inward.

    supraduction The eye turns upward.

    infraduction The eye turns downward.

dynamic retinoscopy Retinoscopy performed while the patient fixates a near target, such as letters, words, or pictures, mounted on the retinoscope.

eccentric fixation Monocular fixation not employing the central foveal area.

electro-oculogram (electromyography) Recording of eye movements and eye position provided by the difference in electrical potential between two electrodes placed on the skin on either side of the eye.

epicanthus A condition in which a fold of skin partially covers the inner canthus. It is normal in infants and may give the impression of an esotropia.

first-degree fusion The ability to superimpose dissimilar targets.

fixating eye The nondeviating eye in strabismus.

fixation disparity A condition in which the images of a bifixated object do not stimulate exactly corresponding retinal points but still fall within Panum's areas, the object thus being seen singly.

forced duction test A procedure performed under local or general anesthesia to test for mechanical restriction of eye movement, in which the eye is rotated by means of forceps pulling on the conjunctiva.

Fresnel press-on prism or lens Trade name for a Fresnel prism, or lens, of thin, transparent, flexible material that adheres to the surface of a spectacle lens when pressed in place.

Haidinger brushes Entoptic phenomenon used to tag the projected location of the fovea; used to determine fixation status in amblyopia.

Hering's law of equal innervation Innervation to the extraocular muscles is equal to both eyes, resulting in movements of the two eyes that are equal and symmetric.

heterophoria (dissociated phoria) A latent condition of the eyes to become misaligned from the orthophoric position, which requires fusional vergence for bifixation to be maintained.

    esophoria Latent tendency for the eyes to turn in.

    exophoria Latent tendency for the eyes to turn out.

    hyperphoria Latent tendency for one eye to turn up.

    hypophoria Latent tendency for one eye to turn down.

Hirschberg test A method for approximating the objective angle of strabismus by noting the position of the reflex of a fixated light on the cornea of the deviated eye.

horror fusionis A specific type of inability to fuse that is characterized by an avoidance of bifoveal stimulation and an absence of suppression.

iatrogenic A condition generated or induced by the clinician.

idiopathic A condition or disease of unknown or indeterminate origin.

incomitant A condition in which the magnitude of deviation is not the same in the different positions of gaze or with either eye fixating. Generally, the magnitude must change by more than 5 PD to be incomitant.

infacility of accommodation The condition in which there is difficulty or sluggishness in changing from one level of accommodation to another.

inferior oblique overaction Elevation, or upturning, of the eye when it adducts.

infranuclear Below the level of the oculomotor, trochlear, and abducens cranial nerve nuclei.

intermittent strabismus A strabismus that is not present at all times.

internuclear ophthalmoplegia Unilateral or bilateral limitation of adduction associated with nystagmus of the contralateral abducting eye. Caused by lesions in the medial longitudinal fasciculus.

Knapp's law A correcting spectacle lens placed at the anterior focal plane of an axially ametropic eye forms an image equal in size to that formed in a standard emmetropic eye.

Krimsky test A method for determining the objective angle of strabismus in which the clinician, with his or her eye directly above a light source fixated by the patient, observes the position of the corneal reflexes. Prisms are placed before the fixating eye until the reflex in the deviated eye appears centered.

lag of accommodation The extent to which the accommodative response is less than the dioptric stimulus to accommodation.

latent nystagmus A jerk nystagmus that occurs only under conditions of monocular fixation. There is no clinically detectable nystagmus with binocular fixation.

lead of accommodation The extent to which the accommodative response is greater than the dioptric stimulus to accommodation.

mechanically restrictive deviation An incomitant deviation resulting from nonparetic causes such as enlargement of an extraocular muscle or scar tissue.

microtropia A strabismus, usually esotropia, in which the deviation is so small that it may not be readily detectable.

monofixation syndrome See microtropia.

motor fusion (fusional reserves) The ability to align the eyes in such a manner that sensory fusion can be maintained.

negative relative accommodation Clinically measured subjectively by the maximum amount of plus lens power, permitting clear, single binocular vision at a given distance, usually 33 or 40 cm.

neutral-density filter test Differentiates between functional and organic amblyopia by measuring visual acuity with or without a neutral-density filter. If acuity is greatly reduced with the filter, the amblyopia is organic, whereas if the acuity is only minimally affected or not affected at all, functional amblyopia is present.

nystagmus A regularly repetitive, usually rapid, and characteristically involuntary movement or rotation of the eye, either oscillatory or with slow and fast phases in alternate directions.

occlusion therapy A method of treating amblyopia by covering the nonamblyopic eye.

ocular myasthenia Severe muscle weakness in the eye that usually results in ptosis and diplopia as a result of involvement of the extraocular muscles.

ocular torticollis Head tilting.

oculomotor nerve Third cranial nerve, which innervates the levator, the superior rectus, the medial rectus, the inferior rectus and the inferior oblique muscles, as well as the sphincter and ciliary muscles.

orthophoria The absence of any tendency of the eyes to deviate.

orthopic fusion Fusion obtained by voluntarily diverging to directly fixate two fusible targets, laterally separated in space, such that the right eye directly fixates the right target and the left eye fixates the left target.

orthoptics/vision therapy The teaching and training process for the improvement and coordination of the two eyes for efficient and comfortable binocular vision.

panoramic vision An extension of the binocular peripheral visual field that exists in some patients with exotropia.

Panum's area An area in the retina of one eye, any point of which, when stimulated simultaneously with a single specific point in the retina of the other eye, will give rise to a single fused percept.

paresis Incomplete or partial paralysis of an extraocular muscle, resulting in an incomitant deviation.

paresis of accommodation Total or almost total loss of accommodation as a result of paralysis of the ciliary muscle.

penalization A method of treating amblyopia in which vision in the nonamblyopic eye is decreased by pharmacologic agents and/or overcorrecting or undercorrecting lenses to get the amblyopic eye to fixate.

Percival's criterion Asthenopia is likely when the vergence demand or stimulus is not in the middle third of the total fusional vergence range.

period of visual immaturity The period in early childhood in which suppression, anomalous correspondence, and amblyopia can develop.

photophobia Abnormal intolerance of light.

physiologic diplopia Normal phenomenon that occurs in binocular vision for nonfixated objects whose images fall on disparate retinal points outside of Panum's area.

pleoptics A method of treating amblyopia in which concentrated and intensive stimulation is provided to the fovea of the amblyopic eye.

positive relative accommodation Clinically measured subjectively by the maximum amount of minus lens power permitting clear, single, binocular vision at a given distance, usually 33 cm or 40 cm.

preferential looking A method of measuring visual acuity in infants in which one target consists of black and white stripes of varying spatial frequency and the other target consist of a clear homogenous field.

primary angle of deviation The deviation, in incomitant strabismus, of the nonfixating eye (the eye with limited motility) from the point of fixation at which the normally fixating eye fixates.

primary position The position of the eyes when looking straight ahead with the head erect and still.

prism diopter (PD) The unit of measurement for heterophoria and heterotropia. One PD is the angle defined by a deviation of 1 cm at a distance of 1 m.

progressive-addition lens A spectacle lens with a gradual and progressive change in power either over the whole lens or over a region intermediate between area of uniform power.

pseudostrabismus The false appearance of having strabismus when actually no manifest misalignment of the eyes exists.

psychometric visual acuity A method used to measure visual acuity in patients with amblyopia, consisting of a series of cards, each with 8 tumbling E's at various orientations.

pursuit Movement of an eye fixating a slowly moving target.

random-dot stereogram A stereogram in which the eye sees an array of little black and white characters or dots of a roughly uniform texture and containing no recognizable shape or contours.

retinal (binocular) rivalry Alternation of perception of portions of the visual field when the two eyes are simultaneously and separately exposed to targets containing dissimilar colors or differently oriented borders.

saccade An abrupt voluntary shift in fixation from one target to another.

saccadic velocity Saccades that are recorded using an electro-oculogram, which gives a graphic record of the speed and direction of eye movement. Used to differentiate extraocular muscle paresis from mechanical restriction of a muscle.

second-degree fusion The ability to fuse targets that have common borders.

secondary angle of deviation The deviation, in incomitant strabismus, of the normally fixating eye from the point of fixation when the normally deviating eye (the eye with limited motility) is made to fixate.

secondary position Any position of the eye represented by a vertical or horizontal deviation of the line of sight from the primary position.

sensory fusion The process by which stimuli, seen separately by the two eyes, are combined, synthesized, or integrated into a single perception.

> **bifoveal fusion (bifixation)** Sensory fusion in which only the foveal images are considered.

> **peripheral fusion** Sensory fusion in which the images in the peripheral portions of the retinae are considered, excluding the foveae.

sensory strabismus Strabismus caused by poor vision in one eye.

shape magnification Magnification resulting from a variation in the curvature of the front surface and thickness of a spectacle lens.

Sheard's criterion The amount of heterophoria should not be less than half the opposing fusional vergence in reserve, or the patient is likely to experience asthenopia.

skew deviation A vertical deviation of the eyes that does not fit the pattern of an isolated cyclovertical muscle paresis and is usually caused by a lesion in the brain stem.

space eikonometer Instrument for measuring aniseikonia.

spasm of accommodation Involuntary contraction of the ciliary muscle, producing excess accommodation.

spasm of the near reflex Intermittent episodes of sustained convergence with accommodative spasm and miosis.

stereopsis Binocular visual perception of three-dimensional space based on retinal disparity.

strabismus (heterotropia) The condition in which binocular fixation is not present under normal seeing conditions, that is, the foveal line of sight of one eye fails to intersect the object of fixation.

> **esotropia** Manifest deviation inward.

> **exotropia** Manifest deviation outward.

> **hypertropia** Manifest deviation upward.

> **hypotropia** Manifest deviation downward.

suppression The lack or inability of perception of normally visible objects in all or part of the field of vision of one eye, occurring only on simultaneous stimulation of both eyes and attributed to cortical inhibition.

supranuclear Above the level of the oculomotor, trochlear, and abducens cranial nerve nuclei.

synergist The muscle in the same eye that acts with another muscle to produce a given movement, that is, the inferior oblique is a synergist with the superior rectus for elevation of the eye.

synoptophore (major amblyoscope) A reflecting mirror haploscopic device consisting of two angled tubes that is held in front of the eyes and can be turned to any degree of convergence or divergence. Used for the measurement of strabismus and the assessment of binocular vision.

tertiary position Any position of the eye represented by an oblique, or a combination of vertical and horizontal deviation of the line of sight from the primary position.

third-degree fusion See stereopsis.

three-step test A test used to isolate a single cyclovertical muscle as being the cause of a vertical deviation.

thyroid myopathy A mechanically restrictive incomitant deviation associated with thyroid dysfunction.

torsion (cyclodeviation) Wheel-like movements of the eye around an anteroposterior axis such as the fixation axis.

extorsion (excyclodeviation) Wheel-like movements of the eye outward.

intorsion (incyclodeviation) Wheel-like movements of the eye inward.

tranaglyphs Trade name of a variety of training and test targets consisting of various red and green details on transparencies to be viewed in combination with a red filter in front of one eye and a green filter in front of the other eye.

trochlear nerve Fourth cranial nerve, which innervates the superior oblique muscle.

TV trainer Used to treat suppression; a plastic sheet attached to a television screen, which the patient views with red-green or Polaroid filters.

unilateral (cover-uncover) cover test An objective test for determining the presence of a deviation and differentially diagnosing a heterophoria from a strabismus, in which one eye is covered and uncovered with an opaque occluder while a target is fixated at a given distance.

unilateral strabismus A condition in which only the nonstrabismic eye can maintain fixation while both eyes are open. In young children it is amblyopiagenic if the strabismus is constant.

V pattern Exotropia in which the deviation increases in straight upgaze, or esotropia in which the deviation increases in straight downgaze.

vectogram A polarized stereogram consisting of two photographic images printed on opposite sides of a gelatin film, with their axes of polarization at right angles to each other and viewed through Polaroid filters so that one image is seen only by one eye while the other image is seen only by the other eye.

vergence A disjunctive rotational movement of the eyes such that the points of reference on the eyes move in opposite directions, as in convergence, divergence, cyclovergence, or sursumvergence.

vergence facility The speed in maintaining fusion with changing fusional vergence demand.

versions A conjugate movement in which the two eyes move in the same direction.

levoversion Movement of both eyes to the left.

dextroversion Movement of both eyes to the right.

supraversion Movement of both eyes up.

infraversion Movement of both eyes down.

visual confusion In strabismus, objects that are physically separated in space are imaged on the foveas of the two eyes and are therefore seen as being superimposed.

visual evoked potential An electrical potential measured at the level of the occipital cortex in response to a light stimulation.

visuoscope An instrument designed to determine the type of monocular fixation in amblyopia, consisting of an ophthalmoscope adapted with a small, central, opaque, fixation target which projects a shadow onto the retina, the position of the shadow in relation to the fovea indicating the type of fixation.

Wheatstone stereoscope A stereoscope with mirrors mounted on an adjustable midline barrier to control what each eye sees when both eyes are open.

Worth four dot test A commonly used test for binocular vision that uses red-green glasses and a hand-held flashlight.

X pattern Exotropia in which the deviation increases as the eyes look straight upward and straight downward.

yoke muscles Muscles of the two eyes that simultaneously contract to turn the eyes equally in the same directions, such as the right lateral rectus and the left medial rectus in turning the eyes to the right.

zone of clear single binocular vision The region determined by the extremes of accommodation and convergence that can be evoked while retaining a clear single image.

From: Cline D, Hofstetter HW, Griffin Jr: *Dictionary of visual science*, ed 4, Radnor, Pa, 1989, Chilton; Millodot M: *Dictionary of optometry*, London, 1986, Butterworth-Heinemann; Stein MA, Slatt BJ, Stein RM: *Ophthalmic terminology speller and vocabulary builder*, St Louis, 1987, Mosby.

Index

A

Abducens nerve paresis, 287, 288, 300-303
Accommodation; *see also specific types, e.g.,*
    Accommodative insufficiency
  AC/A ratios for, 153-154
  amblyopia and, 7, 32
  CA/C ratios for, 154
  in convergence excess esophoria, 164
  in convergence insufficiency, 156
  criteria for, 73
  in equal esophoria, 167
  in equal exophoria, 161
  in esotropia, 217
  excess, 69
  fatigue of, 69
  feedback system for, 173, 174
  function of, 61
  in hyperphoria, 167
  ill-sustained, 69
  inertia of, 75
  infacility of, 75
  in intermittent exotropia, 260
  orthoptics for, 88
  paresis of, 69, 85-86
  pseudoanomaly of, 87
  in refractive esotropia, 218
  secondary anomalies of, 87
  strabismus and, 71
  tests for, 61-68, 149
    reliability with, 64
  tonic, 75
  unequal, 86-87
  weakness of, 71
Accommodative amplitude, 65
  accommodative insufficiency with, 70, 71
  accommodative spasm with, 83
  aging and, 62, 63
  convergence insufficiency and, 155
  definition of, 61
  dynamic retinoscopy for, 62
  expected levels of, 62, 63
  as graphic variable, 170, 171
  Hofstetter's formulas for, 62, 70
  influences on, 62-63
  mean, 74
  minus lens technique for, 62
  push-up technique for, 62
  testing of, 61-63
Accommodative convergence/accommoda-
    tion (AC/A) ratio, 153-154
  in accommodative insufficiency, 71
  CA/C ratio and, 73, 174
  in consecutive esotropia, 239
  in consecutive exotropia, 254, 255
  in convergence excess esophoria, 164, 165
  in convergence insufficiency, 155-156, 158
  definition of, 65
  in divergence excess exophoria, 162, 163
  in divergence insufficiency esophoria, 165,
    166
  in divergence insufficiency exophoria, 236
  in equal esophoria, 167
  in esophoria, 65
  feedback loop for, 174
  as graphic variable, 170, 171
  in inherited strabismus, 191
  in intermittent exotropia, 260-261

Accommodative convergence/accommoda-
    tion (AC/A) ratio—cont'd
  in nonrefractive accommodative es-
    otropia, 227
  in refractive accommodative esotropia,
    218, 220-221
  in strabismus, 198
  in vergence function, 149
  with vergence training, 176, 177
Accommodative demand, 181
Accommodative dysfunction, 61-90
  apparent, 87
  associated conditions with, 87
  case study on, 69
  classification of, 69
  clinical practice for, 334
  in consecutive exotropia, 254, 255
  distribution of, 69
  dynamic retinoscopy for, 66
  fixation training for, 89
  flip lens training for, 63-64, 88-89
  functional, 69
  lenses for, 182
  NRA value for, 87
  organic, 69, 85
  PRA value for, 87
  presbyopia and, 3
  prevalence of, 61
  push-up training for, 89
  secondary, 87
  as sensory anomaly, 2, 3
  symptoms of, 61, 69
  treatment of, 87-90, 175
  vergence anomalies with, 174-175
  vergence training for, 178
Accommodative esotropia, 217-234
  case studies on, 217-219, 222-234
  classification of, 218
  definition of, 217
  infantile esotropia with, 229
  infants with, 206, 218
  liability issues with, 340
  nonrefractive, 226-229
    bifocals for, 227-229
    case studies on, 228-229
    clinical features of, 226-227
    definition of, 226
    drugs for, 325
    onset of, 226
    orthoptics for, 223
    partial, 229
    prisms for, 223
    treatment of, 227-228
  onset of, 206, 217, 218
  partly, 229-234; *see also* Partly accom-
    modative esotropia
    surgery for, 231, 327
  prevalence of, 217
  refractive, 218-226
    AC/A ratio in, 218, 220-221
    acute-onset, 235
    adults with, 223-224
    amblyopia with, 219
      case study on, 225
      treatment of, 220
    bifocals for, 220-221, 224
    case studies on, 219, 222-226

Accommodative esotropia—cont'd
  refractive—cont'd
    clinical features of, 218-222
    consecutive exotropia vs., 255
    course with, 222-225
    cycloplegic retinoscopy for, 220
    definition of, 218
    drugs for, 222, 325
    intermittent phase of, 219
    late-onset, 225-226
    lenses for, 219-221
      contact, 221-222
      progressive-addition, 221
    magnitude of, 218
    muscle paresis with, 219
    ocular motility disorders in, 219
    orthoptics for, 222, 224-225
    partial, 229
    prognosis for, 222
    treatment of, 219-222
      deterioration after, 222-223
  refractive error in, 218
Accommodative excess, 69; *see also* Accom-
    modative spasm
  differential diagnosis of, 83-84
Accommodative facility, 63-65
  aging and, 64-65
  definition of, 63
  dynamic retinoscopy for, 64
  expected levels of, 64-65
  far-near subjective technique for, 64
  flip lens training for, 63-64, 88-89
  flipper test of, 76-77
  MEM technique for, 64
  pass rates for, 64
Accommodative fatigue, 79-80; *see also* Fa-
    tigue
  accommodative insufficiency with, 70, 72,
    74, 80
  associated conditions with, 79-80
  definition of, 79
  diagnosis of, 80
  etiology of, 80
  frequency of, 69
  symptoms of, 79
  treatment of, 80
Accommodative infacility, 75-79
  Adie's syndrome with, 76
  associated conditions with, 76
  case study on, 77
  definition of, 75
  diagnosis of, 76-77
  etiology of, 75
  frequency of, 69
  orthoptics for, 77-79
  prevalence of, 75
  symptoms of, 75
  treatment of, 77-79
Accommodative insufficiency, 69-75
  AC/A ratio and, 71
  accommodative amplitude with, 70, 71
  accommodative fatigue with, 80
  age and, 70
  case study on, 73
  clinical features of, 70-71
  conditions with, 72
  convergence insufficiency with, 157

353

Printed and bound by CPI Group (UK) Ltd, Croydon, CR0 4YY

03/10/2024

01040360-0019